BILIARY TRACT
SURGERY

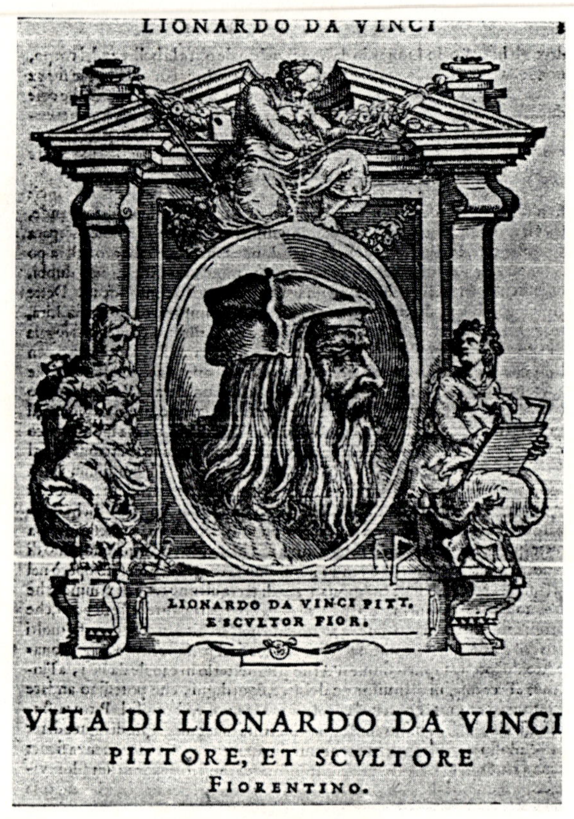

LEONARDO DA VINCI

Born: Vinci, Tuscany, 15 April 1452
Died: Château de Cloux, Amboise, France, 2 May 1519

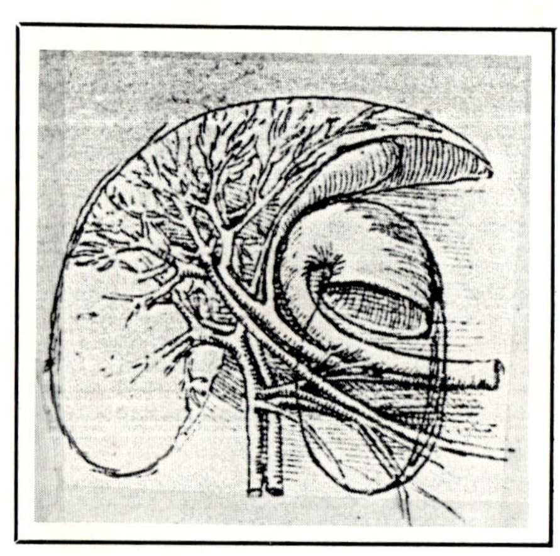

BILIARY TRACT SURGERY

Tactics and Techniques

Jacob A. Glassman, M.S., M.D., F.A.C.S., F.I.C.S., I.B.A.

Formerly

Professor of Post-Graduate Surgery at the Cook County Post-Graduate School of Medicine; Associate Professor of Surgery at The Chicago Medical School; Senior Attending Surgeon at Cook County Hospital in Chicago, Illinois; Chief of General Surgery at St. Francis Hospital in Miami Beach, Florida; Assistant Clinical Professor of Surgery at Miami University of Medicine, Miami, Florida.

Presently

Senior Attending Surgeon at Mt. Sinai Medical Center; Senior Attending Surgeon at St. Francis Hospital, both in Miami Beach, Florida. Research Director at Southeastern Research Foundation, Miami Beach, Florida.

Macmillan Publishing Co., Inc.
New York
Collier Macmillan Canada, Inc.
Toronto
Collier Macmillan Publishers
London

This book is dedicated to
Elinor, Marsha, Stuart, and Dean

Copyright ©1989, Macmillan Publishing Company, a division of Macmillan, Inc.
Printed in the United States of America

Macmillan Publishing Company
866 Third Avenue, New York, New York 10022

Collier Macmillan Canada, Inc.

Collier Macmillan Publishers • London

Library of Congress Cataloging-in-Publication Data

Glassman, Jacob A., 1911–
  Biliary tract surgery.

  Includes index.
  1. Biliary tract—Surgery.   I. Title.   [DNLM:
1. Biliary Tract Diseases—diagnosis. 2. Biliary Tract
Surgery. W1 770 G549b]
RD546.G54   1989   617'.556   89-2723
ISBN 0-02-343741-3

Printing: 1 2 3 4 5 6 7 8   Year: 9 0 1 2 3 4 5 6 7

Preface

Biliary Tract Surgery Tactics, and Techniques has been written to serve as a rapid and precise source of surgical information for the busy surgeon who is confronted by perplexing questions and difficult technical problems that require practical solutions. It also presents the latest information on surgical tricks and techniques not found in other biliary surgical texts. Finally, this book presents the surgical experience of an author who has dealt with clinical and didactic postgraduate teaching for 40 years, during which time he was associated with the late Dr. Raymond W. McNealy, Chief of Surgery at Cook County Hospital in Chicago. Dr. McNealy was one of the great surgeons and outstanding teachers of his time. Together we wrote many articles and two books on pre- and postoperative care of surgical patients, but never a book on biliary surgical technique. The author thought it was time to rectify this omission.

Some surgeons attend postgraduate courses; others do not have the time. It is the latter group of surgeons who depend upon current surgical journals for their continuing education, to which the author is directing his efforts. For these busy surgeons who require rapid, precise, and authoritative answers to their questions and technical problems, this book offers those specific, complete, and germane answers. This author's concepts are based upon his years of teaching experience in the operating room, anatomy laboratory, and lecture room. The author has long felt that a minimum of prose and a maximum of facts are long overdue in surgical publications. In fact, even the major surgical journals have finally reduced the size of their articles so that now more than twice as many shortened articles are published without the loss of factual content. In this book, the author offers the busy surgeon a concise text that will furnish authoritative, precise, and practical answers to his questions, as well as solutions to his technical problems. As in his postgraduate courses, he will speak to the reader directly and personally—one on one.

Our teaching method at the Cook County Postgraduate School was famous for being factual, practical, and complete. If additional information was required, the surgeon was referred to a recent surgical journal, but never to a surgical text, primarily because of the latter's verbosity and lack of factual specificity. The author believes that the format of this book should be based on these same principles of preciseness and completeness, particularly when discussing the more complex and controversial biliary problems based on personal experiences.

The author's latest models of biliary instruments, including his new biliary balloon catheter, are incorporated into this book as exclusive features. The biliary balloon catheter and the modified helix basket instruments are now completely integrated and can be employed interchangeably when dealing with the impacted or recurrent common duct stone. The author's latest contribution to biliary surgical techniques was exhibited at the American College of Surgeons annual meeting in San Francisco and has been included in this book as an exclusive feature. This new concept deals with flexible filiform stone basket and filiform balloon catheter combinations. The filiform combinations have simplified and markedly increased the chances of extracting the resistant and impacted common duct stone. In the last 20 years, the author has focused primarily on the problem of impacted and recurrent gallstones in the common duct, and today his instruments and techniques are recommended when all other methods fail.

For the more formidable operative techniques currently employed for the advanced liver diseases, the author directs the reader to the excellent and authoritative writings of T. E. Starzl, and S. I. Schwartz—both pioneers in this field.

The author wishes to remind the reader that operative failures not infrequently necessitate endoscopic therapeutic intervention. For this reason, the author has included a chapter on endoscopic retrograde pancreaticocholangiography as an adjunct or alternative to surgery.

The author expresses his deep gratitude to all his contributors who have taken time from their busy practices to offer their valuable expertise to this book. It is hoped that this book will serve as an updated ancillary contribution to biliary diagnosis and surgery of the biliary tract.

Jacob A. Glassman, M.D., F.A.C.S., F.I.C.S., I.B.A.
1989

Contributors

John W. Braasch, M.D.
Professor of Surgery, Dept. of Surgery at Harvard School of Medicine; Chief of Surgery, Dept. of Surgery at Lahey Clinic; Boston, Massachusetts

Larry C. Carey, M.D.
Professor of Surgery, Dept. of Surgery, Ohio State University, College of Medicine, Columbus, Ohio

German L. Casal, M.D.
Chief of Gastrointestinal Radiology at Mt. Sinai Medical Center, Miami Beach, Florida; Asst. Professor of Radiology at University of Miami, School of Medicine, Miami, Florida

Robert E. Condon, M.D., M.S., F.A.C.S.
Professor and Chairman of Dept. of Surgery, Medical College of Wisconsin, Milwaukee

Edward L. Cussler, D.Sc.
Professor of Chemistry and Engineering; formerly of Carnegie Mellon University, Pittsburgh, PA; presently Professor of Engineering at the University of Minnesota

Carlos Esquinel, M.D., Ph.D.
Asst. Professor of Surgery, Dept. of Surgery at the University of Pittsburgh, Pittsburgh, Pennsylvania

D. Fennel Evans, D.Sc.
Professor of Chemistry and Engineering, formerly at Carnegie Mellon University, Pittsburgh, PA; presently Professor of Engineering at the University of Minnesota

Scott M. Grundy, Ph.D.
Professor of Medicine, Dept. of Human Nutrition at The University of Texas Health Science Center, Dallas, Texas

Norman B. Javitt, M.D., Ph.D.
New York University Medical Center, New York City, NY; Professor of Pediatrics and Medicine, N.Y. Medical Center; Chief of Div. of Hepatic Diseases, New York City, NY

Oscar Kurzer, M.D.
Attending Urologist at Mt. Sinai and St. Francis Hospitals, Miami Beach, Florida; Instructor in Urology at University of Miami, School of Medicine, Miami, Florida

Louis Lemberg, M.D.
Professor of Clinical Cardiology, Division of Cardiology, Dept. of Medicine at the University of Miami, School of Medicine, Miami, Florida

Luis Martinez, M.D.
Professor of Radiology, University of Miami, School of Medicine, Miami, Florida; Associate Director of Dept. of Radiology at Mt. Sinai Medical Center, Miami Beach, Florida

Charles McSherry, M.D., Ph.D.
Professor and Chairman of Dept. of Surgery, Beth Israel Hospital, New York City, NY

W. Kurt Nichols, M.D.
Assoc. Professor of Surgery, Dept. of Surgery at the University of Missouri; Asst. Chief of Surgery at Harry S. Truman Memorial Veterans Hospital, Columbia, Missouri

Thomas E. Starzl, M.D., Ph.D.
Professor of Surgery, Dept. of Surgery at the University of Pittsburgh and Veterans Administration Medical Center, Pittsburgh, Pennsylvania

Leonard M. Toonkel, M.D.
Chief of Radiotherapy at Mt. Sinai Medical Center, Miami Beach, Florida; Asst. Prof. Radiology; U. of Miami Medical School

Noel R. Zusmer, M.D.
Director of Sonography, Dept. of Nuclear Medicine, Mt. Sinai Medical Center, Miami Beach, Florida; Assoc. Professor, Dept. of Nuclear Medicine at the University of Miami, School of Medicine, Miami, Florida

Contents

1

BRIEF NOTES ON THE ADVANCEMENT OF KNOWLEDGE RELATING TO BILIARY TRACT DISEASES DATING BACK TO THE EARLY HISTORY OF MAN

Parasites were discovered in numerous archaeological digs. The ova of *Ascaris* and *Trichuris* were discovered in preserved bodies about 600 B.C. The ova of *Fasciola hepatica* were found in mollusk shells (intermediate host) about 500 B.C., and calcified *Schistosoma* ova were found in kidney tubules. In a cave near the Dead Sea, fossilized human stool, 1800 years old, revealed cysts of *Entamoeba histolytica*. In Mycenia, a skeleton from about 1500 B.C. was found, revealing cholesterol stones near the costal margin. In the mummy of the Priestess of Amen (21st dynasty), x-rays revealed a gallbladder containing multiple gallstones.

In Assyria and Babylonia, liver abscesses were prevalent; they were believed to have been caused by amebic dysentery. A clay tablet was found describing a sick and weary patient who was jaundiced *(ahhzu)* by *Ascaris*. It is well known that *A. lumbricoides* can obstruct the common duct and cause jaundice. The Egyptians also suffered from parasitic infestations such as ankylostoma and bilhariasis. The latter is still rampant in Egypt. Amenophis IV (pharoah) may have also suffered from the complications of bilhariasis, i.e., ascites, distended abdomen, and thin, emaciated face.

Liver disease is often mentioned in the Bible *(kabed)*. The liver was considered a vital organ capable of uncontrollable bleeding: "My liver is poured upon this earth" *(yeraken)*; jaundice was also recognized, as was amebiasis. The earliest Indian reference to "liver and gallbladder" is found in their religious literature *(Atharvaveda)* in 1500 B.C. Then the liver was considered the seat of the bile *(ranjsksopitta)*. For early ascites *(jalodora)* they prescribed medicines, and for late ascites surgical intervention.

The Chinese considered the liver the storehouse of blood and the soul, as well as the seat of anger. The Chinese also suffered from flukes, i.e., *F. hepatica* and *Clonorchis senensis*. The Greeks learned their medicine from the ancient Egyptians and later passed it on to the Romans. The liver is mentioned in Homer's *Iliad*. Eurypylus speared Apisaon in the liver, under the diaphragm.

Hippocrates was the first to record a case report on cholecystitis with modern clarity. "A man dined well and drank too much. Vomiting, then fever, and pain in the right hypochondrium followed by fever and chills, and on the 11th day, he died." Erasistratus instituted the first study of *pathological anatomy*. He not only described the liver and biliary tract, but associated the liver with ascites. Galen also recognized biliary tract disease and prescribed appropriate diets.

Al Rhaze (Arabian) was influenced by Hippocrates and Galen. He wrote about the causes of jaundice and described tumors, infection, and obstruction. Al-Rhaze described the urine as dark when the bile does not flow into the intestine but goes into the urine. He stressed the affinity of the liver for sweets: "The liver nourishes and flourishes on those foods that are sweet."

Historical Sketches on the Advancement of Surgery of the Biliary Tract

ALEXANDER TRABIANUS (fifth century), a Greek physician, was probably the *first to describe gallstones in the hepatic ducts.*

AVICENNA-IBN-SINA (979–1037) wrote an encyclopedic book (canon), which became the standard medical work through the Middle Ages. Avicenna was a great anatomical dissectionist and recommended puncture for liver abscess.

GENTILE DA FELIGNO (1314) was the *first to describe gallstones.*

LEONARDO DA VINCI (1452–1519) contributed to the advancement of anatomy by his accurate and painstaking dissections. An example of his superb anatomical dissection of the liver, hepatic ducts, cystic duct, and cystic artery is shown by Kenneth Clark in his book on Leonardo da Vinci (Phaidon Press).

ANDREAS VESALIUS (fourteenth century) was first to negate the teachings of Galen. He corrected and replaced Galen's anatomy with realistic human anatomy as revealed by his dissection. *He accurately described the gallbladder and the common bile duct.*

ANTONIO BENINVIENI (fifteenth century) was the *first to replace the humoral theory with more scientific explanations obtained by autopsy findings.* He explained how gallstones were consistent with the clinical signs and symptoms of the patient. He searched for and found the cause of disease at autopsy.

MATTEO REALDO COLOMBO (1559) described gallstones in the body of Saint Ignatius.

WILLIAM HARVEY (1578–1657) established the true role of the cardiovascular circulation. From this point on in medical history, we shall consider the eponyms assigned to those who contributed so much to the advancement of the anatomy and surgery of the gallbladder and common duct.

JEAN FERNEL (1506–88) *was the first to describe gallstones obstructing the common bile duct.*

GABRIELE FALLOPPIUS (1523–62) is credited with providing the *first description of the fallopian tubes.* He was also the first to describe gallstones within the gallbladder and common bile duct.

JOENESIUS (1676) extracted a gallstone from a fistulous tract. He is credited with performing the first cholecystolithotomy.

FRANCIS GLISSON (1597–1677) was *first to describe the hepatic artery, portal vein, and bile ducts.* Glisson was also the first to describe a sphincteric mechanism around the distal orifice of the common bile duct. Glisson was one of the greatest physicians of the seventeenth century, but he is now remembered only for a trivial anatomical feature he didn't feel was significant enough to describe for publication.

JOHANN GEORG WIRSUNG (1600–43), after being shown a pancreatic duct in a rooster by a student (Maurice Hoffmann), proceeded to dissect out the duct in a human pancreas. He described the duct in a letter to Jean Riolan, professor of anatomy at the University of Paris.

ABRAHAM VATER (1684–1751) was the *first to describe a so-called tubercle as "those double ducts [bile and pancreatic ducts]* that come together in no single combination." Paul Gottlob Berger coauthored the term *tubercle or diverticulum,* but only Vater's name lives on.

GIOVANNI DOMINICO SANTORINI (1681–1737) was a brilliant anatomist and professor of medicine. He was the *first to describe a second pancreatic duct.* He named the upper duct the *superior pancreatic duct* and the lower one the *main pancreatic duct.* One hundred years later, Claude Bernard, while studying the physiology of the pancreas in (1856), reaffirmed the priority of Santorini to the eponym.

JAKOB BENIGMUS WINSLOW (1669–1760) held the position of professor of anatomy for 40 years at University of Denmark. Winslow named the anatomical entity he discovered *Duverneys' foramen* after his professor. Other eponyms used were *Scarpa's foramen* and *Winslow's pouch.* Finally, because *Winslow was first to describe the foramen* with such accuracy and clarity, the eponym was bestowed upon him.

LORING HEISTER (1683–1758) was professor of surgery for 38 years at Helmstedt University. He was the *first to illustrate and describe the "valves" in the cystic duct.* Manuel Lichtenstein and Andrew Ivy noted that these valves appeared only in primates, and that they were no more than spiral folds formed embryologically. The valves of Heister are believed to prevent distention or collapse of the cystic duct during pressure changes in the gallbladder and common bile duct.

JEAN-LOUIS-PETIT (1674–1750) demonstrated that the gallbladder could be *aspirated.*

CARRE in 1833 advocated fixing the gallbladder to the abdominal wall in the first stage of surgery, then at the second stage performing a *cholecystostomy.*

THEODORE KOCHER (1841–1915) was professor of surgery in Berne, Switzerland, for 45 years. He won the Nobel Prize in 1909 for his contribution to the *physiology of the thyroid gland. Aseptic technique* is attributed to Kocher. In 1903, Kocher introduced and standardized his *technique for mobilizing the duodenum.* He employed this maneuver to better expedite a gastroduodenostomy. Today the Kocher maneuver is commonly employed to expedite various types of biliary and pancreatic surgical procedures. Kocher is credited with performing the *first successful cholecystostomy for empyema.*

J. L. W. THUDICHUM in 1859 recommended that the gallbladder be marsupialized to the skin, and stones removed.

JOHN BOBBS in 1867 removed gallstones from a hydrops of the gallbladder. It was the first elective cholecystostomy.

CESAR ROUX (1857–1934) was professor of surgery at Lausanne University. In 1897 Roux described his en-Y anastomosis for gastroenterostomy; in 1907 he described the same procedure for bypassing an esophagogastric cancer. Today the term *Roux-en-Y* is often employed in describing numerous bypass procedures.

JAMES RUTHERFORD MORISON (1853–1939) was associated with the Royal Victoria Infirmary in Newcastle, England, for 50 years. In 1894 he described what is now known as *Morison's pouch.* He used this space for biliary drainage postoperatively. The area now known as *Morison's fossa,* also referred to as the *hepatorenal space,* is situated anteriorly and below the right kidney. Penrose or Jackson-Pratt drains are employed in this space to encourage external biliary drainage.

JEAN FRANCOIS CALOT (1861–1944) wrote his doctoral thesis in Paris (1890) entitled "De la Cholecystectomie." He described an isosceles triangle with the common hepatic duct as the base, and the inferior edge of the cystic duct and the superior borders of the cystic artery as the sides. This triangle has since been enlarged so that the liver's edge serves as the superior border. In this important zone are located the cystic artery, hepatic artery, and accessory bile ducts. It is now referred to as *Calot's triangle.* A gland referred to as *Calot's gland* may also be found in this triangle.

HENRI HARTMANN (1860–1952), throughout his long, successful career, meticulously recorded 30,000 operative procedures. At the Hotel Dieu, Paris, Hartmann performed about 1000 operations each year for 30 years. His operation for carcinoma of the rectosigmoid is still referred to as the *Hartmann procedure.* In 1891, Hartmann described the ampulla of the gallbladder as a *vesicle or pouch*. He is now remembered for the eponym *Hartmann's pouch*.

RUGGIERIO ODDI (1864–1913) became director of the Physiology Institute in Genoa at the age of 29. His doctoral thesis, on the workings of the sphincter, demonstrated that removal of the gallbladder resulted in dilatation of the bile ducts. For his accurate observations on the sphincter, the eponym *sphincter of Oddi* was bestowed upon him.

LUDWIG C. COURVOISIER (1843–1918) was the *first to remove a gallstone from the common bile duct*. He wrote, "with stone obstruction of the common duct, dilatation is most common—consequently, we have an important diagnostic point in the differential diagnosis of common duct obstruction." As a result of this work, Courvoisier was awarded the eponyms *Courvoisier's gallbladder* and *Courvoisier's law*.

CARL LANGENBUCH of Germany in 1882 performed the *first successful cholecystectomy for cholelithiasis*.

VON WINIWARTER of Germany in 1882 performed the *first cholecystoenterostomy*.

JUSTUS OHAGE of Minnesota in 1886 performed the *first cholecystectomy in the United States*.

WILLIAM STEWART HALSTED and SIR WILLIAM OSLER in 1897 concluded that common bile duct surgery was feasible, but that it should be undertaken only by the most skillful and experienced surgeons. Halsted's first common duct patient died 10 days postoperatively.

EVARTS GRAHAM and WARREN COLE in 1923 and 1924 reported that they were able *to visualize stones in the gallbladder roentgenologically*; they employed an iodized oral dye. Not too long thereafter, *IV cholangiography* came into use; more recently, *percutaneous transhepatic cholangiography* was introduced. Today ultrasonography, computed tomograph scanning, and magnetic resonance imaging have revolutionized gallbladder and common duct visualization.

C. P. HENRIK DAM and ARMAND J. QUICK in 1929 and 1935, working independently, *discovered a bleeding tendency due to a blood deficiency of prothrombin*.

C. P. HENRIK DAM (1939) independently *recognized that a blood deficiency of prothrombin was relieved by the administration of vitamin K*.

EDWARD A. DOISY (1939) *isolated vitamin K*.

ANSBACHER in 1940 *synthesized vitamin K (menadione)* in the laboratory.

The greatest strides in studying the gallbladder were made in the nineteenth and twentieth centuries. Only through the bold and knowledgeable undertakings of the great surgeons of that era was the rapid progress in gallbladder treatment made possible. It was the great researchers in the laboratories who developed the adjuvant and related medical discoveries that made cholecystostomy, cholecystectomy, and choledochotomy the safe and successful procedures they are today. Though surgery today is the accepted curative treatment, it is conceivable that in the not too distant future the medical treatment of cholelithiasis will become the method of choice. Hopefully, before the year 2000 we may yet witness *its prevention*.

Recommended Reading

Butt HR, Snell AM, Osterberg AE: The use of vitamin K and bile in the treatment of the hemorrhagic diasthesis in cases of jaundice. *Proc Staff Meet Mayo Clin* 13:74, 1938.

Dam H, Schonheyder F: Antihemorrhagic vitamin of the chick. *Nature* 135:652, 1935.

Gadeaz TR, Lillehei K, Zinner M, et al: Common bile duct complications of pancreatitis: Evaluation and treatment. *Surgery* 93:235, 1983.

Garrison FH: *Introduction to the History of Medicine*, ed 4. Philadelphia, WB Saunders Co, 1929, pp 353–354, 395, 504–506.

Glenn F: Historical considerations, in *Atlas of Biliary Tract Surgery*. New York, Macmillan Co, 1963.

Goodman LS, Gilman A: *The Pharmacological Basis of Therapeutics*, ed 2. New York, Macmillan Co, 1955, pp 1746–1751.

Goodwin TW: *Biosynthesis of Vitamins and Related Compounds*. London, Academic Press, 1963, pp 324–326.

Graham E, Cole W: *Diseases of the Gall Bladder and Bile Ducts*. Philadelphia, Lea & Febiger, 1928, pp 142–44, 399–400.

Halsted WS: *Surgical Papers*. Baltimore, Johns Hopkins University Press, 1924, pp 427–462.

Lange F: The surgical significance of gallstone. *Johns Hopkins Hosp Bull* 8:29, 1897.

Littenberg G, Afroudakis A, Kaplowitz N: Common bile duct stenosis from chronic pancreatitis: A clinical and pathologic spectrum. *Medicine* 58:385, 1979.

Osler W: *Principles and Practices of Medicine*, ed 5. New York, D Appleton & Co, 1902, p 569.

Quick AJ, Stanley-Brown M, Bancroft FW: Study of the coagulation defect in hemophilia and jaundice. *Am J Med Sci* 190:501, 1935.

Skellenger ME, Patterson D, Foley NT, et al: Cholestasis due to compression of the common bile duct by pancreatic pseudocysts. *Am J Surg* 145:343, 1983.

Weiss S: History of gall tract and biliary disease, in Selwyn-Brown A (ed): *The Physician Throughout the Ages*, Vol. 2. New York, Capehart Brown Co, 1928, pp 557–562.

Wisloff F, Jakobsen J, Osnes M: Stenosis of the common bile duct in chronic pancreatitis. *Br J Surg* 69:52, 1982.

Yadegar J, Williams RH, Passero E, Jr, et al.: Common duct stricture from chronic pancreatitis. *Arch Surg* 115:582, 1980.

References

1. Saltzsteen, EC, Mercer, LC, Peacock, JB, et al: Report on early operation for acute biliary tract stone disease. *Surgery;* 94(4); 704–8, 1983.

2. Ranson JHC: The timing of biliary surgery in acute pancreatitis. *Ann Surg* 189:654, 1979.

3. Kelly TR: Gallstone pancreatitis: The timing of surgery. *Surgery* 88:345, 1980.

2

A SHORT PRACTICAL REVIEW OF SURGICAL ANATOMY OF THE BILIARY TRACT

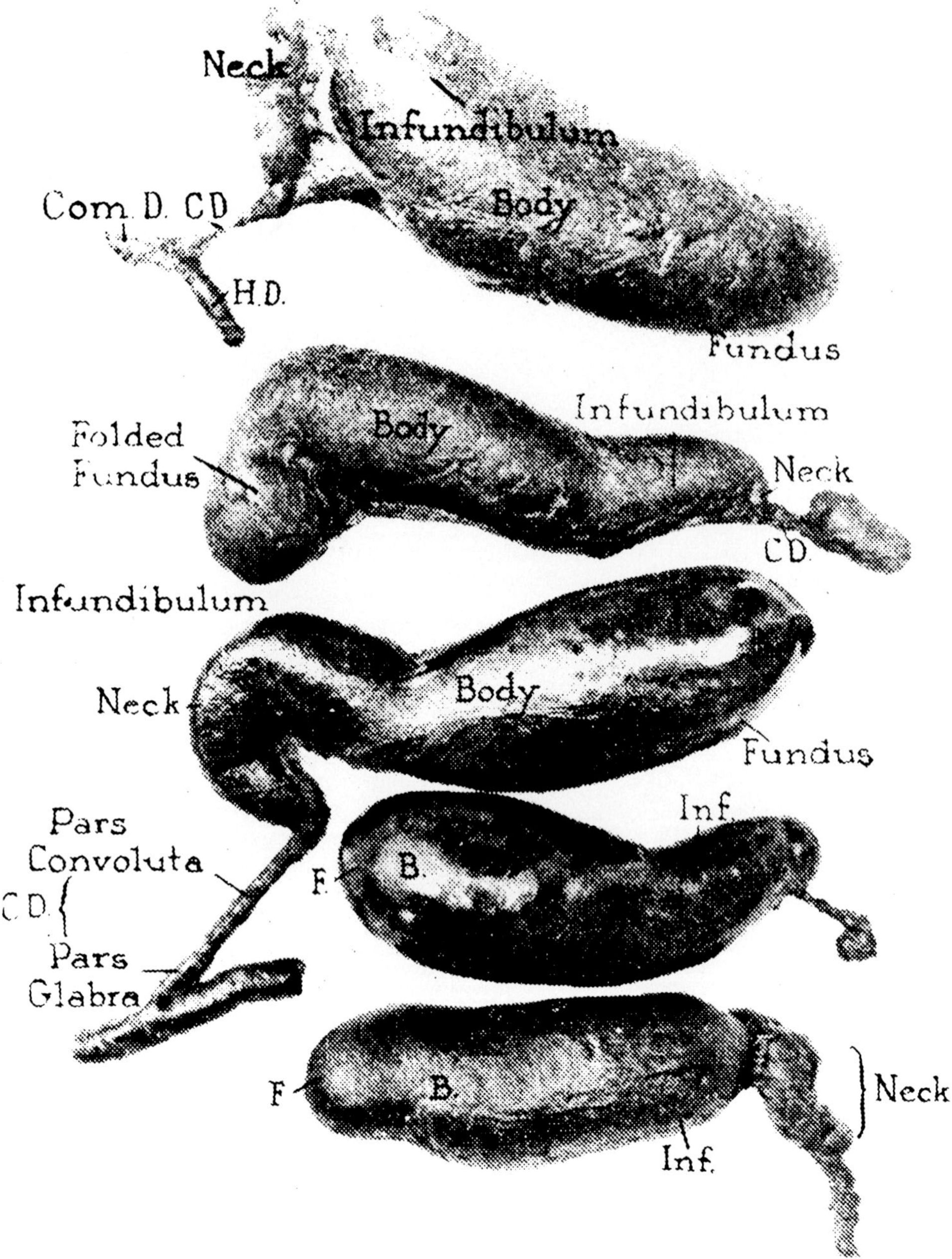

Figure 1. Gallbladders prepared by drying process before being filled with air. Andrew C. Ivy and Manuel Lichten-stein in this illustration show the varying shapes of the body and cystic duct of the gallbladder.

The gallbladder is part of the extrahepatic biliary system. It varies in size, contour, and capacity. Because the fundus (Fig. 1) of the gallbladder is completely invested in the peritoneum, it becomes extremely tender when inflamed; this feature makes it highly diagnostic. The body of the gallbladder tapers to a funnel shape that is referred to as the *infundibulum.* The neck of the gallbladder extends from the first valve of Heister to the cystic duct; it is often kinked, and may be the site of obstruction and acute cholecystitis.

The cystic duct joins the common hepatic duct to form the common bile duct. It varies in size: 50% are between 2 and 4 cm long, about 20% are less than 2 cm long, and about 25% are longer than 4 cm. A small percentage of gallbladders have no cystic duct; the neck of the gallbladder empties directly into the common duct. The diameter of the cystic duct is about 6 mm, sometimes more and often less. Within the lumen of the cystic duct are projections that are arranged spirally; they are called *valves of Heister.* In short cystic ducts they are found along its full length; in long cystic ducts they may be absent at the distal end. After cholecystectomy, this distal nonvalvular portion may enlarge and may be mistakenly diagnosed as regenerated or "reformed" gallbladder.

The function of the valves of Heister is not known; it is conjectured that they prevent the sudden distention of the cystic duct when the pressure in the gallbladder or common duct rises. Their presence decreases the caliber of the cystic duct and thus may impede or modify the flow of thick bile from the gallbladder. The valves of Heister may thicken or swell as a result of inflammation (chemical or bacterial) and possibly allergy; the lumen of the cystic duct then narrows and impedes the flow of bile. Small calculi may become lodged in the small pits or crypts created by the valves. It is probable that gallbladder debris collects in these crypts, becomes impacted, and forms gallstones. Because of its small lumen and peculiar architectural design, the cystic duct becomes a vulnerable site for pathological changes leading to obstruction, cholecystitis, cholelithiasis, and empyema. To prevent gallbladder disease, a free flow of diluted bile is desirable. It is least likely to produce gallbladder disturbances that are usually associated with cystic duct obstruction (Fig. 2).

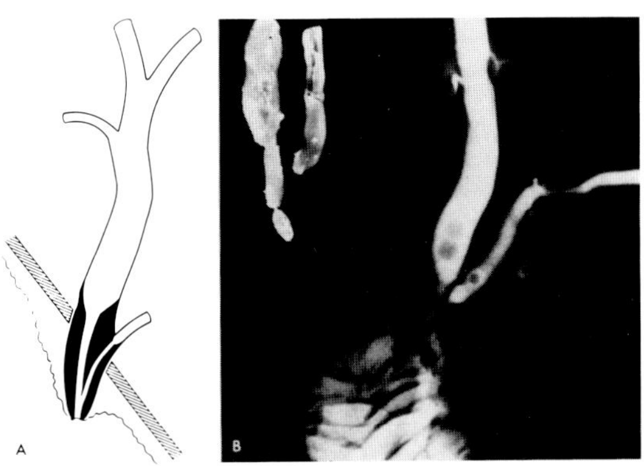

Figure 3.　A. A diagrammatic representation of the common bile duct, showing a notch that divides it into two distinct parts, an upper wide-lumened, thin walled portion and a lower narrow-lumened, thick-walled portion. The lower portion is seen to lie mainly in the submucous layer of the duodenum. B. Cast and cholangiogram of specimen showing a well-marked notch on the bile duct. The narrow-lumened lower portion, called the "thickened segment," and the common channel are well shown. Similar appearances are seen in the pancreatic duct. (From Hand BH: Br J Surg 50:486, 1963. Reproduced with permission.)

Walters and Snell[1] reported that in about two-thirds of a group of cases studied, the head of the pancreas surrounded the distal common duct. In about one-third the distal common duct positioned itself behind the pancreas. In many instances, the common bile duct is joined by the distal pancreatic duct (Wirsung) before terminating in the lower (descending) portion of the duodenum. The point of juncture may be high or low. Not infrequently, the common bile and pancreatic ducts empty separately into the duodenum. It is this varying anatomy that is the underlying cause of bile reflux, either into the common bile duct or the pancreatic duct or both (Fig. 3). The duct of Santorini serves as an accessory duct of the pancreas, emptying into the common duct at a point higher than the termination of the duct of Wirsung. Rarely, the duct of Wirsung becomes atresic or congenitally obliterated, in which case the duct of Santorini becomes the primary outlet for pancreatic juice.

When a stone is impacted at the ampulla, the bile will most often reflux into the pancreas (pancreatitis). If the pressure is great enough, it will continue to reflux into the gallbladder and then onto the liver canaliculi. Jaundice becomes more intense as the serum bilirubin level rises. Carcinoma of the head of the pancreas, or ampulla, will gradually but continuously obliterate the stoma. In the absence of chronic cholecystitis, the gallbladder

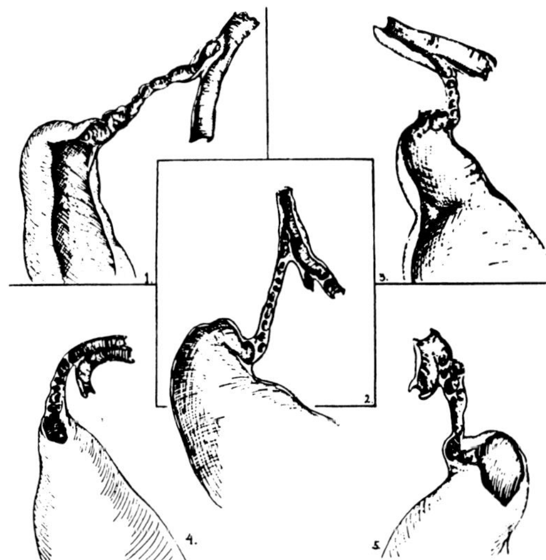

Figure 2.　Ivy and Lichtenstein have dissected the gallbladder and allowed it to dry, then filled it with air. Their purpose was to reveal the valves of Heister.

will become progressively distended until a palpable mass forms.

Because the common bile duct enters obliquely through the duodenal musculature, contractions of the duodenum may seriously interfere with bile passage. The bundle of muscle that encircles the distal end of the common duct (sphincter of Oddi) has a significant physiological function. In great measure, the sphincter of Oddi regulates the filling and emptying of the gallbladder; incompetence or nonfunction will seriously alter this function. It has been reported that postoperatively the sphincter becomes unduly relaxed (paresis). Neoplasms of the sphincter of Oddi (benign or malignant) will obstruct the outflow of bile (partially at first, completely later) (see "Carcinoma of the Ampulla of Vater" in Chapter 16).

The common bile duct, duodenum, and pancreas are intimately related anatomically and physiologically, so that a knowledge of their integrated function may be especially useful during surgical explorations in the area posterior to the duodenum. With a Kocher incision (a curved serosal incision lateral to the duodenal sweep) (See-Kocher Maneuver, Chapter 11, and -Whipple's Operation, Chapter 12), the surgeon with careful blunt finger dissection exposes the retroduodenal common bile duct, head of the pancreas, and pyloroduodenal junction. If the surgeon can palpate the gallstone, he may be able to "milk" it up to a higher and more accessible level where, with simple instrumentation, the stone can be removed via the choledochostomy. Figure 3B illustrates how a stone impacted below the common junction with the duct of Wirsung can produce a reflux of bile, together with a back pressure of pancreatic juice capable of producing serious pancreatitis. The latter can be relieved only by the passage or removal of the obstructing stone. The complications noted above may not occur if the obstructing stone impacts at a point above the site of communication between the common duct and the duct of Wirsung (Fig. 3A,B). Complications can also be avoided if the duct of Wirsung empties directly and independently into the duodenum. The musculature within the choledochoduodenal junction comprises the sphincter of Oddi and helps to regulate the flow of bile. The musculature that encircles the common bile duct before it joins with the ampulla of Vater works synchronously or independently of the encircling musculature of the sphincter of Oddi (Fig. 4). Variations in the biliary system are not uncommon.

Surgeons must be constantly alert for vascular and biliary anomalies to prevent a possible disastrous injury or hemorrhage (Figs. 5, 6). Firstly, the surgeon must dissect, explore, and operate only

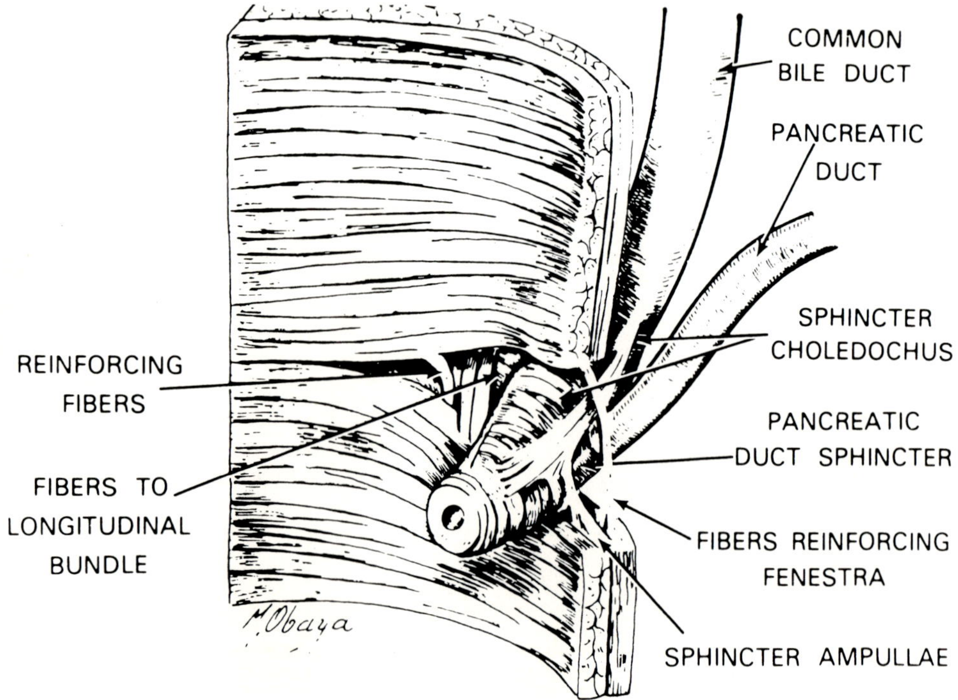

Figure 4. This diagram depicts the musculature involved in the junction of common bile duct and duodenal wall. Note the obliquity of the common duct and pancreatic duct as they penetrate the duodenal wall. Also note the splincter choledochus.

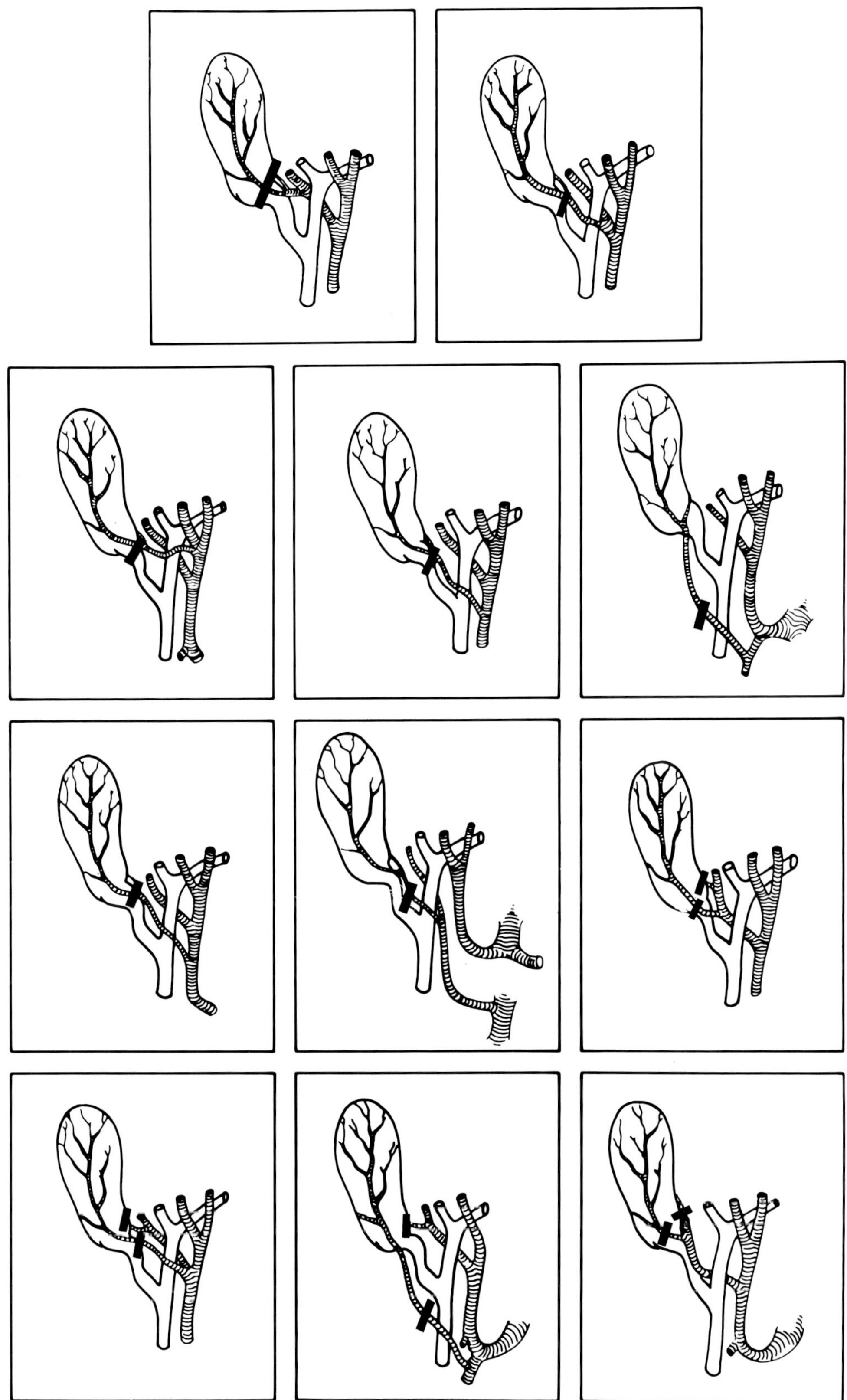

Figure 5. *Sites of cystic artery ligations.*

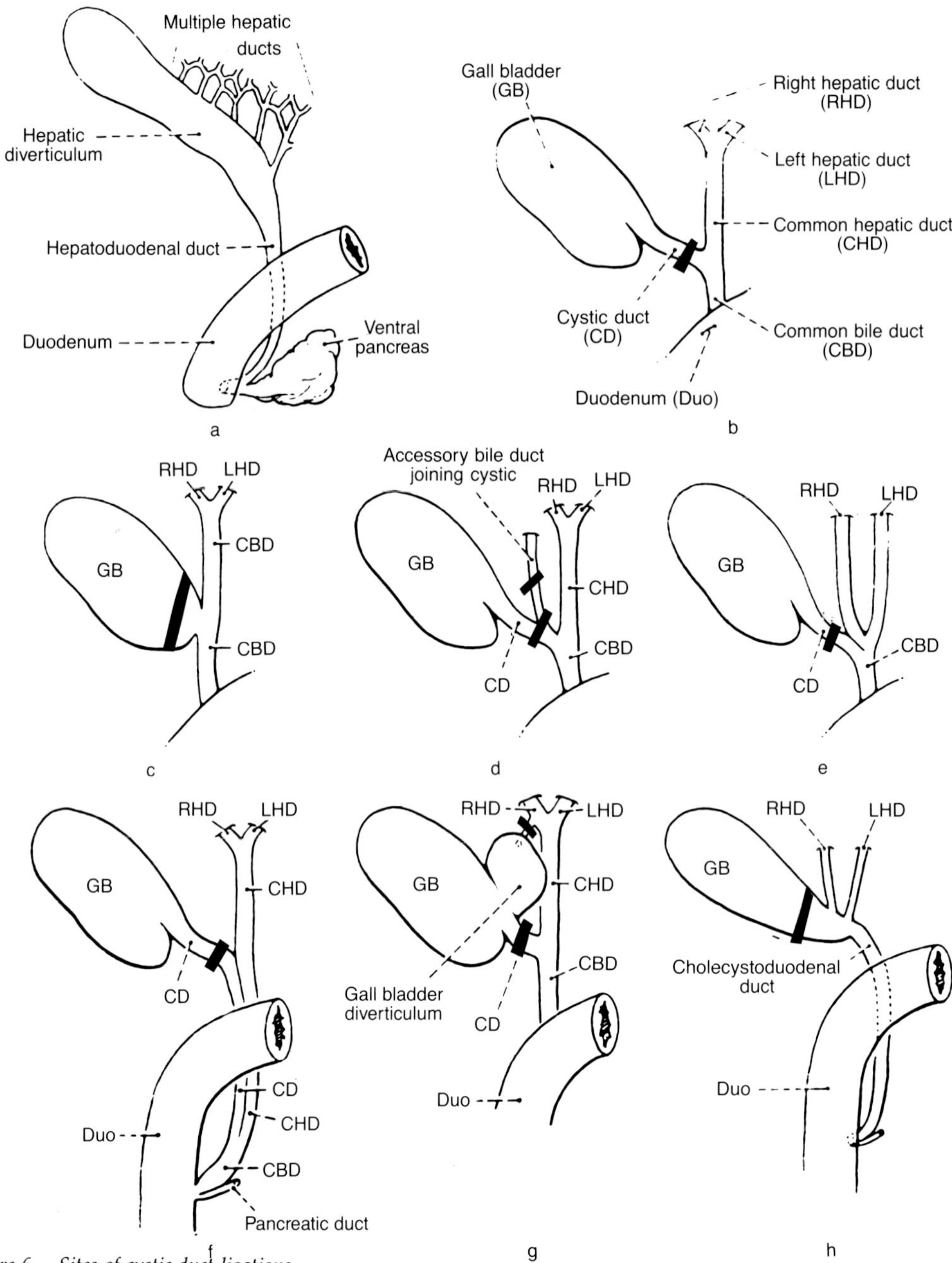

Figure 6.   Sites of cystic duct ligations.

after he has recognized and correctly labeled the anatomy. Gallbladder anomalies are not common; they include congenital absence, intrahepatic location, duplication, and "hourglass" anomalies. The gallbladder may also be "floating"; that is, it may be suspended by an unduly long peritoneal mesentery. The cystic duct too varies on occasion; it may empty into the hepatic duct, the left side of the common bile duct, or very low down and closely adherent to the distal common duct. On occasion one will find accessory small "hepatic" ducts, which, if unobserved and not ligated before closing the abdomen, may continue to leak bile into the peritoneal cavity and produce a biliary peritonitis; the latter does not respond to any known antibiotic. *This is another reason why this writer, despite occasional articles to the contrary, recommends routine drainage of the gallbladder bed (Morison's fossa)* (Fig. 7). (See Chapter 10.)

The blood supply to the liver is derived from the

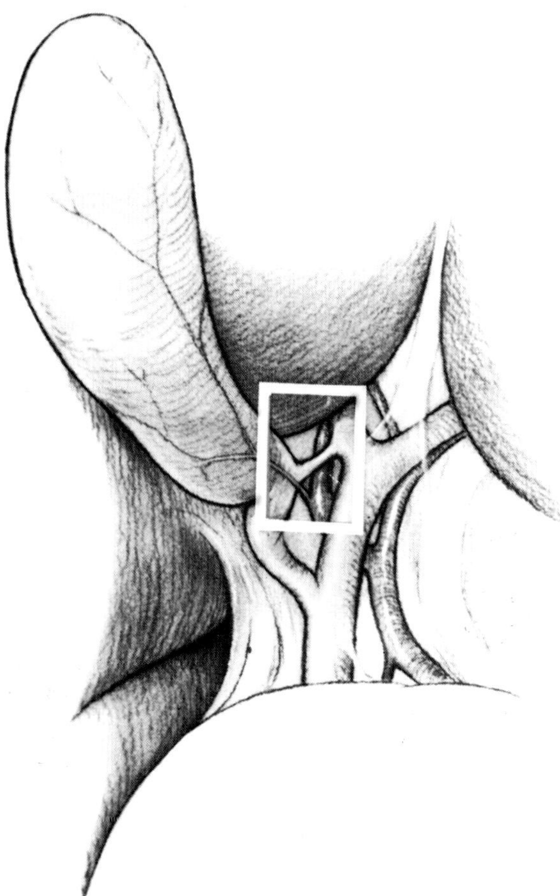

Figure 7.   The cystic duct is shown here joining the common bile duct. The cystic artery is ligated close to the gallbladder wall. An accessory bile duct (small) must also be ligated. Failure to do so may result in postoperative biliary leakage and biliary peritonitis.

hepatic artery, which splits to supply the right and left lobes of the liver. In the majority of instances, the right hepatic artery gives rise to the cystic artery. Certain anomalies do exist (Fig. 8). For example, a cystic artery may originate from either the right or the left hepatic artery; or the main hepatic artery; or even the superior mesenteric artery. It is wise to be aware of these various anomalies, *but only in the individual case must the surgeon identify and correctly label the cystic artery.* Whether or not the cystic artery has an anomalous origin is of no great consequence. What is of great significance is that only the operating surgeon, by his careful dissection, is capable of recognizing the cystic artery as it enters the gallbladder wall. Only then can he safely proceed to ligate and sever the cystic artery, and only then as close to the gallbladder wall as

possible. The surgeon must also be aware of the possibility that on occasion the hepatic artery becomes intimately adherent to the gallbladder wall and can appear as a cystic artery. Careful dissection and observation will reveal this abnormality. On such an occasion the right hepatic artery is carefully separated, and the cystic artery is severed and ligated within the gallbladder wall (Fig. 8).

Venous drainage of the gallbladder is usually into the portal vein but often into the left hepatic vein. The lymphatic drainage from the gallbladder and liver is to the cysterna chyli and the thoracic duct. The lymph glands about the neck of the gallbladder, hepatic ducts, and common bile duct are usually enlarged in inflammatory and neoplastic states. During a cholecystectomy, this writer removed an enlarged lymph gland from the triangle of Calot and sent it to the pathology laboratory for immediate biopsy. The report returned the diagnosis of lymphosarcoma. Chemotherapy was started in the hospital, and today, 30 years later, the patient is alive and working.

Vagal innervation causes the gallbladder and sphincter of Oddi to contract. Cutting the vagal

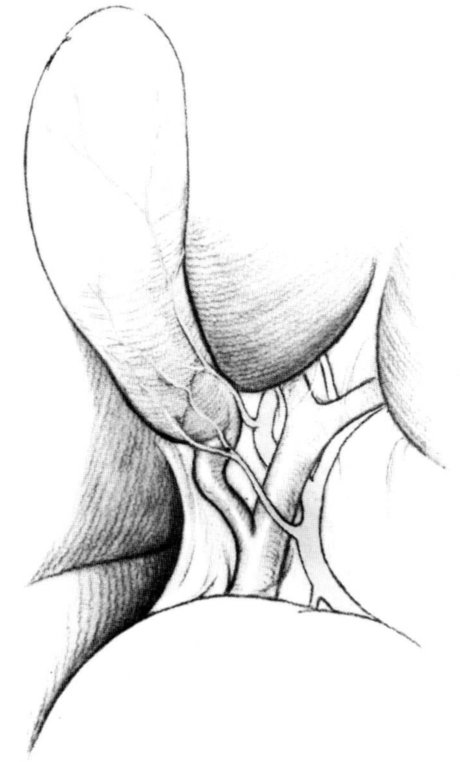

Figure 8.   The cystic duct and cystic artery are ligated close to the gallbladder wall and common bile duct. A separate (or second) cystic is recognized and ligated close to the gallbladder wall.

nerve produces a relaxation of the masculature, further suggesting that the neural control of the gallbladder is dependent on the vagus nerve. Vagotomy may cause the gallbladder to dilate to as much as twice its original size. Because of poor contractions, emptying time is prolonged, with resultant stasis. The latter development appears to be the basis of later stone formation.

Rickles[2] reported on 2 patients he operated on for cholecystitis and cholelithiasis; both had had surgery (for gastrectomy and vagotomy) 4 to 6 years earlier.

Sympathetic innervation produces the opposite effect, namely, contraction. The duodenum may contract independently of the sphincter of Oddi; the reverse is equally true. It is conceivable that these synchronous yet independent functions may be the cause of unreliable data obtained by intraoperative manometry at the operating table (see "Manometry" in Chapter 12).

The Physiology of the Biliary Tract

Bile secreted by the liver flows through the common bile duct into the second portion of the duodenum under 3–10 cm of pressure. When the sphincter of Oddi is closed, the obstructed flow of bile is refluxed into the gallbladder. The capacity of the gallbladder is about 30–90 cc. The liver secretes about 1000 cc daily, but since the body's requirement is not continuous, the bile is backed up into the gallbladder for storage and conservation. If during the interdigestive phase bile for digestion of fat is necessary, the gallbladder contracts and supplies the needed bile immediately. The stimulus for gallbladder wall contraction is the intestinal (duodenal) cholecystokinin that is released when fats enter the gastrointestinal tract. The absorption of fat-soluble vitamins (A, D, E, and K) is facilitated by the bile. Cholecystokinin was originally extracted from the duodenum in pure form by Andrew C. Ivy.[3,4]

The physiologic capacity of the gallbladder can increase 2–10 times greater than its anatomical capacity (30–90 cc). This ability is due to its unique concentrating function. Water absorption can concentrate gallbladder-held bile to about 25% of its total volume; hepatic bile may be concentrated to about 1/10th of its total volume. More concentrated hepatic bile undergoes less concentration. (For a more detailed and more intensive review of bile physiology, see "Pathogenesis of Cholesterol Gallstones," "Cholesterol–Bile Acid Interactions in Gallstone Pathogenesis," and "Physicochemical Considerations in Gallstone Pathogenesis" in Chapter 3.) In the various diseases of liver, there is usually a reduction in the formation of bile salts, which in turn interferes with fat absorption.

Proteins have no direct influence on gallbladder contraction. They stimulate the gastric mucosa to secrete gastric (acid) juice, which, upon entering the duodenum, stimulates the formation of cholecystokinin, causing the gallbladder to contract.

Carbohydrates have no effect on gallbladder contraction. To reiterate:

Fats strongly stimulate gallbladder contraction.
Proteins only mildly stimulate contraction.
Carbohydrates do not stimulate contraction at all.

Diet is most important in the medical management of chronic cholecystitis and cholelithiasis.

Fats are not allowed.
Protein is allowed sparingly.
IV fluids are ordered together with nothing by mouth in acute cholecystitis.

When dealing with a "sluggish" gallbladder, uncooked fats, preferably vegetable oils, are permissible. In obese and pregnant patients, some uncooked fats may be allowed to avoid the development of sluggishness. Bile salts are formed in the liver from amino acids. If the liver does not supply an adequate amount of bile salts, a supplement of oxidized bile salts will help to increase the bile output (hydrochloresis) without increasing the bile salt concentration.

In common duct obstruction, back pressure rises sufficiently to cause distention of the common duct proximal to the obstruction (see Chapter 12). Distention of the noninflamed gallbladder is the cause of pain and spasm. Duodenal spasm is capable of shutting off the outflow of bile from the common duct. A penetrating duodenal ulcer may also cause spasm of the duodenum. Ulcer therapy (i.e., Tagamet) and antacids may relieve the spasm in such cases; antispasmodic drugs may also be helpful. Spasm by the sphincter of Oddi at surgery may be relieved by amyl nitrate and glyceryl trinitrate. In chronic intermittent duodenal spasm, oral medication (i.e., tincture of belladonna, atropine, and Valium) may be effective. Avoid the use of morphine! It will increase spasm and pain.

The Pathology of the Biliary Tract

Gallbladder inflammation may be caused by infection (bacteria) or by chemical toxins (bile salts). It often follows obstruction of the cystic duct or neck of the gallbladder and usually leads to organic changes within the wall. Damage to the mucosa of the gallbladder reduces its ability to concentrate bile; involvement of the masculature interferes with motor function. When the gallbladder fails to concentrate and expel bile, its functional utility is destroyed. When infected, it remains as a focus of disease that may secondarily involve the liver, duodenum, common duct, and pancreas; cancer develops in about 1% of these patients.

A functionless (chronically inflamed) gallbladder that causes recurrent episodes of biliary colic is most unlikely to respond to conservative medical management. Surgery (elective cholecystectomy) is curative in most cases. Bacterial infection causes about 50% of the cases of chronic cholecystitis. Calculus formation is related both to infection and to stagnation of bile. Stones created by preexisting pathology within the gallbladder ultimately produce biliary complications that may or may not require urgent or emergent surgical intervention. Jaundice is usually related to an impacted stone in the lower common bile duct, but it may also be caused by other conditions (see Table 1, "Laboratory Studies in the Differential Diagnosis of Jaundice" in Chapter 6).

Cholesterol stones that result from precipitation of cholesterol crystals in the presence of insufficient bile acids may be single or multiple (see "Pathogenesis of Cholesterol Gallstones," "Cholesterol–Bile Acid Interactions in Gallstone Pathogenesis," and "Physicochemical Considerations in Gallstone Pathogenesis" in Chapter 3). Chronic obstruction and infection of the cystic duct promote mucus secretion and deposition of calcium on preexisting gallstones, creating opaque rings that appear on X-ray. Mixed gallstones include pigment in addition to cholesterol, cellular debris, and calcium; such stones are revealed very clearly on X-ray films and sonography.

We have discussed small stones that often originate in the crypts of the valves of Heister and obstruct the cystic duct. Little has been said about large single stones that completely obstruct the neck of the gallbladder. In the latter instance, bile cannot enter or exit from the gallbladder, and as a result, continued mucus secretion results in marked distention of the gallbladder (hydrops). When the content of a hydrops is aspirated, the aspirate appears white; it is pathognomonic for cystic duct obstruction. When the hydrops ("white bile") becomes infected, the aspirate reveals pus (empyema). In about 1% of the cases, carcinoma of the gallbladder is diagnosed. As a rule, it is established at surgery or on biopsy.

The elective removal of a symptomatic nonfunctioning gallbladder will ultimately avoid the disastrous results that follow urgent or emergent surgery for the more advanced and emergency forms of gallbladder disease.

Recommended Reading

Boyden EA: *Am J Anat* 38:177, 1926.
Brewer GE: Some observations upon the surgical anatomy of the gallbladder and ducts, in *Contributions to the Science of Medicine Dedicated by His Pupils to William Henry Welch*. Baltimore, John Hopkins University Press, 1900.
Browne EZ: Variations in origin and course of hepatic and cystic arteries. *Surgery* 8:424, 1940.
Dennis C, Varco RL: Neoplastic biliary obstruction. *Surgery* 20:72, 1946.
Flint ER: Abnormalities of hepatic and cystic arteries. *Br J Surg* 10:509, 1922–1923.
Jackson RH: Avoidance of injury to the common bile duct. *Surg Gynecol Obstet* 67:769, 1938.
Lander HH, Lyman RY, Anson BJ: *Q Bull Northwest Univ Med School* 15:103, 1941.
Lichtenstein M, Nicosia AJ: The clinical significance of accessory hepato-biliary ducts. *Ann Surg* 195:141:120, 1953.
McWhorter GL: New method of gallbladder dissection. *Surg Gynecol Obstet* 36:256, 1923.
Neuhoff H, Bloomfield S: Surgical significance of anomalous cholecysto-hepatic duct. *Ann Surg* 122:260, 1945.

References

1. Walters W, Snell AM: *Diseases of the Gallbladder and Bile Ducts.* Philadelphia, WB Saunders, 1940.
2. Rickles J: Personal communication.
3. Ivy A, Goldman L: Physiology of the biliary tract. *JAMA* 113:2413, 1939.
4. Ivy A, Oldberg E: A hormone mechanism for gallbladder contraction and evacuation. *Am J Physiol* 86:599, 1928.

Congenital Absence (Agenesis) of the Gallbladder

Agenesis of the gallbladder that is not associated with other anomalies of the extrahepatic biliary system is rare. It is usually difficult, and sometimes impossible, to diagnose this condition preoperatively. It is usually diagnosed at surgery or at autopsy. Danzis[1] reported 25 cases in 1980; Gordon and Gragutsky[2] reported 1 case each. Robertson et al.[3] reported 1 case in which carcinoma of the common duct existed. Talmadge[4] found 18 cases out of 18,350 autopsies; he noted that one-third of the cases of agenesis of the gallbladder were found in infants less than 1 year of age. Gross[5] found 38 cases of true agenesis in 1936. Finney and Owen[6] reported 2 cases. Villareal[7] in 1948 reported 60 cases since 1920; 26 were discovered at autopsy.

Embryologically, there are two common theories regarding the cause of agenesis of the gallbladder:

1. Failure of canalization into a tubular structure from the solid cords phase.
2. Failure of the hepatic diverticulum to develop from the foregut.

At surgery, three criteria are used to establish a diagnosis of agenesis of the gallbladder:

1. There is gross absence of the gallbladder after a thorough study of the biliary tree.
2. Cholecystography with fine needle instillation of 50% Hypaque is performed. Because of suspicious stones in the common bile duct, some surgeons instill the dye via a T-tube. Fifty percent of the time, common duct stones are present.
3. Anomalous (intrahepatic) gallbladder is ruled out.

The diagnosis of agenesis of the gallbladder is most often made by pathologists. Dixon and Lichtman[8] in 1945 reported 10 cases from the Mayo Clinic; 8 were discovered at surgery. The symptomatology associated with congenital absence of the gallbladder varies and is still controversial. Some patients have no symptoms; others have signs and symptoms suggestive of cholecystitis. This writer's patient had signs and symptoms of acute cholecystitis and mild jaundice, but no stones. Other reports state that despite the existence of jaundice, stones were found in 18 of 60 cases. Dixon and Lichtman's patients all had symptoms suggestive of cholecystitis. Preoperative diagnosis is almost impossible; a definitive diagnosis can only be established at surgery or at autopsy. The only preoperative finding is "nonfunctioning gallbladder."

At surgery, it may be recognized that the gallbladder does not exist. Villareal reported on 18 of 60 cases with stones in a dilated common duct. The intrahepatic gallbladder must be ruled out. Aspiration is of no value. The only positive method of establishing the presence of an intrahepatic gallbladder in a live patient is by pre- and postoperative cholangiography. The latter method cannot identify an obstructed gallbladder. Whether a choledochotomy with T-tube decompression would help symptomatic patients is questionable in view of the fact that no stones are found; the size of the common duct is usually within normal limits, and no evidence of jaundice exists.

This writer does not recommend routine common duct exploration without establishing the accepted criteria for choledochotomy and exploration. These criteria are:

1. A history or presence of jaundice.
2. Palpation of gallstones in the common duct.
3. A dilated common duct (no slate blue color) and a thickened wall.
4. Preoperative elevated alkaline phosphatase, bilirubin, or lactic dehydrogenase level.
5. Dilated common duct on the preoperative IV cholangiogram. (See "Choledochotomy and Common Duct Exploration" in Chapter 12.)

To reemphasize, in the differential diagnosis of a nonvisualizing gallbladder in a patient with atypical complaints, the surgeon should consider the rare possibility of an intrahepatic gallbladder or its congenital absence.

Recommended Reading

Bower JO: Congenital absence of the gallbladder. *Ann Surg* 88:80, 1928.

Braasch JW: Congenital anomalies of the gallbladder and bile ducts. *Surg Clin North Am* 38:627, 1958.

Cole WH (ed): *Operative Technic in General Surgery*, ed 2. New York, Appleton-Century-Crofts, 1955, p 537.

Gray H: *The Anatomy of the Human Body*, ed 27, ed CM Goss. Philadelphia, Lea & Febiger, 1959, p 1306.

Mayo CW, Kendrick DB: Anomalies of the gallbladder: A case report of left-sided floating gallbladder. *Arch Surg* 60:668, 1950.

Miller JE: Congenital absence of gallbladder. *Am J Surg* 33:315, 1936.

References

1. Danzis M: Congenital absence of the gallbladder. *Am J Surg* 29:202, 1980.
2. Gordon WC, Gragutsky D: Congenital absence of the gallbladder and cystic duct: Report of a case. *J Lab Clin Med* 27:594, 1942.

3. Robertson HF, Robertson WE, Bower JO: Congenital absence of the gallbladder, with a primary carcinoma of the common duct and carcinoma of the liver. *JAMA* 114:1514, 1940.
4. Talmadge GK: Congenital absence of the gallbladder. *Arch Pathol* 26:1060, 1938.
5. Gross RE: Congenital anomalies of the gallbladder. *Arch Surg* 32:131, 1936.
6. Finney GG Owen JK: The surgical aspect of the congenital absence of the gallbladder. *Ann Surg* 115:736, 1942.
7. Villareal L: Congenital absence of the gallbladder with case report. *Ann Surg* 127:745, 1948.
8. Dixon CF, Lichtman AL: Congenital absence of the gallbladder. *Surgery* 17:11, 1945.
9. Ivy A, Goldman L: Physiology of biliary tract. *JAMA* 113:2413, 1939.
10. Ivy AC, Oldberg E: A hormone mechanism for gallbladder contraction and evacuation. *Am J Physiol* 86:599, 1928.

Torsion of the Gallbladder (Floating Gallbladder)

Torsion of the gallbladder occurs most frequently in the elderly but is also seen in children and young adults. The underlying pathology (congenital and acquired) is an abnormally long mesentery suspending the body of the gallbladder and/or the cystic duct, without any other attachments.

The patient is usually not acutely ill and frequently fails to present an obvious clinical picture of cholecystitis. Yet, to procrastinate in such an instance would run the risk of infarction and necrosis of the gallbladder wall (gangrene), with perforation and peritonitis; empyema is also a possibility. The symptoms may simulate gallbladder colic, and a palpable mass may be present in the right upper quadrant (RUQ); the mass may disappear with relief of the torsion.

Torsion of the gallbladder may be incomplete (chronic form) or complete (acute form). In the incomplete form, the organ may rotate no more than 180° and obstruct the flow of bile but not the integrity of the cystic artery. In the complete form, the organ rotates beyond 180°, and thus obstructs the cystic duct and the cystic artery. Gangrene leads to perforation and peritonitis; the symptoms and signs become more acute.

Symptoms include tenderness in the RUQ, possible rebound, nausea, and vomiting; at the onset, the patient usually does not appear toxic. A blood study may or may not reveal a high leukocyte count, and the fever is usually low grade. The pulse is usually rapid and may remain so. Ultrasound and IV cholangiography may reveal stones in about half of the cases; a thickened gallbladder wall may be seen in most cases.

The surgeon who is visually unaware of torsion of the gallbladder will diagnose acute cholecystitis or a high-lying acute appendicitis. Early surgery is recommended because it will prevent the early complications of infarction and necrosis of the gallbladder wall, with perforation and peritonitis. In elderly patients with markedly constricted arteriosclerotic vessels, even slight distention of incomplete torsion, if unduly prolonged, can result in early infarction, necrosis, and perforation of the gallbladder wall.

Recommended Reading

Ashby BS: Acute and recurrent torsion of the gallbladder. *Br J Surg* 51:182, 1965.
Bothra R: Torsion of the gallbladder in the aged. *Br J Surg* 60:359, 1973.
Caldwell KPS: Torsion of the gallbladder. *Br Med J* 2:1425, 1950.
Carter R, Thompson RJ: Volvulus of the gallbladder. *Surg Gynecol Obstet* 116:105, 1963.
Chilton CP, Mann CV: Torsion of the gallbladder in a nine-year old boy. *JR Soc Med* 73:141, 1980.
Lau WY, Fan ST, Wong SH: Acute torsion of the gallbladder: A reemphasis on clinical diagnosis. *Aust NZ J Surg* 52:492, 1982.
Rawson HD: Torsion of the gallbladder in a child of twelve with a review of the literature. *Aust NZ J Surg* 22:315, 1953.
Schlinkert RT, Mucha P, Farnell MB: Torsion of the gallbladder. *Mayo Clin Proc* 59:490, 1984.
Short AR, Paul RG: Torsion of the gallbladder. *Br J Surg* 22:301, 1934.
Stieber AC, Bauer JJ: Volvulus of the gallbladder. *Am J Gastroenterol* 78:96, 1983.
Wellsted M, Kam J, Funston MR: Radiological pointers to preoperative diagnosis of torsion of the gallbladder. *S Afr Med J* 58:980, 1980.
Wendel AB: A case of floating gallbladder and kidney complicated by cholelithiasis with perforation of the gallbladder. *Ann Surg* 27:199, 1898.

Septate Gallbladder (Double or Triple—Vesica Fellea Duplex)

The intrahepatic biliary tract presents a variety of developmental abnormalities (anomalies).

Double gallbladders are not rare; the incidence is approximately 1 to 2 per 4000 cases.

EMBRYOLOGY

In the 4th to 5th week of fetal growth, the gallbladder arises from a complex endodermal diverticulum at the caudal end of the foregut. From this diverticulum, the hepatic radicles and liver will develop, as well as the ventral pancreas primordium, cystic duct, and gallbladder. By the 6th to 7th week, the solid cystic duct opens, and by the 11th to 12th week the gallbladder becomes hollowed out. A simple gallbladder may develop a true duplication from a splitting of the cystic duct primordium, or it may develop from a second primordium that arises at another site.

The true gallbladder may develop as a double gallbladder with two compartments separated by a complete septum; each compartment has its own cystic duct that drains into the common duct (Fig. 9). The double gallbladder that develops an incomplete septum empties into the common duct via a single cystic duct.

A normally functioning asymptomatic double (or triple) gallbladder without signs or symptoms may not require surgery (Figs. 10, 11). Some surgeons believe that if 1 of the 2 gallbladders becomes involved, the second organ will also ultimately develop cholecystitis and require cholecystectomy. It may be preferable to remove both gallbladders at the initial surgery.

Recommended Reading

Blaine ES: Biliary disease from x-ray viewpoint. *Surg Clin North Am* 6:1004, 1926.

Boni R: Cistifellea triplae bile calcarea. *Radiol Med* 44:833, 1958.

Boyden EA: The accessory gallbladder; an embryological and comparative study of aberrant biliary vesicles occurring in man and the domestic mammals. *Surg Gynecol Obstet* 104: 641, 1957.

Boyden EA, Wrenn EL Jr, Favara BE: Duodenal duplication (or pancreatic bladder) presenting as double gallbladder. *Surgery* 69:858, 1971.

Casey EN: Triple gallbladder. *Proc Coll Radiol Aust* 2:98, 1958.

Croudace WHH: A case of double gallbladder. *Br Med J* 1:707, 1931.

Flannery MG, Caster MP: Congenital abnormalities of the gallbladder; 101 cases. *Int Abstr Surg* 103:439, 1956.

Gross RE: Congenital anomalies of the gallbladder; a review of 148 cases with report of a double gallbladder. *Arch Surg* 32:131, 1936.

Guyer PB, McLoughlin M: Congenital double gall-bladder; review and report of two cases. *Br J Radiol* 40:214, 1967.

Harlaftis N, Gray SW, Olafson RP, Skandalakis JE: Three cases of unsuspected double gallbladder. *Am Surg* 42:178, 1976.

Hause WA: Triplication of gallbladder. *Arch Surg* 79:144, 1959.

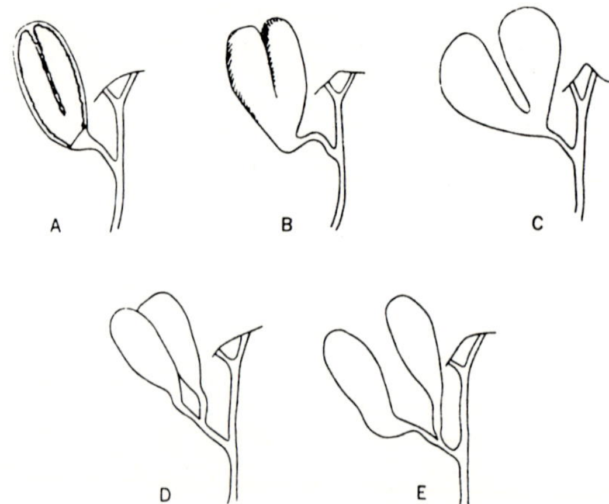

Figure 9.   Septate gallbladder without external groove is shown in part A, with groove and notched fundus in B. Drawing C shows a bi-lobed gallbladder. A Y-type double gallbladder with a common wall is shown in D, and E shows a Y-type double gallbladder divided into two separate organs.

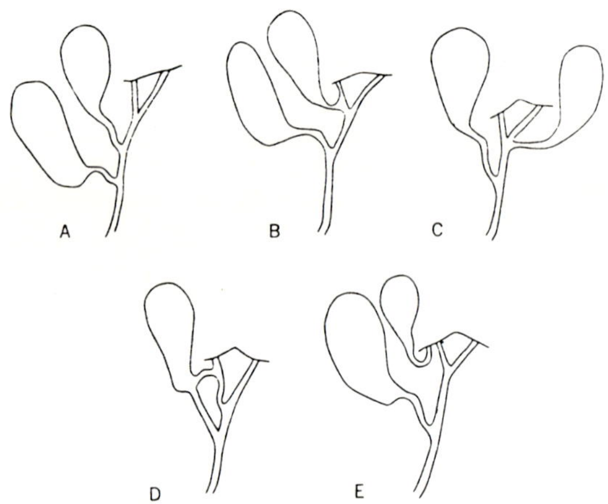

Figure 10.   Types of gallbladder duplication.

Ingegno AP, D'Albora JB: Double gallbladder; roentgenographic demonstration of a case of the "Y" type; classification of accessory gallbladder. *Am J Roentgenol* 61:671, 1949.

Meyer JH, Dowlin WM, Reinglass SS: Double gallbladder. *Am J Surg* 77:117, 1949.

Moore TC, Hurley AG: Congenital duplication of the gall bladder; review of the literature and report of an unusual symptomatic case. *Surgery* 35:283, 1954.

Mulla N, Weintraub S: Accessory liver with double gall bladder. *Arch Surg* 71:202, 1955.

Nichols BH: Double gallbladder. *Radiology* 6:255, 1926.

Papaioannou AN, Bartsokas St K: Problems associated with congenital duplication of the gallbladder. *Int Surg* 53:338, 1970.

Perelman H: Cystic duct reduplication. *JAMA* 175:710, 1961.

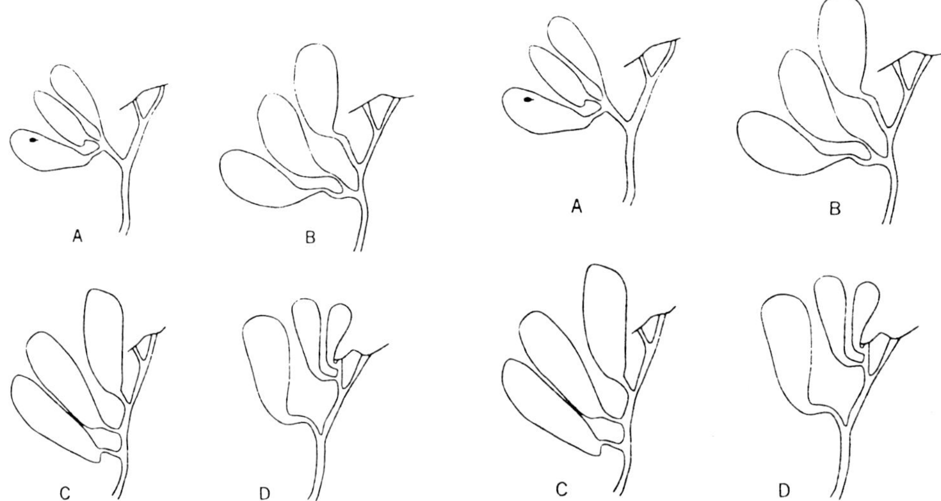

Figure 11.   Types of reported triple gallbladders.

Rabinovitch J, Rabinovitch P, Rosenblatt P, et al: Congenital anomalies of the gallbladder. *Ann Surg* 148:161, 1958.

Ramanathan T: Congenital duplication of the gall bladder; review of the literature and report of a case. *Med J Malaya* 25:305, 1971.

Raymond SW, Thrift CB: Carcinoma of a duplicated gall bladder. *Ill Med J* 110:239, 1956.

Recht W: Torsion of a double gall-bladder; a report of a case and a review of the literature. *Br J Surg* 39:342, 1952.

Roeder WJ, Mersheimer WL, Kazarian KK: Triplication of the gallbladder with cholecystitis, cholelithiasis, and papillary adenocarcinoma. *Am J Surg* 121:746, 1971.

Ross RJ, Sachs MD: Triplication of the gallbladder. *Am J Roentgenol* 104:656, 1968.

Shaw RB, Donato DA, Douglas DD, et al: Multiseptate gallbladder diagnosed during pregnancy. *Am Surg* 41:818, 1975.

Sherren J: A double gallbladder removed by operation. *Ann Surg* 54:204, 1911.

Shibata Y, Wada T, Mitsuiyama T: Surgical cases of formation of the gallbladder wall; review of the literature on cases with double formation of the gallbladder in Japan. *Rinsho Hoshasen* 15:344, 1970.

Skielboe B: Anomalies of the gallbladder—vesica fellea triplex, report of a case. *Am J Clin Pathol* 30:252, 1958.

Slaughter FG, Trout HH: Duplication of the gallbladder. *Am J Surg* 19:124, 1933.

Wren EL Jr, Favara BE: Duodenal duplication (or pancreatic bladder) presenting as double gallbladder. *Surgery* 69:858, 1971.

Reference

Bailby JOW: Stricture of the gallbladder. *J Pathol* 93:175, 1967.

Diameter of the Common Bile Duct

Leslie,[1] from the Department of Surgery of the Royal Melbourne Hospital, Australia, reported on the width of the common bile duct, in which measurements were taken at surgery to ascertain the relationship between the width of the duct and the presence of stones within it. He found that when the common bile duct was less than 9 mm in diameter, there was no disease in the distal portion; in contrast, common bile ducts greater than 17 mm in diameter almost always contained some disease. He concluded that common ducts measuring between 9 and 17 mm may or may not contain disease in the distal portion but that the probability of such disease increases rapidly in common ducts with a diameter of 14 mm or more. Therefore, it would appear from his studies that a common bile duct greater than 14 mm in diameter requires choledochotomy and exploration, and that in a common duct greater than 17 mm in width, exploration is mandatory. Leslie concluded that his method of common bile duct measurement is rapid and of value in assessing the need to explore the duct. This method, Leslie stated, offers a standard procedure that bears a direct relationship to the external diameter of the common bile duct and can easily be measured (Fig. 12).

This writer feels that this investigation has definite merit and fulfills the criteria of surgeons who believe that a common duct should not be opened routinely if its diameter is 10 mm or less. The presence of other criteria mentioned previously—

Level	Average Diameter in Millimeters
A. At entry into pancreas	6·5
B. Above notch	5·7
C. Below notch	3·9
D. In submucosa	3·3
E. At junction with pancreatic duct	1·9
F. Common channel	2·9
G. Orifice of papilla	2·1

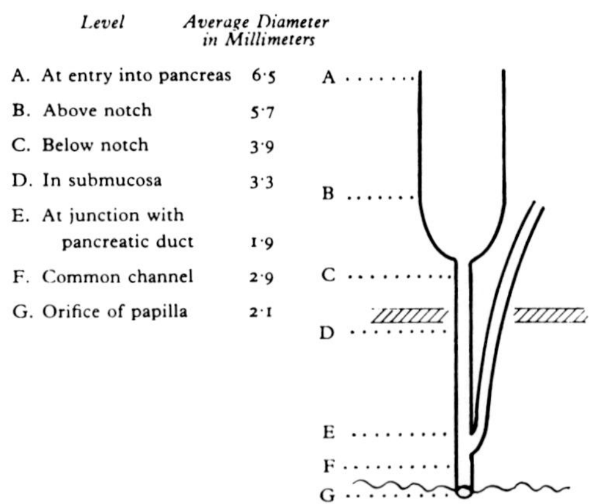

Figure 12. Dimensions and course of the common bile duct. (From Hand BH: Br J Surg 50:488, 1963.)

namely, the color and thickness of the common duct, a history of acholic stool, the presence or history of jaundice, and the size of the cystic duct in relation to the size of the stone found in the gallbladder—all provide additional evidence that may be effectively utilized at the time of surgery in arriving at a decision to open the common duct. Wakim and Mahour,[2] both from the Mayo Clinic, have written on the pathophysiologic consequences of cholecystectomy. They have concluded that uncomplicated cholecystectomy in man is not followed by significant dilatation of the common bile duct. They feel that when a significant dilatation develops, it is associated with a preexisting or concurrent causative disease of the duct wall, its surrounding structures, or both. These writers have carefully studied the anatomical and histological structure of the common bile duct and have found that the smooth muscle fibers in its wall are scattered and disorganized; they do not form a contiguous muscle layer. Consequently, the common duct does not exhibit rhythmic peristaltic activity; it functions as an expansile passive conduit rather than as an active peristaltic organ that rhythmically propels the bile downward. After cholecystectomy the duct wall usually thickens, and the glands in the duct walls proliferate, become more numerous, and spread deeper into the ductal structure. These authors cannot explain the function of these glands. In effect, cholecystectomy deprives the individual of a reservoir with concentrative ability and a pressure regulatory function of the gallbladder organ. This impediment is overcome without difficulty by functional and structural adaptations in which a more frequent delivery of bile into the intestine replaces the hormonal trigger, and the normally timed ejection of bile that occurs during the peak of digestion.

In summary, it should be stated that, according to the findings of these researchers, significant dilatation of the extrahepatic biliary system after cholecystectomy does not develop as a pure compensatory phenomenon; rather, it occurs only when a hepatobiliary complication coexists. In the latter instance, ductal dilatation should not be considered compensatory to the absence of the gallbladder; rather, it should be considered as being due to the disease within the duct wall itself, its contiguous structures, or both.

References

1. Leslie D: The width of the common bile duct. *Surg Gynecol Obstet* 126:761, 1968.
2. Mahour GH, Wakim KG, Soule EH, et al: Chronologic changes in calibre after cholecystectomy. *Arch Surg* 98:239, 1969.

Anatomical Relationship between the Common Bile Duct and the Pancreatic Duct (Duct of Wirsung)

Di Magno et al.[1] studied autopsy specimens to clarify the relationship between pancreatobiliary ductal anatomy and pancreatic ductal parenchymal histology (Fig. 4). Common channel studies revealed that:

74% had a common channel between the common duct and the pancreatic duct
25% had a well-defined ampulla
18% had a long common channel
31% had a short common channel
18% had an interposed septum
19% had separate biliary and pancreatic ducts

Further studies indicated that wherever a common channel between the common and pancreatic ducts existed, no significant histological changes occurred in the mucosa of the pancreatic duct. However, where no common channel existed, definite papillary epithelial hyperplasia took place in the pancreatic ductal mucosa. Di Magno et al. concluded that the lack of a common channel gives rise to ductal epithelial changes that, in turn, suggest the possibility of being precarcinogenic. This theory has not been substantiated.

Reference

1. Di Magno EP, Go VLW, Summerskill WH, et al: Impaired cholecystokinin pancreazmin secretion: Intraluminal dilution and maldigestion of fat. *Gastroenterology* 63:25, 1972.

Pancreas Divisum

Pancreas divisum (PD) is a congenital malformation in which the dorsal and ventral portions of the pancreas fail to fuse. The major portion of the gland drains through the dorsal duct via an accessory papilla. It is claimed that because of the small orifice of the accessory papilla, there is increased resistance to the flow of pancreatic juice; next, the impaired flow and stagnancy of pancreatic juice lead to pancreatitis. Some refer to the latter condition as *idiopathic pancreatitis.* Over a 7-year period, Delhaye[1] performed 9625 endoscopic retrograde pancreatographies (ERCPs) on 6324 patients with biliopancreatic complaints. In 304 patients (5.7%) PD was diagnosed. In patients diagnosed as having acute pancreatitis, PD was found in 7.5%; in cases of chronic pancreatitis the incidence was 6.4%; the average in all pancreatic disease processes was 5.5%. Delhaye was able to cannulate the accessory papilla and obtain dorsal ductograms in 89% of all ERCP patients.

This author believes that Delhaye has made a significant contribution and agrees that idiopathic pancreatitis, or pancreatic-like abdominal pain, should not be diagnosed unless the findings of anomalous ductal anatomy and abnormal biochemical studies support such a diagnosis. CT scan, sonography, and ERCP should be performed to confirm the presence of a dilated dorsal duct before surgical intervention is considered. Sphincterotomy, either via ERCP or by direct surgery, has proven unsuccessful. The author's choice is pancreaticojejunostomy. Delhaye[1] found that the prevalence of PD was similar to that of alcoholic and nonalcoholic pancreatitis.

These authors conclude that (1) PD is not a primary cause of pancreatitis, but rather a coincidental anatomical anomaly seen in about 10% of the population, and that (2) surgical procedures that attempt to improve dorsal duct drainage are not indicated unless a dorsal duct abnormality can be clearly demonstrated.

Delhaye noted that patients with acute biliary pancreatitis were less likely to have PD than those with nonbiliary acute pancreatitis. In fact, PD was more likely to prevent acute biliary pancreatitis.

Reference

1. Delhaye M: Pancreas divisum: Congenital anatomical variance or anomaly? *Gastroenterology* 89:951, 1985.

Anomalous Location of the Papilla of Vater

The location of the papilla of Vater in the third (horizontal) portion of the duodenum has been described only rarely—about once in 1000 cases. It is recognized only on cholangiography. Schwartz and Birnbaum[1] reported an incidence of 8% after studying 122 operative cholangiograms.

Clinically, the anomalous location of the ampulla of Vater may justify some endoscopic failures, as in sphincterotomy and retrograde cholangiopancreatography. A failure to diagnose carcinoma of the ampulla was reported; failure was based upon the anomalous position of the ampulla. Preoperative cholangiography may alert the surgeon to its precise location.

Reference

1. Schwartz A, Birnbaum D: Pancreatic necrosis with gas formation. *Am J Proctol* 21:263, 1970.

3

ETIOLOGICAL CONSIDERATIONS IN THE OVERALL PATHOGENESIS OF GALLSTONES

Pathogenesis of Cholesterol Gallstones

Norman B. Javitt, M.D., Ph.D., and
Charles K. McSherry, M.D., Ph.D.

Around the turn of the century, opinion was clearly divided as to whether the gallbladder or the liver had the predominant role in the formation of gallstones. By that time, it was well recognized that the chief component of gallstones in most instances is cholesterol; any explanation involving the gallbladder or the liver, or both, would have to account for the precipitation of cholesterol to initiate stone formation. Many researchers theorize that the process begins with gallbladder infection, and are convinced that excess cholesterol accumulates as a result of epithelial cell exfoliation associated with inflammation of the gallbladder wall. Other workers, equally sure that infection is not a prerequisite, point to a combination of bile stasis and increased hepatic production of cholesterol.

The authors propose that small pigment particles arising in the liver because of a metabolic defect there, are carried by the bile to the gallbladder, where they serve as a nucleus for cholesterol deposition.

It would be fortunate if we could report that in the intervening years the relative contributions of the gallbladder and the liver to cholelithiasis had become more certain. Recent work may seem to have settled the issue by identifying the culprit as abnormal hepatic bile present only in individuals who develop calculous biliary disease. But another possibility should not be foreclosed, namely, that essentially normal hepatic bile is altered by conditions within the gallbladder that lead to precipitation and crystallization of cholesterol.

Our reasons for urging that the matter be kept open, at least until newer experimental techniques for studying cholelithiasis have been put to fuller use, will become apparent as this discussion proceeds. A greater understanding of the pathogenetic mechanisms in gallstone formation would, of course, be of more than academic interest, considering the major clinical importance of calculous biliary disease (which presently affects some 10 to 15 million persons in the United States alone). Moreover, since the incidence of gallstones increases progressively with age, the number of cases detected yearly (presently about 100,000) can be expected to grow as the mean age of the population increases.

The clinical consequences of cholelithiasis are, of course, amenable to intervention: surgical removal of the gallbladder is curative in more than 90% of the cases so treated, and there is now the prospect of gallstone dissolution by chemical means. But despite its recognized benefits, gallbladder surgery is not without risk, and the potential of medical treatment still awaits definition and proof (we will return to this point later).

Clearly, it would be desirable if enough were known of the mechanisms of gallstone formation to prevent its occurrence. However, the development of an experimental animal model with a fairly close similarity to the human disease proved difficult to achieve, and without such a model, only limited information was obtainable. Until recently, most research in cholelithiasis was performed in species that do not form gallstones spontaneously, permitting little extrapolation to the human situation. Cholesterol gallstones have been produced experimentally in several animals by dietary modification (e.g., in hamsters with a diet free of polyunsaturated fatty acids and containing an easily absorbable sugar), but applicability to human cholelithiasis has remained restricted, since there is little evidence that the nature of man's diet is causally related to stone formation. No other species appeared to share our vulnerability to spontaneous gallstone formation until cholesterol cholelithiasis closely resembling the human disease was found to occur in at least one other primate—the baboon. This long-needed animal model is now providing greater insight into the pathogenesis of cholelithiasis in man.

This discovery—or, more properly, rediscovery—of spontaneous stone formation in the baboon was accidental and was made by one of us (C.K. McS.) in the course of collaborative work with Frank Glenn and Norman B. Javitt[1,2] on hepatobiliary function in nonhuman primates (Fig. 13). Undertaking a literature search, we learned that probably the first example of cholelithiasis affecting a primate—a marmoset that died of acute cholecystitis and calculous obstruction of the common bile duct—had been recorded by Hamerton in 1931. Three decades later (in 1963), other investigators reported the presence of biliary calculi composed chiefly of cholesterol in baboons and marmosets. According to other workers, gallstone formation is a fairly common occurrence among wild baboons in certain parts of Africa.[1]

In any event, development of the primate model provided the opportunity to initiate studies not possible in man with regard to cholesterol chole-

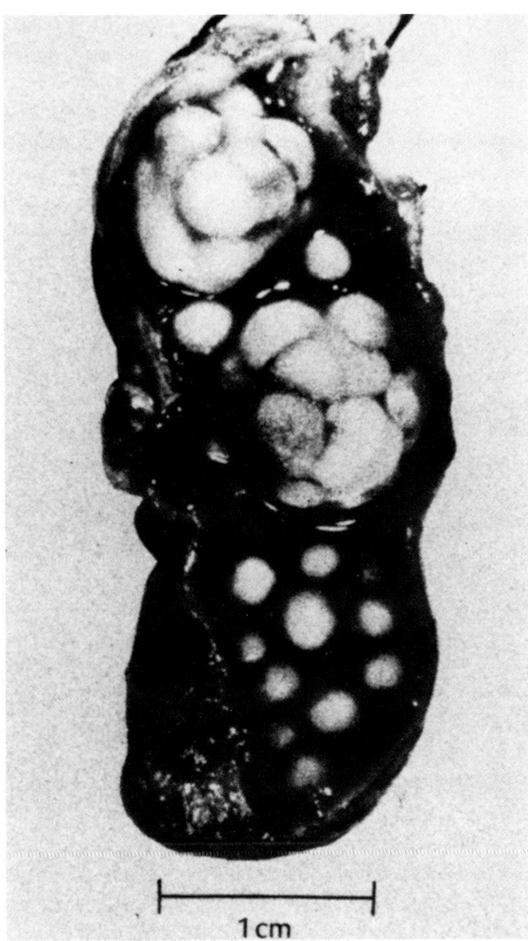

Figure 13. The unexpected finding of spontaneous gallstone formation in the baboon, as shown in excised gallbladder, made available the long-needed animal model for studies or cholesterol cholelithiasis in humans.

lithiasis. Before this work is described in more detail, it would be well to review what is known of the normal mechanisms regulating the production and metabolism of cholesterol, as well as of other bile constituents, and of the conditions (local or systemic) that may underlie stone formation.

A remarkable fact about cholesterol is that, while virtually insoluble in water, it is held in solution in an aqueous medium such as bile by the combined action of the other two major bile constituents, bile salts and phospholipids. The detergency of bile, which makes possible the solubilization of cholesterol, was discovered more than 200 years ago. Informed people recommended the use of bile for cleaning stained wool or linen and for mixing paint colors. The colloidal state of cholesterol in bile, as well as the solubilizing effect of bile salts, was recognized shortly after bile salts were identified in the mid-nineteenth century.

It is significant, of course, that the primary bile acids formed in the liver as products of cholesterol metabolism—and conjugated there with glycine or taurine—in turn dissolve the parent substance, which is then carried in solution through the biliary tract. A point germane to our discussion is that the composition of bile acid in baboons is essentially similar to that in man—the primary bile acids being cholic and chenodeoxycholic acids, both formed from cholesterol and conjugated in the liver; in addition, there is the secondary compound, deoxycholic acid, formed in the intestine through bacterial dehydroxylation of cholic acid.

Evidently, the biliary system in man and the baboon is alike in another respect: under physiological conditions, the bile of both species contains a relatively large amount of cholesterol, noticeably more than that of other species. Indeed, given the high cholesterol content of human bile, it was recognized that solubilization could not be accomplished by bile salts alone. Fatty acids were initially implicated, but the work of Isaksson identified the phospholipid component (chiefly lecithin) of bile as acting in concert with bile salts to maintain the solubility of cholesterol. What is involved is the ability of bile salts, which are water soluble, to form small aggregates, or micelles, in aqueous solutions, and also that of lecithin, which, though insoluble in water, swells to form liquid crystals that incorporate cholesterol. Through the action of bile salts, the insoluble liquid crystals containing cholesterol are formed into small, soluble aggregates, or mixed micelles. (The concept of the micelle, formulated more than 60 years ago in studies of soap solutions, involves spontaneous aggregation in an aqueous medium of molecules having appropriately arranged hydrophilic and hydrophobic regions. The polar ends of the molecules are hydrophilic and oriented toward the center of the micelle. Through micelle formation, as little as 100 ml of bile can hold in solution as much as 1 gm of cholesterol despite the latter's insolubility in water.)

The relative concentrations of the three bile constituents, rather than the absolute amounts present, are the critical factor in keeping cholesterol in solution. This important insight was provided by Small et al.[3] with an in vitro model simulating human bile employed to define the solubility limits of cholesterol. In these studies, dry mixtures of bile salts, lecithin, and cholesterol in varying proportions were mixed with water, allowed to equilibrate, and then examined grossly and microscopically for classification as one-phase (micellar), two-phase (liquid crystal and cholesterol crystal), and three-phase (micellar, liquid crystal, and cholesterol crystal) solutions. With the aid of a triangular phase diagram for depicting the relative concentrations of cholesterol, lecithin, and bile salts in a given mixture in relation to the total quantity of all three constituents, one could predict the maximum amount of cholesterol maintainable in a micellar solution.

Applying the method clinically, Small et al. compared bile samples from patients being operated on for cholesterol gallstones and others without biliary disease undergoing abdominal surgery for other reasons. In reporting their findings, the investigators noted a "clear-cut separation between normal and abnormal bile," attributing the difference to an excess of cholesterol relative to the bile salts and lecithin present. In the patients without gallstones, all bile samples appeared to be less than saturated with cholesterol (i.e., within the micellar zone in the triangular phase diagram); in the patients with gallstones, bile was usually oversaturated with cholesterol, and in some cases contained insoluble cholesterol in the form of microcrystals.

The thesis advanced by Small et al. was that the process of gallstone formation involves, first, the production of abnormal bile—that is, bile oversaturated with cholesterol—followed by a second stage in which excess cholesterol precipitates as cholesterol microcrystals. In a third stage, continued growth of the original crystals or adherence of some small ones results in the formation of macroscopic stones.

These workers moved next to identify the source of the oversaturated bile. Was it the liver, where bile is produced, or the gallbladder, where stones form? Samples of both hepatic and gallbladder bile were obtained from patients undergoing cholecystectomy for symptomatic gallbladder disease; by intent, the study was conducted among Indians of the southwestern United States, a population usually susceptible to cholesterol gallstone formation. Mean values for the composition of hepatic and gallbladder bile differed sharply. In 80 to 90% of the patients studied, gallbladder bile was saturated with cholesterol, and liver bile appeared to be highly supersaturated. These findings strongly suggested to the investigators that the initiating event in stone formation is the production of supersaturated bile by the liver. It was speculated that a metabolic defect involving the canalicular membrane of the liver altered the normal balance of hepatic bile constituents, although the precise nature of the defect remained unknown.

These observations would seem to have put to rest the long-running debate over the primary abnormality leading to gallstone formation—except that other work also bearing on the relationship of the lipid composition of hepatic and/or gallbladder bile to stone formation has failed to show significant differences between individuals with gallstones and those without them. Indeed, when Dam and colleagues[4] in Denmark analyzed bile samples from patients undergoing surgery for cholelithiasis and others being operated on for peptic ulcer, most samples—regardless of their source—appeared to be supersaturated with cholesterol.

Earlier, the Danish investigators had also performed physicochemical studies to define the solubility limits of cholesterol in bile salt solutions to which lecithin was added in varying amounts, plotting the molar ratios logarithmically. In hamsters with induced gallstones, bladder bile samples analyzed for cholesterol solubility proved to be either saturated or supersaturated with cholesterol; in animals without gallstones, bile was consistently unsaturated. On the other hand, with the use of a cholesterol solubility curve calculated according to the Small data, most bile samples from animals with gallstones appeared to be in an unsaturated rather than a saturated state. Similarly, when the Small data were applied to the bile samples obtained from patients with and without gallstones, bile classified as supersaturated by Dam was often unsaturated according to Small. To borrow from Dam's report of these results: "Obviously establishment of a solubility limit to which everybody can agree is called for."

Conceivably, the conditions of the two sets of experiments could have accounted in part for the differences in their findings. In terms of physical chemistry, a given solvent (in this case, bile) becomes supersaturated with a solute when the most stable concentration of the latter is exceeded. With the passage of time, however, a state of equilibrium is reached among molecules going into and out of solution. At that point, some precipitation occurs and the solvent is no longer supersaturated. Thus, depending on how long an interval elapses before a given bile sample is analyzed, it may or may not be supersaturated with cholesterol. Whether the conflicting interpretations in reference to bile composition and cholelithiasis can be explained on this basis is unclear. In any event, more recent work by Holzbach and associates[5] has defined still other

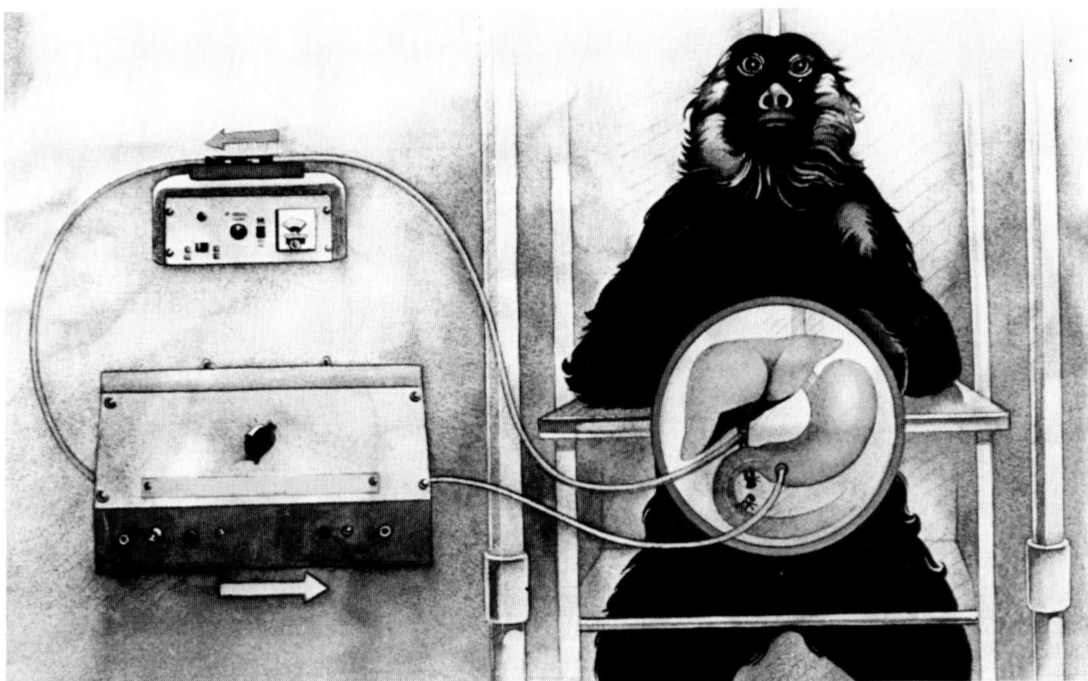

Figure 14.   A baboon (cholecystectomized); hepatic bile is being monitored. For full explanation, refer to Figure 15.

limits for cholesterol solubility in bile, and by these criteria, too, stone formers cannot be distinguished from the rest of the population on the basis of the physicochemical composition of the bile.

If alterations in bile composition do play a role in stone formation, is there a possibility of identifying them in relation to the natural changes occurring with reabsorption of bile salts from the intestine via the portal vein? Or at another phase of the cycle, after excretion of bile from the liver to the gallbladder prior to the return of bile to the intestine? In its general outline, the enterohepatic circulation of bile is well understood, although specific details that could bear on the development of biliary disease have been lacking. Our research in primates with reference to cholelithiasis began with the aim of learning more about normal variations in bile composition that occur in the course of this circulation (Fig. 14). Accordingly, samples of both gallbladder and liver bile were obtained at laparotomy; the relative concentrations of the major components in each bile sample were plotted on triangular coordinates according to the method of Small. Significantly, in about 50% of the cases, values for cholesterol solubility of hepatic bile fell well outside the miceller zone, i.e., hepatic bile was supersaturated with cholesterol. On the other hand, in gallbladder bile samples obtained at the same time, values for cholesterol solubility were usually (in 84.6% of the cases) within the micellar zone, i.e., gallbladder bile was less than saturated with cholesterol.

Since these were presumably normal animals with no evidence of gallstone diseases, was the supersaturation of hepatic bile within normal limits as well? The finding that gallbladder bile was less than saturated with cholesterol also required an explanation. Suppose that at the time of sampling most of the bile salt pool was within the gallbladder awaiting transport to the intestine, as might be expected, since the animals had been fasted overnight prior to surgery. There would be proportionately less cholesterol in gallbladder bile and more in hepatic bile. To extend this line of reasoning, with return of the bile salt pool to the liver, would the cholesterol of liver bile be increased?

In further experiments with baboons, all gallbladder bile was aspirated at laparotomy, hepatic bile was diverted by cannulation of the common hepatic duct, and the aspirated bladder bile was instilled in the terminal ileum on the assumption that it would be promptly transported to the liver. Again, since the animals had been fasted prior to surgery, it was also assumed that the gallbladder bile would be high in bile salts and low in cholesterol. The result? The bile salt content of hepatic

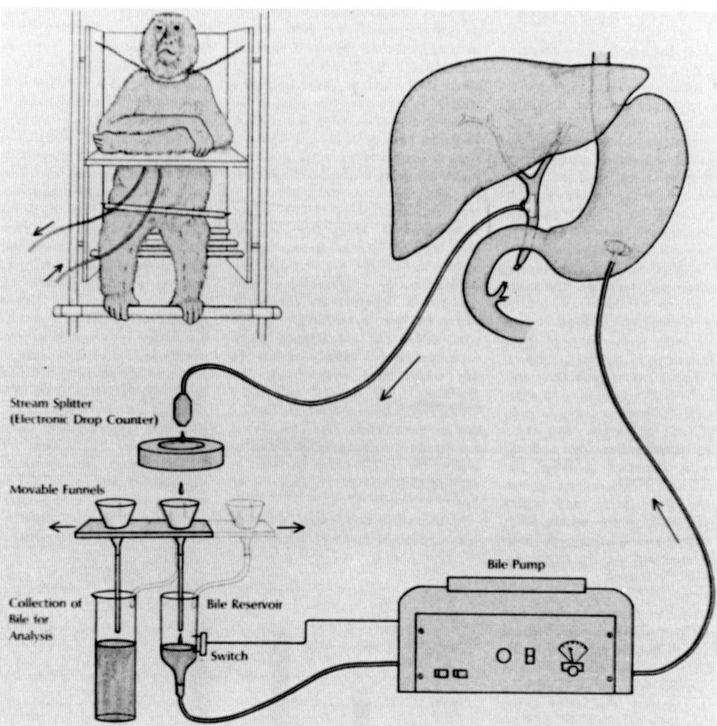

Figure 15.   In primate experiments, hepatic bile composition after cholecystectomy is examined by diverting bile flow through permanent biliary fistula and monitoring it during a 24-hour cycle. With use of electronic fraction collector, a pre-determined percentage of enterohepatic circulation is removed for analysis and the remaining unsampled bile is returned to animal via gastronomy tube.

bile promptly increased, and with it the capacity of hepatic bile to solubilize cholesterol, as evidenced by a shift of coordinate points further into the micellar zone. After an hour, the bile salt content of hepatic bile decreased, and the coordinate points shifted away from the micellar zone (Fig. 15).

In a related experiment, we instilled gallbladder bile into the ileum and, after cholesterol solubility in hepatic bile had reached its maximum, infused bile salt (sodium taurocholate) into the portal circulation. Immediately there was a further increase in the bile salt concentration of hepatic bile, paralleled by a further increase in the cholesterol-solubilizing capacity of bile.

What the experimental findings suggested, of course, was that under physiological conditions the composition of bile may differ significantly, depending on whether or not the bile salt pool is flowing through the liver. Evidently, the demonstration of saturated or supersaturated hepatic bile reflected the fact that sampling had been done when the liver was relatively depleted of bile salts; hence the degree of saturation with cholesterol was high. In the baboon, moreover, the results were similar whether the animal did or did not have gallstones.

Given the experimental conditions up to that point, we could only infer that the observed variations in bile composition were analogous to those occurring during the normal enterohepatic circulation of bile salts. For more direct evidence, a method was needed for monitoring bile flow and composition over a 24-hour period. The technique we adopted (originally devised by Small for studies in rhesus monkeys) involves progressive conditioning of baboons to remain for a prolonged period in a restraining chair after the creation of a permanent biliary fistula. Hepatic bile flowing through the fistula is thus made available as desired for measurement and analysis (Fig. 16).

After training (usually a 3- to 4-week period is required) the animal's gallbladder is excised and a small T-tube is sutured into the common bile duct; the common duct distal to the T-tube is divided, and the ends are closed with sutures. Bile flow is then directed through the T-tube to an electronic fraction collector so that a predetermined percentage of the enterohepatic circulation can be removed for analysis; the remaining unsampled bile is returned to the animal via a gastrostomy tube. Thus far, seven baboons have been trained and studied for periods ranging from 10 to 80 days (Fig. 15).

In representative experiments, animals were allowed both fluids and solid food (standard monkey chow). Liver and hepatic bile remained relatively constant, and cholesterol solubility values were always within the micellar range. Similar results were obtained regardless of the proportion of the flow removed (this ranged from 5 to 25%), indicating that, at least in the baboon, when the need arises, the liver is capable of substantially increasing bile salt synthesis to maintain bile salt secretion and pool size at normal levels.

In light of our earlier discussion, of course, the interesting findings were the constancy of bile composition and the relative balance among bile constituents, whereas under the previously described conditions, hepatic bile had varied greatly in composition and was often supersaturated. A major difference, to be sure, was that the second set of experiments was performed after removal of the gallbladder, which would preclude sequestration of bile salts and its consequences for the liver. In additional experiments, after the biliary fistula was established, human gallbladder bile (obtained by needle aspiration in the course of cholecystectomy) was fed to the animals via gastrostomy tube. In all, there was a prompt increase in bile flow, as in bile salt excretion. With the change in the amount of bile salt relative to cholesterol and phospholipid, the cholesterol solubility of hepatic bile also increased. When pure bile salt (sodium taurocholate) was substituted for human bladder bile, hepatic bile showed a similar increase in flow and in bile salt excretion.

If the experimental findings in animals have their counterpart in man, the bile salt concentration of hepatic bile should normally reach its nadir during the long interval between the evening meal and breakfast the next morning, while most of the bile salt pool remains stored in the gallbladder until required for the digestive process. It should be at its highest after the digestion of a meal, during reabsorption of the bile salt pool from the intestine.

Of necessity, then, the bile composition of a given individual, with or without gallstones, should depend on the location of the bile salt pool at the time of analysis. In sampling a single early morning specimen after an overnight fast—as in patients undergoing gallbladder surgery—the presence of bile with cholesterol in a supersaturated state

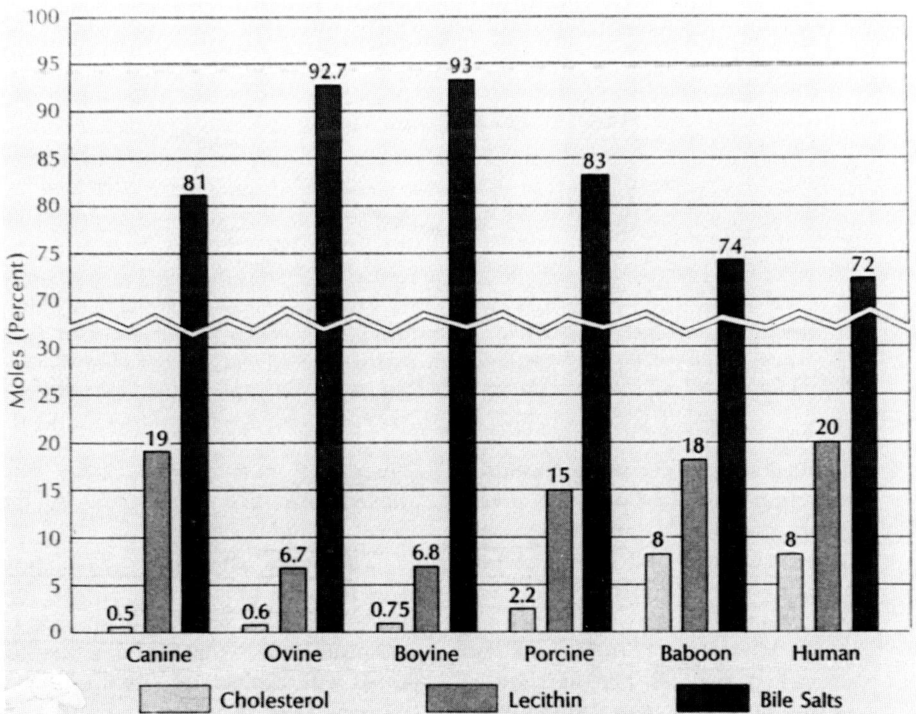

Figure 16.   In both man and baboon, but not in other species, there is a high proportion of cholesterol in bile relative to other components. Spontaneous gallstone formation in both may be partly explained on this basis. Genetic factors, as well as a smaller bile salts pool, may help account for higher incidence of gallstones among primates.

should not be taken to mean that the same physicochemical state is maintained at other times. Nor can it be assumed, on the basis of such sampling, that the hepatic bile of patients with gallstones differs from that of the rest of the population in that it contains more cholesterol than can be kept in solution by the amount of bile salts and lecithin present (Fig. 17).

In this connection, it is worth citing the findings on gallbladder and/or hepatic bile sampling in patients undergoing elective biliary surgery. Most of these patients (51 of 66) were being operated on for cholesterol gallstones; of the remainder, 6 had pigment stones and 9 were free of gallstone disease. The relative concentrations of bile constituents and the degree of bile saturation were calculated according to the criteria of Small. Among the patients with cholesterol gallstones, about half of the bile samples (59% of hepatic bile, 55% of bladder bile) were classified as saturated or supersaturated with cholesterol; in the remainder, values were within the micellar zone. Moreover, there was considerable overlap between these samples and those of patients with pigment stones or without stones of either type.

The investigators noted that, had the criteria of Dam been used instead, a higher proportion of patients with cholesterol gallstones would have had supersaturated bile, but so would more of the others undergoing surgery. In commenting on the relative frequency of unsaturated hepatic bile samples obtained from stone formers, the investigators concluded that secretion of supersaturated bile by the liver must have occurred only intermittently. This was borne out in repeated sampling of hepatic bile from stone formers with T-tubes for drainage after cholecystectomy. Most patients produced both saturated and unsaturated bile, and in no patient did bile remain consistently saturated (Fig. 18).

Most clinical data with regard to biliary lipid composition have been obtained in patients with gallstones. Without more information of a comparable nature on individuals without stones, interpretation of any findings is necessarily limited. The knowledge that the cholesterol content of human bile is relatively high to begin with makes it reasonable to suggest that in the cycling of bile salts through the enterohepatic circulation there might be periods when a relative deficit could leave hepatic bile saturated or supersaturated with cholesterol.

Although thus far we have discussed biliary lipid composition briefly in relation to the bile salt pool, since lecithin secretion in bile appears to be controlled by the rate of bile salt secretion, it is assumed that there is similar diurnal variation in the lecithin concentration of hepatic bile that may also influence the degree of saturation of bile with cholesterol at any time. As for cholesterol itself, according to available evidence, its secretion in bile appears to be independent of bile salt secretion; hence, under physiological conditions, the cholesterol concentration of bile tends to remain relatively constant.

But of course, the important issue in reference to biliary cholesterol and cholelithiasis is less concerned with the amount present than with its physical state (Fig. 17). As we have seen, saturation or supersaturation of bile with cholesterol may be a necessary event in stone formation, but it is scarcely sufficient. The cholesterol must precipitate out of the bile so that microcrystals and then macrocrystals can form.

As a determinant of cholesterol precipitation, how important is the total size of the bile salt pool?

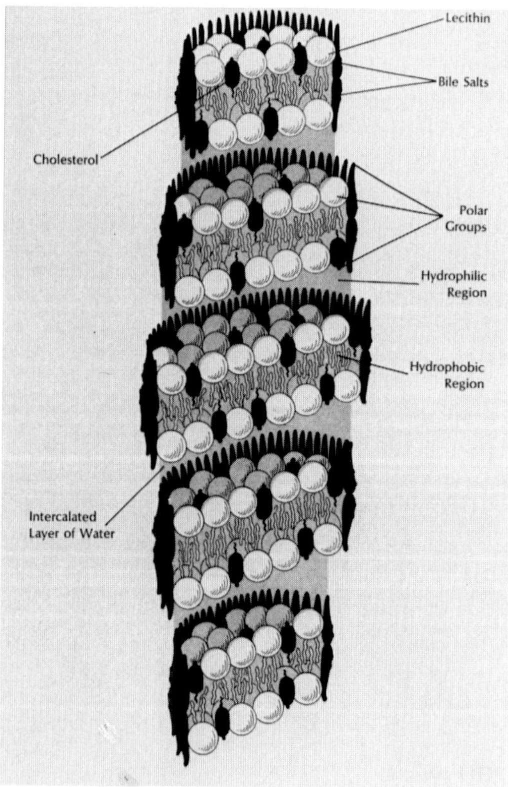

Figure 17. Postulated mechanism whereby cholesterol, although virtually insoluble in water, in held in solution in an aqueous medium such as bile, which entails the formation of mixed micelles comprising cholesterol, lecithin, and bile salts, as schematized above.

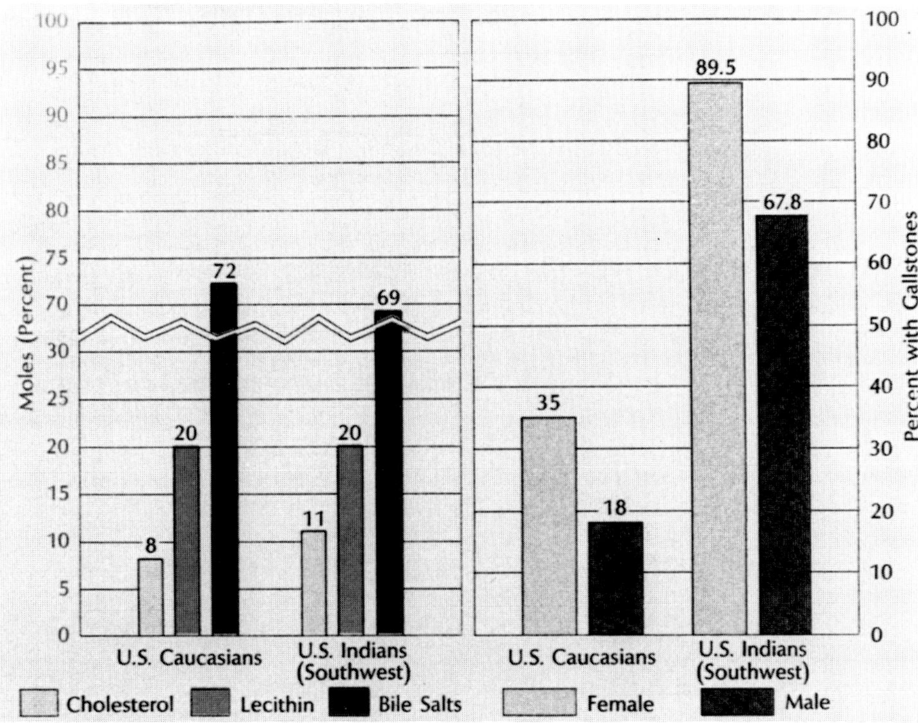

Figure 18.   American Indians of the Southwest as compared with white American population.   Data for Indians are from field study of prevalence by Sampliner et al; those for white Americans represent incidence at autopsy (Newman and Northrup). In both groups percentages compared are those found or estimated among oldest age groups (60 and over).

In theory, if the pool size were greatly reduced for some reason, hepatic bile might remain supersaturated with cholesterol for a longer period, extending the opportunity for precipitation when this supersaturated bile reaches the gallbladder. On the other hand, a large bile salt pool could have a protective effect. Earlier, mention was made of American Indian populations at high risk for symptomatic gallbladder disease (according to Burch et al.,[6] the prevalence rate among Pima Indian women is 60 to 70%). There is some evidence linking the frequency of gallstone formation in the affected tribes to the average size of their bile salt pools, which is relatively small compared with that of the rest of the U.S. population.

On the other hand, consider the Masai, a nomadic African people, among whom gallstone formation is exceptionally rare. Clues were sought in the nature of the Masai diet, but the intake of dietary cholesterol, fat, and carbohydrate proved comparable to that of Western countries, where cholelithiasis is quite common. However, studies among the Masai have turned up significant differences in bile salt pool size. On the average, it is two to three times larger than that of the U.S. groups studied.

In the Masai, as in American Indians, the evidence relating bile salt pool size to gallstone formation seems incontrovertible, and since both populations are genetically relatively homogeneous, a high degree of genetic control over pool size seems likely. But in more heterogeneous populations, this direct correlation between stone formation and either the rate of bile salt secretion or the size of the bile salt pool evidently does not exist. This is not to suggest that the balance of lipid components in the bile is of little importance; it does suggest that there are other variables that we may need to understand better, in particular, those involved in regulating bile salt–cholesterol interaction.

Recent breeding studies in the squirrel monkey have yielded interesting genetic differences that could have a bearing on the problem of gallstone formation. When cholesterol was fed to some animals, it was promptly converted into bile acids; in others, gallstone formation ensued. It would appear that enzyme-regulated processes under genetic control account for the difference, but this can only be a guess until more is known.

Plainly, in seeking the determinants of gallstone formation, we must look not only at the liver and the composition of hepatic bile but beyond, at other aspects of the biliary system. Thus we have come full circle, returning to the thought that gallbladder dysfunction may be a primary factor in cholesterol cholelithiasis. Since among the organs comprising the biliary system the gallbladder is most often the repository of biliary calculi, this would seem a logical prospect. Besides, if the gallbladder is not involved, why should the disease cease with cholecystectomy?

To be sure, if a major role is posited for the gallbladder, the next question is, what might it be? Several possibilities can be suggested. For example, since the production of supersaturated bile by the liver evidently cannot by itself account for stone formation, perhaps we should look at how the rate of physicochemical conversion of supersaturated bladder bile to the saturated state may be related to precipitation and crystallization of cholesterol. Evidence suggests that ordinarily the time required for the shift from supersaturation to saturation is such that bile does not remain in the gallbladder long enough for precipitation and crystallization to occur (Figs. 17, 19). But perhaps because of conditions within the gallbladder, the rate of change may be altered in some individuals so that cholesterol precipitation and crystallization occur sooner and increase the likelihood of stone formation.

The diurnal variations in hepatic bile composition relative to the composition of gallbladder bile may provide another lead. Normally, after contraction and emptying of the gallbladder to provide bile for the digestive process, some residual bladder bile is bound to remain behind, especially when emptying occurs at the end of a fasting period, after the bile salt pool has been sequestered for a time in the gallbladder. The residual bile, of course, is likely to contain bile salts in high concentration and to be less than saturated with cholesterol, whereas "new" bile flowing in from the liver is likely to be low in bile salts and supersaturated with cholesterol. In theory, the two could combine to form either a homogeneous solution or a heterogeneous mixture, and until recently, the assumption has been that the former was more likely. However, in some individuals, IV cholangiograms tend to show streaking of contrast material, suggesting that their gallbladder bile is not uniform in composition. Unless a single homogeneous solution does form, one result may be the layering of bile rich in cholesterol near the gallbladder epithelium, which

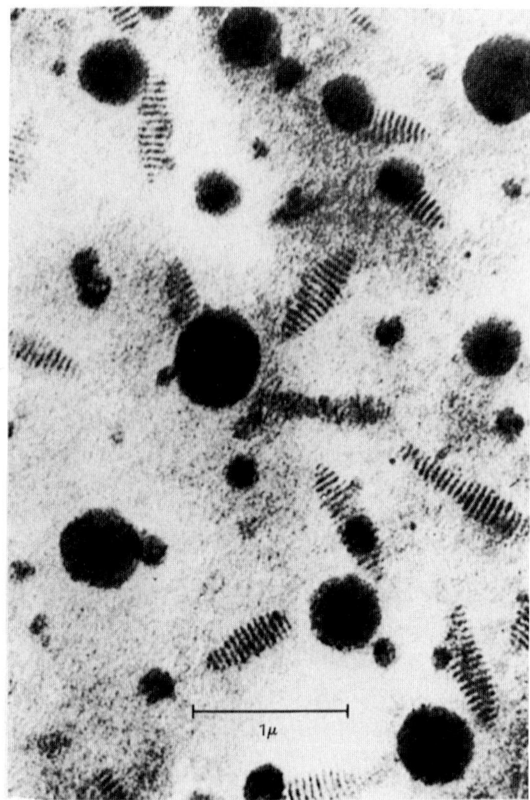

Figure 19. *Artificial mixture simulating human bile, prepared by Howell et al for cholesterol solubility studies, contains cigar-shaped structures identical to those seen on electron microscopy of natural bile. Because of their striped appearance these structures are thought to represent stacked micelles separated by electron-dense water.*

could well contribute to cholelithiasis. Indeed, it has been suggested ("Physicochemical Considerations in Gallstone Pathogenesis" later in this chapter) that heterogeneity in gallbladder bile composition, causing such an accumulation of cholesterol, may be the key factor in stone formation—more important, in fact, than the solubilizing capacity of the bile salt–lecithin complex. To us it seems plausible that at least some cases of cholesterol cholelithiasis may be explainable on the basis of local conditions within the gallbladder that delay the diffusion of cholesterol from a nonmicellar to a micellar phase, so that a single homogeneous solution is never achieved (Figs. 20, 21).

Other processes within the gallbladder might also play a role. For example, in physicochemical terms, for bladder bile to shift in composition so that cholesterol will be precipitated requires a suit-

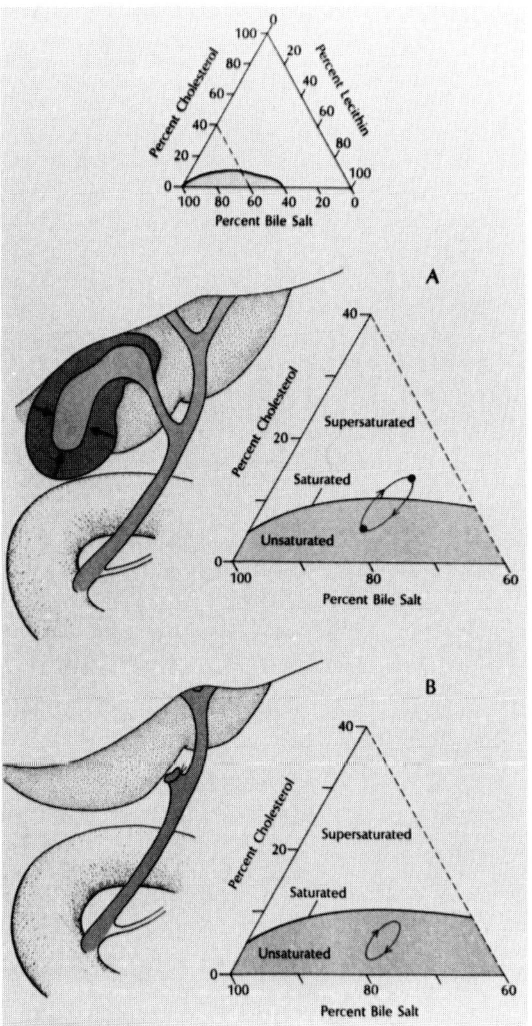

Figure 20.   A. Baboon studies show that normally enterohepatic cycling of bile salts results in supersaturation of hepatic bile with cholesterol during fasting periods, since bile salt pool is sequestered in gallbladder; with food instake and release of bile salts, hepatic bile becomes unsaturated and within the zone of micellar solubility. B. After cholecystectomy, however, hepatic bile maintains relatively constant composition. Cholesterol solubility is plotted as a percentage of the total quantity of bile components on triangular coordinates according to method of Small (representative triangle at top).

able surface on which the change from supersaturation to saturation can occur. Since cholesterol gallstones often contain a pigment center, quite possibly the needed surface could be provided by a nidus of calcium bilirubinate within the gallbladder. Alternatively, the same purpose might be served by epithelial cells loosened from gallbladder mucosa or by bacteria multiplying in bladder bile.

Normally, the gallbladder mucosa is impermeable to bile constituents other than inorganic salts and water, but what would happen if permeability were acutely altered because of local inflammation, or over a longer period for hormonal or other reasons? The consequences could be a reduction in

Figure 21.   In patients with cholelithiasis, Schersten et al found a marked excess of cholesterol in hepatic bile after interruption of the enterohepatic circulation; under physiologic conditions a similar interruption may occur overnight when bile pools in the gallbladder. With duodenal infusion of bile salts most cholesterol was held in micellar solution. Numbers denote hours after start of experiment; infusion began at point 5.

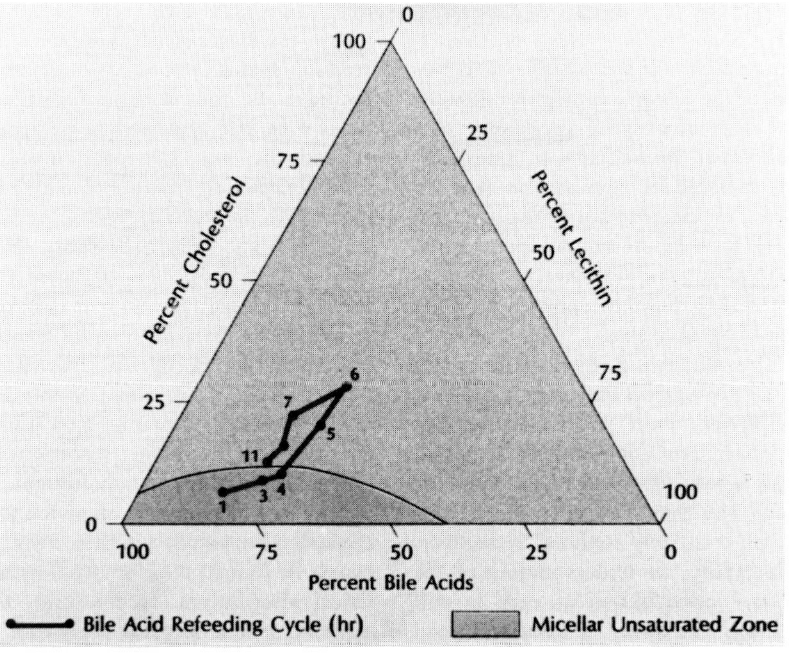

the amount of bile salt relative to cholesterol, which would favor the development of cholelithiasis. It is assumed that in most cases gallstones form in small concretions that grow slowly, as crystals do in vitro. But perhaps stones may also form from an amorphous cholesterol mass, occurring when an acute increase in mucosal permeability causes a rapid rise in the proportion of cholesterol within the gallbladder. Another possibility is that some element of bile stasis could affect the time required for cholesterol to pass from a supersaturated to a saturated state, thus favoring evolution from microscopic crystals to macroscopic stones.

Our understanding of normal gallbladder function is far from complete, yet without this information it is difficult to be sure where in the gallbladder to look for clues to the pathogenesis of cholesterol gallstones. The baboon experimental model is making it feasible to explore aspects of gallbladder function that cannot be directly studied in man. In our work to date, we have used oral and intravenous cholecystography to investigate gallbladder contractility and concentrative ability, in part to see how they are affected by pregnancy. According to the findings, in pregnancy the gallbladder appears no less capable of concentrating the contrast agent than in the nonpuerperal state. Contractility in response to intravenous cholecystokinin appears to be diminished, however.

The preceding discussion is not meant to suggest that only within the gallbladder itself will an explanation for cholesterol cholelithiasis be found. This seems no more likely than the possibility that the underlying abnormality is entirely confined to the liver. Admittedly, an understanding of the relative contribution of each constituent is still lacking. Yet surely, if there was good reason before to learn more about the fundamental mechanisms in gallstone formation, there is even better reason now in light of recent developments concerning the use of chenodeoxycholic acid in treating cholesterol gallstones. When they introduced bile acid therapy experimentally in 1971, Thistle and co-workers [7-9] at the Mayo Clinic took as their premise that decreased bile acid secretion rather than increased cholesterol secretion probably had the primary pathogenetic role in stone formation. Thus, if by feeding bile acid one could expand the bile salt pool, micellar solubilization of cholesterol might be increased. In clinical trials to date, this treatment has reportedly been effective in more than 50% of the cases; dissolution of gallstones or a marked reduction in their size can be demonstrated radiologically. In some cases, it should be noted, stone dissolution has been accompanied by only minor changes in the relative proportions of bile acids, lecithins, and cholesterol.

Any new therapeutic approach to clinically important problem must, of course, be judged in reference to established alternatives. In this case, the alternative is a surgical procedure of proven effectiveness (about 300,000 elective cholecystectomies are performed yearly). Although there is no complete agreement on the management of asymptomatic patients, most physicians agree that stones causing symptoms should be electively removed, with surgery being performed before complications ensue, when the operative risk is minimal.

In the absence of contraindications, we consider surgery in asymptomatic cases to be warranted, since it is sometimes difficult in practice to predict who will remain asymptomatic or to evaluate the likelihood that repeated acute episodes will cause the passage of a stone into the common duct.

Given a choice, of course, any patient would prefer medical to surgical therapy. Before the choice can be offered, both the safety and efficacy of bile acid therapy must be established through properly controlled clinical trials; fortunately a multi-institutional study is getting underway with the support of the National Institutes of Health.

Although the limited clinical work with bile acid therapy to date does not indicate hepatic toxicity, this possibility must not be ruled out. As is known, chenodeoxycholic acid is dehydroxylated by colonic bacteria to lithocholic acid, which is a potent hepatotoxin in animals. Since bile acid administration inhibits endogenous synthesis of bile acid, would prolonged therapy result in an undesirable increase in tissue distribution as well as in the body pool of cholesterol? Might bile acid feeding enhance absorption of cholesterol from the intestine and increase the cholesterol pool?

In considering the potential of bile acid therapy, one must keep in mind that it is feasible only in patients with a functioning gallbladder, one that has the capacity to accept and expel bile; moreover, it probably could not be used in patients with intestinal disease because of the diarrhea induced. And if bile acid therapy does prove to offer a viable option in the management of cholesterol gallstones, as one hopes it will, other questions will arise; for example, how long treatment should be continued. Since the stone dissolution rate appears to be slow, long-term ingestion might be required.

Meanwhile, work aimed at delineating the basic mechanisms underlying gallstone formation will surely be pursued. Certainly, such information will assist in designing the most effective treatment approaches possible. As more answers are awaited, it is comforting to know that cholecystectomy is effective in so high a proportion of cases and that the gallbladder is an organ that apparently any of us can do without.

ADDENDUM
Norman B. Javitt, M.D., Ph.D.

Since this section was written, no new concepts have emerged to explain the formation of gallstones. As the physical chemists refine the concepts of complex mixtures containing components that are in solution above a stable saturation limit, it becomes apparent that cholesterol in human gallbladder bile will always precipitate as a function of time. The periodic flow of bile into and out of the gallbladder is probably the major event that prevents the development of clinically significant calculi.

However, there is considerable variation in the rate at which nidus formation occurs between gallbladder contractions. Gallbladder bile that is highly supersaturated with cholesterol destabilizes more quickly than gallbladder bile containing cholesterol just above the saturation limit. In addition, other components of bile such as mucus secreted by gallbladder epithelium, activation of beta-glucuronidase, and the formation of calcium bilirubinate can all shorten the nucleation time.

The recognition of the critical role of nucleation time in the pathogenesis of gallstones has now directed medical therapy to the development of "stabilizers" that, taken by mouth, will be concentrated in bile and prevent nucleation long enough to allow the periodic cycling of the gallbladder to maintain all of its components in solution.

Recommended Reading

Admirand WH, Small DM: The physicochemical basis of cholesterol gallstone formation in man. *J Clin Invest* 47:1043, 1968.

Howell JI, Lucy JA, Pirola RC, et al: Macromolecular assemblies of lipid in bile. *Biochim Biophys Acta* 210:1, 1970.

Rains AJH: *Gallstones: Causes and Treatment.* Springfield, Ill, Charles C Thomas, 1967.

Schersten T, Nilsson SV, Cahlin E: Current concepts on the pathogenesis of human gallstones. *Scand J Gastroenterol* 5:473, 1970.

References

1. McSherry CK, Javitt NB, de Carvalho JM, et al: Cholesterol gallstones and the chemical composition of bile in baboons. *Ann Surg* 173:570, 1971.
2. McSherry CK, Glenn F, Javitt NB: Composition of basal and stimulated hepatic bile in baboons, and the formation of cholesterol gallstones. *Proc Natl Acad Sci USA* 68:1564, 1971.
3. Small DM, Rapo S: Size and structure of bile salt micelles; influence of structure, concentration, counterion concentration, pH and temperature, in Gould RF (ed), *Molecular Associations in Biological and Related Systems.* Advanced Chemistry Series 84, 1968, pp 31–52.
4. Dam H, Kruse I, Jensen MK, et al: Determinants of cholesterol cholelithiasis in man and animals. *Am J Med* 51:596, 1971.
5. Holzbach RT, March M, Olsewski M: Cholesterol solubility in bile: Evidence that supersaturated bile is common in a healthy man. *J Clin Invest* 52:1467, 1973.
6. Burch TA, Comess LJ, Bennett PH, et al: Prevalence of gallbladder disease in Pima Indians. *N Engl J Med* 277:894, 1967.
7. Thistle JL, Schoenfield LJ: Lithogenic bile among young Indian women; lithogenic potential decreased with chenodeoxycholic acid. *N Engl J Med* 284:177, 1971.
8. Thistle JL, Hoffman AF, Ott B: Effect of varying doses of chenodeoxycholic acid on bile lipid and biliary bile acid composition in gallstone patients; a dose–response study. *Am J Diag Dis* 22:1, 1971.
9. Thistle JL, Schoenfield LJ: Induced alterations in composition of bile of persons having cholelithiasis. *Gastroenterology* 61:488, 1971.

Cholesterol–Bile Acid Interactions in Gallstone Pathogenesis
Scott M. Grundy, Ph.D.

In addition to promoting the digestion of fats in the intestine, the bile acids promote the excretion of excess cholesterol from the body; the bile is in fact the only important pathway in humans for cholesterol elimination. Gallstones are virtually unknown in species in which most cholesterol is converted to bile acids (the dog is an example); in man, however, only about a third of the daily turnover of cholesterol is so utilized. The remaining two-thirds, representing 0.75–1.0 gm/day, must pass through the bile every day, and since cholesterol is insoluble in aqueous media, special mechanisms are needed to keep it from precipitating.

The major mechanism by which this is accomplished—the formation of mixed micelles of bile acids, phospholipids, and cholesterol—was fully described in the previous section. Accordingly, it will not be discussed here beyond recalling that a bile acid-phospholipid:cholesterol ratio of not less than 10:1 (some say 20:1) is needed to solubilize cholesterol, and that if it is not present, bile becomes supersaturated and therefore lithogenic. In most individuals without stones, cholesterol actually accounts for only 3–5% of bile lipids (Fig. 21).

Since the solubility of cholesterol depends on the relative proportions of cholesterol, bile acids, and phospholipids present in the bile, an abnormality in the metabolism of any of these components could be responsible for the development of lithogenic bile. The abnormality may occur in the liver or the gallbladder, but the weight of current evidence implicates the liver. Small[1,2] has suggested that the liver may produce lithogenic bile by one of two general mechanisms: decreased secretion of the solubilizing lipids or increased secretion of cholesterol, with or without a decrease in the other biliary lipids. A third mechanism, the diurnal variation in biliary lipid composition, may also lead to cholesterol precipitation; this will be discussed later.

The size of the bile acid pool—the total amount of bile acids in the enterohepatic circulation—has been considered a critical factor in cholesterol gallstone formation; in turn, pool size depends on the balance between hepatic production and intestinal excretion of bile acids. A low bile acid pool may develop either through underproduction by the liver or excessive loss through the intestines. The amount produced by the liver is a function of several factors, a major one being the availability of cholesterol. In man, unfortunately, an overload of cholesterol does not elicit a marked increase in bile acid synthesis.

Another factor controlling bile acid synthesis is the feedback mechanism of the bile acids themselves. The bile acids circulate from the liver to the gallbladder to the intestines and back to the liver, where their concentration at any given time plays a part in regulating the rate at which bile acids are produced from cholesterol. It is apparent that an abnormality in this mechanism, such as a defect in the liver cell, could result in failure to regulate synthesis that might be expressed through a reduction in the pool. Another possibility is that extremely rapid cycling of bile acids through the enterohepatic circulation, by increasing the amount that fluxes in the liver at any given time, may overrepress bile acid synthesis.

In the intestinal phase of the cycle, depletion of the bile acid pool may occur because of an inability to return bile acids to the enterohepatic circulation. This has been observed in patients who do not have normal ileal function as a result of disease or surgery, since the ileum is the site or reabsorption.

The amounts of phospholipids in the bile may also be reduced in some individuals; in fact, there is some indication that phospholipids tend to be decreased when bile acids are low. If the amount of bile acids is borderline and the amount of phospholipids is borderline or even normal, the problem of keeping cholesterol in solution clearly becomes more difficult.

While Small popularized the concept that persons with gallstones have lithogenic bile, it was Vlahcevic et al.[3] and their team at the Medical College of Virginia who first observed that bile acid pools were reduced in individuals with gallstones and lithogenic bile. The natural conclusion was that bile acid deficiency leads to gallstone formation.

In their studies, Vlahcevic et al. found that in American Indian women, almost 80% of whom develop gallstones, the pool of bile acids is indeed deficient. Most investigators would now agree that the presence of a low bile acid pool contributes to the lithogenesis in Indian women. The disease usually has its onset between the ages of 20 and 30. It appears to occur in all tribes, and probably in South America as well as North America, making it an enormous health problem for a single population group.

At the time of the studies of Vlahcevic et al., the contribution of cholesterol to stone formation was not clear. Was there an excess production of cholesterol by patients with gallstones, or was the biliary cholesterol excessive only relative to the bile acid deficiency?

This question could only be answered by measuring the lipid composition of the bile and the hepatic secretion rates of the various bile components, specifically cholesterol, bile acids, and phospholipids. For this purpose, we devised a three-lumen tube to sample bile in the duodenum (Figs. 22, 23). The procedure is as follows: Market chemicals and a liquid formula diet are introduced into the duodenum through one of the lumens. Two outlets are positioned near the ampulla of Vater, where bile enters the duodenum, and a distal outlet is about 10 cm beyond it, just past the ligament of Treitz. The patient swallows the tube the night before the study. On the following morning, the tube is positioned in the proper place under X-ray visualization, and the patient is given something to stimulate gallbladder contraction, either liquid for-

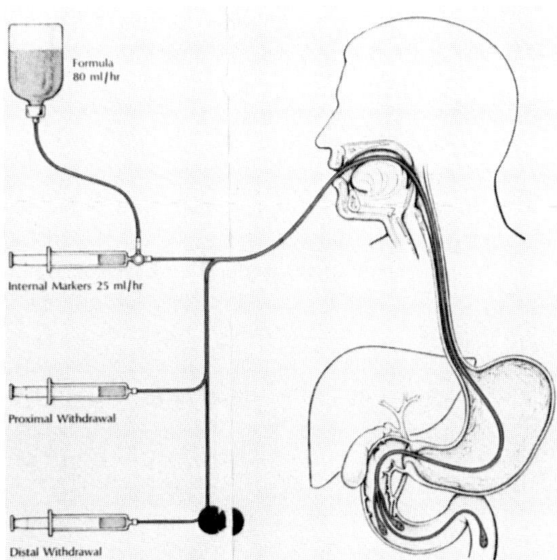

Figure 22. Lipid composition of both gallbladder and hepatic bile is studied by means of a tube having three lumens with perforated tips. The tube is swallowed by the patient and positioned in the duodenum under x-ray visualization. A food formula plus specific lipid marker substances is infused through one lumen situated near the ampulla of Vater. Gallbladder bile is sampled through a second lumen nearby after the gallbladder contracts in response to formula infusion. Since the gallbladder remains contracted during the infusion, samples withdrawn later through the distal lumen contain pure hepatic bile mixed with the markers.

mula diet or cholecystokinin intravenously. The gallbladder contracts, emptying its contents into the duodenum, and a sample is collected from one outlet near the ampulla of Vater and analyzed for cholesterol, bile acid, and phospholipid composition, with the results plotted on triangular coordinates to determine whether the bile is lithogenic or normal.

The bile sampled initially is gallbladder bile. After the first sample is obtained, infusion of the liquid formula diet is begun through the other proximal outlet. During the first few hours after the infusion begins, some gallbladder bile continues to enter the duodenum, but thereafter, as long as the infusion continues, the gallbladder remains contracted; it no longer fills and empties, and for practical purposes is removed from the enterohepatic circulation. Since the bile produced by the liver is now entering the duodenum directly through the bile ducts, it is possible to obtain an unadulterated sample of hepatic bile. By adding market substances to the formula infusion, one can measure the flow rates of the various bile components into the duodenum. These estimates are made, as described below, from a thoroughly mixed sample obtained at the distal outlet. The markers used are beta-sitosterol, a nonabsorbable plant sterol, or radioactive labeled cholesterol.

For the determination of cholesterol output in milligrams per hour, duodenal contents are aspirated through the distal tube. The aspirate contains cholesterol secreted in bile that has been completely mixed with the marker. Since the rate of marker infusion is known precisely, the rate of cholesterol secretion can be determined simply by measuring the ratio of cholesterol to marker. In turn, bile acid output equals the cholesterol output in milligrams per hour multiplied by the bile acid:cholesterol ratio. The latter ratio is determined by analysis of the duodenal contents aspirated from the proximal tube. Phospholipid output equals cholesterol output multiplied by the phospholipid:cholesterol ratio. By using radioactive bile acids, it is also possible to measure the size of the total bile acid pool.

We have used this technique to study biliary lipid output in patients without gallstones. These studies were carried out under the auspices of the National Institute of Arthritis, Metabolism, and Digestive Diseases and the Indian Health Service of the U.S. Public Health Service. They were performed at the Phoenix Indian Medical Center in Arizona. Our first report compared the results in American Indian women with gallstones with those of both Indian and non-Indian subjects without stones.

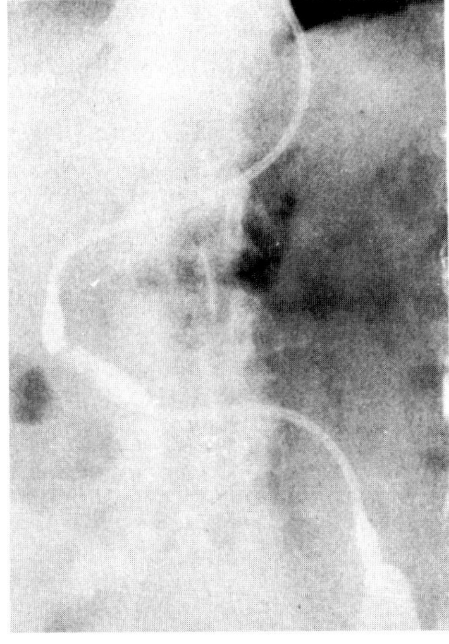

Figure 23. X-ray shows actual position of the lumens in procedure described in Figure 22.

Hepatic secretion of biliary lipids was studied by the intubation method in 17 American Indian women with gallstones and in 6 Indian women, 7 Indian men, and 12 Caucasian women without gallstones. The mean age of the Indian women with gallstones was 29, and they were generally overweight, a frequent finding in Indian women over the age of 20. The Indian women without gallstones had a slightly higher mean age, but they tended to be less overweight. The Indian men had a mean age of 34 and were not overweight. The ages of the Caucasian women ranged from 19 to 25 years; their weights were normal, with the exception of one individual who was obese. During the several weeks of the study, all subjects received a part-food, part-formula diet in which 40% of the calories were supplied as fat. Average hourly output of biliary lipids was obtained for each person, as well as the molar percentage of each lipid component. The output of cholesterol in the Indian women with gallstones—47 mg/hr—was not much greater than that of the Indian men and women without gallstones, but was significantly greater than that of the nonobese Caucasian women, who had a mean output of 29 mg/hr. The gallstone patients' cholesterol output differences appeared even greater when the values were corrected to normalize ideal weight and body surface area in order to eliminate the effects of obesity and the differences in body size.

Bile acid output by the Indian women with gallstones (mean, 440 mg/hr) was not greatly different from that of Indian women without gallstones (551 mg/hr) but was considerably less than that of Indian men (1,013 mg/hr) and Caucasian women (868 mg/hr). No difference in phospholipid output was observed among any of the groups.

As stated earlier, the 10:1 ratio is considered the maximum ratio of solubility. If the hourly outputs for cholesterol are plotted against the hourly outputs of bile acids and phospholipids along a line representing the 10:1 molar ratio, the relative importance of the secretion rates of bile components can be seen. Points above the line are in the lithogenic zone. Most Indian women with gallstones were protected from developing lithogenic bile either because their cholesterol output was relatively low or their bile acid and phospholipid secretion rates were relatively high. In Indian men, protection from the development of lithogenic bile depended mainly on a relatively high output of bile acids. In Caucasian women, low cholesterol output appeared to be the major factor in preventing lithogenic bile development. In some, bile acid-phospholipid output was in the low range found in Indian women with stones, but the bile was not lithogenic because the cholesterol output was low. The two women with the highest percentage of cholesterol in bile in the Caucasian group also had the highest cholesterol outputs in the group. Although neither had lithogenic bile, their bile lipid excretion pattern closely resembled that of the Indian women with gallstones.

In the gallstone patients, cholesterol and bile acids were not secreted together in a single fixed ratio. The ratio was considerably greater than in patients with stones. The cause of lithogenic bile in the Indian women, therefore, appeared to be a combination of two factors: a high output of cholesterol and a low output of bile acids and phospholipids.

To determine the mechanism for these abnormalities, cholesterol balance studies were done on Indian women with gallstones and on normal Indian men. The results were compared with those of previous cholesterol balance studies done on the Caucasian patients. The Indian women with stones were found to excrete about twice the quantity of fecal steroids derived from cholesterol as non-Indians from other studies. Most of the cholesterol increase was in the neutral steroid fraction and was probably derived in large part from the increased biliary cholesterol secretion observed in these women.

At least part of the increased cholesterol synthesis could be attributed to obesity. Cholesterol synthesis is generally increased in obesity, and both the Indian women and men in the study were inclined toward obesity, especially the women. However, the balance data suggested that cholesterol synthesis by Indian women might be greater than normal even after correction of the values obtained for obesity. A greater synthesis of cholesterol might be simply a genetic characteristic of Indians, but it might also be related to bile acid metabolism. As mentioned before, cholesterol synthesis in the intestines, and possibly in the liver, is regulated by feedback inhibition by the bile acids. A decreased recirculation of bile acids might enhance cholesterol synthesis in the liver and intestines, leading to increased cholesterol secretion into the bile; Indian women show a slight increase in fecal excretion of bile acids, which might be offered as an explanation for the depletion of bile acids in the enterohepatic circulation. However, this mechanism does not give a completely satisfactory explanation because non-Indians can sustain much greater intestinal losses of bile acids and nevertheless replenish bile acid pools rapidly. The Indian women with gallstones do not seem to be able to convert increased cholesterol into bile acids, since their bile acid pools remain depleted in the face of excess cholesterol synthesis.

A recent report by Small and Repo[1] has indicated that cholecystectomy results in the transformation of lithogenic bile to normal in Caucasians with gallstones suggests another mechanism: that the presence of the gallbladder in the enterohepatic circulation influences the secretion of biliary lipids. For instance, a diseased gallbladder might be the cause rather than the effect of lithogenic bile in the Indian women. Such an explanation seems unlikely for at least three reasons: (1) Indian women without gallstones, and presumably without gallbladder disease, have abnormally low biliary lipid secretion rates compared with Caucasian women; (2) a high percentage of young, nonobese Indian women have lithogenic bile due to a relative decrease in bile acids; and finally, (3) we have noted that in six of seven Indian women who underwent cholecystectomy, eliminating the gallbladder did not result in the conversion of lithogenic bile to normal—in contrast to the effect of cholecystectomy on Caucasian patients. Therefore, gallstones and biliary tract disease do not seem to be the cause of lithogenic bile in Indian women. The observations cited above suggest, rather, that lithogenic bile in these patients is due to more generalized abnormalities in the metabolism of cholesterol and bile acids, with the key abnormality appearing to be a defective regulation of bile acid synthesis by the liver.

However, while such a mechanism may explain the high prevalence of gallstone formation and the early onset of the disease in Indian women, it may be asked whether the same mechanism operates in non-Indian women. To answer this question, we studied 10 young Caucasian women with gallstones who were comparable in age, body build, and degree of overweight to the Indian women previously studied and to 14 normal Caucasian women without gallstones.

The hourly output of hepatic biliary lipids was studied in these two groups by the intubation method (Fig. 24). The gallstone patients' bile was consistently more lithogenic. Their mean hourly output of cholesterol was 56 mg/hr compared with 29 mg/hr for the women without gallstones. While the mean hourly output of bile acids was higher for the women without stones than for the gallstone patients (1098 vs. 742 mg/hr), the difference was not significant.

The striking difference between the gallstone patients and the controls in the study was the greatly increased secretion rates of biliary choles-

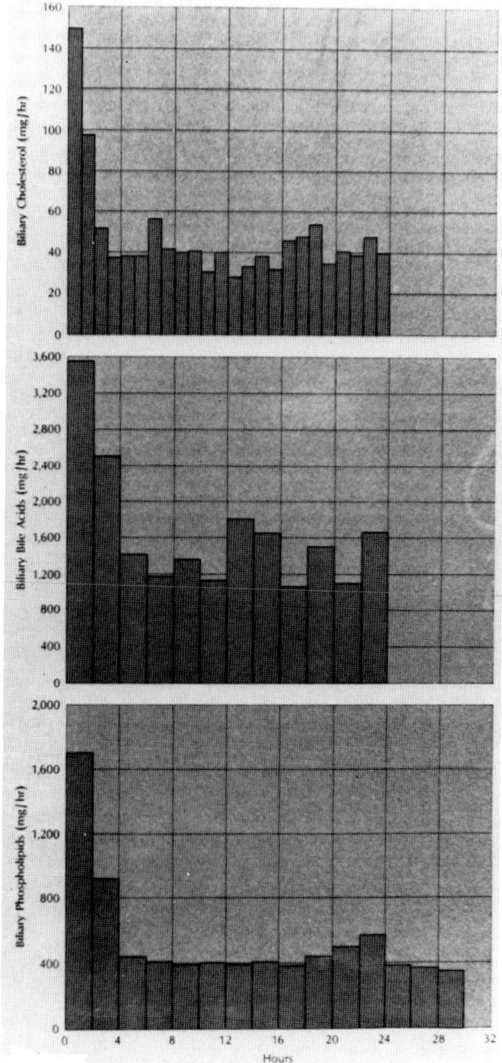

Figure 24.　When hepatic output of bilary lipids is studied by the method of intubation plus infusion of liquid formula, patterns like those shown in are obtained in persons with intact gallbladders. The initial high outputs of cholesterol, bile acids, and phospholipids are thought to result from gallbladder contraction. A steady state of cholesterol output is reached thereafter, while that of bile acids and phospholipids is more likely to fluctuate.

terol in the gallstone patients, which was almost twice that of the controls. It was this factor that contributed most to the greater lithogenicity of the gallstone patients' bile. Anything that resulted in abnormally high synthesis of cholesterol could account for an increase in biliary cholesterol, but in these patients, as well as in the Indian women with gallstones, the obvious cause was obesity. Several studies have shown that cholesterol production is roughly proportional to total body weight. As more cholesterol is synthesized by the body in obesity, the total amount of cholesterol secreted into the bile tends to increase.

However, not all obese individuals develop gallstones, and it may be that if the excess production of cholesterol in obesity is matched by an increase in bile acid production, the bile will not become lithogenic. Indeed, we have observed increased bile acid production in obese individuals without gallstones. Clearly, such a mechanism was not functioning in the patients in this study, since, despite the production of an increased amount of cholesterol to serve as substrate for conversion into biliary acids, they were unable to expand their bile acid pool sufficiently to solubilize the excess biliary cholesterol. This fact may help explain the frequency of gallstone disease among obese young women, regardless of their racial background.

The investigation of gallstone disease in Indian women was undertaken on the assumption that a metabolic defect of genetic origin underlay the extraordinarily high prevalence of disease in this particular population group. In Indian women, the cause of gallstone disease now appears to be a genetically determined low bile acid pool probably related to a defect in bile acid synthesis on which is superimposed a cultural factor expressed as a common tendency to become obese in early adulthood (Fig. 25). The apparent correlation between onset of obesity and onset of gallbladder disease has added another dimension to the problem, which may be very important in determining the prevalence of gallstones because it suggests than an abnormality in cholesterol metabolism may also be a very important element in gallstone formation.

Excess biliary cholesterol secretion, therefore, seems to be one mechanism for the development of lithogenic bile and gallstones. It is not unique to Indians but occurs in other groups as well, especially young, obese Caucasian women. There remains a group of middle-aged, nonobese individuals who develop gallstones for reasons not entirely understood at present. Bile acid deficiency may be an explanation, but 30–40% of those who develop gallstones do not have lithogenic bile on a single sampling. One other possible mechanism, the diurnal variation in bile composition, deserves consideration. The results of our investigations indicate that during fasting, the bile, even in normal individuals, becomes lithogenic. In the studies described above, hepatic bile samples were aspirated at the end of an overnight fast of 10–12 hours, again after the steady state was reached during infusion of a liquid-formula diet, and again at 2-hour in-

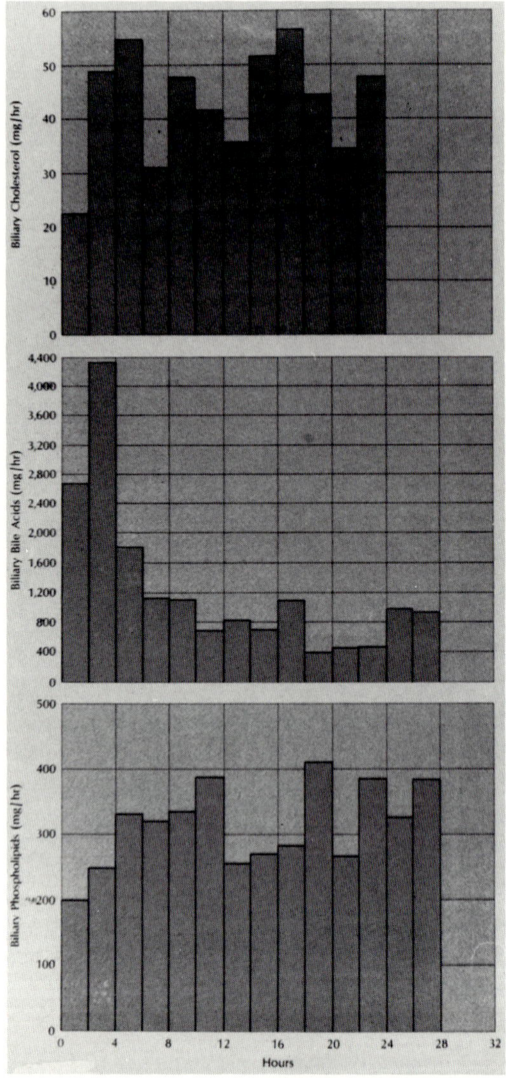

Figure 25. The patterns change after removal of the gallbladder, as illustrated by the findings in a patient who had previous cholecystectomy. The initial surge of cholesterol output resulting from gallbladder contraction is typically absent. Bile acid output may be high early following food intake; this initial increase is probably the result of mobilization of the bile acid pool from the distal small intestine. Phospholipid output, like that of cholesterol, shows no early increase.

tervals during fasting after completion of the infusion. Gallbladder bile was sampled immediately after fasting by infusing amino acids, which stimulate cholecystokinin release and cause the gallbladder to contract and empty.

The patients with and without gallstones both developed lithogenic bile during fasting, and in all subjects hepatic bile was more lithogenic during fasting than gallbladder bile or bile obtained during

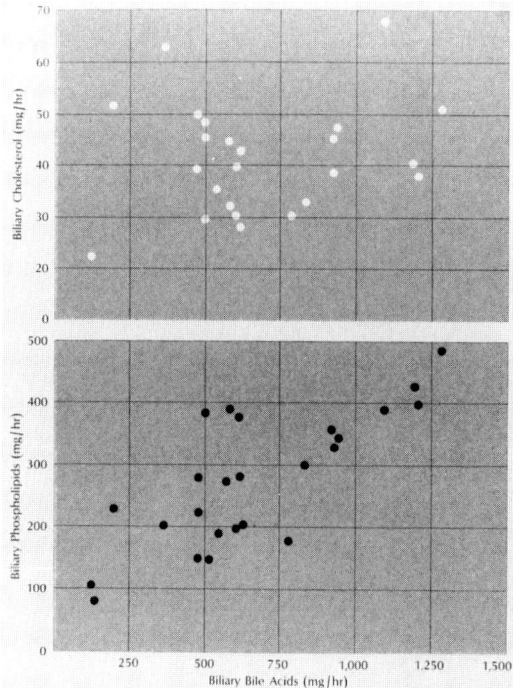

Figure 26.   The relationship among hepatic outputs of the three bilary lipids is suggested in this graph, in which each dot represents the results of one patient. Hepatic cholesterol secretion shows no correlation with bile acid output, whereas phospholipid output increases as bile acid output increases.

the infusion of formula. The continued independent secretion of cholesterol during fasting appeared to be the cause of lithogenicity. While the ratio of cholesterol to bile acids increased threefold in all three groups, it was three times greater in the Indian women with stones than in the normal Caucasian women.

The lipid composition of hepatic and gallbladder bile during fasting was compared in three normal subjects by sampling both types of bile concurrently at different times during fasting. At each interval, i.e., after 6, 9, and 12 hours of fasting, hepatic bile was more lithogenic than gallbladder bile, and was supersaturated at 12 hours in all three individuals. Gallbladder bile became progressively more lithogenic throughout fasting and was supersaturated in two subjects at 12 hours (Fig. 26).

These findings in humans are consistent with those of McSherry (see the previous section), who demonstrated that infusion of gallbladder bile into the ileum of the baboon during fasting reduces cholesterol saturation of hepatic bile. Our results show that feeding reduces the lithogenicity of hepatic bile in humans. Fasting represents a physiological interruption of the enterohepatic circu-

lation that leads to storage of bile acids in the gallbladder (Figs. 27, 28).

Fewer bile acids are then available for secretion by the liver, which nevertheless continues to secrete cholesterol, at least in man. The longer the individual fasts, the more lithogenic the bile becomes, and if the person has a slight abnormality in bile lipid composition—either a deficiency of bile acids or an excess of cholesterol—the defect can become quite pronounced. It has been suggested that failure of the lithogenic bile produced during fasting to mix with more normal gallbladder bile could result in precipitation of cholesterol in localized regions of the gallbladder. Gallstones might then gradually develop in spite of an overall bile composition that is nonlithogenic (Figs. 29, 30).

Studies on the bile composition of patients being treated for hyperlipidemia support our findings on the factors underlying the development of lithogenic bile in patients with gallstones. Some of the drugs and diets used in the treatment of hypercholesterolemia act by changing the metabolism of cholesterol and bile acids in the liver and the enterohepatic circulation. For example, one means of lowering plasma cholesterol is to interrupt the enterohepatic circulation of bile acids and promote the excretion of bile acids from the body. This may be done by giving cholestyramine, a quaternary ammonium anion exchange resin that binds bile acids through exchange with chloride and prevents their reabsorption by the intestine, or by ileal bypass, which removes the ileum from the fecal stream and thus prevents the reabsorption of bile acids and cholesterol. The resulting increase in excretion of bile acids reduces the feedback inhibition by bile acids on their own production. More cholesterol becomes converted to bile acids, which in turn causes a drain on body cholesterol pools and reduces plasma cholesterol. However, while the treatment is effective in reducing plasma cholesterol, it could eventually lead to depletion of the bile acid pool and development of lithogenic bile.

Another drug used in the treatment of hyperlipidemia, clofibrate, enhances cholesterol output in the bile. We have demonstrated in several patients that the bile becomes lithogenic during clofibrate treatment, and, in fact, some patients have developed gallstones during treatment. The cause of lithogenic bile during clofibrate treatment appears to be an excess cholesterol output and a block in the formation of bile acids. Sturdevant et al.[4] have reported that men on a serum-cholesterol-lowering diet high in unsaturated fats had a greater prevalence of gallstones than individuals on saturated fat diets, which again suggests that excess choles-

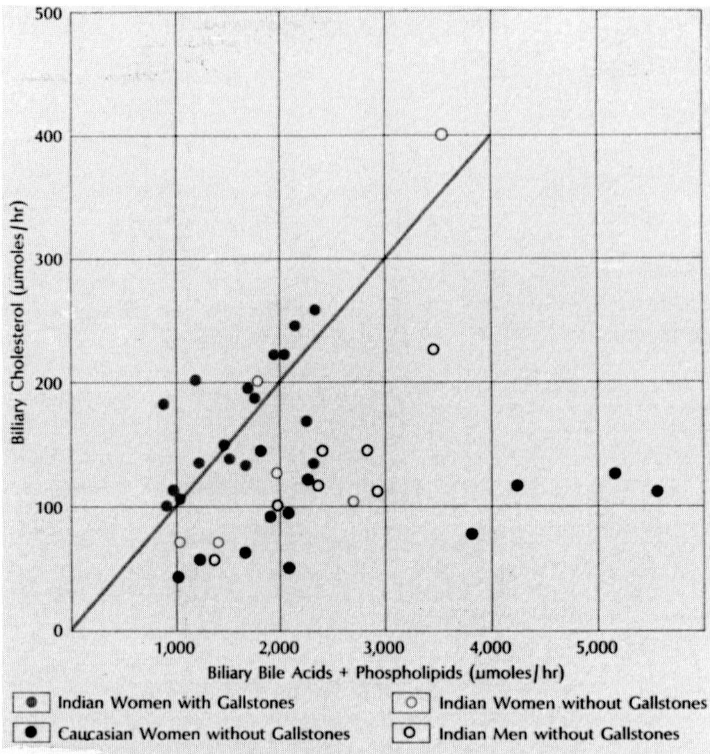

Figure 27.   The relative importance of the secretion rates of the three biliary lipids is illustrated in this graph in which the line at 45° represents the 10:1 molar ratio of bile acids + phospholipids to cholesterol. This line corresponds closely to the solubility of cholesterol. Most Indian women with gallstones fall above the line, i.e., in the lithogenic zone.

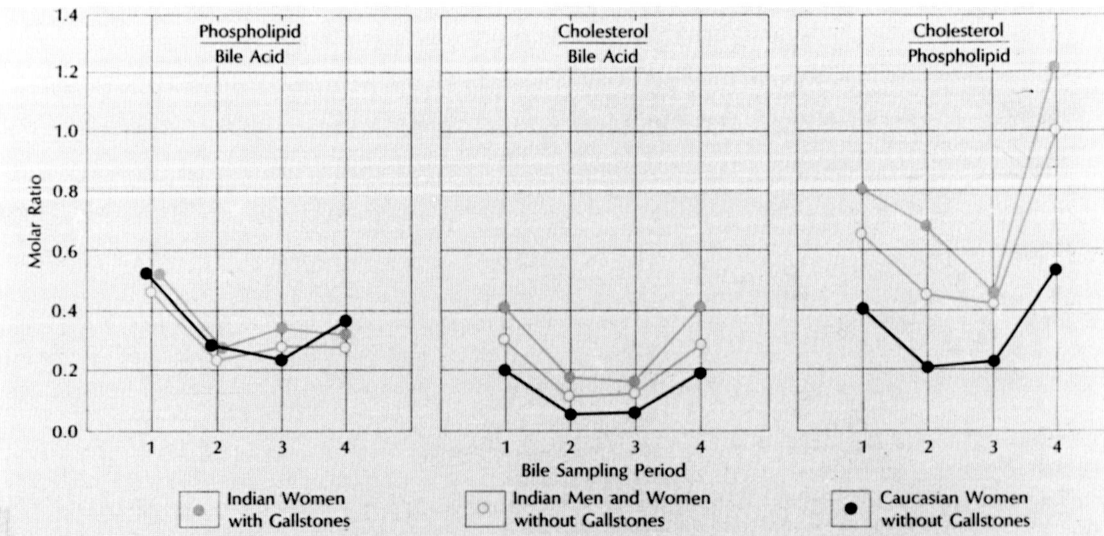

Figure 28.   Diurnal variations in the ratios of the three biliary lipids was also plotted for each of the three groups: 1) during fasting; 2) after gallstone stimulation; 3) during food infusion; 4) during postinfusion fasting. The ratio of the bile acids to phospholipids remained comparable in all three groups throughout the cycle, but the ratio of cholesterol to the solubilizing lipids increased threefold during fasting, indicating that cholesterol secretion continued independently of the bile acid and phospholipid secretion.

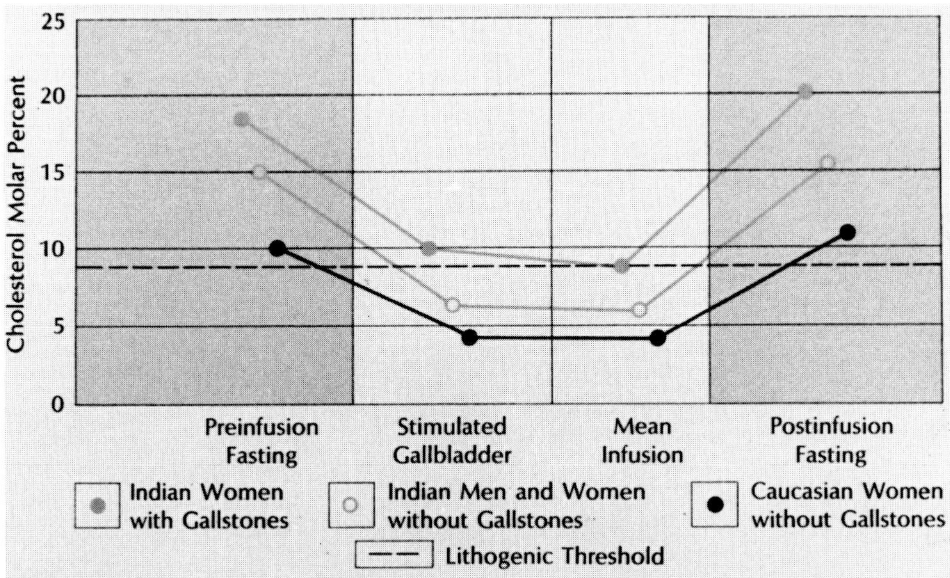

Figure 29.   Diurnal variation in biliary lipid composition occurs in normal individuals as well as in those with gallstones. Shown above is the molar percentage of cholesterol in bile obtained during various periods of study; it is apparent that fasting bile (hepatic) obtained before the study was lithogenic in all groups. In contrast, gallbladder bile and bile obtained during constant fusion of formula were less lithogenic. Again, after formula infusion was discontinued, bile returned to its previous high level of lithogencity. Although all individuals studied showed this pattern, Indian women with gallstones had the most lithogenic bile in any period of the study.

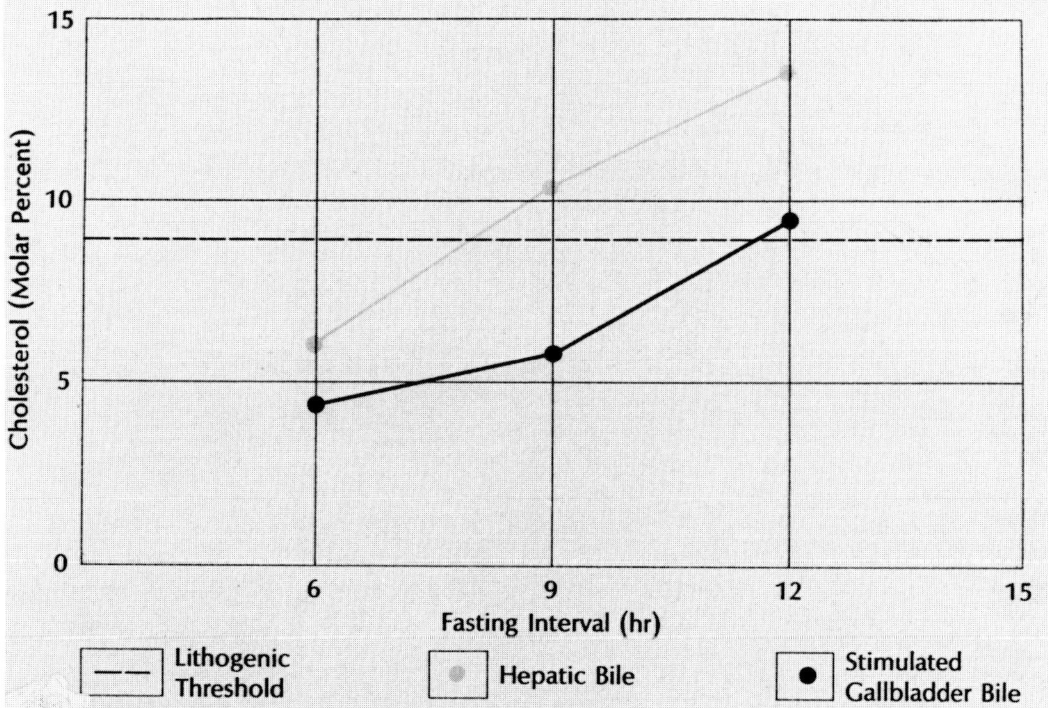

Figure 30.   Analysis of the lipid composition of both hepatic and gallbladder bile at intervals during fasting in an individual without gallstones revealed that the percentage of cholesterol in both types of bile increases with the duration of fasting.

> *Bile Acid Deficiency*
>   A. Defect in synthesis
>   1. Defective regulation of bile acid synthesis in liver cell (Indian women)
>   2. Overrepression of bile acid synthesis by excessive recycling of bile
>   acid pool (some Caucasian patients)
>   B. Defect in bile acid reabsorption
>   1. Ileectomy patients
>
> *Excess Cholesterol Secretion into Bile*
>   A. Overproduction of cholesterol
>   1. Due to obesity (Indian women, young obese white women)
>   2. Due to bile acid deficiency (Indian women, young obese white women)
>   3. Excessive dietary cholesterol (?)
>   B. Defective conversion of cholesterol into bile acids
>   1. Human beings in general
>   2. Indian women
>
> *Diurnal Variation in Bile Lipid Composition*
>   A. Storage of bile acids in gallbladder
>   B. Bile acid–independent secretion of cholesterol
>   C. Accentuated by combinations of bile acid deficiency and excess
>   cholesterol secretion

Figure 31.   Patho-physiologic causes of lithogenic bile.

terol secretion in bile tends to promote lithogenic bile. We have observed the development of lithogenic bile in several patients on an unsaturated fat diet, but it has not been proved that such a diet increases the risk of gallstone formation (Fig. 31).

Research on the pathogenesis of gallstone disease indicates that gallstones develop when the bile becomes lithogenic, i.e., when the ratio of biliary cholesterol to bile acids and phospholipids exceeds the limits of cholesterol solubility. The mechanisms underlying the development of lithogenic bile appear to be an excess secretion of cholesterol into the bile, a decrease in the bile acid pool, or a combination of both factors.

This writer (S.M.G.), in collaboration with Dr. Abbas Sedaghat,[5] published a paper entitled "Cholesterol Crystals and the Formation of Cholesterol Gallstones." In it we confined our study to the relationship of cholesterol crystallization to the formation of gallstones. We studied 54 patients; 8 asymptomatic patients had gallstones and 17 had had cholecystectomy for gallstones. Hepatic bile was obtained from nine patients with stones in the common bile duct. The bile samples were studied for cholesterol monohydrate crystals and analyzed to determine the percentage of cholesterol saturation. In the eight asymptomatic patients who had gallstones, the bile aspirate revealed a cholesterol saturation of 142 ± 42%; in five patients, crystals were found. Thirty-six patients with supersaturated bile (cholesterol saturation of 166 ± 44%) had no crystals; 10 patients with unsaturated bile 81 ± 24%, showed no crystals. Of 26 patients with sympto-

matic stones in the gallbladder and/or common duct, cholesterol crystals were not found in 7; these latter patients had pigmented stones. *In all of the 19 patients with cholesterol stones, crystals were found.* In some instances, the cholesterol crystals did not appear until after 24–48 hours of incubation. We concluded that, in all probability, there is a prerequisite for the formation of cholesterol gallstones. Not fully understood is why so many patients had no cholesterol crystallization despite the presence of marked supersaturation. This, of course, indicates that supersaturation in itself may not be the sole cause of gallstone formation.

Scanning electron microscopy and X-ray diffraction studies have shown that the cholesterol component of pure or mixed cholesterol stones consists primarily of cholesterol monohydrate crystals. Thus, the precipitation of cholesterol monohydrate crystals in bile may be a necessary prelude to the formation of cholesterol gallstones.

Clearly, a mechanism exists to maintain cholesterol in solution in the bile. This mechanism is probably defective in patients who develop cholesterol gallstones. There were repeated instances in which crystals were absent in the supersaturated gallbladder bile but appeared after 24 hours of incubation. There were also instances in which patients with cholesterol gallstones in the common bile duct, in whom no crystals were found developed crystals after a 24-hour incubation period. At surgery, Holan et al.[6] removed bile from gallbladders with cholesterol stones and ultracentrifuged it to remove all existing cholesterol crystals. After standing for a period at 37°C, crystals formed. The results indicated that although supersaturation of bile with cholesterol may be a prerequisite for the formation of cholesterol gallstones, it is not the only factor involved. Supersaturated bile must yield cholesterol monohydrate crystals before they can adhere to each other and enlarge to form macroscopic stones. Crystallization apparently occurs in patients with cholesterol stones, but not in patients with noncholesterol stones (or no stones), even when the bile is supersaturated with cholesterol. What, then, is the mechanism that resists cholesterol crystallization? One possibility is that the bile may contain factors (possibly proteins) that solubilize the excess cholesterol of the supersaturated bile and thereby inhibit the formation of cholesterol monohydrate crystals. Two significant practical applications emerge from this research. First, the finding of cholesterol monohydrate crystals in the bile of patients with gallstones implies the presence of cholesterol stones. Second, future research may reveal a subgroup of patients with cholesterol crystals without stones but in whom stones may develop at a later date. If this is so, the finding of cholesterol crystals in the bile may prove to be a more accurate indicator of stone formation than bile saturation. Most important, the finding of cholesterol monohydrate crystals may well become a prerequisite for the selection of the ideal patient for chenodeoxycholic acid therapy.

Small[2] believes that there are five stages in the formation of cholesterol gallstones, each step being a prerequisite for the next. *First,* there is a genetic and/or *metabolic stage;* in this stage, the bile may become supersaturated and eventually lead to supersaturated abnormalities. *Second,* there is a *chemical stage* in which the gallbladder bile develops a supersaturation of cholesterol. *Third,* there is a *physical stage* in which the supersaturated bile is nucleated and the growth of cholesterol monohydrate crystals is initiated. This stage is diagnosed by the finding of microscopic crystals of cholesterol monohydrate in patients who do not have stones. In the *fourth stage,* microscopic crystals grow or agglomerate into macroscopic stones. In the *fifth stage,* the stones produce symptoms by initiating cholecystitis, cystic, and/or common bile duct blockade.

Small selected the Pima Indians to illustrate his five stages. About 70% of the Pima women ultimately develop gallstones. The *chemical stage* he claimed develops at the time of puberty. By approximately 18 years of age, these Indian women develop supersaturated duodenal bile, but no stones. By 25 years of age, over 50% of these women reveal gallstones that can be demonstrated on

cholecystography. Finally, after about 10 years from the time of gallstone recognition, about 50% will complain of symptoms.

Susann et al.[7] studied the bile of 100 patients with abdominal pain (suspected cholecystitis and/or cholelithiasis). The bile collections were studied for cholesterol and calcium bilirubinate crystals. Sixty patients had negative oral cholecystograms, negative sonograms, and no objective findings of gallbladder pathology. These 60 patients were selected to be the subject of their report.

Susann et al. believe that endoscopic collection of bile with analysis for crystals is indicated in those patients with symptoms suggestive of gallbladder disease with negative gallbladder series and oral cholecystography or in whom the only positive radiographic finding is a positive cholecystokinin cholangiogram. The endoscopic collection of bile provides a simple means of obtaining a specimen while at the same time evaluating the entire upper gastrointestinal tract. An additional 38% of patients with symptoms suggestive of gallbladder disease but with negative radiographic studies will show either cholesterol or calcium bilirubinate crystals in their bile, and 88% of this group will respond favorably to cholecystectomy. The response to medical treatment in patients with bile crystals is poor.

Recommended Reading

Admirand WH, Small DM: The physico-chemical basis of cholesterol gallstone formation in man. *J Clin Invest* 47:1043, 1968.

Grundy SM, Metzger AL: A physiologic method for estimation of hepatic secretion of biliary lipids in man. *Gastroenterology* 62:1200, 1972.

Grundy SM, Metzger AL, Adler RD: Mechanisms of lithogenic bile formation in American Indian women with cholesterol gallstones. *J Clin Invest* 51:3026, 1972.

Grundy SM: Effects of polyunsaturated fats on lipid metabolism in patients with hypertriglyceridemia. *J Clin Invest* 55:269, 1975.

Grundy SM, Mok HYI: Colestipol, clofibrate, and polysterols in combined therapy of hyperlipidemia. *J Lab Clin Med* 89:354, 1977.

Holzbach RT, Marsh M, Holan K: Cholesterol solubilizing capacity: A direct assessment of lithogenic potential in bile. *Gastroenterology* 60:777, 1971.

Metzger AL, Adler R, Heymsfield S, et al: Diurnal variation in biliary lipid composition. *N Engl J Med* 288:333, 1973.

Northfield TC, Hofmann AF: Biliary lipid secretion in gallstone patients. *Lancet* 1:747, 1973.

References

1. Small DM, Repo S: Source of abnormal bile in patients with cholesterol gallstones. *N Engl J Med* 283:53, 1971.
2. Small DM: Cholesterol nucleation and growth in gallstone formation (editorial). *N Engl J Med* 302:1305, 1980.
3. Vlahcevic AR, Yoshida T, Juttijudata P, et al: Relationship of bile acid pool size to the formation of lithogenic bile in female Indians of the Southwest. *Gastroenterology* 62:73, 1973; 64:298.
4. Sturdevant RAL, Pearch MD, Dayton S: Increased prevalence of cholelithiasis in men ingesting a serum-cholesterol-lowering diet. *N Engl J Med* 288:24, 1973.
5. Grundy S, Sedaghat A: Cholesterol crystals and the formation of cholesterol gallstones. *N Engl J Med* 1980: 5:302:(23)274–7.
6. Holan, et al: Supersaturation of bile not the only factor in gallstone production. Gastroenterology; 77(4 Pt.) 611–617; 1979.
7. Susann PW, Sheppard F, Baloga AJ, et al: Detection of occult gallbladder disease by duodenal drainage collected endoscopically. *Am Surg* 51:162, 1985.

Physicochemical Considerations in Gallstone Pathogenesis

D. Fennell Evans Ph.D., and Edward L. Cussler, Ph.D.

A few years ago, two pieces of a "Rosetta Stone" were discovered that apparently clarified the mechanisms responsible for cholesterol gallstone formation. One "piece," epitomized by a triangular phase diagram, provided a scientific rationale for this disease. This phase diagram summarized the solubilities of bile salts, lecithin, and cholesterol. The second "piece" was the apparent clinical identification of two populations, one with high bile cholesterol and a tendency to form stones, and the other with low cholesterol and few stones. The coupling of a simple scientific rationale with the clinical observations suggested that an understanding of gallstone pathogenesis was at hand.

This promise of scientific and clinical understanding greatly accelerated research efforts. Significant progress was made in many areas, some of which have been described in this chapter. Paradoxically, these efforts have shown that the first two Rosetta Stone findings were being misinterpreted. What is now clear is that dynamic factors in both liver and gallbladder function must be explicitly considered.

Recognition of the importance of dynamic factors requires consideration of scientific phenomena that have not been a principal focus in medicine. The phenomena to which we refer are those involving rate processes, such as rates of stone growth and gallbladder emptying. Similar phenomena are important in many other physiological processes, such as blood oxygenation and digestion.

This section delineates the rate processes involved in cholelithiasis. First, we attempt to show why the original two pieces of the Rosetta Stone became limiting. Then we discuss other rate processes that are important in this context. Finally, we present one example: the kinetics of stone dissolution.

In order for gallstones to form and grow, a prerequisite is that the cholesterol in bile must be supersaturated. There had been considerable disagreement as to where this supersaturation begins. Although this disagreement has now been resolved, the reasons for it will be explored, since they provide considerable insight into some of the factors controlling gallstone formation.

CHOLESTEROL SOLUBILITY

The solubility of cholesterol in the bile salts and lecithin is shown schematically in the triangular phase diagram in Figure 32 (line A). The water content is fixed at 90% by weight, since the solubility of cholesterol in bile does not change appreciably with water content. The region of interest is the one representing solutions with high concentration of bile salts relative to cholesterol. For ex-

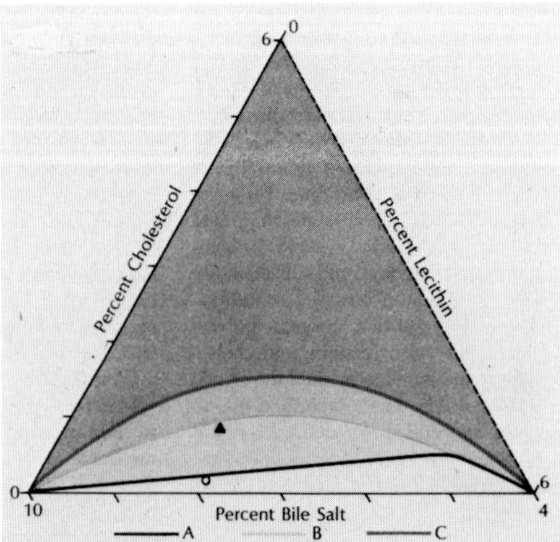

Figure 32. Triangular phase diagram gives the solubility of cholesterol in bile, with line A representing the equilibrium solubility; line B, an apparent solubility line resulting from metastability; and line C, the upper limit of apparent solubility.

ample, the small circle represents a solution containing 7.8% bile salts, 1.9% lecithin, and 0.3% cholesterol, while the triangle represents a solution containing 7.3% bile salts, 1.8% lecithin, and 0.9% cholesterol. Below the solid line, cholesterol will not precipitate; it solubilizes in the mixed micellar solution.

Holzbach et al.,[1] in their study of cholesterol solubility, demonstrated two different ways of reaching this line. First, he added cholesterol crystals to a bile salt–lecithin solution, stirred the solution for several days, and subsequently determined the cholesterol concentration in the solution. Second, he dissolved bile salts, lecithin, and cholesterol in methanol, a method developed by Small. He then evaporated the alcohol and added the desired amount of water. With this procedure, one can prepare solutions with a cholesterol concentration considerably above the solid line in the triangular phase diagram (Fig. 33) that still appear clear and homogeneous. However, when these solutions are forced through Millipore filters, their cholesterol concentrations drop to the values given by the solid line. Thus Holzbach et al. were able to approach this line from above and from below, strongly indicating that it represents the true equilibrium solubility. In addition, he showed that the solubility of cholesterol in these model systems is essentially the same as that in human and canine bile. These values have been obtained independently by Dam and by Carey and Small.

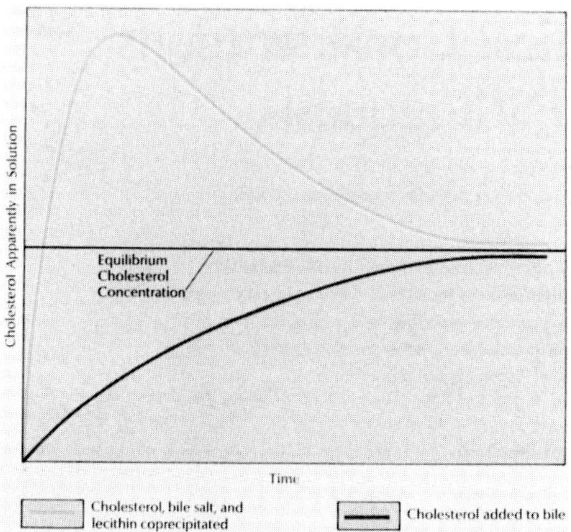

Figure 33. This figure demonstrates that with time, the amount of cholesterol in solution approaches the equilibrium solubility value, i.e., the curve labeled as line A in Figure 32, regardless of the history of the sample. The maximum in the curve for the coprecipatated solution corresponds roughly to line B in Figure 32.

Prior to these studies, the accepted values for the solubility of cholesterol in bile were determined using the methanol coprecipitation procedure described above, but without filtration. The solubility values obtained were reproducible and are given by line B in Figure 32. In the region of physiological interest, these apparent solubility values can be almost twice as high as the lower ones now generally accepted. Studies by Mufson et al.[2,3] provide a partial explanation for this discrepancy. They show that solutions originally prepared with methanol having a cholesterol concentration above line A of Figure 32 gradually approach the lower equilibrium line but require days or weeks to do so. However, when cholesterol crystals were dissolved in bile salt–lecithin solutions, the equilibrium solubility line was directly attained (Fig. 32). This type of behavior is consistent with the existence of a metastable state in which supersaturated cholesterol is retained in solution for long periods of time.

These results show that cholesterol gallstones may not form even if bile is supersaturated with cholesterol. One must also explicitly consider the rates at which precipitation occurs, which is one of the dynamic factors that must be taken into account in reinterpreting the Rosetta Stone of cholelithiasis.

DIURNAL VARIATION

More clinical evidence that rate processes are important comes from a growing body of evidence that the composition of hepatic bile and, consequently, of gallbladder bile varies with the state of the enterohepatic circulation, i.e., during feeding and fasting. As described by Grundy et al.,[4] this has been documented in humans, baboons, and monkeys. This variation in composition can result in the gallbladder bile's becoming periodically subsaturated and then supersaturated with respect to cholesterol.

As the cholesterol concentration varies back and forth across line A in Figure 32, say, from the circle to the small triangle, gallstones can grow and dissolve on a periodic basis. For example, if the growth rate is much slower than the dissolution rate, bile can be supersaturated for long periods without stone formation. If the growth rate is much faster than the dissolution rate, only occasional supersaturation may produce stones. Thus, a more correct interpretation of this second piece of the Rosetta Stone is that the solubilizing power of gallbladder bile varies continuously with time. Consequently, one cannot relate the possibility of gallstone formation to the composition of bile determined at a single time; rather, one must use a weighted average that explicitly considers the relative rates of growth and dissolution.

A third factor that focuses attention on the time-dependent processes involved is the successful dissolution of gallstones by the oral administration of chenodeoxycholic acid or phenobarbital. Chenodeoxycholic acid appears to achieve this effect by lowering the rate of cholesterol synthesis in the liver, so that hepatic bile contains less cholesterol. The typical dissolution rates are slow, and months or years may be required to dissolve a particular gallstone completely. As we show in the section entitled "Accelerating Gallstone Dissolution," detailed consideration of the kinetics of this process allows one to determine under what conditions this process may be accelerated.

RATE PROCESSES

Let us now consider how the potential for significant advances in our understanding of the pathogenesis of cholesterol gallstones can be augmented by considering the dynamic and kinetic factors—the rates—that control this process.

The physicochemical processes involved are conveniently organized into three categories: stone origin, stone growth, and gallbladder function. Stone origin is primarily a function of the type and nature of nucleation. Stone growth includes both growth by precipitation of the cholesterol from supersaturated micelles and growth by the aggregation of smaller gallstones to form a compound stone. The gallbladder wall and degree of gallbladder emptying are also significant. The importance of all these factors had been mentioned in past studies, but the scientific framework underlying each has not yet been fully or sufficiently utilized.

Stone Origin

To originate, a gallstone must be nucleated. The existence of several distinct families of stones rather than a continuous range of sizes in many patients undergoing cholecystectomy suggests that the genesis of stones is occasional and coincides with infrequent nucleation. This initial nucleation can result from either of two mechanisms: heterogeneous or homogeneous nucleation (Fig. 34). Either process occurs only when bile is supersaturated.

Heterogeneous nucleation requires small particles consisting of, e.g., bacteria, calcium carbonate, or bilirubinate around which cholesterol can accumulate. The number of stones that begin to form equals the number of particles, or nuclei, suspended in bile. To eliminate precipitation, one need only eliminate these particles. Indeed, the presence in a supersaturated solution of a detergent-like bile does much to disguise these particles as micelles and thus reduces the rate of nucleation.

However, nucleation can occur even when the supersaturated bile contains no suspended particles. This dynamic process of homogeneous nucleation takes place whenever several cholesterol molecules combine spontaneously to form a nucleus consisting only of cholesterol. The rate of this combination, which is determined by statistical chance, increases sharply as the degree of supersaturation increases. This mechanism produces the maximum degree of supersaturation possible in bile. In other words, it represents the highest apparent "solubility" (line C in Fig. 32).

There are, therefore, two lines in Figure 32 that are conceptually well defined. These are the equilibrium solubility (line A), below which stones will always dissolve, and the homogeneous nucleation (line C), above which the cholesterol will always precipitate. Between these two extremes may lie many apparent solubility lines, determined by the way in which the solution is prepared. The concentration at which the precipitation rate becomes significant is reproducible. Below this critical concentration, the solution is metastable and may remain unchanged for long periods of time. Since it has been observed in many surfactant solutions, line B in Figure 32 is probably representative of such behavior in bile.

Stone Growth

After nucleation occurs, stones will grow when the bile is supersaturated and will dissolve when it is below saturation. Both growth and dissolution rates can be most conveniently discussed in terms of the three-step mechanism shown in Figure 35. For stone growth, cholesterol in a micelle first diffuses to the surface of the stone; next, cholesterol diffuses away from the stone. The rate of growth is determined by the rates of all three steps but is dominated by the slowest step. A useful way of thinking about this process is to represent each step in terms of a resistance not unlike an electrical resistance. Another analogy is that of traffic flow. The speed at which one drives to work can be viewed as a rate process consisting of a series of steps. For example, getting from the garage to the street, getting onto an interstate highway, going through a tunnel and over a bridge, and, finally, parking the car. Each of these steps can be thought of as a resistance

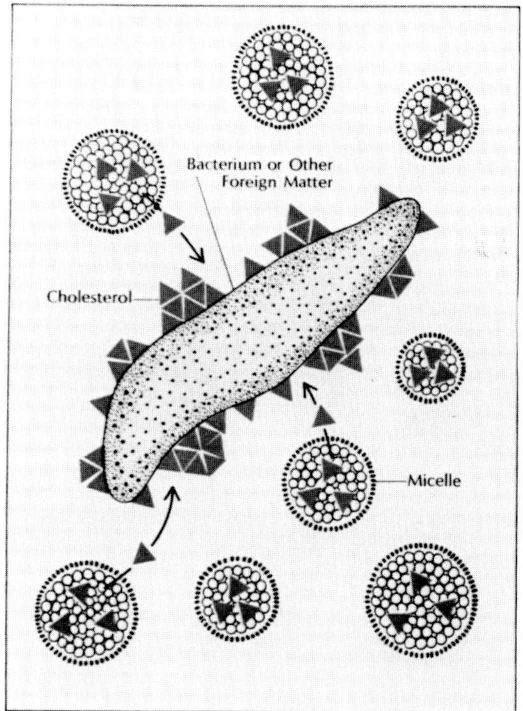

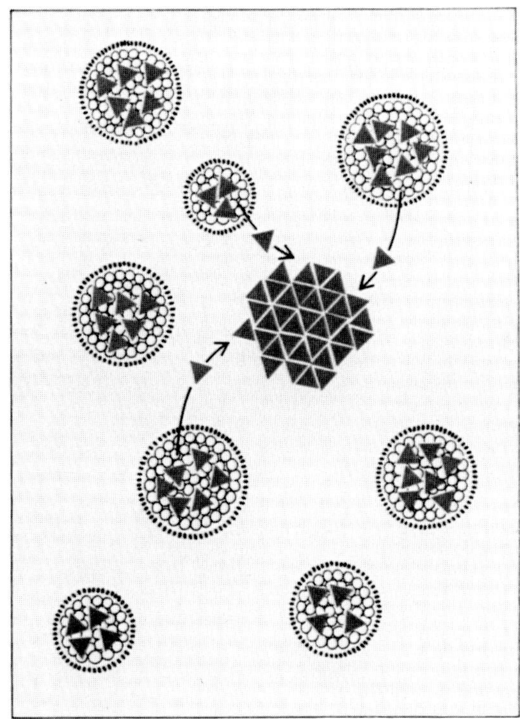

Figure 34. Two mechanisms of nucleation in supersaturated solutions are illustrated, heterogeneous (left), in which precipitation occurs around foreign matter, and homogeneous (right), in which precipitation occurs spontaneously at very high supersaturation.

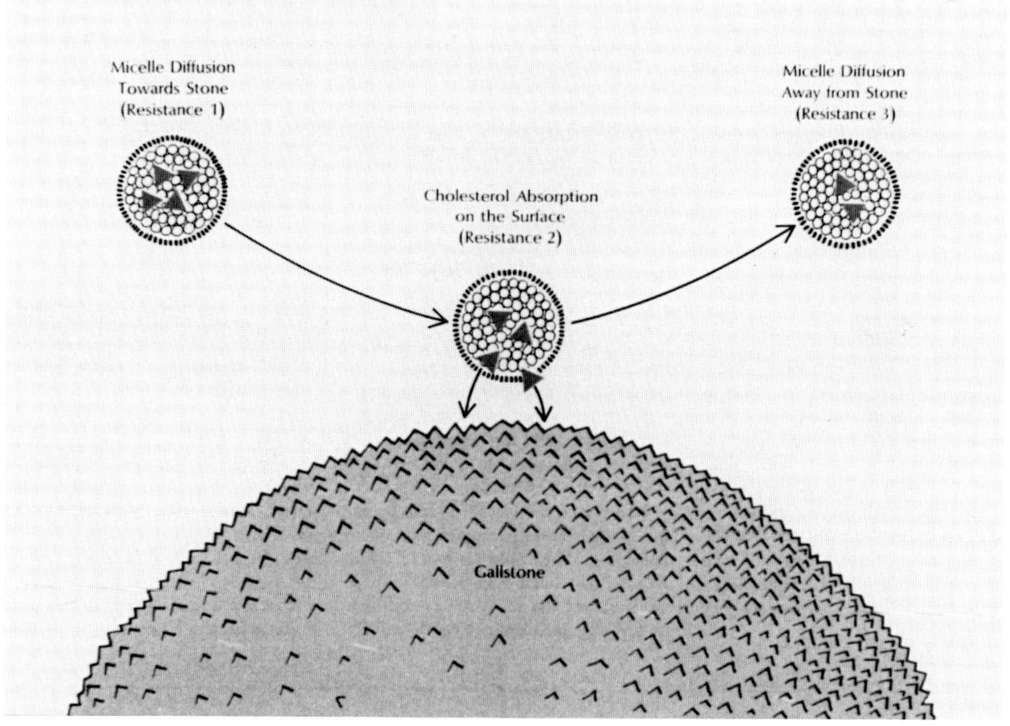

Figure 35. The speed of each of the steps by which stone growth proceeds involves a characteristic resistance; the speed of the overall process depends on the sum of these resistances. The same mechanism with the sequence of steps reversed describes dissolution.

to traffic flow. The rate at which one makes this trip is determined by how long each step takes; a longer time equals a higher resistance. If one is interested in decreasing the travel time, i.e., increasing the rate of the process, one must identify where the bottlenecks occur and alter those parts of the route. Modifying only a part where delays never occur will not materially alter the travel time.

A similar series of steps accounts for gallstone growth. The overall rate is governed by the sum of three resistances; the largest one dominates the rate. One might be able to decrease the rate of growth by creating a roadblock at a strategic point. However, alternating or blocking a less critical step is less likely to have a significant effect.

Two of the steps shown in Figure 35 are determined almost entirely by properties of the solution. These are the diffusional steps—1 and 3—which are strongly dependent upon the fluid velocity of the bile flowing past the stone. The other step, step 2, is determined by properties of the cholesterol surface at low flow and the micelle in bile. At low flow, the diffusion steps will provide the greatest resistance and will limit the overall growth rate. At high flow, the surface deposition step will be slowest, so its resistance will be greatest. In the gallbladder, the growth of a single stone will probably be controlled by diffusion at low bile flow.

During this growth, two other phenomena occur that can dramatically alter the nature of the gallstones formed. The first of these phenomena, Oswald ripening, occurs because small cholesterol particles (i.e., less than about 1 μm in size) are more soluble in bile than larger ones. The result is that large stones tend to grow at the expense of small ones, as shown schematically in Figure 36. This is the process commonly used in organic chemistry laboratories for digesting a precipitate, i.e., boiling it to produce larger particles. In most cases, it occurs slowly and so will be important over many cycles of gallbladder operation.

The second phenomenon that alters the course of gallstone growth is aggregation. This rapid process occurs when many small cholesterol crystals agglomerate to form a single composite stone. Aggregation rates vary with the sixth power of the counter-ion change in the system, and so are strongly affected by small amounts of ionic calcium in bile. They can also be strongly affected by traces of polyelectrolytes and proteins; indeed, such macromolecules are used as flocculent bile in many water treatment processes. Since traces of these macromolecules can have such a large effect, they should be included in any complete study of the rates of gallstone pathogenesis.

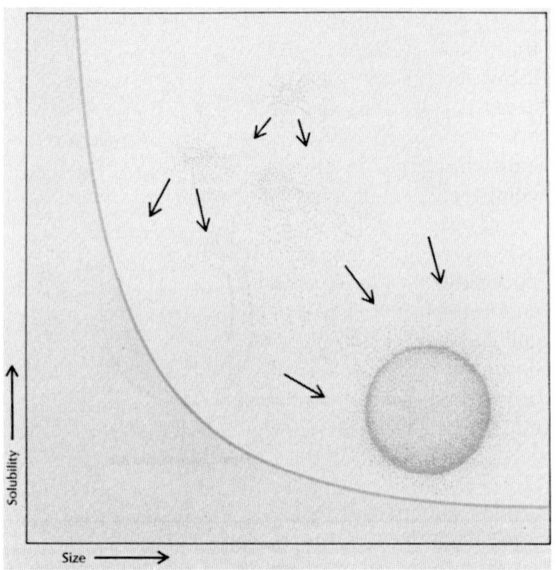

Figure 36. 1In "Oswald ripening," large stones grow at the expense of small ones because the solubility of cholesterol increases as the stones become smaller.

The rates of gallstone destruction occur by mechanisms that are the reverse of those responsible for stone growth. Dissolution by cholesterol solubilization involves the reverse of the growth mechanism diagrammed in Figure 35. This is discussed quantitatively later. Dispersion, the fragmentation of an existing stone into smaller stones, is the reverse of the aggregation mechanism shown in Figure 37. Because dispersion offers the potential for very rapid nonsurgical therapy, it deserves much more careful attention than it has received in the past.

Gallbladder Function

The dynamics of gallbladder function contribute to gallstone formation in several ways. Bile is sequestered in the gallbladder until one eats a meal containing fats or proteins. This induces the synthesis of cholecystokinin. This hormone causes the sphincter of Oddi to relax and the gallbladder to contract and expel the bile into the small intestine. The bile recirculates through the enterohepatic system approximately 10 times a day.

If emptying were complete in each cycle, large gallstones would not form because the maximum total amount of cholesterol in the bile above saturation is only about 0.1 gm, not enough to form much of a stone even if it were all in one piece. Small particles that did form would be removed during emptying. However, estimates of the extent to which the human gallbladder empties suggest that the maximum degree of emptying in normal individuals is only 84%. (Some studies have shown it to be 80% in males and 65% in females.) Significantly different half-times and smaller degrees of emptying occur in groups at high risk for the development of gallstones. For example, human and animal experiments have documented that the efficiency of gallbladder contraction is greatly reduced during the latter half of the menstrual cycle and in the last trimester of pregnancy. Since normal gallbladder function probably always involves some degree of incomplete emptying, the characteristics of residual bile are probably important in the formation of gallstones.

Another aspect of gallbladder function that may influence stone formation is layering, or stratification. When bile enters the gallbladder from the liver, it contains 1.4–1.7% solids by weight. In the gallbladder, water and salts are removed until the bile contains about 14% solids by weight. This removal results in a concentrated layer at the gallbladder wall that, because it has a higher density, can flow down the wall by free convection and collect in the bottom of the gallbladder. The resulting layering, or stratification, was first observed in vivo in the gallbladders of patients undergoing cholecystectomy. These layers contain approximately the same relative amounts of bile salt and lecithin as are found in the bulk, and so do not result in different solubilities at different positions in the gallbladder. However, the different densities do alter the fluid mechanics involved, and many lead to the retention of some supersaturated bile over

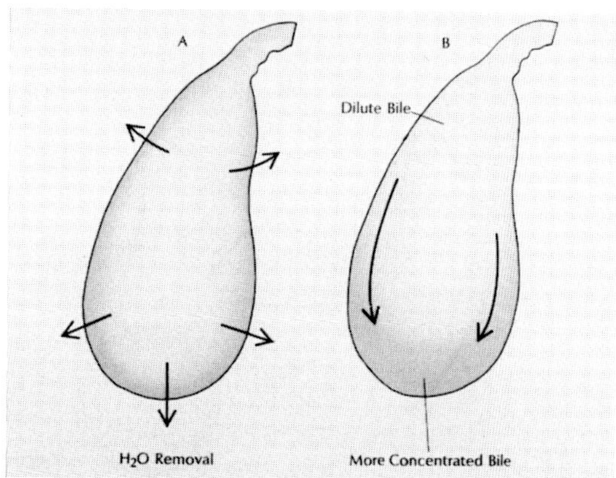

Figure 38.   A. As the bile becomes more concentrated in the gallbladder, layers of greater density occur close to the wall. B. These denser layers may flow down the wall and result in stratification of the bile.

many cycles that allows long-term stone growth (Fig. 38).

Thus, the overall picture that emerges is a dynamic one, based on a wide variety of time-dependent processes. Bile can be periodically lithogenic, oscillating between subsaturation and supersaturation. Nucleation rates are only occasionally significant. Once nucleation occurs, growth and dissolution take place sequentially in the periodically supersaturated bile. Aggregation and dispersion can result in the rapid formation or destruction of composite stones, while Oswald ripening always tends to eliminate the smaller stones. All these processes are affected by the fluid dynamics in the gallbladder and, in particular, by the rate and extent of gallbladder emptying. Whether stones collect and continue to grow depends on the sum of this entire sequence of time-dependent processes.

ACCELERATING GALLSTONE DISSOLUTION

Now for the promised example of the importance of considering dynamic factors. In the in vivo situation, gallstone dissolution is a slow process; 6 months to 2 years are required to dissolve a stone 1 cc in volume. A means of accelerating this dissolution rate by, for example, a factor of 5 would obviously provide a highly attractive alternative to surgery.

To seek this potential acceleration, we studied the dissolution rates of cholesterol pellets and actual gallstones in model bile solutions of sodium taurocholate, lecithin, and sodium chloride. The key feature of these experiments is that the bile

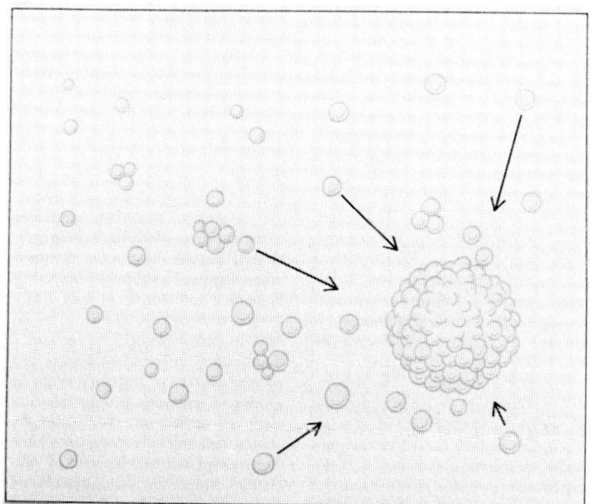

Figure 37.   Aggregation can result in very rapid stone growth. Both aggregation and its opposite—dispersion— depend strongly on the presence of ionic charges and very small amounts of polyelectrolytes in the solution.

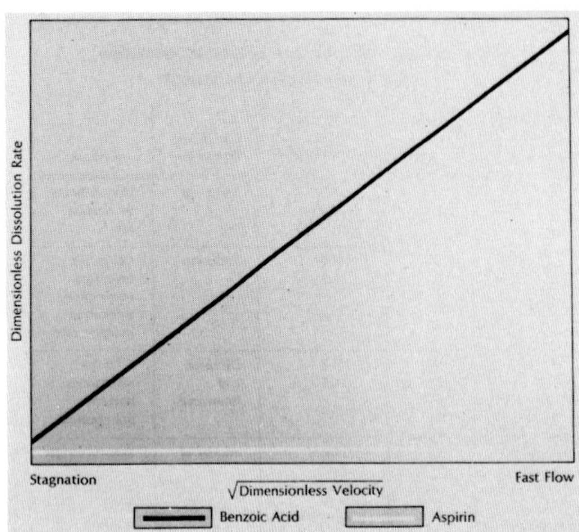

Figure 39.   Dissolution rates of benzoic acid and of aspirin are very different in water. Benzoic acid dissolution is affected by the fluid velocity and can be predicted from the diffusion coefficient, fluid velocity, and other solution properties. Aspirin dissolution is governed by a surface reaction and hence is unaffected by solution properties.

flow is exactly known; this known flow allows us to compare the experimentally measured dissolution rates with those calculated a priori from independent physicochemical measurements. Moreover, we used three different experimental methods suitable at different flows, and paralleled all measurements of cholesterol dissolution with measurements of benzoic acid dissolution, which has been completely studied by others. These three independent experimental methods and the benzoic acid comparisons provide quantitative cross-checks on the phenomena being studied.

Before discussing cholesterol dissolution, we describe the dissolution behavior of benzoic acid and aspirin because these two compounds illustrate two limiting cases of Figure 39. The dissolution rate of benzoic acid is linear in the solution velocity to the one-half power and is diffusion controlled over the entire velocity range. On the other hand, the dissolution of aspirin is independent of flow and is controlled by an interfacial reaction. In other words, the dissolution of benzoic acid is controlled by diffusional steps like steps 1 and 3 in Figure 35, while that of aspirin is controlled by an absorptional step like step 2 in the same figure.

Typical dissolution rates for two bile compositions are plotted in Figure 40 vs. the square root of bile velocity. These rates, which result from a mechanism like that in Figure 35, are most easily discussed in terms of stagnant bile, slowly flowing bile, and rapidly flowing bile. For stagnant bile, we assume that steps 1 and 3 are more important

than step 2 and are governed only by diffusion. From diffusion measurements on bile salt–lecithin solutions we can then calculate a predicted dissolution rate, which is 1.04 ± 0.08 of that actually observed. For slowly flowing bile, we again assume that steps 1 and 3 are more important than step 2 but are influenced by bile velocity. We can then calculate a priori the dotted line shown in Figure 40. The agreement of this line with the measured dissolution rates supports our contention that steps 1 and 3 are most important in this region.

Dissolution in rapidly flowing bile is dominated by the interfacial resistance, R_2 (cf. Fig. 35). While we have not made a completely independent prediction of R_2, we do know that it can be increased by the addition of bile salts or sodium chloride and that it is decreased by the addition of lecithin. This behavior is consistent with the hypothesis that this interfacial step depends strongly on the rates of micelle adsorption.

The increased values of R_2 on the addition of lecithin, which result in slower dissolution rates, are an excellent example of the importance of rate processes in bile.

On the basis of solubility alone, one would expect stone dissolution in bile salt–lecithin solutions to be up to 10 times faster than in bile salt solutions; in fact, the observed dissolution rate is three times faster in bile salt solutions. In other words, at high flow, stones dissolve more slowly in bile salt–lecithin solutions than in bile salt solutions, although cholesterol is less soluble in bile salt solutions. Such

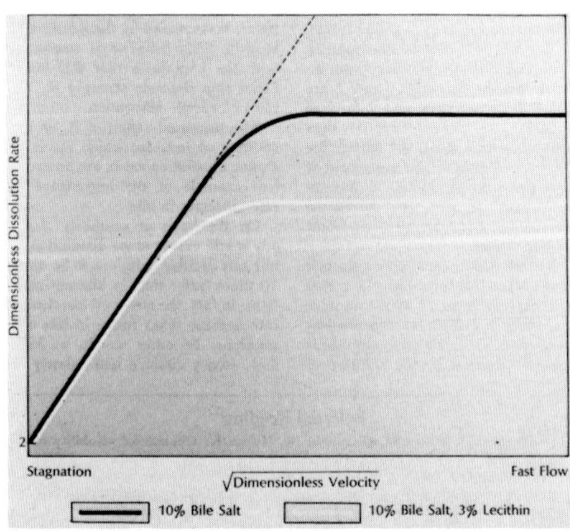

Figure 40.   Dissolution of cholesterol in model bile solution has characteristics of both benzoic acid and aspirin dissolutions. At low flow it is controlled by the properties of the solution; at high flow, it is controlled by the characteristics of the cholesterol surface. While lecithin increases the amount of cholesterol that can be dissolved, it slows the dissolution rate.

a discrepancy can only be explained by differences in rate processes.

Stone dissolution rates vary widely as a function of bile flow even in bile containing no cholesterol. Rates in stagnant bile are less than 2% of those in rapidly flowing bile. If the bile were 50% saturated with cholesterol, dissolution rates would be 50% of those reported here; if bile were 90% saturated, the rates would drop to 10% of those reported here. While the dissolution rates per unit area are greater for small stones than for larger ones, the total mass of cholesterol removed per unit time is greater for larger stones.

Gallstone dissolution can be increased by increasing the solubility of cholesterol in bile. Whether it can be increased by other physicochemical changes depends on the rate of bile flow. In stagnant bile (velocity = 0 cm/sec), increases in dissolution will be almost impossible because increases in diffusion are so difficult to achieve. In slowly flowing bile (velocity < 0.1 cm/sec), a fourfold increase in bile velocity is required to double the dissolution rate (cf. Fig. 40). In rapidly flowing bile (velocity > 0.1 cm/sec), the dissolution is independent of bile flow. Interfacial resistance controls the dissolution; such resistance can be decreased by adding another component; thus, dissolution rates can be increased up to the diffusion-controlled limit (the dotted line in Fig. 40). However, we have found that these new components are effective only at high bile flow.

These studies of dissolution will give clinically useful information only when the flows in the gallbladder are known more exactly. Available evidence does suggest that these flows are small, which is not surprising for an organ with only one way in and no way out (Fig. 41).

Recommended Reading

Evans DF, Tarr EW, Cussler EL: Cholesterol monohydrate growth in model bile solutions. *Proc Natl Acad Sci USA* 75:6630, 1978.

Evans DF, Tarr EW, Cussler EL: The nucleation of cholesterol monohydrate crystals in model bile solutions, in Fisher MM, Govsky GA, Shaffer SM, et al (eds): *Gallstones.* New York, Plenum, 1978.

References

1. Holzbach RT, March M, et al: Cholesterol solubility in bile; evidence that supersaturated bile is common in healthy man. *J Clin Invest* 52:1467, 1973.

Bile Velocity (cm/sec⁻¹)	Stone Diameter (cm)	Dissolution Rate (gm/cm⁻²/sec⁻¹)	Controlling Resistances	Remarks
0	0.1 1.0	4.5 0.45	Diffusion	Very difficult to increase rate
0.01	0.1 1.0	6.0 2.5	Diffusion	Velocities from free convection; difficult to increase rate
0.1	0.1 1.0	8.4 6.6	Diffusion and Interfacial	All three resistances become unimportant
1.0	0.1 1.0	11.0 11.0	Interfacial	Rate no longer varies with bile velocity; larger increase possible

*Bile composition: 10 wt % sodium taurocholate and 3 wt % lecithin; units: bile velocity [=] cm sec⁻¹; stone diameter [=] cm; dissolution rate [=] g cm⁻² sec⁻¹.

Figure 41. Examples of the kinetics of gallstone dissolution in bile containing no cholesterol. Bile composition is 10 wt % sodium taurocholate and 3 wt % lecithin.

2. Mufson D, Meksuwan K, et al: Cholesterol solubility in lecithin–bile salt systems. *Science* 177:710, 1972.
3. Mufson D, et al: Sterile incubation apparatus for cholesterol solubility studies. *Gastroenterology* 63:1090, 1972.
4. Sedaghat A, Grundy SM, et al: Cholesterol crystals and the formation of cholesterol gallstones. *N Engl J Med* 5:302(23) 1274, 1980.

Cholelithiasis and Acalculous Cholecystitis: Possible Complications of Prolonged Parenteral Nutrition

Anderson[1] in 1972 was the first to associate total parenteral nutrition (TPN) with acalculous cholecystitis. In 1979 Peterson and Sheldon[2] reported eight patients who developed acalculous cholecystitis while receiving TPN management. Pitt et al.[3] in 1982 reported on 71 patients who had received TPN. These patients underwent prolonged periods of fasting, which the writer felt altered their bile composition and led to gallstone formation. They found that of 60 selected at-risk patients (with ileal disorders) who received TPN for 3 months or longer, 21 (35%) developed cholelithiasis. *Pitt et al. concluded that patients who receive long-term TPN— especially those with ileal disorders—suffer the risk of developing cholelithiasis.*

It should be remembered that the great majority of patients (both children and adults) who developed gallstones during the course of TPN therapy had coexistent ileal disorders. When the stones of the children's group were studied by spectroscopy, they were found to consist mainly of calcium bilirubinate. When the stones of the adult group were studied, they were found to contain more cholesterol.

Pitt et al.[3] and Roslyn et al.[4,5] recommend that patients on TPN be carefully monitored with ultrasonography and that absolute fasting be avoided if possible. These patients should be encouraged to take some food by mouth in order to stimulate gallbladder emptying. Pitt et al. further believe that gallstone formation during TPN therapy is conceivably a reversible process—but not a predictable one. They are of the opinion that gallbladder stasis is related to gallstone formation, and that in the future gallbladder stasis may be eliminated by continued small oral feedings.

Recommended Reading

Adler N, Pieroni PL, Takeshima T, et al: Effects of parenteral hyperalimentation on pancreatic and biliary secretion. *Surg Forum* 26:445, 1975.

Hamilton RF, Davis WC, Stephenson DV, et al: Effects of parenteral hyperalimentation on upper gastrointestinal tract secretions. *Arch Surg* 102:348, 1971.

References

1. Anderson DL: Acalculous cholecystitis; a possible complication of parenteral hyperalimentation. *Med Ann DC* 41:448, 1972.
2. Peterson ER, Sheldon GF: Eight cases of gallbladder disease following IV nutritional feedings. *Am J Surg* 138:814, 1979.
3. Pitt HA, KingnW III, Mann L, et al: Increased risk of cholelithiasis with prolonged total parenteral nutrition; UCLA, School of Medicine, Los Angeles, California. *Am J Surg* 145:106, 1983.
4. Roslyn JJ, Pitt HA, Mann LL, et al: Long-term parenteral nutrition induces gallbladder disease (abstracted). *Gastroenterology* 80:1264, 1981.
5. Roslyn JJ, Pitt HA, Ament ME, et al: Gallbladder disease in patients on long term parenteral nutrition. *Gastroenterology* 1982.

dence of hepatic duct stones is approximately 1.5%. In the Eastern countries such as Japan, China, Malaysia, Hong Kong, and Taiwan, the incidence varies from 3% to as high as 30%. It is interesting that the incidence of intrahepatic duct stones in the Chinese and Japanese who have been living in the United States is the same as that of the broader U.S. population. This same pattern also exists with regard to carcinoma of the stomach. That is, the incidence of stomach carcinoma is highest in Japan; however, the Japanese who have migrated to the United States and have lived there for many years show the same low incidence as the general population. Apparently socioeconomic as well as environmental factors play an important etiological role in this marked difference. The true etiological factors are as yet undetermined. The high incidence of hemolytic anemia and biliary parasites apparently plays an important role in hepatic duct stone formation.

According to Juttijudata et al.,[1] biliary parasites, liver flukes *Opisthorchis viverrini* and its ova, were documented as the nidus of biliary calculi, as well as *Ascaris lumbricoides* and its ova. In pediatric cases, giardiasis has been implicated as the cause of cholecystitis. In Thailand the prevalence of *O. viverrini* was 22%; it was as high as 90% in endemic areas. The overall incidence of ascariasis was 19.6%. The incidence of choledochal cysts and other congenital anomalies of the biliary system is believed to be higher than in the United States. Juttijudata et al. conclude that the high prevalence of congenital anomalies of the biliary system probably explains the high incidence of intrahepatic stones in Thailand. There, of 109 cholestatic patients with acute acalculous cholecystitis, 17 (15.6%) were documented as having intrahepatic stones.

Reference

1. Juttijudata P, Prichanond S, Churaratanakul, et al: Opisthorchiasis and its associated diseases. *J Med Assoc Thai* 68:222, 1985.

The Incidence of Intrahepatic Stones in the Oriental Races

By definition, an intrahepatic stone is one that is lodged in the biliary system within the liver proximal to the cystic duct's junction with the common hepatic duct. In the Western countries, the inci-

The Changing State of Gallstones in Japan

In 1970 Nakayama and Miyake[1] of Fukuoka, Japan, reported on the "Changing State of Gallstone Disease in Japan," and described the difference in composition between gallstones in the East and those in the West. In the Chinese of Hong Kong, bile pigment stones predominate, whereas in the United States the stones consist almost exclusively of cholesterol. In Japan the findings were intermediate; that is, both types of gallstones were found. These writers believe that cholesterol stones are metabolic in origin and originate within the gallbladder, and on many occasions are not necessarily accompanied by fever, liver damage, nonfunctioning gallbladder, or inflammatory signs. Gallbladder disease that harbors stones of bile pigment is closely associated with bacterial infection and is found mainly in the biliary tract, especially in the common bile duct. The latter usually results in fever, severe liver damage, and a nonfunctioning gallbladder. The writers believe that when cholesterol stones exist, cholecystectomy and occasional choledochotomy are indicated, but that whenever pigment stones are found, treatment invariably requires common duct exploration. Rapid re-formation of gallstones is a common occurrence. The authors present 12 criteria for common duct exploration:

1. Common duct dilated beyond 10 mm.
2. Existence or history of jaundice.
3. Cystic duct dilated and joining the common duct at a right angle.
4. Presence of cholangitis.
5. Repeated attacks of gallbladder colic.
6. Existence of cirrhosis of the liver.
7. Hardening of the head of the pancreas.
8. Multiple small stones in the gallbladder.
9. Stones or mud in the cut cystic duct.
10. Palpable stones in the common duct, with corroboration by cholangiography.
11. Presence of anomalies in the bile duct.
12. In Hong Kong, Ong[2] has recommended that whenever pigment stones are found in the common duct, exploration should be carried out and the gallbladder preserved for later anastomosis. Nakayama et al. believe that Ong's recommendation is not valid; they prefer choledochoduodenostomy or choledochojejunostomy.

Nakayama et al. conclude that the pigment gallstones of the East are gradually changing to the cholesterol stones of the West. They attribute this change to environmental alteration (i.e., urbanization) and changes in food habits, especially after World War II.

References

1. Nakayama F, Miyake: Changing state of gallstone disease in Japan. *Ann Surg* 120:974, 1970.
2. Ong GB: A study of recurrent pyogenic cholangitis. *Arch Surg* 84:409, 1962.

Gallbladder Disease in the Pima Indians

According to Burch et al., the prevalence of gallbladder disease among the Pima Indians was found to be significantly higher than that of the Framingham, Massachusetts, test population. Gallbladder disease was associated with a higher number of pregnancies in both the Pima Indian women and the Framingham test women. Pima Indians between the ages of 30 and 60 years, with two pregnancies or less, had a greater prevalence of gallbladder disease than the women in the Framingham test population (4.5 times greater). In the male group of Pima Indians, aged 50 to 62 years, the incidence was greater than that of the Framingham male population.

Serum studies in the Pima Indians revealed that their serum cholesterol levels were not related to the incidence of gallstone formation.

References

1. Burch TA, Camess LJ, Bennett PH, et al: Prevalence of gallbladder disease in Pima Indians. *N Engl J Med* 277:894, 1967.
2. Small DM, Rapo S: Source of abnormal bile in patients with cholesterol gallstones. *N Engl J Med* 283:53, 1971.

4

OPERABLE CONGENITAL ANOMALIES

Atresia of the Biliary Ducts

Atresias of the biliary ductal system are congenital defects in which the biliary lumen fails to develop. Atresia may involve the intra- and/or extrahepatic ductal systems, including the gallbladder. Atresias proximal to the right and left hepatic ducts, or distal to the hepatic duct itself and involving the common bile duct, result in marked dilatation of the proximal biliary tree, with severe jaundice in the newborn. Atresia of the biliary tree is not a rare congenital disorder. Just as extrahepatic atresia may result in obstruction, intrahepatic atresia may result in jaundice as well as eventual parenchymatous atrophy; the latter may take place without jaundice. It is well known that jaundice of a physiological nature occurs in the majority of newborn infants and spontaneously disappears. However, this physiological jaundice is not diagnosed as atresia of the biliary ducts until the patient is several weeks of age and beyond the usual period for spontaneous regression. The obstructive jaundice that follows congenital atresia is unrelenting and is usually associated with enlargement of the liver, bile in the urine, and acholic stools.

Blood studies will show increased bilirubin levels. Every infant suspected of having atresia of the biliary system should receive an abdominal exploration for the following reasons: (1) It will be possible to determine the presence or absence of the specific type of congenital defect. (2) Given the limited experience with this problem throughout the world, a certain amount of relief may be offered that could possibly prolong the life of the infant. (3) On occasion, an infant may be cured if the atresia is of a simpler and milder form. The majority of these infants die within the year because of the wide extent and noncorrectability of the disease process or the impossibility of surgery.

Unfortunately, congenital atresia of the biliary system is a genetic process, and unless the cause or the pathogenesis is discovered and prevented, surgery per se, though it offers the only hope of relief, is at present inadequate. The possibility of surgery to help or correct atresia of the biliary system will depend upon the limitation and location of the defect; the latter will determine the ultimate prognosis. The cases of biliary atresia that have experienced the best results to date are those in which the disease has been found distal to the common hepatic duct in which the gallbladder is a remnant and the common duct merely a cord. The other form of atresia that is amenable to effective correction is atresia of the common duct beyond the cystic duct in which the cystic duct empties itself into the gallbladder; this anatomy offers the possibility of gallbladder anastomosis to the jejunum, thus bypassing the site of obstruction. Atresias that call for procedures that extend into the liver hilus offer the poorest prognosis and offer little or no opportunity for corrective surgery.

The latest possibility, of course, is a liver transplantation with a completely new hookup of the common hepatic duct to the gastrointestinal tract. Starzl* has been a pioneer in this field, and his results will be referred to subsequently. The cardinal sign of congenital atresia is progressive jaundice that fails to disappear spontaneously after 2 weeks and increases in intensity. Additional signs and symptoms are a slowly enlarging liver that is hard to the touch and is associated with a palpable spleen; accompanying acholic stool and dark brown urine, both with a high bile content. Gallbladder studies usually indicate evidence of obstructive jaundice, and the picture of a secondary microcytic anemia is not conclusive. Nevertheless, in the differential diagnosis at this time, jaundice of a hemolytic nature (hemolytic anemia) must be considered, as well as erythroblastosis fetalis hepatitis, obstruction of the biliary system with debris; congenital syphilis and familial hemolytic anemia are also possible.

SURGICAL TECHNIQUE

Percutaneous intrahepatic cholangiography may be considered prior to laparotomy. The mortality in this type of patient is usually extremely high, approaching 100%. The majority die within the first 12 months, while others survive for 1 or 2 years. There are some patients who, after surgery, have survived for 2 to 10 years, and there have even been a few who did well into the teenage period, but such cases are extremely rare.

Only general anesthesia should be employed. A large exploratory incision, either paramedian or subcostal, is preferred, and a careful search under good light and magnification should be conducted for the specific congenital defect. The gallbladder should be searched for to see if it exists, and whether or not there is a communication with the common bile duct. If the gallbladder is collapsed, fibrotic, or nonexistent, this indicates that obstruction, stenosis, or atresia exists at a higher level than

---

*Thomas E. Starzl, Professor of Surgery at the University of Pittsburgh, is a world authority on liver transplantation and to date has published the best prognostic results in cases of congenital biliary atresia.

the junction of the cystic duct with the common hepatic duct. If the gallbladder is normal in size, has a patent cystic duct, and communicates with the common bile duct, the obstruction or atresia exists beyond the cystic duct junction. In the latter instance, a bypass procedure can be considered palliative and possibly even curative. Even if the gallbladder is found to be present with a lumen and a normal cystic duct continuous with the common duct, the ductal system proximal to the hepatic duct may still be absent or atretic.

Whenever a gallbladder is patent and its cystic duct communicates with the common hepatic duct, a needle cholangiogram may help to outline the entire biliary tree. If a patent biliary system proximal to the cystic duct's junction with the common duct is shown to exist, a bypass procedure would most likely be successful, and this should be carried out at once. A choleocystojejunostomy (side-to-side) or a Roux-en-Y end-to-end anastomosis between the gallbladder and jejunum are the palliative procedures of choice. A good procedure when the extrahepatic ductal structures are visible is to inject them further, using a small hypodermic needle; warm saline solution is injected under slight or moderate pressure to cause further distention of the ducts. This aids in recognizing the more available and workable anatomy that is associated with the specific anomaly.

Many times the duct is opened and found to be filled with mud and gravel; irrigation with further distention may clean out the entire common duct and produce a cure. Figure 42 illustrates the various types of anomalies of the gallbladder that may develop and the surgical options for possible palliation or cure. In the routine surgical exploration of patients with biliary atresia, the duodenum should be routinely mobilized with the Kocher maneuver. That is, the duodenum is bluntly freed and rolled medially to help display more of the common duct and expose more of whatever involvement may exist. The liver itself should be carefully evaluated because now and then an intrahepatic cyst may be found to exist; in this case, all other extrahepatic ducts are atretic. In such an instance, if only a small portion of the cyst can be dissected free without excessive bleeding, a Roux-en-Y anastomosis may help to drain the liver of its bile. The latter procedure is the ideal treatment.

Finally, in atresias of the biliary system, the operative procedure selected will depend in great measure upon the type and extent of the atretic process that is found after careful exploration and dissection of the entire extrahepatic ductal system; when possible, the existing intrahepatic ductal system should be visualized. Three practical procedures are available to the surgeon when favorable lesions are recognized: (1) A cholecystogastrostomy, though possibly unphysiological in the adult, can be a lifesaving operation in the infant. (2) A cholecystoduodenostomy can be performed when a normal gallbladder is available with a patent cystic duct communicating with an intact common duct and hepatic duct. An end-to-side cholecystoduodenostomy can be carried out especially when the duodenum has been made more mobile by the Kocher maneuver. (3) A cholecystojejunostomy is an effective procedure whenever possible and indicated; it can be made side-to-side with a supplemental jejunojejunostomy. (4) Another acceptable procedure is an end-to-side cholecystojejunostomy, using a Roux-en-Y procedure. A one-row anastomosis should be adequate because of the small anatomy and the possible obliterative effect of a second row. Still, whenever an extra stitch is required, it should certainly be employed. There is still a difference of opinion regarding the type of suture to be used. Some surgeons prefer a (00000) silk atraumatic needle type of suture, while others prefer a similarly fine suture made of chromic catgut. A polyethylene tube may be ideal; it is inserted into the hepatic duct, whenever possible, to connect or anastomose the end of the hepatic duct to the duodenum. When this is possible, an end-to-end or end-to-side anastomosis is performed with the polyethylene tube utilized as a splint left in place, halfway into the hepatic duct and halfway into the duodenum. The suturing or anastomosis takes place around it. The tube will pass at a later date in the postoperative period.

PROGNOSIS OF BILIARY ATRESIA

The obstructive jaundice that accompanies congenital atresia of the biliary system leads to progressive, irreversible biliary cirrhosis. The liver enlarges and becomes green, nodular, and hard. Though the cellular degeneration is followed by extensive cellular regeneration, the ultimate change is that of progressive biliary cirrhosis and death. In time, bleeding tendencies develop because of the lowered prothrombin levels. It may be possible for the infant to develop normally for 1 or more years, but progressive liver degeneration and liver failure usually result in death.

Every infant with obstructive jaundice should have an abdominal exploration in the hope that an anomalous atresia will be found that can be corrected with surgery. Even with indicated surgery, however, the prognosis remains guarded and difficult to predict. The

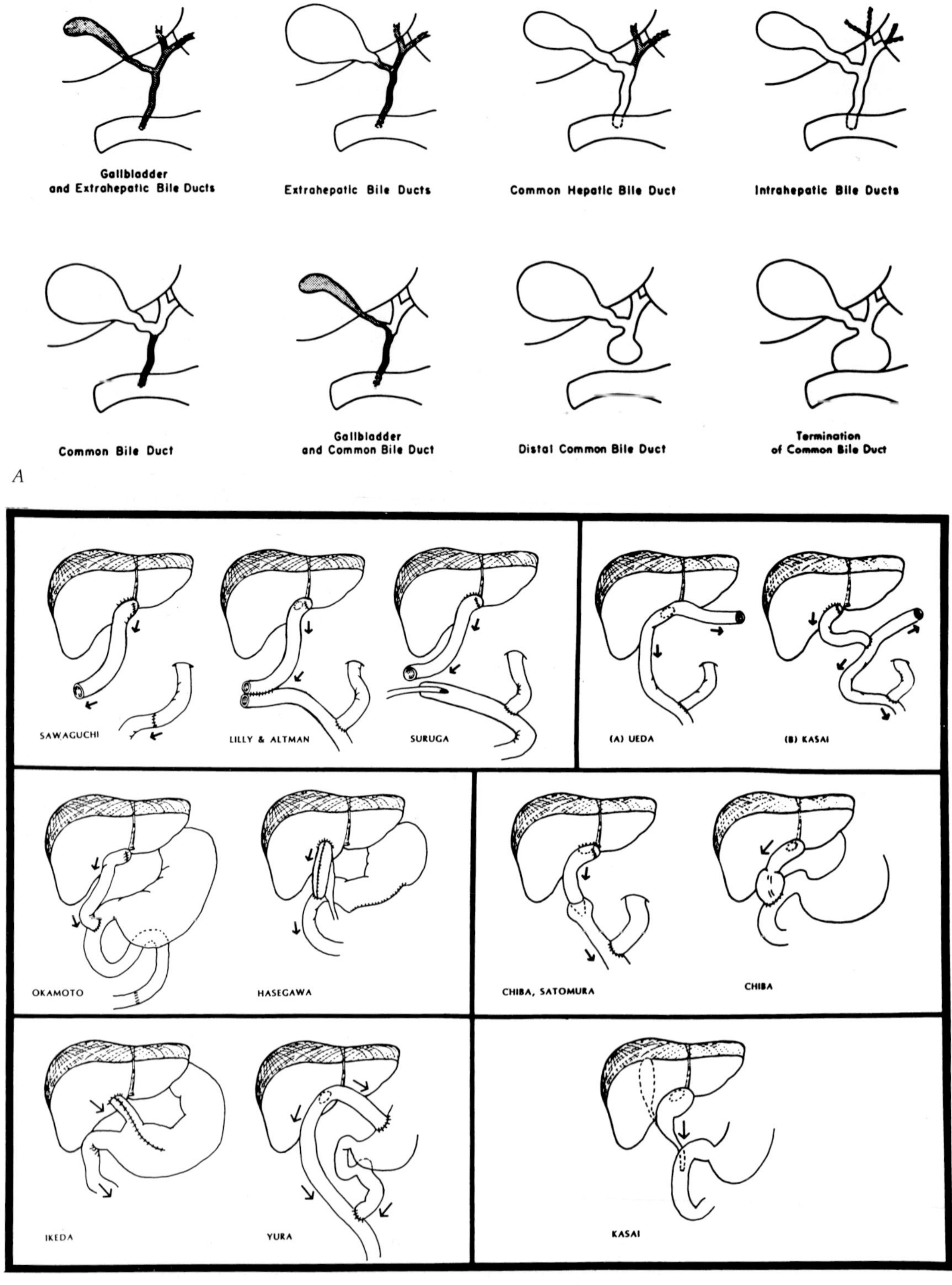

Figure 42.   A. Diagrammatic illustrations depicting the many varieties of atresia, as well as their many locations. B. Variety of surgical approaches for correcting the abnormalities.

Longmire procedure (hepatojejunostomy) has been tried, but with little success, and many do not recommend it because even in adult cases where carcinoma is the underlying obstructive factor, the result obtained with the Longmire procedure is invariably poor and short-lived. The final cure will ultimately be in the hands of the geneticist, who must prophylactically reduce the number of congenital atresia cases that come before the surgeon. Figures 42 and 50 show the various operative techniques for congenital atretic lesions amenable to surgery.

Liver Transplantation for Biliary Atresia*

Thomas E. Starzl, M.D., Ph.D.
Carlos O. Esquivel, M.D., Ph.D.

INTRODUCTION

Orthotopic liver transplantation is the treatment of choice for patients with end-stage liver disease. The increasing enthusiasm for hepatic transplantation during the last decade is the result of better immunosuppression, particularly with the introduction of cyclosporine in the early 1980s and of monoclonal antibodies more recently. New improvements in technique have made the operation more practical. For these reasons, liver transplantation is no longer considered an experimental procedure but rather an accepted mode of therapy for patients with hopelessly advanced hepatic disease.

The indications for liver transplantation are changing constantly in order to benefit more patients who otherwise would inevitably die of complications of liver disease, as in fulminant hepatitis. Still, an absolute indication for hepatic transplantation in children is biliary atresia.

CLINICAL TRIALS

The first attempt at hepatic transplantation in a human was in 1963. The patient, a 3-year-old boy

with biliary atresia, died on the operating table from hemorrhage. It was not until 1967 that the first long-term survival was obtained. A 1.5-year-old girl with hepatocellular carcinoma survived for 13 months before succumbing to metastatic disease.

Three years later, a 4-year-old girl with biliary atresia and an incidental hepatoma underwent a liver transplant; this patient is alive and attending college more than 16 years later.

During the precyclosporine era from March 1963 to February 1980, 86 children underwent liver replacement, of whom 51 had biliary atresia (Table 1).

Cyclosporine was introduced in March 1980 and since then, there has been a progressive increase in the number of liver transplants performed. The series began at the University of Colorado and continued until 1981, when the program was transferred to the University of Pittsburgh. Five hundred patients received liver transplants from March 1980 to November 1985. There were 203 pediatric recipients, of whom 99 had biliary atresia, the most common indication. Other indications for hepatic transplantation under cyclosporine therapy are listed in Table 2.

Almost all of the children undergoing liver transplantation for biliary atresia had had at least one portoenterostomy procedure (Kasai). Since these patients had failed with a biliary drainage procedure, the decision for transplantation was easy. The children rapidly developed progressive hepatic disease manifested by failure to thrive, increasing jaundice, and complications of portal hypertension.

Table 1. Indications for Liver Transplantation in Pediatric Patients in the Precyclosporine Era

Main Indication	No. of Patients (March 1, 1963– February 29, 1980)	Percent
Biliary atresia	51	59.3
Inborn metabolic errors	13	15.1
Nonalcoholic cirrhosis	13	15.1
Primary liver malignancy	3	3.6
Neonatal hepatitis	2	2.3
Congenital hepatic fibrosis	2	2.3
Secondary biliary cirrhosis*	2	2.3
Total	86	100%

*Trauma or choledochal cyst.

From the Department of Surgery, University of Pittsburgh Health Center, University of Pittsburgh, and the Veterans Administration Medical Center, Pittsburgh, Pennsylvania.

*Supported by Research Project Grant No. AM-29961 from the National Institutes of Health, Bethesda, Maryland.

SURGICAL TECHNIQUES

Donor Operation

The technical aspects of the donor hepatectomy and preservation have been discussed in detail elsewhere. A significant problem in the procurement of organs for children is the limited availability of small pediatric donors. In extreme circumstances, adult livers have been used in children after partial resections at the "back table."

In small donors, it is advisable to leave the celiac axis in continuity with the thoracic or abdominal aorta or both. This is particularly important when the recipient or donor hepatic artery cannot be used for the reconstruction, as in the presence of anomalous vessels. If the donor abdominal aorta cannot be retrieved, the thoracic aorta may be turned down 180° for anastomosis to the recipient's aorta. A useful technique is to transect the thoracic aorta, reanastomose it to the aortic cuff below the celiac axis, and tailor the transected end of the thoracic aorta to form a smooth funnel. This avoids a blind pouch, which could be the source of thrombus formation (Fig. 43). It must be emphasized, however, that in the presence of a recipient hepatic artery of good quality, the best results are obtained when an end-to-end anastomosis is carried out between the recipient hepatic artery and the donor celiac axis.

Recipient Operation

In children, a bilateral subcostal incision, often using the previous incision, will suffice. The dissection is then continued in the hilum of the liver, attempting to identify the Roux-en-Y limb of the

Table 2. Indications for Liver Transplantation in Pediatric Patients in the Cyclosporine Era

Main Indication	No. of Patients (March 1, 1980– December 1, 1985)	Percent
Biliary atresia	99	48.8
Inborn metabolic errors	45	22.2
Nonalcoholic cirrhosis	21	10.3
Familial cholestasis	14	6.9
Neonatal hepatitis	6	3.0
Acute hepatic necrosis	5	2.5
Congenital hepatic fibrosis	3	1.5
Secondary biliary cirrhosis	3	1.5
Sclerosing cholangitis	2	1.0
Toxic hepatic injury	2	1.0
Trauma	1	0.5
Inflammatory pseudotumor	1	0.5
Budd-Chiari syndrome	1	0.5
Total	203	100%

portoenterostomy. This is useful in patients with dense adhesions, since dissection of the portoenterostomy will aid in exposing the hilar structures for proper identification. The hepatic artery should be ligated early to minimize bleeding. Then the portal is ligated deep into the hilum in order to obtain a long vessel. It is better to trim a long portal vein during the reconstruction than to come out short, necessitating interposition grafts.

Hepatectomy in children is usually easier than in adults, and this is often the case in patients with biliary atresia and a single portoenterostomy pro-

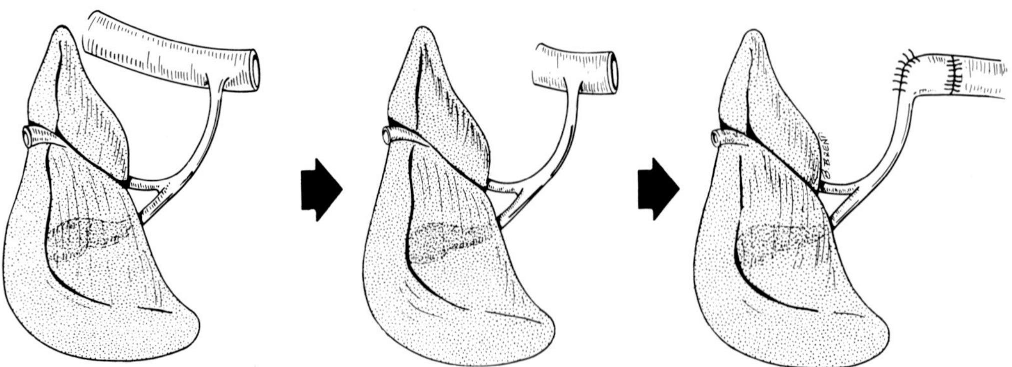

Figure 43. The thoracic aorta is transected above the celiac axis and anastomosed below it. The suraceliac cuff is tailored and closed to form a smooth funnel avoiding a blind pouch that could be the source of thrombus formation.

cedure. However, numerous attempts at biliary drainage, creation of stomas, and infection in the right upper quadrant can make the hepatectomy extremely difficult. Recently, venous bypass has been used more frequently and successfully in children. Decreased blood loss, stable hemodynamic physiology during the anhepatic phase, and less renal insult are some of the advantages of venous bypass. It also facilitates the hepatectomy and allows more time for hemostasis during the anhepatic phase, since the latter is better achieved with venous bypass.

If dissection of the hilar structures is impossible because of dense adhesions, encircling the hepatoduodenal ligament (Pringle's maneuver) will permit en bloc clamping of the portal triad. The ligament is then transected, and the vascular structures are identified so that they may be dissected more safely. Another valuable maneuver employed when adhesions preclude a safe hepatectomy is to clamp the suprahepatic vena cava, divide it, and insert one or two fingers into the intrahepatic cava to minimize blood loss. The liver is then dissected free from above until the infrahepatic cava is encountered. Finally, a clamp is placed on the infrahepatic cava to obtain vascular control.

The sequence and techniques of the vascular anastomoses have been reported elsewhere. Prevention of anastomotic strictures is of the utmost importance. A running suture of monofilament material is used, and excessive traction of the suture should be avoided. The "growth factor" technique is a practical method for eliminating purse string at the anastomosis. Upon termination of the anastomosis, the suture is tied away from the vessel, allowing the anastomosis to expand to its normal diameter. The extra suture will work its way into the suture line as the anastomosis grows (Fig. 44).

The biliary reconstruction is performed last when satisfactory hemostasis has been accomplished. End-to-side anastomosis of the donor common bile duct to a Roux-en-Y loop of jejunum with an internal stent is the technique of choice. This method of biliary reconstruction has provided excellent results even in small bile ducts, as in livers from newborns. As previously mentioned, the majority of these patients have had portoenterostomies with Roux-en-Ys which may be reused if they have not been damaged during the dissection. However, the old Roux-en-Y has had to be resected in most instances because, with previous revisions, the limb has been rendered unsuitable for biliary reconstruction.

IMMUNOSUPPRESSION

Precyclosporine Era

The current immunosuppression therapy for liver transplantation was derived from experience with renal transplantation, since the latter provided a much simpler model with which to work. Combination therapy with azathioprine and prednisone was the first widely used immunosuppressive regimen. However, most of the liver recipients from 1963 to 1980 in our series were treated with azathioprine, prednisone, and antilymphocyte (ALG). Occasionally, cyclophosphamide was substituted for azathioprine. Other additions to the immunosuppressive therapy, such as thoracic duct drainage, had no obvious benefit in hepatic transplantation.

The overall survival with the triple-drug therapy was 32.9% and 20% at 1 and 5 years, respectively.

Cyclosporine Era

Cyclosporine A is derived from two strains of fungi, *Cylindrocarpomlucidum* and *Tolypocladium inflatum* Gams. Cyclosporine was introduced to transplantation based on the experimental work of Borel et al, and the first clinical trials were performed by Calne et al. Better understanding of its mechanism of action has minimized complications such as the development of lymphomas and nephrotoxicity. Patient mortality has been reduced (Fig. 45).

In March 1980, cyclosporine and prednisone were introduced to the liver transplant program. There was a dramatic improvement demonstrated by an overall actuarial survival of 69.7% and 62.8% at 1 and 5 years, respectively. During the last year, a 2-week course with the monoclonal OKT3 (Ortho) was added to the immunosuppression regimen. The first clinical trials with OKT3 showed reversal of steroid-resistant rejection in a high percentage of kidney and liver transplant recipients.

RESULTS (SURVIVAL)

Precyclosporine Era

Eighty-six out of a total of 170 patients underwent liver replacement from 1963 to 1980. Fifty-three of the 86 died within a year after transplantation. The main causes of death are listed in Table 3. There was a high incidence of bacterial, fungal, and viral infections. Technical complications played an important role and, in part, were the cause of the poor results obtained in patients with biliary atresia compared to children with inborn errors of metab-

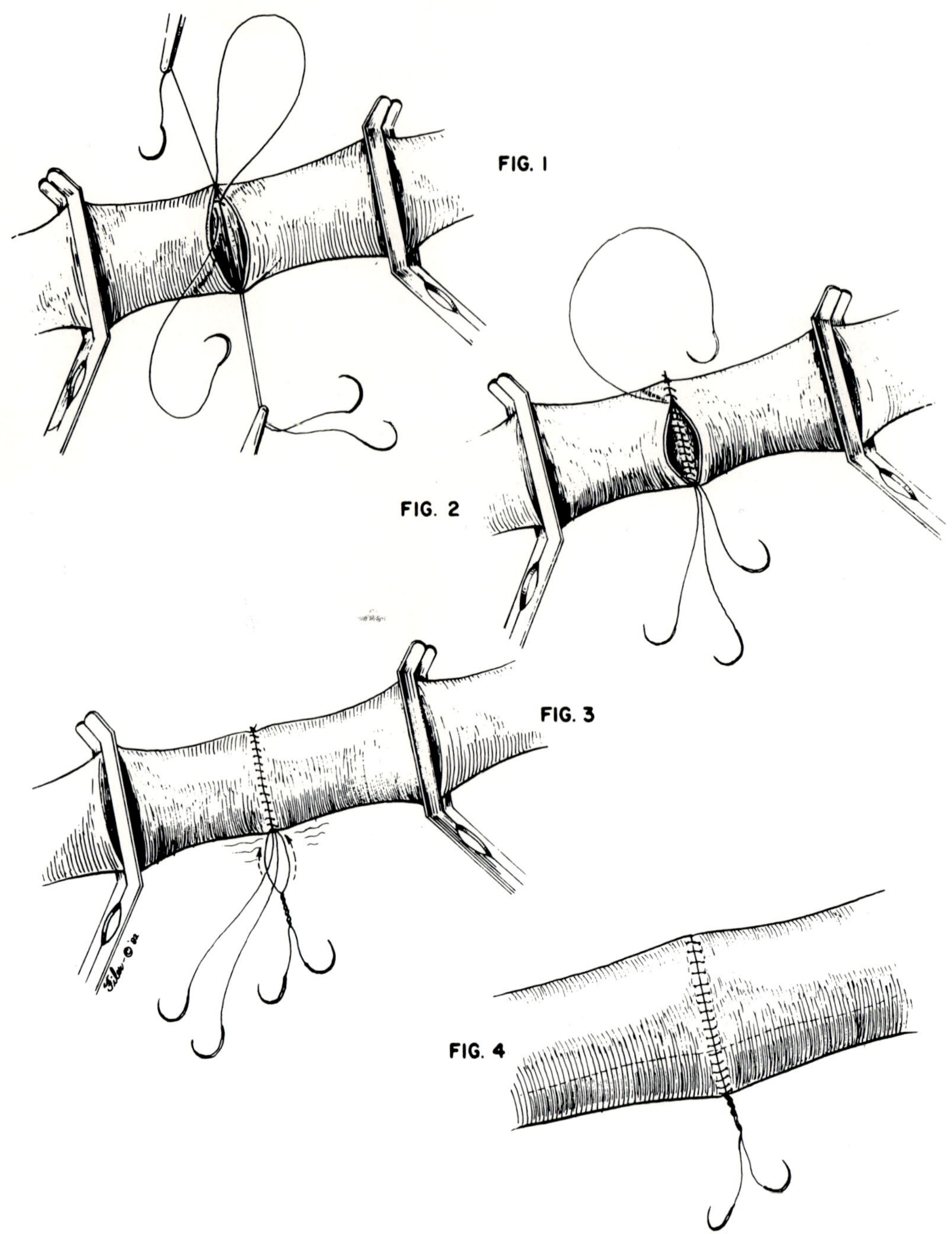

Figure 44. "Growth factor" technique used with continuous Prolene suture of small vessels. Note that anastomosis of half the circumference of the vessels is performed with each half of the original suture. Where the two halves meet, the knot is tied at a considerable distance away from the vessel wall, providing an excess of Prolene that is secondarily drawn into the suture line.

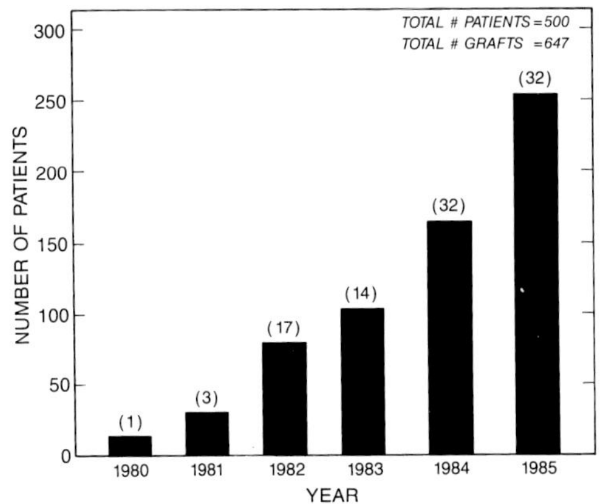

Figure 45. Number of patients receiving orthotopic liver transplants during the cyclosporine era. The number in parentheses represent retransplants per calendar year.

olism (Fig. 46). As mentioned before, previous surgical procedures in the right upper quadrant made the operation more difficult. Additionally, anomalies of the portal vein, including thrombosis, are frequently observed in patients with advanced biliary atresia. The 5-year survival in patients with biliary atresia was 14%.

Cyclosporine Era

The 5-year actuarial survival for the entire series (500 patients) is 60.6%. Of these patients, 203 were children (less than 18 years); the 5-year actuarial survival in this group is 67.7%. The 5-year actuarial survival in patients with biliary atresia is shown in Figure 47. The period of observation in patients

Table 3. Chief Causes of Death Within a Year After Hepatic Transplantation Among 86 Pediatric Patients in the Precyclosporine Era

	No. of Patients	Percent of Total
Infection	20	23.3
Technical complication	15	17.4
Rejection	9	10.5
Intra- and perioperative death	3	3.5
Primary graft dysfunction	3	3.5
Other	3*	3.5
Total	53	61.7%

*One patient died of recurrent malignancy, another from pulmonary embolism, and the third from respiratory failure secondary to an oversized graft.

less than 2 years of age is only 3 years, and the actuarial survival is slightly better than that of patients older than 2 years (Fig. 48). In contrast to the precyclosporine experience, there was little difference between patients with inborn metabolic errors and those with biliary atresia. The narrowing of the gap between these two groups of patients is explained by the fact that patients on cyclosporine seem to tolerate the perioperative trauma better than those on conventional immunosuppression. Further, there has been more familiarization with the procedure and better understanding of the perioperative metabolic changes as the number of transplants increased during the last

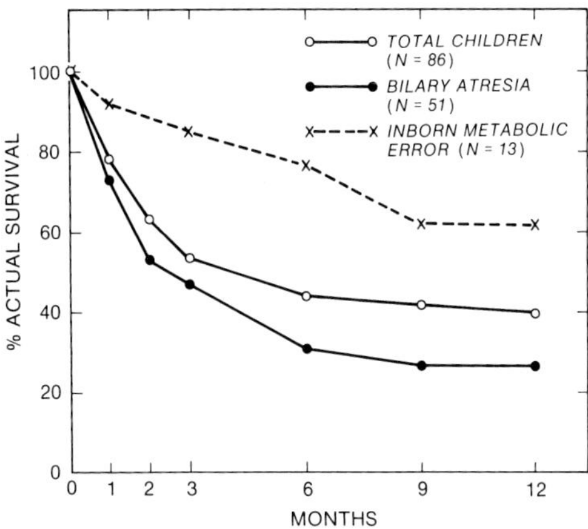

Figure 46. Pediatric liver transplantation: precyclosporin era. Influence of original liver disease on 1-year survival under conventional immunosuppression.

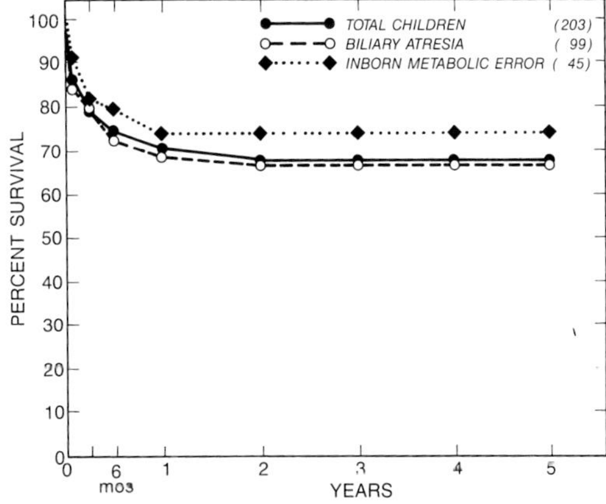

Figure 47. Five-year actuarial survival in pediatric patients receiving orthotopic liver transplants during the cyclosporine era.

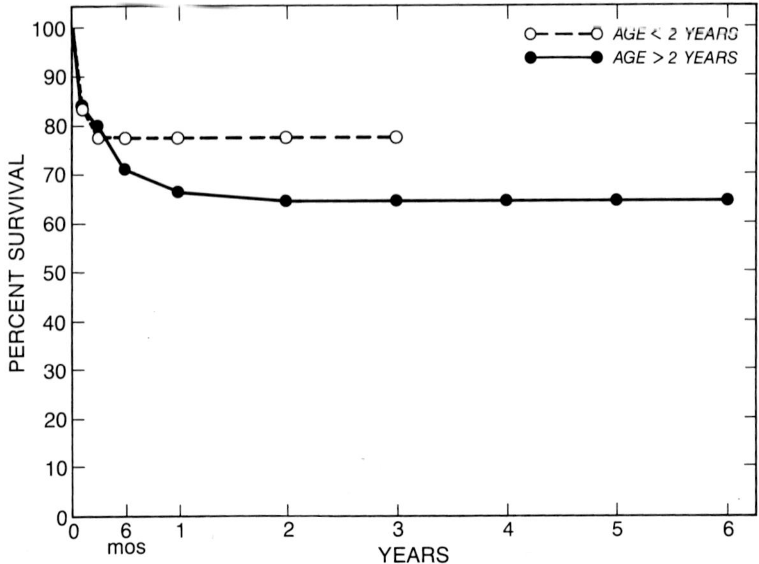

Figure 48.   Actuarial survival of liver transplant recipients for biliary atresia under 2 years compared to patients over 2 years of age.

few years. Although there was an immediate improvement in survival when cyclosporine was introduced, there were some early deaths which could have been avoided by more effective dose control of cyclosporine and by aggressive retransplantation. At present, cyclosporine blood levels are monitored daily until the patient is discharged, and then twice a week for several weeks until the best dosage is reached in order to prevent irreversible rejection or overimmunosuppression.

Retransplantation

Retransplantation should be strongly considered when the allograft is failing. Failure of the graft is due to rejection, primary graft dysfunction, or technical complications. The most common problems in the pediatric population are technical, and of these, arterial thrombosis is by far the most frequent reason for retransplantation. The causes of arterial thrombosis are multifactorial: technical errors, small size of the vessels, overcorrection of bleeding with clot-promoting products, infection, and rejection. Rejection with swelling of the liver may create a low-flow state, which in turn could lead to thrombosis.

The 5-year actuarial survival in children who received more than one hepatic transplant is 55.3%. Although this survival is not as good as that of patients with the first graft, it is high enough to justify such efforts when the primary graft has failed or is failing.

Growth

In a recent report, Urbach et al.[1] showed that 76% of 29 children who received liver replacement and were followed for at least 2 years had excellent growth patterns. This response is explained in part by the small doses of steroids needed for immunosuppression when cyclosporine is used in conjunction. Biliary atresia accounted for 13 out of the 29 patients.

Effect of Age on Survival

The influence of age on survival in the pediatric patient population was reviewed by Iwatsuki et al.[2] In the precyclosporine era, 53% of infants and preschool children (less than 6 years), 50% of those between 6 and 12 years, and 76% of those between 12 and 18 years lived for more than 3 months. In the cyclosporine era, 76% of infants and preschool children, 67% of children between 6 and 12 years of age, and 86% of the adolescents lived for more than 3 months. The 3-month survival was not influenced by age either before or after cyclosporine therapy (Fig. 49).

CONCLUSIONS

Biliary atresia is the most common indication for hepatic transplantation in the pediatric population. Liver replacement is the treatment of choice for biliary atresia, and there is no limitation of age or weight. Transplantation should be performed as soon as the patient begins to show signs of hepatic decompensation.

The scarcity of small pediatric donors is a most important practical factor. Adequate biliary drainage may stabilize the patient and buy valuable time. A single attempt at portoenterostomy may not add any risks to liver transplantation; however, surgical procedures of questionable benefit such as revisions of portoenterostomies and portosystemic shunts should be avoided, since they may jeopardize the final option of a hepatic replacement.

The progress in liver transplantation during the last few years has not been explained by better patient selection. Improvements in surgical techniques in the donor and recipient, aggressive retransplantation, and better immunosuppression have all played a role. Of these factors, cyclosporine has had the greatest impact in improving survival following hepatic transplantation.

A Consensus Development Conference held in 1983 in Maryland concluded that liver transplantation was a service rather than an experimental procedure. Liver transplantation is the most appropriate treatment for biliary atresia. If successfully treated, these patients can grow and function normally.

Recommended Reading

Bismuth H, Houssin D: Reduced sized orthopic liver graft in hepatic transplantation in children. *Surgery* 95:367, 1984.

Borel JF, Feurer C, Gubler HU, et al: Biological effects of cyclosporin A: A new antilymphocyte agent. *Agents Actions* 6:468, 1976.

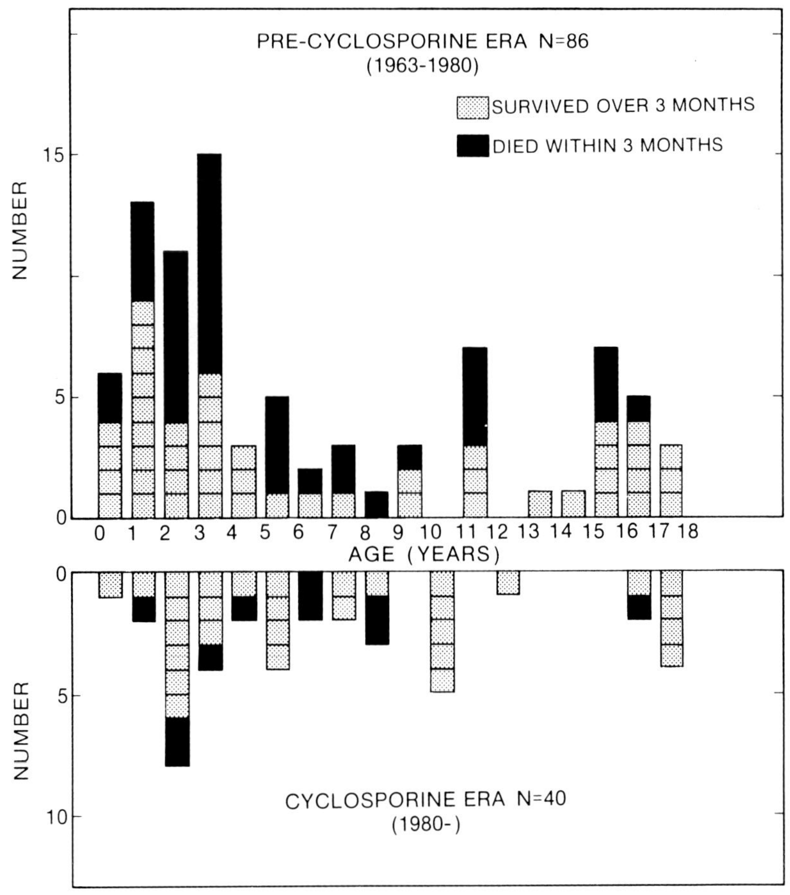

Figure 49.   Age distribution of 126 childhood liver recipients. A shaded square represents a child who survived more than 3 months, and a black square represents a child who died within 3 months. All of the surviving patients treated with cyclosporine have follow-ups of at least 15 months.

Calne RY, Rolles K, White DJG, et al: Cyclosporin A initially as the only immunosuppressant in 34 recipients of cadaveric organs, 32 kidneys, 2 pancreases, and 2 livers. *Lancet* 2:1033, 1979.

Fung JJ, Demetris AJ, Porter KA, et al: Use of OKT3 with cyclosporine and steroids for reversal of acute kidney and liver allograft rejection. *Surg Gynecol Obstet* (in press).

Iwatsuki S, Shaw BW Jr, Starzl TE: Liver transplantation for biliary atresia. *World J Surg* 8:51, 1984.

Iwatsuki S, Shaw BW Jr, Starzl TE: Biliary tract complications in liver transplantation under cyclosporine-steroid therapy. *Transplant Proc* 15:1288, 1983.

Kam I, Lynch S, Todo S, et al: Low flow veno-venous bypasses in small animals and pediatric patients undergoing liver replacement. *Surg Gynecol Obstet* (in press).

National Institutes of Health Consensus Development Conference Statement: Liver transplantation—June 20–23, 1983. *Hepatology* 4:107S, 1984.

Shaw BW Jr, Iwatsuki S, Starzl TE: Alternative methods of arterialization of the hepatic graft. *Surg Gynecol Obstet* 159:490, 1984.

Shaw BW Jr, Gordon RD, Iwatsuki S, et al: Hepatic transplantation. *Transplant Proc* 17:264, 1985.

Shaw BW Jr, Martin DJ, Marquez JM, et al: Venous bypass in clinical liver transplantations. *Ann Surg* 200:524, 1984.

Starzl TE, Iwatsuki S, Van Thiel DH, et al: Evaluation of liver transplantation. *Hepatology* 2:614, 1982.

Starzl TE, Marchioro TL, von Kaulla K, et al: Homotransplantation of the liver in humans. *Surg Gynecol Obstet* 117:659, 1963.

Starzl TE, Groth CG, Brettschneider L, et al: Orthotopic homotransplantation of the human liver. *Ann Surg* 168:392, 1968.

Starzl TE, Hakala TR, Shaw BW Jr, et al: A flexible procedure for multiple cadaveric organ procurement. *Surg Gynecol Obstet* 158:223, 1984.

Starzl TE (with the assistance of Putnam CW): *Experience in Hepatic Transplantation.* Philadelphia, WB Saunders Co, 1969.

Starzl TE, Koep LJ, Weil R III, et al: Development of a suprahepatic recipient vena cava cuff for liver transplantation. *Surg Gynecol Obstet* 149:76, 1979.

Starzl TE, Iwatsuki S, Esquivel CO, et al: Refinements in the surgical technique of liver transplantation. *Semin Liver Dis* 5:349, 1985.

Starzl TE, Iwatsuki S, Shaw BW Jr: A "growth factor" in fine vascular anastomoses. *Surg Gynecol Obstet* 159:164, 1984.

Tzakis AG, Gordon RD, Shaw BW Jr, et al: Clinical presentation of hepatic artery thrombosis after liver transplantation in the cyclosporine era. *Transplantation* 40:667, 1986.

References

1. Urbach AH, Gartner AC Jr, Malatack JJ, et al: Linear growth following pediatric liver transplantation. *J Pediatr. Am J Dis. Child.* 141:(5):547–9; 1987.
2. Iwatsuki S, Starzl TE: Liver transplantation for fulminant hepatic failure. *Sem Liver Dis* 5:325, 1985.

Congenital Cyst of the Common Bile Duct (Choledochal Cyst)

Congenital cyst or choledochal cyst is, as the name implies, of congenital origin, idiopathic in nature, and rare. It may be small or large, ovoid or round, and usually presents in the supraduodenal portion of the common bile duct. The cyst may or may not involve the right and left hepatic ducts. The background for this congenital formation has many etiological and theoretical explanations, but none has yet been found universally acceptable. We speak of a choledochal cyst, recognize it, and deal with it as best we can. This condition is more frequent in the female than in the male, and its size may vary from that of a small orange to a grapefruit. No one has established any relationship between the size of the cyst, its duration, and the severity of the symptoms. There is no constant relationship between the size of the cyst and the patient's age. The larger cyst, however, is more often seen in the teenage or adult patient. The wall of the cyst is usually thick and firm, and is almost invariably composed of epithelium; the lining of the cyst may be entirely absent, and on frozen section the wall may contain fibrous tissue. The size of the distal common duct may vary and, more often than not, is narrowed. The gallbladder is usually of normal size. Regardless of the dilatation of the common duct, it is uncommon for stones to be found in the gallbladder or cyst; however, stones in the cyst have been reported (see Fig. 50). As a rule, the intrahepatic ductal system is of normal size, but this too may be dilated on occasion. The

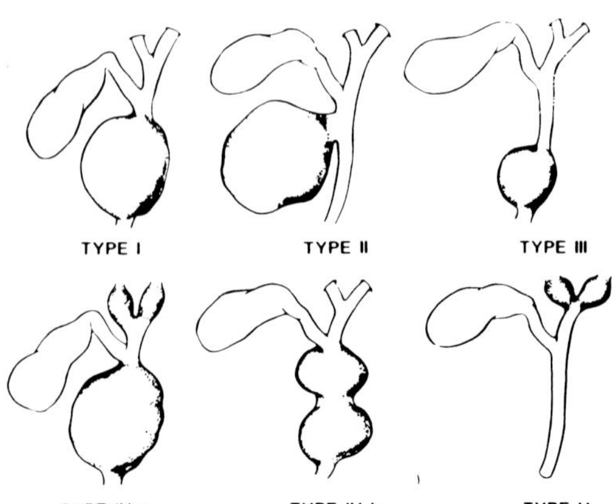

Figure 50. Classification of bile duct cysts. Refer to chapter on Congenital Cysts of the common bile duct. T. Todani describes his classifications of bile duct cysts.

liver may be altered, depending upon the nature and extent of the induration of the biliary stenosis at the common duct outlet; the terminal change in the liver is usually cirrhosis, and associated with it may be cholangitis. In some cases splenomegaly may coexist, but this has not yet been explained. The average case reported usually occurs prior to the 15th year, and the great majority of patients are under 25 years of age.

Diagnosis

Pain may be the first sign of a congenital cyst of the common duct. It may be associated with an epigastric mass that may or may not be tender. Jaundice may be an accompanying sign. The signs and symptoms of biliary obstruction may result from the expansion and pressure effect on contiguous organs, as well as slow, progressive degenerative changes in the liver, namely, those of biliary cirrhosis. In making the differential diagnosis, we employ several diagnostic tools, including the upper gastrointestinal study, cholecystogram, IV cholangiogram, ultrasonic scan (sonogram), and computed tomography scan. Kasai et al.[1] recommend gastrointestinal barium X-rays as an ideal diagnostic aid. They expand the duodenal loop in the anteroposterior view, and with forward displacement of the descending portion, a characteristic view of the lesion is obtained. We must consider hydrops of the gallbladder, carcinoma or cyst of the head of the pancreas, hydronephrosis, and kidney tumor; and finally, liver pathology such as hamartoma, liver abscess, and hydatid cyst. The patient may give a history of intermittent jaundice associated with low-grade fever and malaise. The physical examination will invariably reveal a mass in the upper right quadrant or in the epigastrium. Final evaluation of this pathological entity is established at laparotomy, and surgery can then be effectively carried out to relieve the specific condition.

Complications

The complications of choledochal cyst are usually secondary to the distal obstruction, and, as indicated previously, suppurative cholangitis may occur, with the ultimate development of biliary cirrhosis. Multiple hepatic abscesses and stone formation are also a possibility. Spontaneous or traumatic rupture of the cyst has been reported, and in a few cases, rupture of the cyst has occurred during pregnancy.

Operative Treatment

This condition requires early surgical decompression of the dilated cyst. This is the most widely accepted method today. One approach is a choledochocystoduodenostomy, which is preferable only when the anatomy lends itself to this procedure. A dependent type of drainage, similar to that utilized in pancreatic cysts, is best. In choledochocystojejunostomy with a supplemental enteroenterostomy, we select a jejunal loop approximately 12 to 14 inches distal to the ligament of Treitz. The anastomosis should be placed at the most dependent portion of the cyst to assure dependent or gravitational drainage. Two rows of sutures should preferably be employed, and the outer row should consist of 000 interrupted black silk with an atraumatic needle. Just as in a pancreatic cyst, prior to a choledochocystojejunostomy anastomosis, the contents of the congenital cyst should be evacuated, and stones, sand, mud, or gravel should be searched for and removed. Attempts should be made to probe the common duct in order to find the distal stones within the cyst, and then the duct should be followed with a flexible metal dull-tipped probe. The ampullary stoma should be evaluated. If found to be stenotic, it may be dilated, utilizing Bakes dilators.

Another surgical procedure is choledochocystojejunostomy employing the Roux-en-Y technique. Here again, the most dependent portion of the cyst is selected as the ideal site for the anastomosis. Gravitation or dependent anastomosis assists evacuation and drainage of the cyst and in great measure minimizes regurgitation of gastrointestinal contents into the choledochal cyst. The Roux-en-Y procedure utilizes the same amount of bowel, i.e., approximately 12 to 14 inches of jejunum distal to the ligament of Treitz. The bowel is divided between two Glassman noncrushing clamps, and in order to establish a larger cystenterostomy between the cyst and jejunum, the Roux-en-Y's distal end is closed. Two layers may be utilized to close it effectively, and the closed end should be brought up to the lowest portion of the choledochal cyst and a side-to-side anastomosis performed. In this procedure, the reflux of intestinal, gastric, and pancreatic juices into the cystoenteric anastomosis should be prevented because a reflux of the latter juices and contents can result in intermittent attacks of cholangitis.

Another technique is a choledochocystoduodenostomy. This should be done only when the anatomical position of the cyst allows it to be anastomosed easily to the second portion of the duodenum. A side-to-side anastomosis is carried out, as in a choledochoduodenostomy. Decompression in the postoperative period rapidly ameliorates the back pressure, jaundice, and inflammation. On occasion, in certain well-prepared patients in whom a smaller cyst is found, it may be possible to dissect it out and excise it completely. Dissecting out a choledochal cyst is not a small procedure. It can be tedious and prolonged, and not without risk. One may easily injure the hepatic artery, the portal vein, or possibly the pancreatic duct. If it can be done with minimal risk, however, excision is believed to produce a more lasting result.

The incision must be large enough to accommodate a complete exploratory operation of the cyst before the actual surgery is undertaken. Where one congenital anomaly exists, several others may be present as well; they too should be looked for. Such anomalies include duplication of the small intestine, malrotation of the small bowel, and possibly other anomalies in the genitourinary tract. A choledochal cyst is recognized as it begins below the level of the liver margin. Here it is usually found displacing the right colon downward. The degree of displacement of all contiguous organs depends on the site of the cyst and its duration. The cyst site is related to the degree of obstruction, supportive structures, and wall thickness; back pressure plays an important role here. Usually in the younger age group, the cyst wall is thinner than that in the older age group, and calculi are more often found in the adult cyst. This writer is not enthusiastic about searching out these cysts for resection, because this procedure carries with it a higher morbidity and mortality. Because of the rarity of this problem and the infrequency with which the surgeon has to work with such a pathological entity, the ideal procedure should be the safest, the one that has the smallest morbidity and mortality. That procedure is a palliative decompressive operation. The reported results are best when resection of the cyst can be carried out without undue risk to the patient.

Operative Technique

The incision should be large, preferably midline from xiphoid to symphysis, but not to open up the peritoneum until it is necessary to do so, making use of the desired amount of exposure. The incision should always be ready for a complete opening. A midline incision is not the only incision. A right oblique incision, if made long enough, may also be utilized in a direction from the xiphoid to the right anterior-superior iliac spine. Depending upon

the existing pathology, the surgeon should have his choice in selecting one of these two incisions. A transverse incision is also acceptable in certain patients with a transverse habitus, but a longitudinal incision, if made long enough, can readily be retracted laterally in any desired transverse position. The writer recommends "incise" drapes.

Choledochal Cysts in Adults

Choledochal cyst is a surgical disease mainly of infancy, but about 20%, according to Mayo Clinic,[2] are delayed until adulthood. Some adults come to surgery because of problems that arise from previous failures, i.e., cystenterostomy. In their study of 29 males, the Mayo Clinic team found the following:

1. Management of choledochal cysts is complex because the clinical symptoms do not accurately reflect the underlying hepatobiliary disease.
2. Pancreaticobiliary disease, ductal anomalies, pancreatitis, and malignancy are often associated with choledochal cysts, and these are the outside influences that dictate the surgery and the outcome of the patient.
3. The signs and symptoms in adults are quite similar to those of pediatric patients.
4. Whenever unexplained weight loss is observed, malignancy must be suspected.
5. In adults the association of hepatobiliary disease approached 80%.
6. Twenty of 29 patients were reoperated on for revision of prior procedures.
7. Failures of prior surgery were usually due to anastomotic stricture that led to bile stasis, stone formation, pancreatitis, biliary cirrhosis, and possible cancer. Patients with other anomalies appeared to be at greater risk.
8. Pancreatitis was caused by reflux of combined pancreatic juice and bile and by stone formation either in the cyst or the common duct; stone removal and the restoration of a free flow of bile were effective treatments. Cyst excision, when possible, is considered a prophylactic procedure.
9. When excision of the cyst is not possible or feasible, the Mayo Clinic recommends transduodenal sphincterotomy.
10. During cystenterostomy, where feasible, the base of the cyst can be closed intraluminally.
11. The incidence of malignancy approached 30% and was most likely related to the advancing age of the patient.
12. When cancer did develop, it was located inside

or outside of the cyst, was intra- or extrahepatic, or occurred in any combination. Excision of the cyst did not prevent cancer from occurring.

13. Postoperative results were considered to be excellent.
14. In a few cases, it was possible to do an enterostomy of an intrahepatic cyst. Conditions that preclude definitive surgery include secondary biliary cirrhosis, portal hypertension, and extensive intrahepatic cyst disease.

CHOLEDOCHAL CYSTS IN INFANTS

Todani et al.[3,4] classify choledochal cysts into five types (see Fig. 50):

Type I: accounts for 90% of the cases; the cyst is fusiform and extrahepatic.
Type II: accounts for 3% of the cases; it is a lateral saccule.
Type III: occurs as a duodenal choledochocele; it involves the common and pancreatic ducts.
Type IV: occurs as multiple intrahepatic and extrahepatic dilatations.
Type V: occurs as a single (or multiple) intrahepatic duct cyst.

The majority of cases have an elongated channel about 2–3.5 cm long. One etiological theory proposes that pancreatic enzymes reflux into the common duct and are activated by the bile, which in turn erodes and weakens the duct wall. Inflammation, ulceration, and cholangitis further weaken the duct wall. This theory is favored because an elevated amylase level exists in the cyst; by contrast, pancreatitis may develop when bile refluxes into the pancreatic duct.

The frequency of occurrence is as follows:

20% occur at 1 year or less.
60% occur at less than 10 years; girls outnumber boys by a ratio of 4:1.

The majority of surgeons believe that most choledochal cyst patients present a triad: (1) right upper quadrant pain, (2) jaundice, and (3) right upper quadrant mass. Other signs and symptoms include elevated amylase, fever (cholangiohepatitis), vomiting, and possible gastrointestinal tract bleeding. The last may be caused by compression of the portal vein by a mass. In older children, the complaints may precede the diagnosis by several years. The diagnostic approach in infants is quite similar to that of older children. It is discussed in detail under

"Congenital Cyst of the Common Bile Duct (Choledochal Cyst)."

Most surgeons believe that choleductal cysts need to be removed because of their complications (biliary obstruction, cholangitis, liver abscesses, and stone formation). Cirrhosis, portal hypertension, perforation, and carcinomatous changes (adenosquamous) are also considerations. Carcinoma generally occurs in 3% of the patients; 0.7% under 10 years; and 2.3% in adults. The survival rate is 5% at 2 years.

After an ultrasonogram or an intraoperative gallbladder cholangiogram is taken, the cyst must be removed. Type I cysts (most common) should have as much of the cyst wall as possible excised; the mucosa should be stripped. A choledochojejunostomy is recommended. Stevenson advises that the anastomosis be mucosa to mucosa and that the distal common duct be oversewn as far down as possible. Cholecystectomy should be done. The writer describes a method that is still not fully accepted; it consists of a jejunal interposition between the duct and the duodenum. This procedure may avoid ulceration and fat malabsorption. The medical mortality is 100%; if at all feasible, surgery should be carried out. The mortality rate is under 9%. Type II cysts may be excised; type III requires some anastomotic procedure.

REOPERATING CHOLEDOCHAL CYSTS IN YOUNG PATIENTS

Takiff et al.,[2] from the UCLA Medical Center, reported their experience with 23 young patients with choledochal cysts over a 28-year period. All patients had saccular or fusiform extrahepatic cysts; one patient had a diverticular cyst. Thirty-nine operations for biliary drainage were performed: 17 had Roux-Y choledochojejunostomy; 7 had choledochoduodenotomy; 7 had excision; and 8 received miscellaneous procedures. The morbidity was 17% with the primary operation. The mortality was 31%. Biliary calculi were found in 2 of 23 primary operations (9%) and in 6 out of 16 reoperated cases (37.5%). All stones were primary bile duct stones. After cyst excision, no reoperation was required. In one patient after drainage surgery, an intrahepatic cholangiocarcinoma developed. Three of 10 patients who did not undergo choelcystectomy at the primary operation required it at a later date. The authors recommend cyst excision and cholecystectomy in young patients, when feasible, as the primary operation for choledochal cysts.

Recommended Reading

Alonso-Lej R, Rever WB Jr, Pessagno DJ: Congenital choledochal cyst, with a report of two and an analysis of 94 cases. *Surg Gynecol Obstet* 108:1, 1959.

Babbitt DP, Starshak RJ, Clemett AR: Choledochal cyst: A concept of etiology. *AJR* 119:57, 1973.

Chaudhuri PK, Chaudhuri B, Schuler JJ, et al: Carcinoma associated with congenital cyst dilatation of bile ducts. *Arch Surg* 117:1349, 1982.

Deeg HJ, Rominger JM, Shah AN: Choledochal cyst and pancreatic carcinoma demonstrated simultaneously by endoscopic retrograde cholangiopancreatography. *South Med J* 73:1678, 1980.

Dexter D: Choledochal cyst with carcinoma of the intrahepatic bile ducts and pancreatic ducts. *Dr J Cancer* 11:18, 1957.

Flanigan DP: Biliary cysts. *Ann Surg* 182:35, 1975.

Flanigan DP: Biliary carcinoma associated with biliary cysts. *Cancer* 40:880, 1977.

Fonkalsrud EW, Boles ET: Choledochal cysts in infancy and childhood. *Surg Gynecol Obstet* 121:733, 1965.

Gallagher PJ, Millis RR, Mitchinson MJ: Congenital dilatation of the intrahepatic bile ducts with cholangiocarcinoma. *J Clin Pathol* 25:804, 1972.

George PA, Maingot R: Choledochus cyst associated with carcinoma in the liver. *Br J Surg* 50:339, 1962.

Han BK, Babcock DS, Gelfand MH: Choledochal cyst with bile duct dilatation: Sonography and ^{99m}TcIDA cholescintigraphy. *AJR* 136:1075, 1981.

Harris V, Ramilo J, Radhakrishnan J: Choledochal cyst with cholelithiasis: 15-year follow-up. *J Pediatr Surg* 14:191, 1979.

Ikada A, Okjuchi Y, Kamata S, et al: Jejunal interposition hepaticoduodenostomy for congenital dilatation of the bile duct (choledochal cyst). *J Pediatr Surg* 18:588, 1983.

Joseph WL, Fonkalsrud EW, Longmire WP Jr: Cystic dilatation of common bile duct in adults. *Arch Surg* 91:468, 1965.

Kagawa Y, Kashihara S, Kuramoto S, et al: Carcinoma arising in a congenitally dilated biliary tract. *Gastroenterology* 74:1286, 1978.

Kim SH: Choledochal cyst: Survey of the surgical section of the American Academy of Pediatrics. *J Pediatr Surg* 16:402, 1981.

Lilly JR: The surgical treatment of choledochal cyst. *Surg Gynecol Obstet* 149:36, 1979.

Lorenzo GA, Seed RW, Beal JM: Congenital dilatation of the biliary tract. *Am J Surg* 121:510, 1971.

Matsumoto Y, Uchida K, Nakase A, et al: Congenital cystic dilatation of the common bile duct as a cause of primary bile duct stone. *Am J Surg* 134:346, 1977.

Nagorny DM, McIlrath DC, Adson MA: Choledochal cysts in adults: Clinical management. *Surgery* 96:656, 1984.

Nunez-Hoyo M, Lees CD, Hermann RE: Bile duct cysts: Experience with 15 patients. *Am J Surg* 144:295, 1982.

Powell CS, Sawyers JL, Reynolds WH: Management of adult choledochal cysts. *Ann Surg* 195:666, 1981.

Rattner DW, Schapiro RH, Warshaw AL: Abnormalities of the pancreatic and biliary ducts in adult patients with choledochal cysts. *Arch Surg* 118:1068, 1983.

Rustad DG, Lilly JR: The surgery of choledochal cyst. Presented at the Fifth Annual Pediatric Surgical Residents' Conference, Pittsburgh, Pennsylvania, November 10, 1984.

Todani T, Tabuchi K, Watanabe Y, et al: Carcinoma arising in the wall of congenital bile duct cysts. *Cancer* 44:1134, 1979.

Todani T, Watanabe Y, Narusue M, et al: Congenital bile duct cysts: Classification. Operative procedures and review of 37 cases including cancer arising from choledochal cyst. *Am J Surg* 134:263, 1977.

Trout HH III, Longmire WP Jr: Long-term follow-up study of patients with congenital cystic dilatation of the common bile duct. *Am J Surg* 121:68, 1971.

Tsuchiya R, Harada N, Ito T, et al: Malignant tumors in choledochal cysts. *Ann Surg* 186:22, 1977.

Venu RP, Geenen JE, Hogan WJ, et al: Role of endoscopic retrograde cholangiopancreatography in the diagnosis and treatment of choledochocele. *Gastroenterology* 87:1144, 1984.

Yamaguchi M: Congenital choledochal cyst: Analysis of 1,433 patients in the Japanese literature. *Am J Surg* 140:653, 1980.

References

1. Kasai M, Asakura Y, Taira Y: Surgical treatment of choledochal cyst. *Ann Surg* 172:844, 1970.
2. Takiff H, Stone M, Fonkalsrud EW, et al: Choledochal cysts: Results of primary surgery and need for reoperation in young patients. *Am J Surg* 150(1), 1985.
3. Todani T, (see-p.188) for reference detail.

Miscellaneous Congenital Biliary Diseases

CAROLI'S DISEASE

Caroli's disease[1] is a congenital condition in which cystic dilatations of the intrahepatic bile ducts are the predominant feature. Clinically, there is pain, cholangitis, stasis, and stone formation. Generally the main ducts are also dilated. Patients usually present a history of chronic abdominal pain, fever, chills, and mild jaundice. Symptoms and signs often begin in childhood, and the great majority of patients develop symptoms before the age of 30. Caroli's disease patients may have other associated congenital conditions such as congenital hepatic fibrosis, which can ultimately lead to portal hypertension, variceal hemorrhage, and hepatic encephalopathy.

The diagnosis is established by a good history with early onset of pain, stone formation, stasis, and infection. Valuable diagnostic modalities such as ultrasonography, endoscopic retrograde choledochopancreatography, and percutaneous transhepatic cholangiography have increased the number of diagnosed cases of Caroli's disease.

The treatment is surgical and usually involves one or more abdominal procedures, primarily to remove stones and establish better drainage in the dilated, stagnant, and infected bile ducts. Resection of a liver segment with stagnant and infected bile ducts has been tried.

The prognosis is poor and the morbidity is high; however, utilizing the more exotic diagnostic modalities mentioned above, earlier recognition and intervention may improve the survival rate. It is more likely that surgery will still be concerned with the complications of dilated, stagnant, and infected intrahepatic bile ducts, i.e., obstruction, stones, and cholangitis. Tompkins and Pitt[2] report the experience at UCLA with Caroli's disease; in their series of 142 cases, 10 reported by Dayton et al.,[3] carcinoma occurred in 7%. This is comparable with an incidence of bile duct cancer in the general population. This leads these authors to conclude that Caroli's disease may well be a premalignant condition, presumably related to stagnation, infection, and irritation of the biliary ductal epithelium.

GILBERT'S SYNDROME

Gilbert's syndrome is the commonest form of familial nonhemolytic jaundice. A hyperbilirubinemia develops, most likely due to faulty bilirubin metabolism and probably caused by familial inheritance. In one case, a 17-year-old male with intermittent yellow discoloration of his skin and sclera developed jaundice that became more persistent and intense. The boy's family history, physical findings, and jaundice were due entirely to an increase in unconjugated serum bilirubin without evidence of hepatic dysfunction or hemolysis; a diagnosis of Gilbert's syndrome was established. In this condition, a normal life is expected; not uncommonly, the patient may reveal an associated cholecystitis or cholelithiasis. Because preexisting Gilbert's syndrome may complicate a diagnosis of hepatobiliary disease in later life, this possibility should be borne in mind. It has been shown that oral administration of iopanoic acid can make the gallbladder visible on X-ray despite the fact that the bilirubin concentration at the time is 2.8–4.5 mg/100 ml. The patient this writer has in mind was reported as having a normal cholecystogram and common bile duct. The latter finding pointed to the presence of a defective bilirubin metabolism within the liver. The prognosis is good to excellent.

CRIGLER-NAJJAR SYNDROME

This disease is rare and represents a familial disturbance in bilirubin conjugation. The unusually high serum levels of unconjugated bilirubin results in damage to the central nervous system. The prognosis is usually one of early death.

NEONATAL JAUNDICE

This is disturbance of bilirubin conjugation due to a fetal enzyme deficiency in conjugating bilirubin.

HEPATITIS

Abnormal bilirubin uptake and conjugation may occur in viral hepatitis and toxic hepatitis; cholestasis and hemolysis also contribute to the development of jaundice.

Recommended Reading

Mercardier M, et al: Caroli's disease. *World J Surg* 8:22, 1984.

Nagasue N: Successful treatment of Caroli's disease by hepatic resection: Report of six patients. *Ann Surg* 200:718, 1984.

References

1. Caroli J: Diseases of the intrahepatic biliary. *Clin Gastroenterol* 2:147, 1973.
2. Tompkins RK, Pitt HA: Surgical management of benign lesions of the bile ducts. *Curr Probl Surg*, vol 29, no 7, Chicago, Year Book Medical Publishers, 1982.
3. Dayton MT, Longmire WP, Tompkins RK: Caroli's disease: A premalignant condition? *Am J Surg* 145:41, 1983.

5

THE ROLE OF RADIOLOGY IN THE DIAGNOSIS OF BILIARY DISEASES

Luis Martinez, M.D.

The proper clinical management of patients with biliary tract disease requires a total understanding of the radiology of gallbladder and bile ducts. The many different radiological procedures used for the evaluation of the biliary tract may encompass simple procedures, and may vary from plain films of the abdomen to sophisticated techniques such as computed tomography of the biliary tract.

Plain Films of the Abdomen

The oldest and simplest radiological method for the detection of disease of the biliary tract is a plain radiograph of the abdomen. These films may demonstrate the presence of opaque stones, calcification of the wall of the gallbladder, or the presence of milk of calcium. Abnormal gas patterns may also be detected by such films. In the last category, we will discuss gas in the biliary tract, particularly fistula formation between the biliary tract and the gastrointestinal (GI) system. Air in the wall and/ or in the lumen of the gallbladder with acute gangrenous cholecystitis; so-called emphysematous cholecystitis, will also be discussed. Another abnormal gas pattern that may be present in acute cholecystitis is the *sentinel loop.*

Opaque Cholelithiasis

Only 10 to 30% of gallstones are radiopaque. However, it is common to find cholelithiasis incidentally in patients who have radiographic studies of the stomach, colon, or urinary tract. It is important to understand that the number and size of the stones in the gallbladder do not in any way reflect the size and/or number of stones in the common duct. Consequently, a patient shown to have cholelithiasis may or may not have choledocholithiasis as well. Occasionally, perforations of the gallbladder can be detected when gallstones are noted in the peritoneal cavity. When either hydrops or empyema of the gallbladder occur, a mass adjacent to the liver may become visible on the plain abdominal radiograph. Calcification in the gallbladder wall is known as *porcelain gallbladder.* Plain radiographs of the abdomen show an irregular ring of calcium in the right upper quadrant which often resembles a large single gallstone. There is enough evidence in the literature to suggest that patients with calcification of the gallbladder wall have a higher than normal incidence of carcinoma of the gallbladder;

the latter diagnosis is sufficient to warrant a prophylactic cholecystectomy.

When a gallstone obstructs the cystic duct, calcium may be deposited in the lumen or in the wall of the gallbladder. Calcium within the gallbladder, termed *milk of calcium,* is visible in the plain abdominal radiograph. In these cases, the appearance of the gallbladder on the plain radiograph is sometimes identical to that on a normal cholecystogram. In patients with acute cholecystitis, plain films of the abdomen may reveal a dilated loop of the small bowel with air-fluid levels in the right upper quadrant. In these cases, *localized ileus* results from impaired motility in a loop of the bowel adjacent to the inflammatory reaction.

Gas in the biliary tract may be seen in acute or chronic conditions. Erosion of a gallstone into the intestinal tract produces typical findings on X-ray films of the abdomen. If the gallstone is large enough to produce intestinal obstruction, *gallstone ileus* develops. In these circumstances, the usual triad of X-ray findings are air in the biliary tree; gas-filled, distended loops of small bowel; and a gallstone in an ectopic location, provided that the gallstone is radiopaque. Very often gallstone ileus will reveal dilated small bowel loops and air in the biliary tract, but without visualization of a stone in the abdomen. On rare occasions, we have seen gallstone ileus without evidence of air in the biliary tree. This occurs when the gallstone that has produced the fistula becomes fragmented and one of the fragments seals off the communication between the biliary tract and the upper GI tract.

In chronic conditions, air may be seen in the biliary tract of patients with fistulous formation due to malignancies of the upper GI tract perforating into the common duct; any form of surgical communication between the two systems may take place, i.e., choledochoduodenostomy, choledochojejunostomy, and choledochocolostomy. Occasionally, Crohn's disease involving the descending duodenum may produce a patulous sphincter of Oddi that may permit the retrograde passage of gas from the duodenum into the common bile duct. Rarely, malignancies of the common duct may erode into the duodenum to produce a fistula with visualization of air in the biliary tract. Acute cholecystitis with gas formation resulting from anaerobic bacteria, typically shows air in the wall and in the lumen of emphysematous the gallbladder, (see "Emphysematous Cholecystitis" in Chapter 8). If the patient is X-rayed in the upright or lateral decubitus position, an air-fluid level may be demonstrated within the gallbladder. Under these circumstances, the air does not go beyond the cystic duct because acute emphysematous cholecystitis (or gangrene of the gallbladder) usually implies an acute obstruction of the cystic duct. Occasionally, the air may dissect along the wall of the cystic duct, and may extend into the common duct and farther into the intrahepatic radicles.

Oral Cholecystography

With the recent development of new imaging techniques, the diagnosis of gallbladder disease is currently changing at a prodigious rate.

As a result of the availability of ultrasound, there is less reliance on nonopacification of the gallbladder with oral cholecystography after two consecutive contrast doses as indirect evidence of disease. This finding was judged to be 90% accurate only when an extrinsic cause of nonopacification could be excluded. Unfortunately, in the usual hospital patient population, extrinsic causes of nonopacification cannot be excluded on clinical grounds alone. It is this uncertainty which had reduced the reliability of oral cholecystography, since completion depends too heavily on clinical impressions rather than on anatomical evidence.

Today, direct morphological data are so readily obtainable by real-time ultrasound that we no longer repeat the oral cholecystogram the following day; instead we proceed immediately to ultrasound if visualization is poor the first day, thus avoiding a day's delay in establishing the presence of gallstones. Ultrasound reduces the possibility of extrinsic causes accounting for poor opacification. It may be argued that the significance of nonopacification, even with the second dose of contrast, is being judged unfairly because patients operated on on the basis of this indirect evidence of gallbladder disease are nearly always found to have chronic cholecystitis, with or without cholelithiasis. Nevertheless, the accuracy of the pathological diagnosis on which these impressions are based must be questioned. In fact, the histological criteria for the diagnosis of cholecystitis, especially the chronic form, are rather ambiguous. Histologically, inflammatory cellular infiltrates can be identified in the wall of the gallbladder in many asymptomatic patients of middle age. Certainly, the pathologist is unhappy to have to report that a normal gallbladder has been removed. It is universally accepted that gallstones are the only objective indication of the disease. Therefore, it is appropriate to order ultrasonography as a follow-up procedure when a single-dose oral cholecystogram fails to show opacification.

Ultrasonography has revealed that oral cholecystography has a significantly elevated false-negative rate, perhaps as high as 6 to 8%. Sonographic and surgical data from numerous studies have shown that small calculi were often overlooked on oral cholecystography; presumably they were obscured by the contrast material in the gallbladder, even on upright views. Several modifications of oral cholecystography have been introduced in recent years, but interest in them is now waning. One such modification is tomography of the gallbladder during oral cholecystography. Similarly, neither fractionated dosage of cholecystographic agents nor magnification cholecystography has won many converts. The issue at stake here is not how to perform oral cholecystography or which contrast medium to use, but whether to do it at all. For the first time, there is a choice of primary imaging modalities of the gallbladder.

For a patient with chronic symptoms localized to the right upper quadrant, normal liver function tests, and the ability to follow the preparation schedule, cholecystography, is still an acceptable initial screening procedure. On the other hand, ultrasound is an efficient primary screening examination, not only for patients with chronic complaints but also for those with acute symptoms or abnormal liver function tests. It is especially useful in unreliable patients, i.e., the very elderly and the very young.

If gallstones are found on ultrasound examination, no further studies are necessary. Reports indicate that the false-negative rate for ultrasonography is about 5% or less; this is about the same range as in oral cholecystography. Consequently, a normal ultrasound examination of the gallbladder has the same significance as a negative oral cholecystogram, and if symptoms persist, a follow-up examination with either sonography or oral cholecystography is indicated. In oral cholecystography, the contrast medium of choice is iocetamic acid (Cholebrine). We have used this contrast medium for about 10 years and have never encountered a significant reaction or side effects. At present, it is probably the most reliable contrast medium available. Our preparation consists of the following routine:

1. A heavy, high-*fat* lunch on the day prior to the examination; this is avoided if an attack can be provoked.
2. A light evening meal on the day prior to the examination; it is fat free, with no dairy products, and is given between 6 and 7 PM.
3. Four Cholebrine tablets with water are given immediately following this meal.

4. Nothing by mouth after midnight; the patient may have some water.

Cholecystokinin Cholecystography

Cholecystokinin oral cholecystography has been a popular test in some centers for a number of years, and there have been claims of symptomatic improvement in the majority of patients undergoing cholecystectomy on the basis of a positive examination. Some writers claim that cholecystokinin cholecystography is a useful test for acalculous cholecystitis. These claims can be challenged for many different reasons. Ferruci et al.[1] have commented on the questionable reliability of the pathological diagnosis of cholecystitis. As early as 1945, McDonald and McKibben[2,3] indicated that inflammation is often seen in a normal gallbladder. In 612 consecutive autopsies of nonsymptomatic patients, inflammatory changes in the gallbladder, which could have been considered pathological, were present in 75%. In 25% of the surgical cases in which an apparently normal gallbladder was removed, 92% of the patients revealed inflammation that could have been considered pathological. Thus the chances of finding some histological abnormality in normal gallbladders are high.

Another criticism of cholecystokinin studies is that the initial relief of pain following cholecystectomy in patients with a positive cholecystokinin oral cholecystogram does not necessarily imply that removal of the gallbladder per se was responsible. Recent studies by Berk et al.[4-6] showed that cholecystokinin cholecystography was not helpful in predicting the histological findings in the gallbladder. Histological evidence of chronic inflammation has been observed in as many patients with normal cholecystokinin studies as in those with abnormal tests. *This writer concludes that this test is not helpful in the diagnosis or management of acalculous gallbladder.*

Intravenous Cholangiography

The utilization data from the Radiology Department of the Massachusetts General Hospital show a decrease from 262 examinations using intravenous cholangiography in 1976 to 39 in 1980—a decline of more than 80%. Intravenous cholangiography is still a reliable method of detecting retained common duct calculi following cholecystectomy, es-

pecially in thin patients with no impairment of liver function. (See the author's technique summarized in the following list.) The sensitivity of the examination has recently been questioned, so patients with persistent symptoms, dilated bile ducts on ultrasonography, and/or elevated alkaline phosphatase levels should have direct transhepatic or endoscopic cholangiography even if the intravenous cholangiogram is normal. The declining popularity of intravenous cholangiography is due to the following factors: (1) greater awareness of the high mortality rate compared with retrograde urography; (2) the frequent equivocal or false-negative results; and (3) the reliability of newer techniques for direct opacification of the biliary tree, i.e., transhepatic and endoscopic cholangiography. It appears that the intravenous cholangiogram will not long survive as a useful clinical tool. The acceptable indications for this procedure are (1) nonvisualization of the gallbladder on oral cholecystography; (2) previous surgery and nonvisualization of the gallbladder, with a need to know the status of the common bile duct; and (3) in postcholecystectomy patients suspected of having residual biliary tract disease. The technique has changed throughout the years, and most writers agree that infusion technique is safer than direct injection, the incidence of reactions being much lower. In the United States, the contrast medium of choice for intravenous cholangiography is iodipamide meglumine (Cholografin Meglumine).

The author's technique for intravenous cholangiography is as follows:

1. Routine: A dose of 40 ml of contrast medium diluted in 250 cc of D5W is infused over a 1-hour period. The first tomograms are taken at the conclusion of the infusion. Upon visualization of the common duct, delay films are taken an hour later for evaluation of the gallbladder; the latter provide adequate time for mixing of contrast medium with bile. At this point, filming of the gallbladder consists of taking routine supine right posterior oblique films and upright spot films of the gallbladder. Post-fatty meal films may be taken if no evidence of cholelithiasis is detected in the initial gallbladder studies.
2. Postcholecystectomy: In patients evaluated after previous cholecystectomy, the technique is identical to that of individuals with intact gallbladder, except that the examination is concluded following the tomograms taken after the infusion.
3. Emergency: In individuals with acute colicky pain, the objective of this procedure is to dem-

onstrate the presence or absence of cystic duct obstruction. The examination is modified as follows: If the gallbladder opacifies early, the examination should be stopped. Cystic duct obstruction has been ruled out. If gallbladder opacification does not occur early, the procedure is continued routinely as described. Recently, glucagon has been advocated for intravenous cholangiography. The dose used may range from 0.5 to 1.0 mg. Glucagon may be used when there is an unsatisfactory demonstration of the choledochoduodenal area. We have used it successfully when the distal duct has been inadequately visualized; however, we do not employ it routinely. *With our infusion technique, visualization of the distal common duct is usually adequate.*

Computed Tomography in the Evaluation of Biliary Tract Pathology

CHOLEDOCHOLITHIASIS

Computed tomography (CT) is a clinically useful method for evaluating patients with obstructive jaundice, especially when sonography fails to demonstrate the level or etiology of the obstruction. CT has made an important contribution to the noninvasive imaging of common duct stones. Even small bilirubinate duct stones can be readily diagnosed by CT.

In studies of cholelithiasis in the United States, it has been found that about 73 to 85% of calculi are primarily cholesterol; the rest are calcium bilirubinate. It is rare to encounter pure cholesterol stones because they invariably contain a small admixture of calcium bilirubinate. In-vitro studies have shown that cholesterol stones may be slightly less than water density with CT. Such stones usually show a faint rim or increased density along the periphery, or punctate areas of increased density within the central portion of the stone. These findings may not always be apparent on routine 1-cm scans; consequently, high-resolution scans at 5-mm intervals are sometimes necessary to demonstrate these findings. *Oral and intravenous cholangiographic contrast studies are useful adjuncts to conventional CT in defining the extrahepatic biliary tree.*

Cholesterol stones leading to extrahepatic obstruction in the common duct usually produce the following CT findings: (1) There is evidence of distal common bile duct obstruction without an adjacent mass. (2) The dilated common bile duct comes to an abrupt termination at the level of the ampulla or the intrahepatic portion of the common duct. (3) Malignant masses produce an irregular termination of the common duct and biliary stricture (as in chronic pancreatitis), a succession of gradually tapering ring shadows representing the narrowing of the common duct lumen. (4) Patients with an abrupt termination of the common bile duct at the level of the ampulla without an obvious obstructing mass, should be suspected of harboring cholesterol calculi.

Recent reports have shown that CT is effective in imaging common duct stones and is superior to sonography. CT correctly diagnosed 9 out of 49 patients with choledocholithiasis; its sensitivity rate is 18%. The accuracy rate for sonography was 19%. There were five false-positive examinations. CT correctly identified common duct stones in 26 of 30 patients, for a sensitivity rate of 87%. The accuracy rate was 84%. There was only one false-positive result. Sonography is limited in its ability to image calculi in the distal common bile duct. The more distal common bile duct passes posterior and medial to the duodenum, and it is this relationship that obscures the distal duct. Even when the distal duct is clearly seen, including the tapered intrapancreatic segment, an ampullary stone may exist and be missed. The role of sonography is primarily to demonstrate the status of the biliary tract. *Most patients with choledocholithiasis have dilated extrahepatic ducts, yet the demonstration of a dilated duct is not specific for choledocholithiasis. Conversely, incomplete, intermittent, or early obstruction of the common bile duct may occur without ductal dilatation.*

CARCINOMA OF THE GALLBLADDER

Primary carcinoma of the gallbladder is the fifth most common malignancy of the gastrointestinal tract, yet the diagnosis is often difficult to establish preoperatively. CT has been found most useful in suggesting this diagnosis. The most common CT finding in carcinoma of the gallbladder is a mass that replaces the gallbladder; the latter finding is present in approximately 42% of these patients. A mass protruding into the gallbladder is seen in approximately 23% of patients; diffuse, asymmetric thickening of the wall is seen in approximately 15%.

Carcinoma of the gallbladder is very difficult to detect in its early stages because patients are often asymptomatic and do not present signs or symptoms of chronic cholecystitis and/or cholelithiasis. Gallstones are found in 73 to 98% of the cases, and calcification of the gallbladder (*porcelain gallbladder*) in 25%. Gallbladder carcinoma is often a coincidental finding with cholecystectomy, but it is not always recognized at the time of surgery. At present, the 5-year survival rate for this disease is 4 to 12%. Intraductal spread of carcinoma occurs in at least 4% of the cases of gallbladder malignancy. This lesion can clinically mimic carcinoma of the pancreas or a bile duct tumor. When a soft tissue tumor is seen within the common bile duct, its origin may not necessarily be from the bile duct or pancreas; rather, it may be from the gallbladder itself.

Careful examination of the gallbladder is essential in jaundiced patients with a mass near the head of the pancreas or in the common duct, in order to detect unsuspected primary tumors of the gallbladder. Nonvisualization of the gallbladder by sonography and/or CT in a patient with a mass in the right upper quadrant is suggestive of a neoplasm of the gallbladder. It is important to examine the right upper quadrant carefully to be sure that no other fluid-filled structures in relation to the gallbladder can be identified. Decubitus views of the gallbladder during a sonographic or CT examination may be helpful in determining whether or not the soft tissue density seen with the gallbladder represents a mass or sludge. Sludge moves to the most dependent part of the gallbladder when the patient's position is changed.

PRIMARY INTRAHEPATIC BILIARY MALIGNANCY

Primary carcinomas of the liver are histologically classified as hepatocellular carcinomas, cholangiocellular carcinoma, and a combined type. Hepatocellular carcinoma is about 10 times as frequent as cholangiocarcinoma; it has been well investigated by various diagnostic modalities, including CT. Cholangiocarcinoma is also known as *bile duct carcinoma*. It can originate in a small intrahepatic bile duct (peripheral type) or in major intrahepatic ducts including the hepatic hilus; it is also found in extrahepatic ducts, as well as near the papilla of Vater.

CHOLANGIOCARCINOMA OF THE LIVER

Bile duct carcinoma of the liver arises predominantly in noncirrhotic livers. These carcinomas may have the same gross configurations as hepatocellular carcinomas: massive, nodular, or diffuse. The nodular type is the most frequent. Sometimes polypoid or papillary carcinomas arise from the larger peripheral bile ducts, though on occasion, carci-

nomas arising from the hilar region extend along the intrahepatic bile ducts to fan out widely into the liver. The exact site of origin cannot be determined from the extent of the histological type of the tumor, according to Itai et al.[7] The male:female ratio in cholangiocarcinoma is 1.7:1, while in hepatocarcinoma it is 7.2:1. Hyperbilirubinemia is significantly more frequent in cholangiocarcinoma, and may be the initial symptom as well as the chief complaint. On the other hand, hepatomegaly, elevation of serum glutamate, and positive tests for hepatitis B surface antigen are more frequently noted in hepatocellular carcinoma. The radiological diagnosis of cholangiocarcinoma is made very reliably on direct cholangiography, percutaneous transhepatic cholangiography, or endoscopic retrograde pancreatography (ERCP). A massive amount of mucinous substance is occasionally found in the biliary tree and may mimic cholelithiasis. Angiography is especially useful in differentiating cholangiocarcinoma from hepatocellular carcinoma. Typical angiographic findings in the liver hilum include tiny, thin neoplastic vessels with irregular or obstructed arteries. There are no unusual hypervascular tumor vessels, arteriovenous shunts, or tumor thrombi in the veins, so frequently seen in hepatomas.

The CT findings of primary intrahepatic biliary malignancy are classified into three types: (1) a well-defined round, cystic mass with internal papillary projections; (2) localized intrahepatic biliary dilatations without a definite mass lesion; and (3) miscellaneous low-density masses. Two of four cases revealed biliary cystadenocarcinomas, with internal septa and papillary projections. The remaining two patients were diagnosed as having papillary cholangiocarcinoma with lesions consistent with a papillary tumor located in the well-defined mass. Daughter cysts were noted in each of the patients with biliary cystadenocarcinoma and papillary cholangiocarcinoma. All patients showed dilatation of intra- and extrahepatic biliary trees.

Dilated intrahepatic biliary radicles were mainly confined to one hepatic lobe or segment, which also showed a decrease in size. Dilatation of the extrahepatic biliary tree was moderate in one case, equivocal in another, and absent in the third. The surgical specimens revealed dilatation of the intrahepatic biliary tree without gross tumor, and the microscopic studies demonstrated diffuse spread of cancer along the dilated biliary tree.

Eight cases showed various patterns of a low-density mass (type C), with wide variation in density, homogenicity, shape, and reduced contour. Of these eight cases, two showed Thorotrast deposits in the liver, spleen, and peripancreatic lymph nodes; three cases revealed masses with markedly low attenuation and irregular shape. On CT contrast films, enhancement was usually slight; marked enhancement was noted in only one case. In the type C category, four patients had diffuse intrahepatic biliary dilatation; one showed equivocal dilatation of the extrahepatic duct.

BILIARY CYSTADENOCARCINOMA

This is a rare biliary ductal neoplasm, and only a small number of cases have been reported. The gross appearance is that of a well-defined cystic mass, most often multilocular, having internal papillary projections as in biliary cystadenoma. This carcinoma is more commonly seen in females than in males. The major signs and symptoms include abdominal swelling and pain. The prognosis is relatively good compared with that of other primary hepatic malignancies. Angiographic evaluation of this tumor reveals a hypervascular mass, except for minimal neovascularity and staining of septa and/or projections. ERCP is not very useful, since most cases do not have a communication between the tumor and the biliary tree. Differentiation of cystadenocarcinoma from cystadenoma is made microscopically.

Intraoperative Cholangiography

The purposes of intraoperative cholangiography are (1) to avoid unnecessary exploration of the common duct; (2) to detect residual common and hepatic duct calculi after duct exploration; (3) to identify congenital anomalies, strictures, and tumors of the biliary tree; and (4) to determine the presence of a cystic duct remnant. The successful use of intraoperative cholangiography is based on teamwork between the surgeon, the radiologist, the anesthesiologist, the X-ray technician, and the operating room nurse. If good teamwork is developed, some of the theoretical problems (e.g., too time-consuming, too many false positives) do not occur. To achieve consistent, satisfactory cholangiographic examinations, intraoperative cholangiography should be performed routinely. *The frequency of overlooked common duct stones remains high—16 to 25% in most institutions.* To depend on the clinical history or evidence of common duct dilatation alone as an indication for common duct exploration is not reliable. The routine use of intraoperative cholangiography has markedly diminished the number of patients who have to undergo choledocholith-

otomy. Several authors have found to 3 to 10% of gallstones noted on intraoperative cholangiography were clinically asymptomatic.

Success with intraoperative cholangiography depends on careful attention to the technical aspect of the procedure. A scout film of the abdomen should always be taken before the injection of contrast medium. Precise radiographic technique using proper collimation, a short exposure time, and correct kilovoltage is essential. All surgical instruments and lap pads must be removed from the field during X-ray exposure. The contrast material should be properly diluted so that it is neither too radiopaque nor too radiolucent. A 50% sodium diatrizoate solution diluted to one-half is generally recommended; the concentration may be changed depending on the size of the common duct. If the common duct is very dilated, further dilution of the contrast medium is recommended. A determined effort should be made to fill both the right and left hepatic ducts in order to avoid overlooking stones within the intrahepatic radicles. Air bubbles must be carefully removed from the injecting tubing.

The patient should be positioned 15° to the right posterior oblique position so that the common duct is not obscured by the spine. This may be achieved by placing the patient in the oblique position prior to surgery. During surgery the patient is turned supine. If the table cannot be turned, the proper obliquity for the radiograph can be obtained with the X-ray tube. A radiologist should be available to assure ideal radiographic technique, as well as to review and interpret the radiographs as they are made. If there is any doubt about the results, the X-ray examination should be repeated until clarified. A common error occurs when there is a question of functional or organic obstruction at the ampulla. A pseudocalculus sign, gas bubbles within the lumen, and failure to obtain complete opacification of the biliary tree are common equivocations. Visualization of the pancreatic duct takes place frequently and is not indicative of pathology of the ampulla of Vater. Opacification of the pancreatic duct is obtained when the intraluminal pressure within the biliary system exceeds 35 to 40 cm of water and provided that a common channel exists. The demonstration of secondary intrahepatic ducts during cholangiography requires an injection pressure of approximately 35 cm of water. With pressures of 40 to 60 cm of water, smaller hepatic radicles, common duct distention, and narrowing of the sphincter segment become evident (pseudocalculus sign). Above a pressure of 60 cm, the sphincter is usually occluded with demonstrable terminal bile ducts. *Operative cholangiography plays a major role in reducing the incidence of overlooked calculi in the common and hepatic ducts.*

The surgeon has no other effective way of knowing whether intrahepatic calculi are present; *there is a reported incidence of 17.3% of associated intrahepatic duct calculi with common duct stones.* The calculi are usually nonopaque, and are single or multiple. They may assume any size or shape, and appear at any level in the biliary duct system. The stones may have different shapes: regular, irregular, or spherical. Faceted stones overlap, so that it may be difficult to determine their number. Common duct obstruction due to calculi is not rare. Obstructing large stones may result in a common duct dilatation of 30 mm without complete occlusion. However, it is common for the contrast medium to trickle around and outline a stone. The common duct dilatation due to a stone is frequently passive and elastic; it will recoil as soon as the calculus is removed. A small stone lodged in or near the ampulla may produce spasm with occlusion of the common duct. If a common channel exists, there may be reflux into the pancreatic duct. On occasion the intraoperative cholangiogram may detect the presence of a congenital anomaly such as a choledochal cyst. Sometimes it may reveal the presence of pancreatitis. In acute or chronic pancreatitis, the common duct is usually displaced laterally and appears compressed externally. There may be some degree of proximal dilatation of the biliary duct system. Mild stasis occurs in the dilated proximal common duct, where sludge and calculi may form. Occasionally, it is possible to see pancreatic calcifications confined to the head and tail. Sclerosing cholangitis usually produces multiple areas of segmental stenosis without significant proximal dilatation. Occasionally, sclerosing cholangitis may produce just one area of localized stenosis; this may require a differential diagnosis with stenotic lesions of a different etiology.

Clinical correlation (history) and the evaluation of signs and symptoms are always helpful in establishing the final diagnosis. Cholangiocarcinoma is a consideration in the presence of concentric stenosis of the ductal system. It is more frequently found at the bifurcation of the right and left hepatic ducts. The latter is associated with significant proximal dilatation of the hepatic radicles. Cholangiocarcinoma may, in fact, involve any part of the biliary system, and in rare cases it has been described as multicentric, producing multiple stenotic areas. On rare occasions, hepatomas may produce intraluminal defects within the common duct by external infiltration into its lumen.

Recently, the use of nondiluted contrast medium for T-tube cholangiography with high kilovoltage technique has been advocated. We have used this technique with great success. The removal of residual stones in the common duct has changed the management of this condition, and patients who were once required to undergo surgery to remove residual stones are now handled by the radiologist, who can extract these stones from the common duct, employing the long wire basket and balloon that are now available. This subject will be discussed elsewhere under "Special Procedures" by G. Casal in Chapter 5.

Celiac Angiography

Celiac angiography to evaluate the biliary tract or the gallbladder is not performed routinely. The gallbladder is often visualized by angiography, especially with the use of superselective methods. In the arterial phase, the cystic artery is usually seen arising from the right hepatic artery. Generally two branches of the cystic artery encircle the gallbladder and, together with secondary branches, outline its position, size, and shape. The capillary phase distinctly outlines the gallbladder by outlining its wall as a 2- to 3-mm radiopaque line. Chronic inflammation of the gallbladder usually produces diminished vascularity. The gallbladder wall opacifies intensely in the capillary phase.

Carcinoma of the gallbladder usually produces tumor neovascularity and arterial encasement. Extension of the tumor into the hilum of the liver is determined by the presence of abnormal vessels and neovascularity in the porta hepatis. In jaundiced patients, the detection of an enlarged gallbladder on angiography suggests obstructive jaundice. When jaundice is due to carcinoma of the pancreas, tumor encasement of the divisions of the celiac artery is a common finding, as well as obstruction of the splenic vein. These findings do not indicate the nature of the process involving the pancreas, but do serve as valuable indicators of inoperability.

Magnetic Resonance Imaging (MRI) of the Gallbladder

In this writer's experience, MRI has not been as accurate as CT scanning in gallbladder diagnosis. One of the major drawbacks of MRI is that breathing induces diaphragmatic movements, which in turn cause undue gallbladder movements. CT scanning and ultrasonography are considered superior to MRI for diagnosing biliary disease.

A recent paper by Hricak et al.[8] suggests that MRI provides physiological information about the gallbladder and that it may prove to be a simple and safe clinical test for gallbladder physiology. Hricak et al. state that MRI promises to be the first imaging modality to evaluate the physiology of the gallbladder, as well as its anatomy, and could become a fast, simple, and safe test. Many cases are now being studied along these lines. They include both normal individuals and symptomatic gallbladder patients. See MRI under "What's New."

Recommended Reading

Beneventano TC, et al: The pseudocalculus sign in cholangiography. *Arch Surg* 98: 1969.

Berk RN: Cholecystokinin cholecystography in the diagnosis of chronic acalculous cholecystitis and biliary dyskinesia, a critical appraisal. *Gastrointest Radiol* 1:325, 1977.

Berk RN, Barnhart JL, James L, et al: The potential of iosulamide meglumine as a contrast material for intravenous cholangiography: An experimental study in dogs. *Invest Radiol* 16:240, 1981.

Berk RN, Robert N, Barnhart JL, James L, et al: Does glucagon enhance opacification of the bile ducts during intravenous cholangiography? An experimental study in dogs. *Invest Radiol* 17:50, 1978.

Burgener FA: Intravenous cholangiography: Experimental evaluation of the time-density-retention concept. *AJR* 134:665, 1980.

Burhenne HJ, Morris DE, Groeb DA, et al: Single-visit oral cholecystography for inpatients. *Radiology* 140:505, 1981.

Cannon P, Legge D: Glucagon as a hypotonic agent in cholangiography. *Clin Radiol* 30:49, 1979.

Cheung LY, Chang FC: Intravenous cholangiography in the diagnosis of acute cholecystitis. *Arch Surg* 113:568, 1978.

Doran J, et al: Iotroxamide studies in man—biliary iodine levels following bolus injection and slow infusion. Comparison with ioglycamide. *Clin Radiol* 31:651, 1980.

Eubanks B, Martinez ER, Carlos R, et al: Current role of intravenous cholangiography. *Am J Surg* 143:731, 1982.

Evans AF, Whitehouse GH: The effect of glucagon on infusion cholangiography. *Clin Radiol* 30:499, 1979.

Evans AF, Whitehouse GH: Further experience with glucagon enhanced cholangiography. *Clin Radiol* 31:663, 1980.

Flannigan BD: Intra-arterial digital subtraction angiography: Comparison with conventional hepatic arteriography. *Radiology* 148:17, 1983.

Fuchs WA, Preisig R: Prolonged drip-infusion cholangiography. *Br J Radiol* 48:539, 1975.

Goodman MW, Ansel HJ, Vennex JA, et al: Is intravenous cholangiography still useful? *Gastroenterology* 79:642, 1980.

Hricak H, Roy AF, Margulis AR, et al: Work in progress: Nuclear magnetic resonance imaging of the gallbladder. *Radiology* 147:481, 1983.

Jarrett LN, Bell GD: Effect of intravenous glucagon on the biliary secretion of a cholangiographic agent. *Clin Radiol* 31:657, 1980.

Jarrett LN, Doran J, Clifford K, et al: Glucagon and infusion cholangiography. *Br J Radiol* 55:269, 1982.

Loeb PM: Biliary excretion of iodipamide. *Gastroenterology* 68:554, 1975.

Loeb PM, Barnhart JL, Berk RN, et al: Iotroxamide—a new intravenous cholangiographic agent, comparison with iodipamide and the effect of bile salts. *Radiology* 125:323, 1977.

Lucaya J, Gomez JL, Molino E, et al: Congenital dilatation of the intrahepatic bile ducts (Caroli's disease). *Radiol* 127:746, 1978.

Madayag MA: Combined hepatic angiography and percutaneous aspiration biopsy in the evaluation of primary hepatic neoplasm. *Gastrointest Radiol* 7:159, 1982.

Martinez LO: Technique of intravenous cholangiography. *Proceedings of the XIII International Congress of Radiology,* Vol. 1. Amsterdam, Excerpta Medica, 1974, pp 170–175.

Martinez LO, Viamont M, Gassman P, et al: Present status of intravenous cholangiography. *Am J Roentgenol Radiother Nucl Med* 113:10, 1971.

Musante F, Derchi LE, Bonati P, et al: CT cholangiography in suspected Caroli's disease. *J Comput Assist Tomogr* 6:482, 1982.

Nelson JA, White GL Jr, Nakashima EN, et al: Iosulamide: Human tolerance study of a new intravenous cholangiographic drug. *Invest Radiol* 15:511, 1980.

Robbins AH: Successful intravenous cholecystocholangiography in the jaundiced patient using meglumine iodoxamate (Cholovue). *AJR* 126:70, 1976.

Rosenberg FJ: Iosulamaide: A new intravenous cholangiocholecystographic medium. *Invest Radiol* 15:S142, 1980.

Sargent EN, et al: A new contrast medium for cholangiocholecystography: Meglumine Iodoxamate. *AJR* 125:251, 1975.

Shehadi WH: Adverse reactions to intravascularly administered contrast media: A comprehensive study based on a prospective survey. *AJR* 124:145, 1975.

Sherman M: Intravenous cholangiography and sonography in acute cholecystitis: Prospective evaluation. *AJR* 135:311, 1980.

Taenzer V, Volkhardt V: Double blind comparison of meglumine iotroxate (Biliscopin), meglumine iodoxamate (Endobil), and meglumine ioglycamate (Biligram). *AJR* 132:55, 1979.

The Radiologic Clinics of North America, Vol. IV, No. 3, Philadelphia, WB Saunders Co, 1966.

Thorpe CD, Olsen WR, Fischer H, et al: Emergency intravenous cholangiography in patients with acute abdominal pain. *Am J Surg* 125:46, 1973.

Ulreich S, Foster K, Stier S, et al: Acute cholecystitis: Comparison of ultrasound and intravenous cholangiography. *Arch Surg* 115:158, 1980.

Wallers CJ, McDermott P, James WB, et al: Intravenous cholangiography by bolus injection of meglumine iotroxamate: A comparative trial of two new contrast media. *Clin Radiol* 32:457, 1981.

Wittenberg J, Maturi RA, Williams LF Jr, et al: Intravenous cholangiography in the rhesus monkey. *Invest Radiol* 11:45, 1976.

References

1. Ferrucci JT Jr, Joseph T, Wittenberg J, et al: Hypotonic cholangiography with glucagon. *Radiology* 118:466, 1976.
2. MacDonald JH: Perforation of the gallbladder associated with acute cholecystitis. *Ann Surg* 164:849, 1966.
3. McKibben JT, Hall WW: Hypertopic gastric mucosa in gallbladder wall. *Ann Surg* 140:242, 1954.
4. Berk RN, Clemett AR: *Radiology of the Gallbladder and Bile Ducts.* Philadelphia, WB Saunders Co, 1977.
5. Berk RN, Ferrucci JT, Cooperberg JS, et al: The radiological diagnosis of gallbladder disease; Imaging Symposium. *Radiology* 141:49, 1981.
6. Berk RN: Radiology of the gallbladder and bile ducts. *Surg Clin North Am* 53:973, 1973.
7. Itai Y, Aroki T, Yoshikawa K, et al: Computed tomography of gallbladder carcinoma. *Radiology* 137:713, 1980.
8. Hricak H, Filly RA, Roy A, et al: Work in progress: Nuclear magnetic resonance imaging of the gallbladder. *Radiology* 147:481, 1983.

Interventional Radiological Techniques in the Liver

German L. Casal, M.D.

POSTCHOLECYSTECTOMY PROCEDURES

Repositioning of a Dislodged T-Tube

The replacement of a prematurely dislodged T-tube under fluoroscopic control has become a routine urgent procedure. It is urgent because successful repositioning of the tube depends upon the time elapsed between dislodgement and repositioning. Other factors affecting success are the size of the T-tube and its location. Anteriorly located T-tubes are more difficult to reposition because of the acute angulation between the T-tube and the common duct. At times, it is not possible to reposition a T-tube. In such instances, a straight tube is used, with its distal end placed into the common duct in a manner that does not obstruct the flow of bile around it. Because the T-tube is usually repositioned through a tender or soft tract, the original long limb of the tube cannot be used and a shorter-limb T-tube or straight tube is employed. This procedure usually requires sedation, as the patient is very tender in the right upper quadrant area. It is not advisable to merely push a T-tube back into place. It is preferable to use a guidewire or interchangeable catheter system that will provide a

The author is indebted to Sheldon A. Roen, M.D., who graciously consented to review the original manuscript for this chapter.

guide for the final insertion of the tube into the common duct.

Removal of Retained Calculi

The removal of retained calculi (Fig. 51) employing the T-tube tract and using fluoroscopic control became popular in the early seventies, particularly after the extensive work of Mazzariello and Burhenne.[1-3] Mazzariello[4] used the Mondet[5] stone extraction forceps, a specifically designed slender but rigid instrument, while Burhenne relied on the Dormia basket. The basket was originally designed for the cystoscopic removal of a urinary calculus, and was first used by Lagrave in the biliary tract[6] (Fig. 52).

The fundamental maneuver consists of engaging the retained calculus within a helix basket instrument for extraction. Larger calculi may require fragmentation before extraction. The radiologist applies the skills gained in selective arterial catheterization such as the use of different guidewires and catheters to establish a path for the Dormia

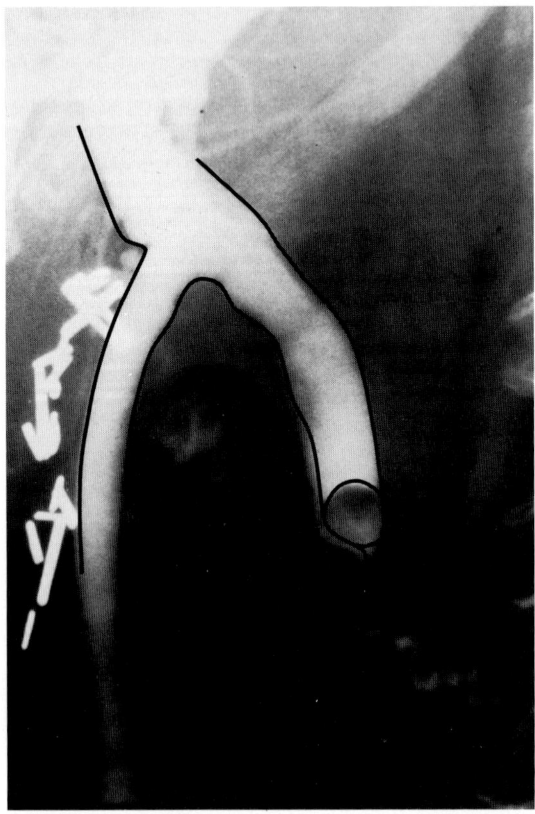

Figure 51. *A T-tube cholangiogram shows a retained common duct calculus.*

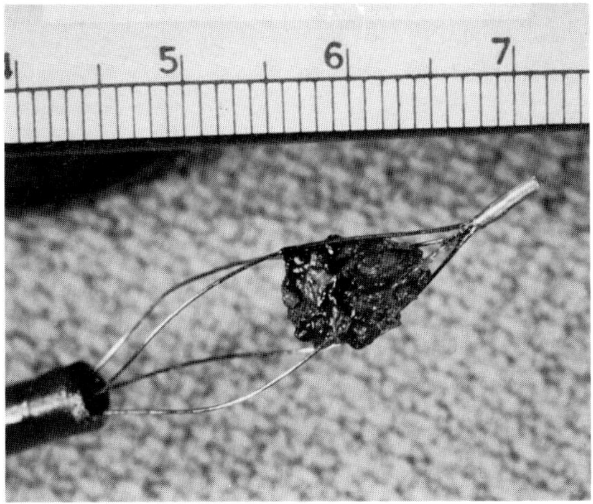

Figure 52.   Dormia basket with extracted calculus.

basket. The removal of a calculus consists of the following steps:

1. Insertion of a guidewire through the T-tube and into the distal part of the common bile duct.
2. Withdrawal of the T-tube for a wider fistulous tract.
3. Advancement of a steerable or straight catheter into the distal common duct.
4. Manipulation of stones so that they may be captured in the distal common duct.
5. Advancement of a Dormia basket for the final entrapment of the calculus.
6. Withdrawal of the calculus.
7. Exploration for further stones.
8. Replacement of a temporary T-tube.

The procedure described above is greatly improved if a large T-tube (minimal 14 F) is inserted at surgery to facilitate the later extraction of stones, particularly when insertion is toward the lateral position. A ventral insertion of the T-tube results in an acute angle with the common duct, and difficulty is encountered in manipulating the catheter and the stiffer Dormia basket. The time for extraction of the retained calculus is no less than 4 to 6 weeks after the initial surgical procedure; this allows a fistulous tract lined with granulation tissue to develop. A lined tract reduces the possibility of bleeding and even perforation. A minimal period of 4 to 6 weeks also allows better healing with less patient discomfort. Specific technical problems develop when a calculus migrates upward into a biliary radicle. For this reason, it is best for the patient to be ambulatory in order to encourage gravitational migration of the calculus down into the common duct, where it is much easier to retrieve. At times

it may be necessary to continue the procedure another day due to the number of calculi to be removed, the inaccessibility of the calculi, or the extreme discomfort of the patient. A very large calculus that cannot be crushed and cannot be delivered intact through the T-tube tract might require ampullary dilatation or even sphincterotomy. Though the ampulla can be dilated with a Gruntzig balloon catheter, sphincterotomy is probably superior and is best accomplished by retrograde endoscopic technique. Once the sphincter of Oddi has been dilated, the calculus can be retrieved by employing an endoscopic Dormia basket. The calculus may also be pushed through the sphincter with a suitable catheter via the T-tube tract.

COMPLICATIONS. The most common complication is sepsis. Removal of a calculus should not be attempted in a septic patient. The procedure is routinely performed on an outpatient basis; however, due to the need for various manipulations, most patients are given an oral antibiotic. The most commonly used antibiotic is ampicillin. A patient requiring extensive manipulation should be admitted to the hospital so that intravenous antibiotics can be instituted 24 hours prior to the procedure. In outpatient cases, oral antibiotic coverage is continued for 48 hours, but the patient may be switched to an intravenous antibiotic if signs of cholangitis or pancreatitis develop. Even after the removal of all calculi, it is wise to continue T-tube drainage for at least an additional 48 hours to help maintain a route of drainage and minimize the danger of infection. It may be wise to remove the T-tube at another time, when all debris and small stones have passed, thus giving complete assurance of an obstruction-free common duct. The patient should be well hydrated at all times to avoid further obstruction by inspissated bile.

It is important to practice aseptic technique when performing either the initial or final T-tube cholangiography in patients with suspected retained calculus. It is essential to use a tilting table to obtain a position as erect as possible, thus allowing the calculus to migrate and gravitate into the distal common duct, where it can be differentiated from a retained air bubble. We prefer to connect a three-way plastic disposable stopcock to the T-tube via a Christmas tree adapter and to one of the ports of the stopcock extension tubing (Fig. 53). Connected to the extension tubing is a syringe containing the diluted contrast. Aspiration is performed first to evacuate the air from the T-tube and common duct. The stopcock is then closed toward the patient, and by gentle injection of contrast, the

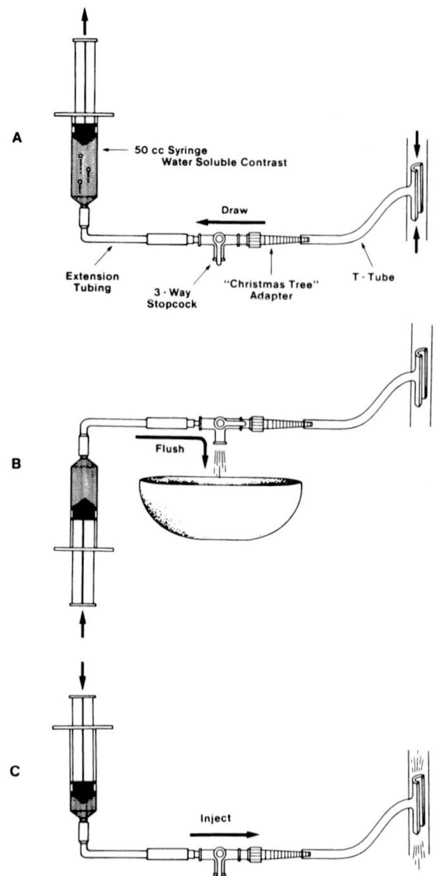

Figure 53. Technique for T-tube cholangiography. (Casal GL: A technique for postoperative cholangiography. Appl Radiol 15:161, 1986.)

extension tubing is drained of air. After this is accomplished, contrast is allowed to flow, but under fluoroscopic control to avoid filling of the pancreatic duct. The latter technique accomplishes complete filling in a sequential manner: first the common duct, and then the hepatic duct radicles. The first views are obtained with the patient in the upright position; sequential views are then obtained in the recumbent right and left posterior oblique positions in order to fill the right and left hepatic ducts completely. The kilovoltage and contrast material concentration are chosen to minimize the possibility of masking a calculus in the opacified biliary system.

Removal of a Calculus in the Absence of a T-Tube

The removal of a calculus via a percutaneous transhepatic approach has been described. This procedure is not the procedure of choice because it may necessitate the creation of a large tract through the liver parenchyma to remove the calculus. Also, undue traumatic manipulations might be required, further damaging a rather soft liver parenchyma. If surgery is not contemplated due to advanced age or poor condition of the patient, a more expedient approach would be an endoscopic papillotomy (Fig. 54A,B).

Management of Strictures

A choledochoduodenostomy or choledochojejunostomy may occasionally become stenosed at the site of anastomosis. With the advent of the transhepatic approach, it is now possible to introduce dilators of increasing size or a balloon catheter of the type devised for percutaneous angioplasty. Stenotic areas, however, tend to recur; they respond only temporarily to percutaneous dilatation. It might be necessary to maintain a dilating catheter for a long period of time (up to 6 months) before a permanent result is attained. As with any longtime indwelling catheter, the possibility of a permanent fistulous tract requiring surgical intervention should be considered.

DRAINAGE OF THE OBSTRUCTED BILIARY SYSTEM

The first question to be answered in a patient with jaundice is whether the problem represents an obstructive process or hepatocellular disease. Initially, ultrasonography or computed tomography is used to investigate the size of the biliary ducts. In most patients with dilated ducts, and even in those with nondilated ducts, the next step is endoscopic retrograde pancreatocholangiography (ERCP) or percutaneous transhepatic cholangiography (PTHC). The latter procedure is more commonly performed because of its safety record. Safety has been further assured since the introduction of the Okuda[7] needle (also known as the *Chiba* or *skinny needle*) (Fig. 55A). If it is determined that the process is obstructive, a decision must be made as to whether or not it is surgically correctable.

Older patients with extensive metastatic disease and no pruritis require only adequate analgesia. The problem is quite different in a younger jaundiced patient with obstruction of the common duct secondary to pancreatic carcinoma. Although a carcinoma of the pancreas might be in a stage beyond surgical resection, the possibility of palliative surgery or a drainage procedure may be considered. Before evaluating for percutaneous drainage,

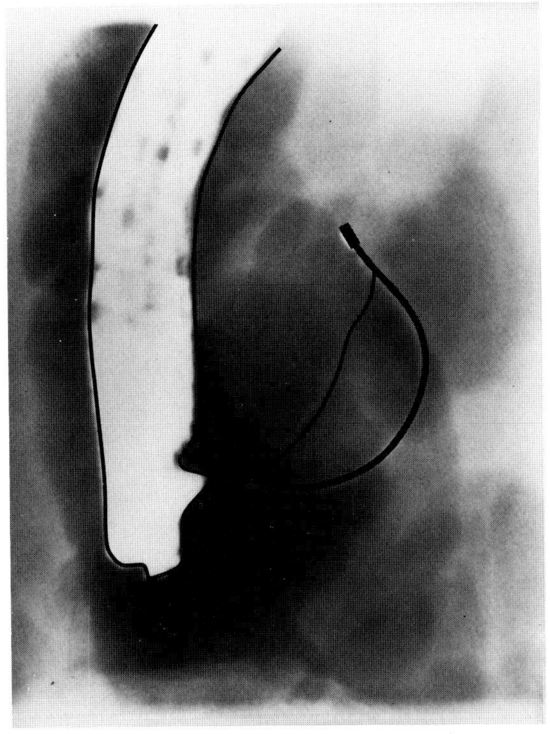

A

Figure 54.   A. Olympus fiberoptic endoscope with papilloto-my (sphincterotomy) cautery open in the papilla. B. After papillotomy, a small Fogarty catheter can be advanced from the endoscope into the common duct to help withdraw calculi into the duodenum.

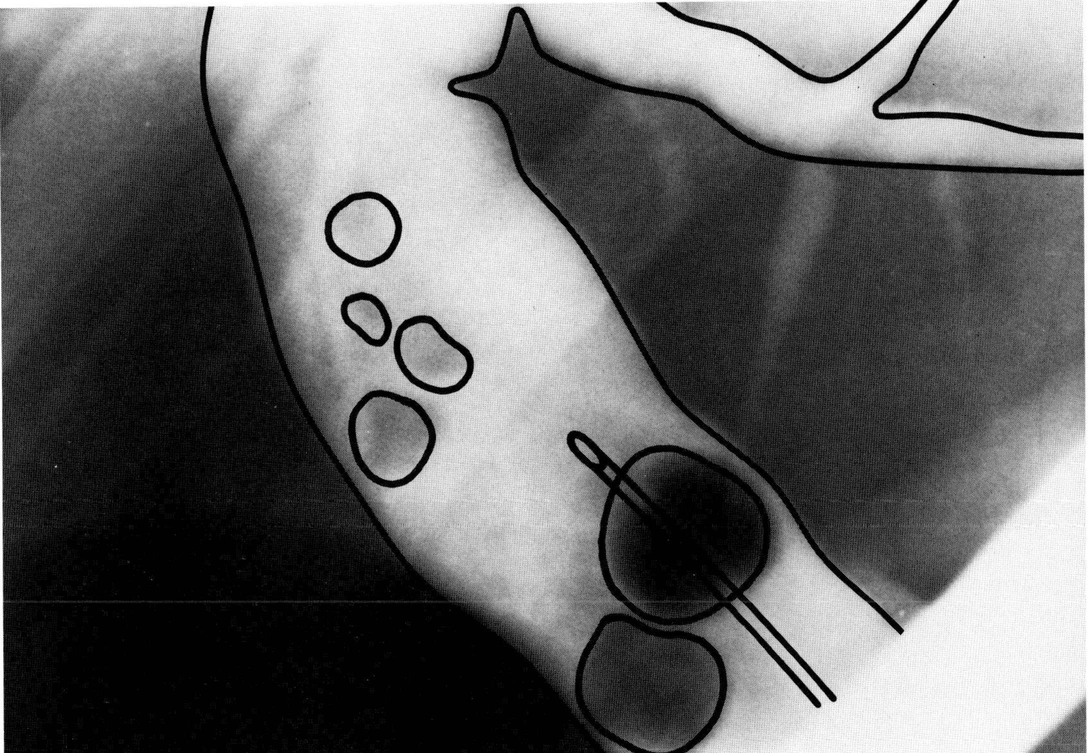

B

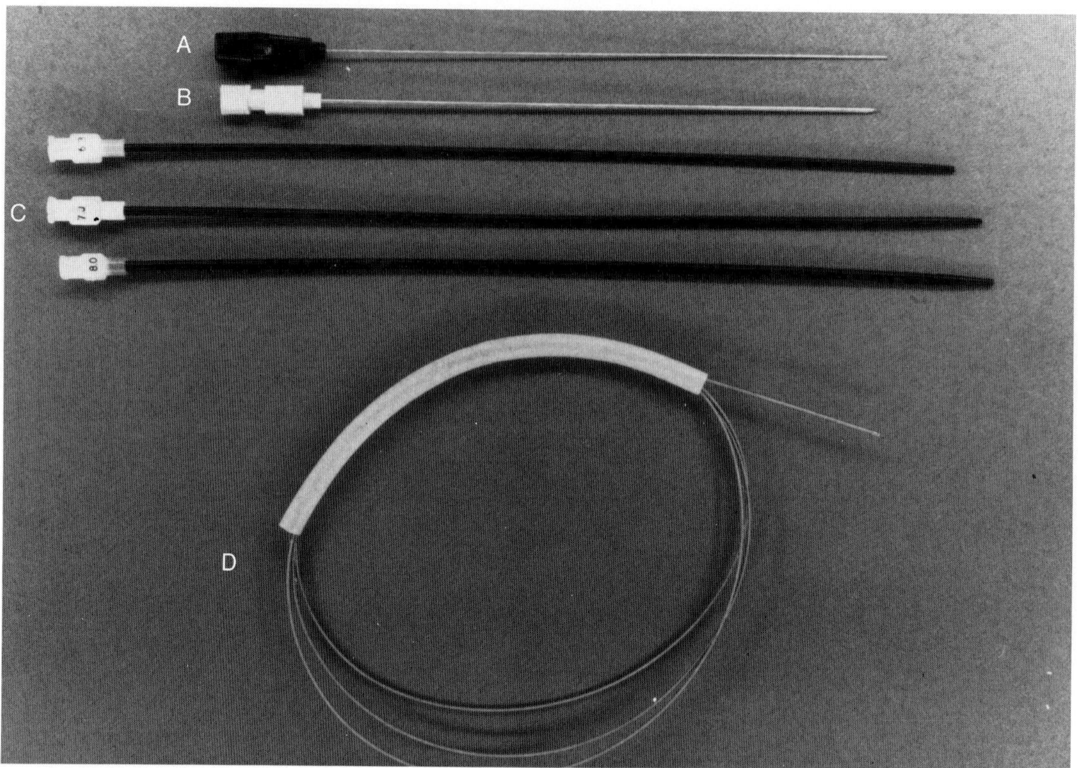

Figure 55.   A. Chiba needle, 22 French gauge. B. Bilary cannula, 18 French gauge. C. Dilator set (6.3, 7.0, 8.0 French gauge). D. Ring-Lunderquist guidewire (0.038 inch).

a diagnosis should be firmly established. It would be most unfortunate if palliative treatment were given for a potentially correctable condition such as impacted stone in the ampulla. A diagnosis can be established by cytological evaluation of a bile aspirate made during PTHC, a brush biopsy through a transhepatic catheter, or a thin needle biopsy of a suspected tumor. At this time, no consensus has been established as to the best approach (surgical or nonsurgical) for pancreatic carcinoma; the final plan of treatment will always require an analysis of the individual case. Due to the poor prognosis in advanced pancreatic carcinoma, older patients are usually treated with the percutaneous approach to avoid serious major surgery. Patients who are relieved by this approach might require surgery at a later period if gastric outlet obstruction develops. However, the majority of our patients who had been relieved by the percutaneous approach ultimately died without any gastric outlet obstruction. Only in two cases has gastric outlet obstruction occurred. One of these involved our longest-surviving patient with percutaneous drainage (14 months); obstruction was secondary

to a slow-growing pancreatic carcinoma that finally required a gastroduodenostomy. The possibility of complications such as bleeding during percutaneous drainage is not a deterrent, since the overall complications appear to be less than those resulting from surgical procedures. Percutaneous biliary drainage should be performed only when the patient and the surgeon are fully aware of the risks of the procedure; the surgeon orders adequate antibiotic premedication.

Another alternative form of nonsurgical drainage is now available: the endoscopic placement of an endoprosthesis or an external nasobiliary catheter. This consists of placing a long, thin (usually 6 F) catheter into the common duct with extension into the duodenum. In nasobiliary drainage, a thin catheter extends into the oropharynx, esophagus, stomach, and duodenum for external drainage. This latter method is only a temporary measure and may also be employed in cases of cholangitis. Internally placed stents are limited in size and therefore have not gained wide acceptance, especially since they tend to become easily obstructed by inspissated bile.

PERCUTANEOUS DRAINAGE

Three types of percutaneous drainage can be employed: strictly external, internal-external, and strictly internal (stents) or endoprosthesis. Each of these will be discussed.

Strictly External Drainage

This is the least desirable type of drainage, since it deprives the patient of biliary fluids and electrolytes, which require oral replacement. It is, however, the only procedure when there is a complete obstruction that cannot be bypassed. This type of drainage should be reserved for patients who are symptomatic, especially those with severe pruritis. It probably serves no function in the asymptomatic patient other than to lower the blood bilirubin level, with resultant lightening of the skin. The type of catheter used for this drainage is usually a 6 to 8 F "pigtail" (Fig. 56). The pigtail, or curved-end, configuration helps to anchor the catheter and to avoid the possibility of trauma and perforation

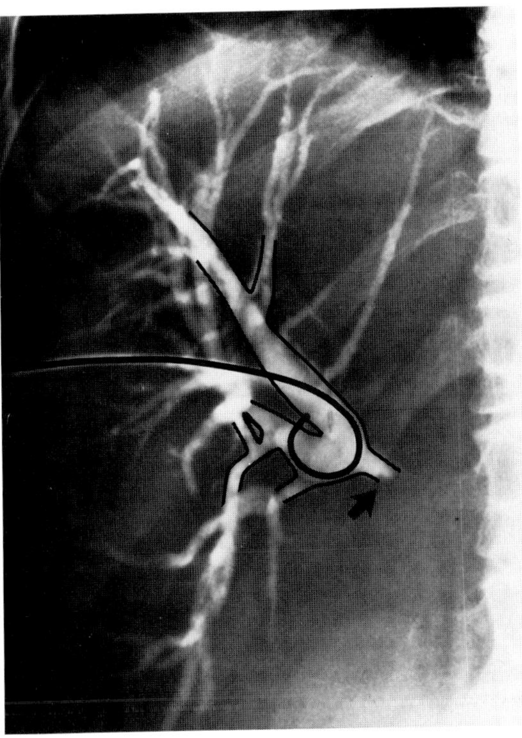

Figure 57. "Pigtail" catheter for external drainage in a carcinoma obstructing the common bile duct (arrow).

(Fig. 57). The catheter may also be straight or gently curved if further manipulations are planned. It must be secured to the skin by suture or adhesive tape to prevent accidental dislodgement during respirations and bodily motions.

Internal-External Drainage

This type of drainage is the most common. Ideally, it is used when the internal flow of bile into the distal common duct and duodenum is assured, while an external avenue for irrigation and even replacement is also secured. The type of catheter employed might be straight or preferably pigtail, depending upon the length needed to bypass the obstruction (Fig. 56). If the obstruction is high in the biliary tree, as in a cholangiocarcinoma close to the confluence of the hepatic ducts, all that is required is a straight catheter extending into the common duct but not beyond the ampulla (Fig. 58A–E). The catheter should have an adequate number of proximal side holes to allow drainage of the biliary tract, but there should be no side holes within the liver parenchyma itself. The caliber of

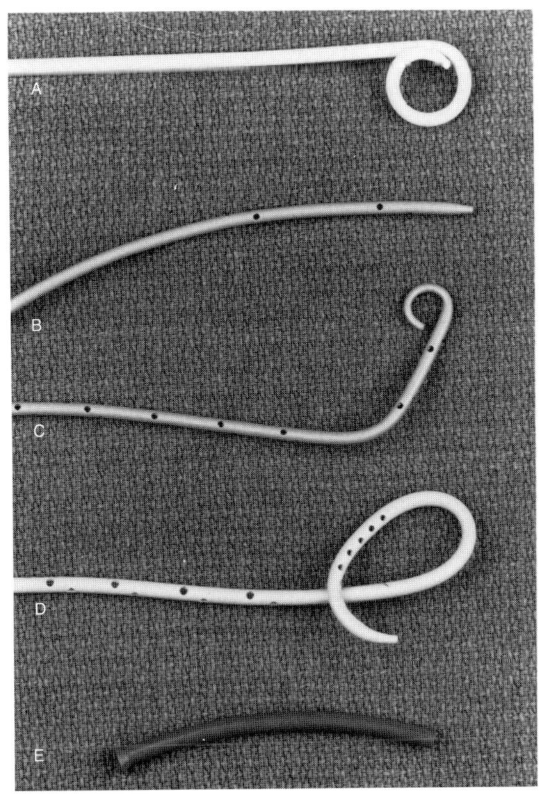

Figure 56. Bilary drainage catheters: A. "Pigtail." B. "CSL" straight. C. Ring "internal-external." D. Cope system. E. Internal prosthesis (Stent).

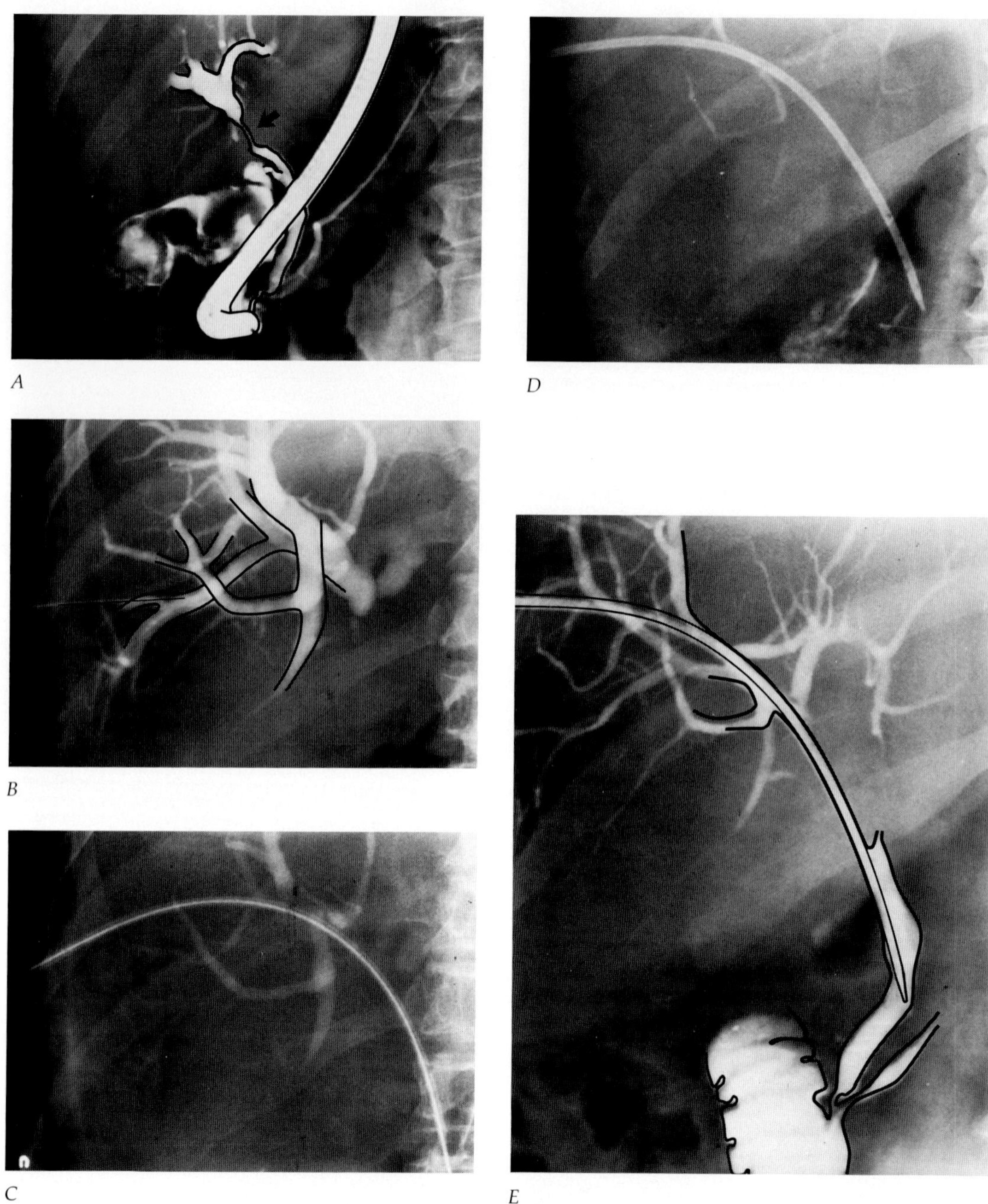

A

B

C

D

E

Figure 58.   A. Cholangiocarcinoma producing stricture in the proximal common duct demonstrated by ERCP (see arrow). B. Same patient as in part A. A few days later the stricture has become more severe as demonstrated by thin (Chiba) needle PTHC. C. A Ring-Lunderquist guidewire has been advanced via a second puncture using an 18 g straight needle. A straight CSL catheter is advanced over the guidewire. D. A catheter with multiple side holes is now in place across the stenotic area. E. Injection of contrast material demonstrates the internal drainage advantage with external "back up" possibility. The biliary system has been decompressed.

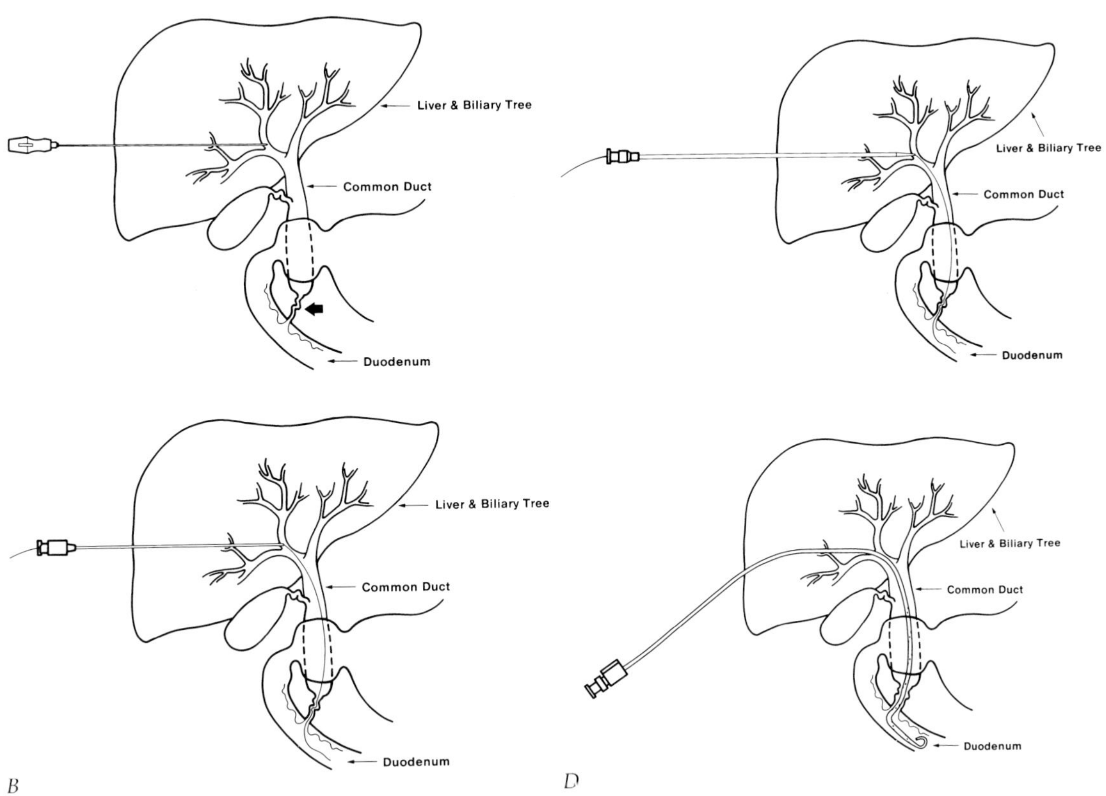

Figure 59. A and B represent the main steps required in the placement of an internal-external type of bilary decompressing catheter. A. Initial opacification of of the bilary system using a Chiba needle. The arrow points toward a stenotic area. B. After the bilary radicals are opacified a larger needle is used to advance a guidewire through the stenotic lesion and the duodenum. C. Dilators increasing in diameter from 6 through 8 French are serially advanced over the guidewire. D. In the last step and internal-external decompressing catheter of the Ring type is introduced over the guidewire. The guidewire is then withdrawn.

this type of catheter is usually between 8 and 12 F. Available catheters at present are 8.3 and 12 F. The initial catheter is usually the smaller one; larger catheters are reserved for future replacements. When the obstructive site is in the distal common duct, as with a pancreatic carcinoma, it is best to use a catheter such as the one designed by Ring (Fig. 56C); this catheter's distal end has a pigtail configuration that extends beyond the ampulla into the duodenum (Fig. 59). This configuration does little to help anchor the catheter; however, it does render it safe, as duodenal perforation is less likely to occur. The number of side holes or ports in this catheter permits an easier flow proximal and distal to the obstructive site. It is important to place the catheter so that the proximal holes are not outside the biliary tract. If necessary, extra holes may be added at the time of catheter placement. A more effective internal anchoring effect is provided by the Cope catheter (Figs. 56, 60).

When the catheter is first inserted into the common duct, it is kept on external drainage for approximately 48 hours in order to evacuate any debris and clots. It may also be flushed with 3 to 5 cc of normal physiological saline to aid the dissolution and clearing of clots. After 48 hours, the external port is usually closed off and drainage continues internally. For maintenance of drainage, these catheters should be irrigated once a day with 5 cc of normal physiological saline. This procedure may be safely performed by the patient. As there is no further need for continuous external drainage, the patient approaches a more normal life pattern. With time, the catheter may become brittle or occluded, or leakage may develop around the catheter. We believe that it is best to replace the catheter on a routine 3-month basis rather than to wait until occlusion or leakage occurs. If an occlusion occurs, it is easily relieved by the use of a guidewire aided by flushing with physiological saline. If leakage develops around the catheter, it may be related to catheter occlusion, which is easily demonstrated

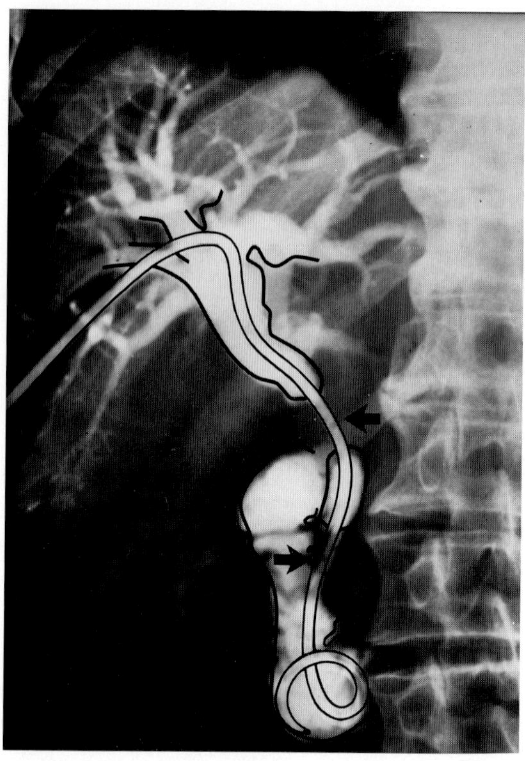

Figure 60.   The "Cope" internal-external catheter in place bridging two stenotic areas produced by a pancreatic carcinoma.

and corrected, as described above. Necrosis of liver parenchyma immediately about the tract of the catheter may also be a cause of leakage. When necrosis occurs, it is necessary to replace the catheter with a larger one, e.g., from 8.3 to 10 F. Most patients do well with an 8.3 or 10 F catheter; an occasional patient will require a 12 F catheter.

Cholangitis is an infrequent complication. Pancreatitis may be related to the passage of draining catheters through the ampulla; however, we have not personally encountered this complication. Either cholangitis or pancreatitis may require the temporary withdrawal of the catheter into the distal common duct just above the ampulla.

Strictly Internal Drainage (Stent or Endoprosthesis)

The most physiologic result of a bypass procedure is attained by strictly internal catheters that drain the occluded region (Figs. 56, 61A–D). Such stents were originally developed by Hoevels et al. [8–10] and Pereiras[11] to bypass short stenotic areas within the common bile duct. This type of catheter is especially important for patients who cannot either manage or tolerate the internal-external type of drainage. One significant drawback is the possibility of migration of the catheter or an occlusion which might be impossible to resolve by the transhepatic route and might involve surgical correction. Another drawback to this type of drainage is that the larger (12 F) catheter has a higher incidence of complications, such as bleeding and perforation. These stents are therefore used only in very specific instances. We believe that when such a catheter is required, it is best to perform a two-stage procedure. A temporary internal-external catheter is kept in place and maintained for a few days; then an internal drain is introduced.

Either type of biliary drainage requires the use of needles and dilators much larger than the 22-gauge Chiba needle (Fig. 55A) used for transhepatic *diagnostic* cholangiography. The possibility of complications such as bleeding and infection is increased. Percutaneous drainage should not be attempted until there has been a surgical consultation, and the patient and family are fully advised that the procedure is performed primarily to avoid surgery, but that if it is unsuccessful or if complications set in, emergency surgery might be required.

AVOIDANCE OF COMPLICATIONS DURING PERCUTANEOUS TRANSHEPATIC CHOLANGIOGRAPHY AND REPLACEMENT OF BILIARY DRAINAGE CATHETERS

Standard coagulation studies including prothrombin time (PT), partial thromboplastin time (PTT), and platelet counts must be performed. The platelet count should preferably be over 20,000/mm^3. The PT and PTT values should be less than 1.5 times normal. Serious contraindications to the study are the presence of a bleeding diathesis or a vascular tumor in the liver (which can be diagnosed by ultrasonography, computed tomography, or angiography). Ascites is also a serious contraindication. The presence of ascites is a contraindication because separation of the liver surface from the abdominal wall can contribute to serious leakage of bile into the peritoneal cavity. An absolute contraindication to the procedure is an allergy to the iodinated contrast material used in visualization of the biliary ducts. The possibility of bleeding or the establishment of an arteriovenous fistula is sometimes unavoidable. The procedure is at best considered to

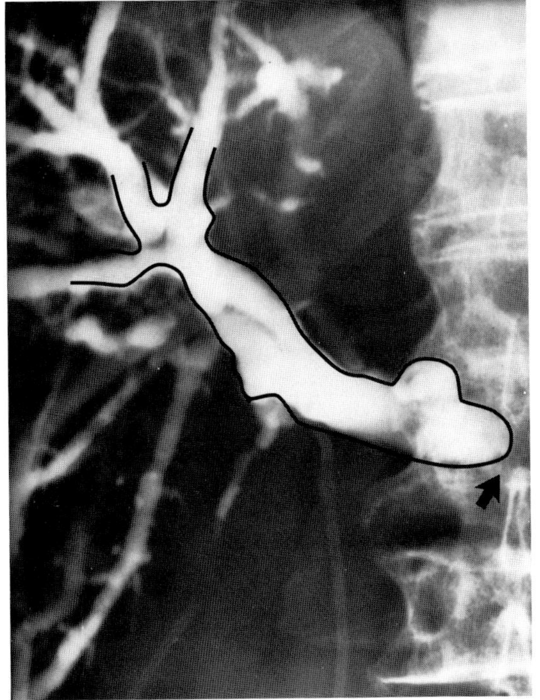

A

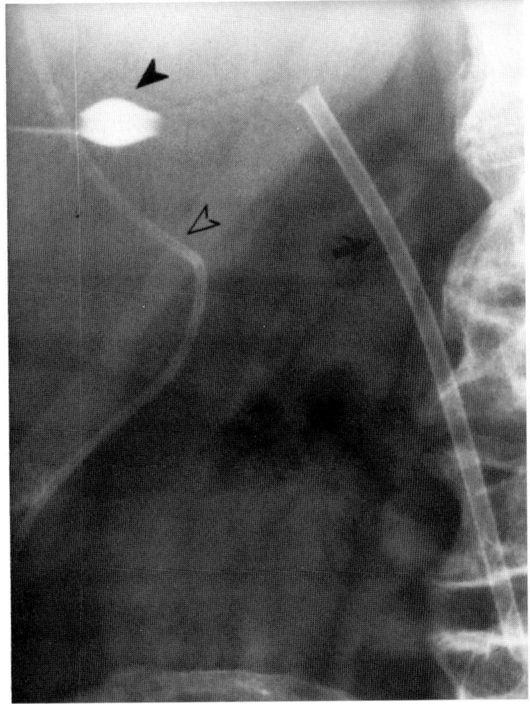

C

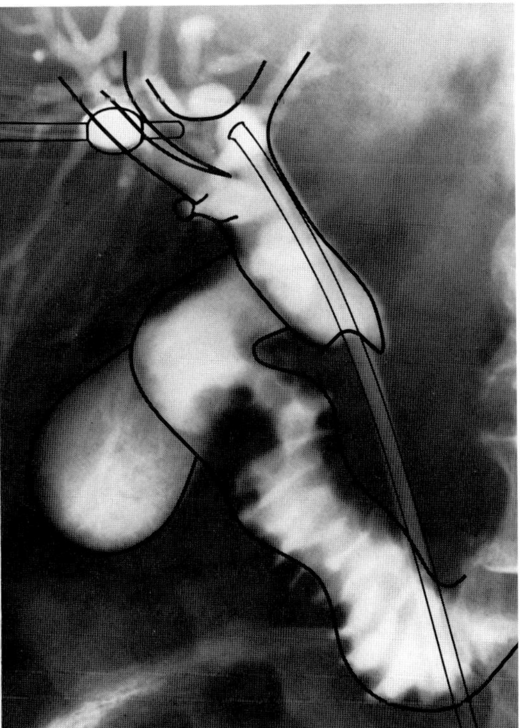

B

D

Figure 61.   A. A complete or almost complete obstruction of the common duct demonstrated by PTHC. Biopsy proven pancreatic carcinoma. B. Same patient as in part A after placement of a ''Ring'' internal-external drainage catheter; however, the patient would not tolerate a permanent catheter protruding from his abdomen. C. The Ring catheter was withdrawn over a Ring-Lunderquist guide and after progressive dilation a French 12 internal prosthesis (see arrow) man-

ufactured from thin-wall Teflon tubing was advanced in place. The black arrowhead points toward a small Foley catheter left in the liver tract on a temporary basis. The open arrowhead points to a ventricoperitonal shunt. D. Internal prosthesis decompressing the biliary system. Duodenal irregularity secondary to tumor and/or manipulation. Injection was performed via the small Foley catheter; this catheter was withdrawn 72 hours later.

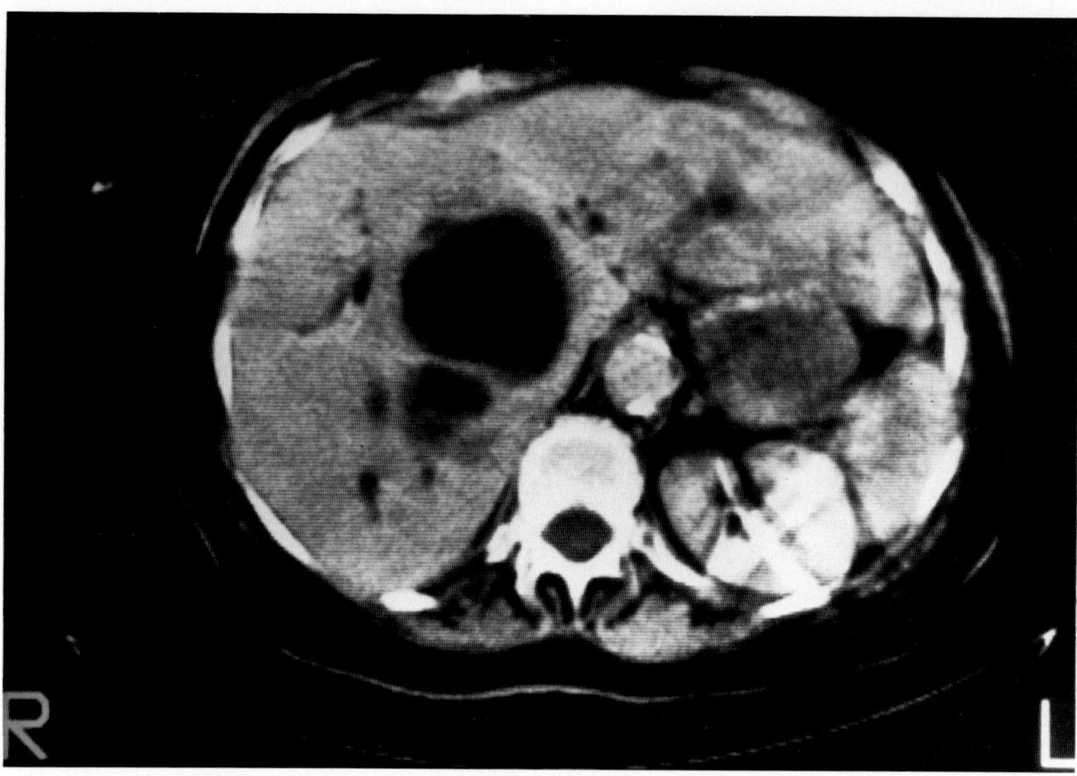

Figure 62.   A. A lucent defect in the liver was demonstrated by CT in a patient who presented with fever of unknown ori-gin (see arrows).

be blind, even though guidelines under fluoroscopy such as the dome of the diaphragm and gas in the duodenal bulb are effectively utilized. The catheter is inserted via the intercostal space of the lower ribs in the anterior axillary line. It is important to avoid the vascular lower border of the rib and the lower aspect of the pulmonary lobes. Of necessity the catheter must traverse the pleural space. These considerations should be kept in mind, since on occasion we have encountered partial dislodgement of the biliary catheter with resultant spillage of bile into the pleural space. If multiple punctures are required to enter the biliary system and undue bleeding results, the procedure should be discontinued and rescheduled for a later date.

THE USE OF ANTIBIOTICS

It has been repeatedly demonstrated that a distended biliary ductal system has a higher probability of being or becoming infected. Therefore, the patient should be placed on intravenous antibiotic coverage before puncturing the biliary system. To minimize the possibility of septic shock (which is often related to the release of endotoxins), adequate antibiotic coverage should begin 24 hours before manipulation of the biliary system. Antibiotic coverage should be continued for not less than 48 hours after the procedure is completed. In our experience, ampicillin, 1 gm IV every 6 hours, has proven adequate. Patients who are allergic to ampicillin might best be given gentamicin or cefamandole, since these antibiotics are excreted into the bile.

When multiple stenotic areas exist in the biliary system, drainage of only one or two of these areas may not contribute sufficiently to the overall improvement of the patient. To drain the left hepatic duct more effectively, a subxyphoid approach may be used.

Every needle puncture must be performed most carefully. The liver parenchyma must be treated with extreme care, being certain not to place the needle into the portal circulation outside the liver. The unprotected portal veins are prone to extensive, life-threatening hemorrhage. The patient's vital signs must be monitored. Intravenous fluids

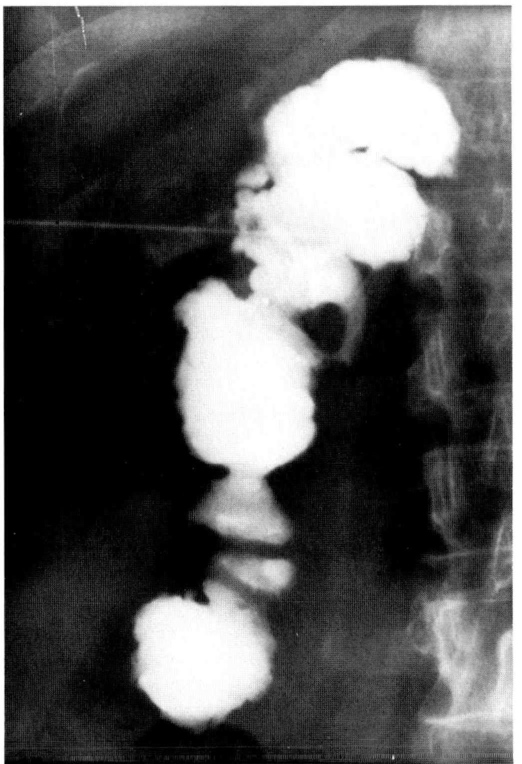

B

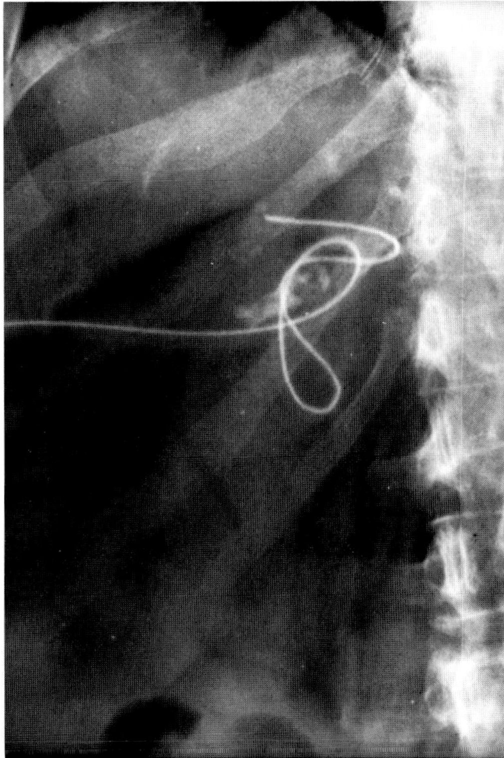

D

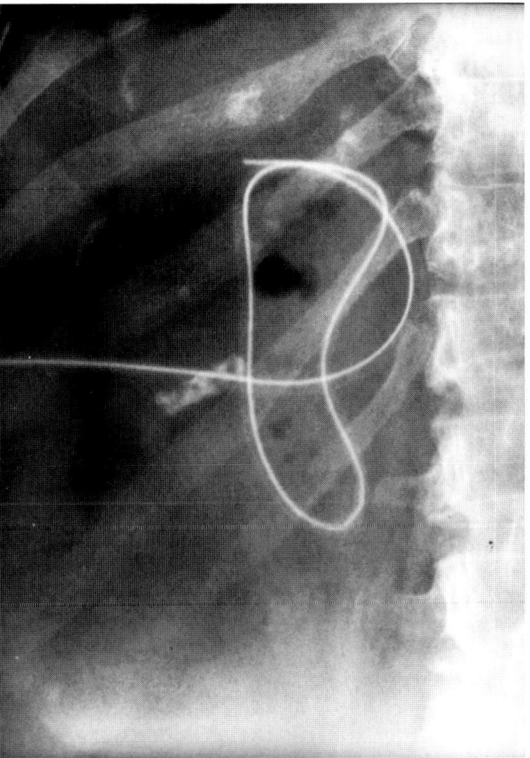

C

Figure 62.   B. Fluoroscopy-guided puncture of the lucent defect yielded pus which was cultured and grew E. coli and enterococci. Injection of water soluble contrast material demonstrates the abscess cavity. C. A thin radiopaque catheter with multiple side holes was coiled into the abscess cavity to provide a route for drainage and irrigation. Medication could be instilled at the discretion of the surgeon. D. After four weeks of drainage and antibiotic therapy, the abscess cavity has become smaller, as shown here by the effect on the coils of the draining catheter (compare with part C.)

are administered during the procedure, and the patient is well sedated. The surgeon must be on constant alert for serious changes in the vital signs and responsiveness of the patient.

PERCUTANEOUS DRAINAGE OF HEPATIC ABSCESSES

Abscesses can develop in the liver following rupture of a gastric ulcer, perforation by foreign objects, postsurgical procedures, and even after percutaneous procedures. Once an abscess has been sited by ultrasonography, computed tomography, radionuclide scanning, or any combination of these diagnostic procedures, it is mandatory to establish a bacteriological diagnosis as well as a plan for effective drainage and irrigation. Antibiotics are of limited value unless drainage is successfully accomplished. Employing the same principles and precautions used with diagnostic transhepatic cholangiography and biliary drainage, a catheter is advanced into the abscess cavity to secure a specimen and to provide drainage. The draining catheter need not be large; usually a 6 to 8 F catheter will suffice. When the needle is initially introduced into the abscess cavity, the first sample is sent for bacteriological culture and sensitivity study. A guidewire is then introduced and gently moved into the abscess cavity to break down all soft loculations and to secure a good position within the abscess in order to permit replacement of the needle with progressive dilators. A selected draining catheter is finally put in place, and extensive irrigations are carried out with normal physiological saline while the patient is still in the radiology unit. When the patient is returned to the surgical unit, adequate written instructions should be given for sterile irrigations to be carried out on every shift for several days. Usually no further irrigations are required after 7–10 days. The presence of pus in the irrigating fluid dictates the need for further irrigations. Ultimately, the catheter is left in for continued drainage.

The reduction in the size of the abscess cavity can be monitored by sterile injections of contrast material at periodic intervals. Based on the size and character of the abscess, 2–4 weeks may be necessary for complete closure of the abscess. The patient continues to receive adequate intravenous antibiotics. The catheter is withdrawn when the patient is asymptomatic and afebrile, and when no residual abscess cavity can be demonstrated. The catheter may be withdrawn over a period of 2 or 3 days to close the fistulous tract. If there are multiple or multiloculated abscesses, therapy by percutaneous drainage may not be adequate. If no improvement is noted in 48–72 hours, the abscess or abscesses may require surgical drainage.

The same precautions used with transhepatic cholangiography in the placement of catheters for biliary drainage are also employed in cases of hepatic abscesses. The possibility of an ecchinococcus cyst should be considered, since this type of cyst must never be punctured. Diagnostic studies should establish the presence of hydatid cyst first. Amebic cysts are usually treated without drainage; however, with a large, nonresponsive amebic cyst, percutaneous drainage has been used, with a favorable outcome.

EMBOLIZATION

Embolization of hepatic arteries for trauma or for the treatment of primary or metastatic hepatic tumors can be accomplished via a transfemoral approach using standard angiographic techniques. Embolization of the hepatic artery or its branch usually produces no deleterious effect, since approximately 75% of the blood supply to the liver is provided by the portal circulation. This is not true in the cirrhotic patient, in whom the portal circulation is severely impaired and the only residual source of oxygenation and nutrition is the arterial supply. Temporary embolization can be accomplished with blood clots or Gelfoam. Permanent embolization can be accomplished by (among other agents) Gianturco[12] stainless steel wire coils. Embolization may be carried out for the correction of an arteriovenous or biliary fistula caused iatrogenically by hepatic procedures such as biopsy.

Hepatic perfusion catheters for chemotherapy can be introduced via a surgical approach. On a temporary basis, the femoral artery may be selected, with the catheter advanced into the hepatic artery. Because it is important to perfuse only the liver, the catheter should be advanced beyond the origin of the gastroduodenal artery. If there is an accessory hepatic artery (that on occasion arises from the superior mesenteric artery), this accessory artery should be embolized before chemotherapy is started in order to avoid collateral circulation to the tumor.

MISCELLANEOUS PROCEDURES INVOLVING THE LIVER

Thin needle aspiration biopsies of liver tumors may be performed under ultrasonographic, computed tomography, or fluoroscopic control. Two lesions that should not be biopsied are the hydatid cyst (to be suspected in the presence of calcifications) and the cavernous hemangioma (which may require a liver arteriogram to rule it out).

A percutaneous transportal approach might be used in the embolization of esophageal veins for correction of life-threatening hemorrhage in cirrhotic patients. Embolization may be completed by Gianturco coils, alcohol, or other agents.

The portal system also provides a source for the venous sampling localization of small pancreatic tumors such as insulinomas. This procedure is performed by advancing a catheter into the splenic vein and obtaining samples at several sites within this vein or its pancreatic branches. This procedure, though diagnostic, can result in complications such as arteriovenous fistula that may require corrective embolization.

The development of diagnostic and interventional procedures involving the liver has opened up avenues for further therapies and different approaches in the treatment of inflammatory and neoplastic diseases of the liver. The procedure must be chosen in relation to the clinical diagnosis and the condition of the patient. Close cooperation must exist between the internist, the surgeon, and the radiologist. Symptomatic improvement and increased longevity of the patient must remain the paramount goals of the therapist. The ultimate aim must be to improve the patient's quality of life, with minimal discomfort and few side effects.

Recommended Reading

Anderson JH, Wallace S, Gianturco C, et al: "Mini" Gianturco stainless steel coils for transcatheter vascular occlusion. *Radiology* 132:301, 1979.

Berenstein A, Kricheff II: Catheter and material selection for transarterial embolization: Technical considerations. *Radiology* 132:631, 1979.

Centola CA, Jander HP, Stauffer A, et al: Balloon dilatation of the papilla of Vater to allow biliary stone passage. *Am J Roentgenol* 136:613, 1981.

Chuang VP, Wallace S: Hepatic artery embolization in the treatment of hepatic neoplasms. *Radiology* 140:51, 1981.

Cook Incorporated, Bloomington IN: Catalog number RBD-1, Casal 110281.

Cotton PB: Duodenoscopic sphincterotomy and bile duct stone retrieval, in Bennet JR (ed): *Therapeutic Endoscopy and Radiology of the Gut.* London, Chapman and Hall, 1981. pp 169–183.

Dotter CT, Bilbao MK, Katon RM: Percutaneous transhepatic gallstone removal by needle tract. *Radiology* 133:242, 1979.

Elyaderani MK, Gabriele OF: Brush and forceps biopsy of biliary ducts via percutaneous transhepatic catheterization. *Radiology* 135:777, 1980.

Gerzof SG, Robbins AH, Johnson NC, et al: Percutaneous catheter drainage of abdominal abscesses. *N Engl J Med* 305:653, 1981.

Goldstein HM, Zornoza J, Wallace S, et al: Percutaneous fine needle aspiration biopsy of pancreatic and other abdominal masses. *Radiology* 123:319, 1977.

Irish CR, Meaney TG: Percutaneous transhepatic cholangiography: Comparison of success and risk using 19 versus 22 gauge needles. *Am J Roentgenol* 134:137, 1980.

Juler GL, Conroy RM, Fuellman RW: Bile leakage following percutaneous transhepatic cholangiography with the Chiba needle. *Arch Surg* 112:954, 1977.

Marwan U, Hagop K, Maher O, et al: Cefamandole bile levels in patients with hepatobiliary disease. *Antimicrob Agents Chemother* 22:1087, 1982.

McLean GK, Ring EJ, Freiman DB: Therapeutic alternatives in the treatment of intrahepatic biliary obstruction. *Radiology* 145:289, 1982.

Molnar W, Stockum AE: Transhepatic dilatation of choledochoenterostomy strictures. *Radiology* 129:59, 1978.

Mura A, Mueller PR, Ferrucci JT Jr, et al: Bile cytology: A routine addition to percutaneous bile drainage. *Radiology* 149:846, 1983.

Ring EJ, Husted JW, Oleaga JA, et al: A multihole catheter for maintaining long term percutaneous antegrade biliary drainage. *Radiology* 132:752, 1979.

Van Sonnenberg E, Ferrucci JT, Mueller PR, et al: Percutaneous drainage of abscess and fluid collections: Techniques, results and applications. *Radiology* 142:1, 1982.

Viamonte M Jr, LePage J, Lunderquist A, et al: Selective catheterization of the portal vein and its tributaries. *Radiology* 114:457, 1975.

References

1. Burhenne HJ: Nonoperative retained biliary tract stone extraction: A new roentgenologic technique. *Am J Roentgenol* 117:388, 1973.

2. Burhenne HL: Nonoperative roentgenologic instrumentation techniques of the post-operative biliary tract. Treatment of biliary stricture and retained stones. *Am J Surg* 128:111, 1974.

3. Burhenne HJ: Nonoperative extraction of retained biliary tract stones requiring multiple sessions. *Am J Surg* 128:288, 1974.

4. Gianturco C, Anderson JH, Wallace S: Mechanical devices for arterial occlusion. *Am J Roentgenol* 124:428, 1975.

5. Hoevels J, Ihse I: Percutaneous transhepatic insertion of a permanent endoprosthesis in obstructive lesions of the extrahepatic bile ducts. *Gastrointest Radiol* 4:367, 1979.

6. Hoevels J, Lunderquist A, Owman T, et al: A large-bore Teflon endoprosthesis with side holes for nonoperative decompression of the biliary tract in malignant obstructive jaundice. *Gastrointest Radiol* 5:361, 1980.

7. Hoevels J, Nilsson U: Intrahepatic vascular lesions following nonsurgical percutaneous transhepatic bile duct intubation. *Gastrointest Radiol* 5:126, 1980.

8. Lagrave G, Plessis JL, Pougeard-Dulimbert G, et al: Lithiase biliaire residuelle: Extraction a la sonde de Dormia par le drain de Kehr. *Mem Acad Chir* 95:431, 1969.

9. Mazzariello R: Review of 220 cases of residual biliary tract calculi treated without reoperation: An eight-year study. *Surgery* 73:299, 1973.
10. Mondet A: Technica de la extraccion incruenta de los calculos en la litiasis residual del coledoco. *Bol Soc Cir B Air* 46:278, 1962.
11. Okuda K, Tanikawa K, Emura T, et al: Nonsurgical, percutaneous transhepatic cholangiography–Diagnostic significance in medical problems of the liver. *Am J Dig Dis* 19:21, 1974.
12. Pereiras RV, Rheingold OJ, Hutson D, et al: Relief of malignant obstructive jaundice by percutaneous insertion of a permanent prosthesis in the biliary tree. *Ann Intern Med* 890 (Part I):589, 1978.

A Statistical Comment on Preoperative Drainage of the Obstructed Biliary Tree

(*Percutaneous Transhepatic Cholangiography*)

At the University of Michigan a controlled study on 50 patients with unusually high bilirubin readings who underwent percutaneous transhepatic cholangiography (PTHC) for 9 days before having surgery. Serum bilirubin levels averaged about 14.9 mg/ml in the non-PTHC patients and 1.65 mg/ml in the PTHC patients. The morbidity and mortality rates in the two groups showed a significant difference. In the non-PTHC group, two patients (8%) died from sepsis, abscess formation, bleeding, or renal failure. Of the patients who had had preoperative biliary drainage (PBD), one (4%) died; five (20%) patients who had not had PBD died. The hospital stay was shorter in the patients who received PBD. Gundry et al. *conclude that preoperative PBD reduces morbidity and mortality. Hyperbilirubinemia is also more rapidly improved in the pre- and postoperative periods* (see Chapter 5).

Reference

1. Taplin GV, Meredith OM Jr., Kade H: "Radioactive I[131] tagg rose bengal up take-excretion test for liver function using external gamma-ray scintillaton counting techniques". *J of Lab and Clin Med* 45:665:May 1955.

Ultrasound and Scintigraphy in the Diagnosis of Biliary Diseases

Noel R. Zusmer, M.D.

In the past 10 years, there has been a marked increase in the ability of the radiologist to evaluate hepatobiliary disorders. The rapid developments in the nuclear medicine field, as well as the competing claims of accuracy by ultrasonographers and nuclear medicine physicians, have led to some confusion among radiologists and clinicians.

The impetus of diagnosis-related groups (DRGs) and other government efforts at cost containment will exert significant pressure to improve the efficacy of examinations, as well as to reduce the number of procedures performed, especially those that report similar information. It is therefore important to understand fully the value and limitations of the information obtained from the various imaging modalities when evaluating heptatobiliary disease.

The magnitude of this problem can be appreciated by looking at the statistics of biliary disease in this country. It has been estimated that approximately 20 million Americans have gallstones. Of these, 30% are asymptomatic, 30% will develop acute cholecystitis, and 40% will develop chronic cholecystitis. Cholelithiasis and its complications are the common indications for abdominal surgery and account for more than 500,000 procedures annually. Assuming an average cost of $300 per day, a reduction of 1 day's stay in the hospital of these 500,000 patients could result in a saving of $150 million.

Up to the mid-1970s, the primary techniques for the evaluation of the gallbladder and biliary tree were oral cholecystography, intravenous cholangiography, and percutaneous cholangiography. The oral cholecystogram was considered the standard technique for detecting cholecystolithiasis. The drawbacks of this technique were the time delay between administration of the oral contrast material and visualization of the gallbladder, the frequent necessity to employ double-dose studies, (prolonging the test for 1 day), the nonspecific nature of nonvisualization, and finally, the difficulty of administering oral contrast material to patients with acute cholecystitis.

Intravenous cholangiography permits more rapid visualization of the biliary tree and gallbladder, and is often used in suspect acute cholangitis. This procedure is frequently accompanied by adverse reactions and occasional fatalities. It has therefore been superseded by hepatobiliary scintigraphy and ultrasound studies. An elevated serum bilirubin level will significantly interfere with the results and does not permit adequate biliary tree visualization when the bilirubin level is above 3–4 mg%.

ULTRASOUND OF THE BILIARY TREE

The use of diagnostic ultrasound to detect gallstones was first reported in 1973 by Leopold and

Sokolof.[1] Since that time, there has been a marked improvement in ultrasonic imaging techniques that has led to the development of high-resolution, real-time imaging devices. Reported accuracy for the detection of gallstones in nonacute situations is about 95%. The rapidity and accuracy of ultrasound have made it the procedure of choice, and the use of oral cholecystography has progressively declined.

TECHNIQUE

High-resolution, real-time imaging has largely replaced static gray scale ultrasound imaging because real-time technique is more flexible and results in more rapid visualization of the gallbladder and the biliary tree. The fluoroscopic nature of the examination produces multiple images in rapid succession and requires a highly trained technician. Although these studies can be performed by a well-trained technologist, physician supervision is desirable. Real-time imaging enables the operator to assess rapidly the anatomy of the gallbladder, liver, and biliary ducts, as well as their relationship to adjacent upper abdominal and retroperitoneal structures. The ease of the procedure often enables pathological conditions outside the gallbladder to be detected during the examination, particularly if a diligent search is undertaken to exclude contiguous pathology.

The usual examination is performed in a supine position; the patient is forbidden to eat or drink for at least 4 hours. The gallbladder is looked for in the right upper quadrant, employing a longitudinal plane of section; most often it appears as a characteristic pear-shaped, fluid-filled structure. If the gallbladder is not readily identified, we attempt to locate the right kidney as a landmark, since the gallbladder lies anteriorly in the same sagittal and transverse planes as the kidney. In those instances where the liver is high-riding in position, examination of the patient during deep inspiration may help to visualize the gallbladder more effectively. Another maneuver that may help to visualize a gallbladder that is not seen in the supine position is to rotate the patient into the left posterior oblique or left lateral position. These positions assist the gallbladder to descend from behind the costal margin. In some instances, this may be accomplished by having the patient stand. Even if the gallbladder cannot be identified despite the fact that the patient was on nothing by mouth, with no history of gallbladder surgery, presumptive evidence for gallbladder disease still remains.

Once the gallbladder has been identified, it is carefully examined in both the sagittal and transverse planes, employing both the supine and lateral decubitus positions. An effort is made to examine the entire gallbladder carefully, particularly the region of its neck. Echoes arising from duodenal contents that are adjacent to the gallbladder must be distinguished from intraluminal gallbladder abnormalities. The presence of echodensities associated with classic acoustic shadowing arising from within the gallbladder that change with position, is pathognomonic for cholecystolithiasis.

It has been stated that all gallstones cause acoustic shadowing, regardless of the composition or shape of the calculus. The lack of demonstration of acoustic shadowing is most often due to the physical properties of the ultrasonic beam, the most common difficulty being the width of the beam in relation to the size of the calculus. Real-time scanning has improved the accuracy of gallbladder visualization but still presents diagnostic difficulties. Interpretation can also be difficult when acoustic shadowing is seen secondary to adjacent gas collections; examples are junctional folds of the gallbladder and refractor shadows arising from the region of the cystic duct.

In 15–25% of the patients with cholecystolithiasis, the gallbladder lumen may not visualize ultrasonically. In such instances, the gallbladder is usually contracted or filled with calculi, and the diagnosis may be suggested by the identification of high-level echoes and shadowing in the region of the gallbladder fossa. Occasionally, the double-arc shadow sign may be observed. The proximal arc represents the near wall of the gallbladder, with an anechoic space representing bile in the gallbladder lumen; a distal arc represents gallstones that are responsible for the acoustic shadowing. When the patient is placed in the left lateral decubitus position and this double-arc sign remains unchanged in its relationship to the liver, the confidence level for diagnosing cholecystolithiasis should approach 100%. With real-time scanning, there are virtually no indeterminate results for nonvisualization of the gallbladder.

Echogenic bile, commonly called *sludge*, has been found in medical conditions such as cholestasis and acalculous cholecystitis. It is often seen as a nonshadowing, dependent, echogenic layer within the gallbladder. Echogenic bile most likely originates from sedimented calcium bilirubin and cholesterol crystals. When the patient is placed in the decubitus position, the sludge will shift to the more dependent portion of the gallbladder lumen. Echogenic bile is different from pseudosludge, which is due to an averaging of the echoes from the adjacent liver. This appearance can also be seen in any other curved, fluid-filled structure adjacent to an echogenic structure, such as the aorta, urinary bladder, and renal cysts. The appearance of pseudosludge is dependent on beam direction and will remain perpendicular to the incident beam regardless of patient positioning. The finding of sludge in a symptomatic patient is nonspecific and must be studied further with biliary scintigraphy to evaluate cystic duct patency.

HEPATOBILIARY SCINTIGRAPHY

Nuclear medicine techniques for evaluating hepatobiliary function have been available since their introduction in 1955 by Taplin et al.[2] [131]I rose bengal found its greatest use in differentiating hepatocellular disease from common bile duct obstruction in patients with clinical jaundice. Other ^{131}I-labeled compounds have been evaluated for their use in hepatobiliary imaging since that time but have not performed better than ^{131}I rose bengal to justify their continued use. Only with the development of the technetium(Tc)-labeled hepatobiliary imaging agents has the clinical usefulness of this technique been markedly expanded.

Pyridoxylidine amino acid complexes of ^{99m}Tc were first reported in 1974 by Baker et al.[3] and were found to be clinically useful hepatobiliary agents. They were clinically supplanted by the ^{99m}Tc-labelled chelates of iminodiacetic acid (IDA). Other IDA compounds have been evaluated, but diisopropyl IDA (DISIDA) is the only agent that has thus far received Food and Drug Administration approval for hepatobiliary imaging. Further information concerning the pharmacokinetics of hepatobiliary imaging agents can be obtained in an excellent review by Chervu et al.[4]

^{99m}Tc (DISIDA) has the advantages of high extraction efficiency by the liver, rapid excretion into the biliary ducts, and high concentration in the gallbladder; it also has a low renal excretion rate in patients with normal hepatocellular function and the ability to image the biliary system with an elevated bilirubin level (as high as 30 mg%). Several studies have suggested that DISIDA is the agent of choice in hepatobiliary imaging because of its high uptake and rapid clearance by the liver; we do not necessarily find this to be the case. In instances of abnormal gallbladder function, as in chronic cholecystitis, there may be delayed visualization of the gallbladder for 3–4 hours after the injection of ^{99m}Tc (IDA); the duodenum and common bile duct visualize normally within 60 minutes. Recent kinetic data have shown that the excretion half-times of the ^{99m}Tc-labeled IDA compounds vary greatly: from 18.8 minutes for DISIDA to 59.3 minutes for paraisopropyl IDA to 108 minutes for parabutyl IDA. Most early studies on the accuracy of hepatobiliary scintigraphy employed the slower clearing agents that showed high overall diagnostic accuracy, specificity, and sensitivity, as well as a low number of false-positive results. More recent studies employing the rapidly clearing agents have shown them to have a higher incidence of false-positive results. The latter may be related to the fact that less than 1.5% of the liver activity at injection time is retained when imaging is performed 2 hours postinjection with ^{99m}Tc (DISIDA). In instances where there is slow filling of the gallbladder, the activity remaining in the lines is probably insufficient to visualize the gallbladder. More important, it appears that the faster clearing agents are preferable for visualizing the intrahepatic biliary and common bile ducts. The latter may be inferior to the slower clearing agents in visualizing the gallbladder when its filling is impaired. Some caution should therefore be exercised in evaluating claims concerning the efficacy of the various agents. The most desirable situation may be the availability of agents with different clearance time, permitting a choice of agents depending upon the particular clinical situation.

To evaluate the cystic duct effectively, the patient should be on nothing by mouth; 5–10 mCi of ^{99m}Tc (DISIDA) are injected, and serial images are obtained over the liver and upper abdomen. In our institution, we routinely obtain images every 5 minutes after injection for the first half hour, and then obtain subsequent images at variable time intervals until the study is terminated. A normal study is shown in Figure 63. There is prompt uptake of the pharmaceutical, and it is cleared from the blood pool within 5–10 minutes. The intrahepatic biliary radicles, as well as the common bile duct, are seen shortly thereafter, and the gallbladder is visualized within 1 hour. Activity in the small bowel should be recognized within this period, although the significance of delayed bowel visualization is uncertain. If the gallbladder has not been visualized by 1 hour postinjection, we continue to obtain images until at least 2 hours and preferably 4 hours have passed. If the liver activity has essentially cleared and most of the activity is found within the bowel prior to 4 hours, the study is terminated.

If the gallbladder has not visualized at the completion of the study, and there has been adequate visualization of the common bile duct, there is a high probability of cystic duct obstruction. Delayed

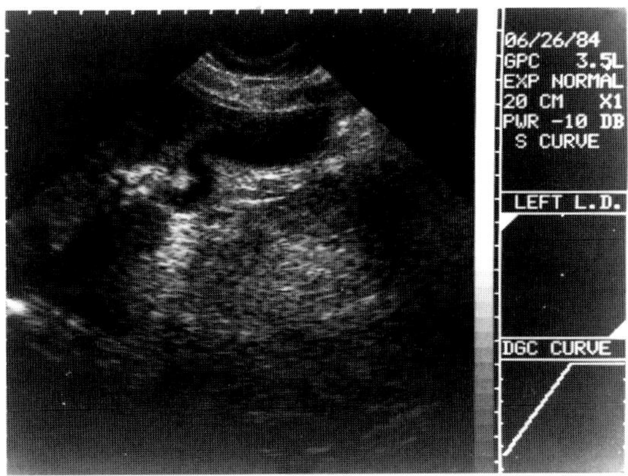

Figure 63.   Longitudinal view of the gallbladder. Normal appearance to the gallbladder. No internal lumenal echodensities are demonstrated. Arrowheads point to the body of the gallbladder and the arrow points to the neck of the gallbladder.

visualization of the gallbladder beyond 1 hour is most often seen in chronic cholecystitis. A normal study, however, does not exclude the possibility of cholecystolithiasis; approximately one-third to one-half of the patients with gallstones may show a normal DISIDA study. If there has been no excretion into the biliary ducts, as in complete common duct obstruction, or if the hepatocellular function is too poor to visualize the biliary ducts adequately in spite of some activity in the bowel, the presence or absence of cystic duct obstruction cannot be established with certainty and the study must be considered indeterminate.

Occasionally, there may be difficulty in deciding whether or not an imaged structure represents the gallbladder or bowel. In such instances, a left anterior oblique or right lateral view of the abdomen may be useful in differentiating between the gallbladder and the duodenum.

Small stones within the gallbladder are seen infrequently; large stones are visualized more easily. It is quite difficult to reach conclusions concerning the presence or absence of biliary dilatation; even in cases of grossly dilated ducts, comments concerning the presence of biliary duct dilatation should be made with caution.

ACUTE CHOLECYSTITIS

Cholecystolithiasis and its complications, most notably acute cholecystitis, are the most common causes of abdominal surgery in the United States. The ability to rapidly evaluate patients presenting with suspected acute cholecystitis is desirable; delay in treatment is a common cause of increased

morbidity and mortality. Early cholecystectomy is usually recommended for patients with acute cholecystitis. The clinical signs and symptoms are variable; the patient most often complains of right upper quadrant pain that radiates to the back or right shoulder. The pain is colicky and persistent, and often progresses to secondary distention of the gallbladder. Laboratory findings are nonspecific. Blood studies reveal leukocytosis with mild elevations of liver enzymes; an elevated serum amylase level often accompanies acute cholecystitis. On physical examination, patients are often found to have a low-grade fever with variable physical findings; right upper quadrant tenderness is commonly present. Elderly patients often present diagnostic difficulties; their physical and laboratory findings may be minimal or absent.

Ultrasound has proven to be most useful in obtaining a rapid evaluation of a patient with suspected acute cholecystitis. The diagnostic accuracy of ultrasound in acute cholecystitis has improved remarkably with the development of high-resolution, real-time scanners. Recent studies have shown that the sensitivity of ultrasound may be as high as 97% when real-time sector scanners are employed.

The most common finding in the setting of acute cholecystitis is the presence of gallstones within the gallbladder. Unfortunately, the presence or absence of cholecystolithiasis per se does not necessarily indicate the presence of acute cholecystitis or specify it as being the cause of the patient's signs and symptoms. The high prevalence of nonsymptomatic gallstones in the population must be kept in mind. Acalculous cholecystitis and single stones in the cystic duct are difficult to detect sonographically. For the latter reasons, other sonographic signs of gallbladder inflammation are helpful in indicating the presence of acute cholecystitis. The most commonly seen sign is increased thickness of the gallbladder wall due to inflammation and edema. A thickening of the gallbladder wall greater than 5 mm has been seen in about 50% of patients with acute cholecystitis.

It is, however, a nonspecific finding which can be seen in patients with heart failure, alcoholic liver with hypoproteinemia, hepatitis, renal disease, and chronic cholecystitis. A thickened wall can also be seen following contraction of the gallbladder in a patient who has eaten. A more significant sign than homogeneous thickening of the gallbladder wall is the presence of sonolucency within the wall, which is seen as a hyporeflective layer between the inner and outer layers of the gallbladder wall; it is highly suggestive of subserosal edema. The hyporeflective layer may be interrupted or continuous around the gallbladder, and the presence of a sonolucent layer is more significant than homogeneous thickening. The presence of fluid collections adjacent to the gallbladder is highly significant and may indicate the presence of a pericholecystic abscess.

Laing et al.[5,6] have suggested that improved sensitivity in the detection of acute cholecystitis can be obtained by eliciting the sonographic Murphy's sign. Up to 85% of patients with acute cholecystitis will demonstrate direct tenderness over the sonographically determined position of the gallbladder. This is a nonobjective test which requires the subjective evaluation of the patient's response to palpation. With the advent of real-time scanning, calculi may be demonstrated in the neck of the gallbladder or the cystic duct; the latter cannot be done with complete reliability. In some patients with acute cholecystitis, the sonogram may be entirely normal, with a false-negative rate ranging from 30% to less than 5%.

Hepatobiliary scintigraphy, while not providing the anatomical detail that is available with ultrasound, is still a highly accurate technique for determining the patency of the cystic and common ducts. In acute cholecystitis, the vast majority of patients have obstruction of the cystic duct due to stone, edema, and inflammation. Three basic patterns may be seen in the DISIDA studies. In the first category, there is normal visualization of the gallbladder within 1 hour and delayed visualization in a significant number of patients with chronic cholecystitis. The biliary ducts and bowel are clearly seen. In the second category, there is nonvisualization of the gallbladder, which is usually indicative of cystic duct obstruction. The latter is the finding most indicative of acute cholecystitis, with some exceptions. The third category is seen in total common duct obstruction; there is visualization of the liver without excretion into the biliary ducts and bowel. In this instance, the patency of the cystic duct cannot be evaluated with complete accuracy.

A comparison of the accuracy of hepatobiliary scintigraphy with ultrasound in the detection of acute cholecystitis is difficult. Differences in sonographic technique, equipment used, technical expertise of the sonographer, and patient populations studied result in wide variability in reported figures for accuracy. In regard to hepatobiliary imaging, various investigators have employed different protocols which differed primarily in the radiopharmaceuticals used. Other detracting factors included the time of termination of the study and whether or not patients with indeterminate scan findings were included in the data. The differences

Table 1. Scintigraphic Findings in Postcholecystectomy Patients ($n = 125$)

	No. of Patients	Accuracy (%)
Normal ^{99m}Tc-IDA	35	98
Dilated ducts with functional patency	20	85
Partial ductal obstructive pattern		
Dilated ducts with delayed B-BT*	5	100
Abnormal ductal time activity dynamics	24	96
Nonvisualization of ducts with delayed B-BT	1	100
Complete ductal obstructive pattern	19	95
Persistent cystic duct remnant	12	92
Biliary leakage	9	100

Source: Adapted from Weissman et al.[7–11]
*B-BT = biliary-bowel transit.

in pathological criteria also introduced variables which made comparison between reported results difficult. Table 1 presents a summary of the results of several of the larger series. Several conclusions can be drawn from these data concerning the current state of ultrasound and hepatobiliary scintigraphy. First, the sensitivity of ultrasound has improved due to a range similar to that of hepatobiliary imaging. However, the detail of hepatobiliary scintigraphy appears to be superior to sonography. By applying Baysian analysis, we can look at the predictive value of an abnormal test result. In the study by Samuels et al.,[52] the predictive value of an abnormal scintogram was 77% vs. 40% for an abnormal sonogram. The latter results were obtained by employing state-of-the-art ultrasound techniques. The major advantage of hepatobiliary scintigraphy is its ability to determine the patency of the cystic duct accurately.

Nonvisualization of the gallbladder in hepatobiliary scintigraphy can occur in several clinical states other than acute cholecystitis. The most common cause of nonvisualization resulting in a false-positive diagnosis is premature termination of the study prior to gallbladder visualization. This error is minimized by carrying out studies in which the gallbladder is not seen for at least 4 hours, provided that adequate liver activity is present. The majority of patients with delayed visualization usually show evidence of chronic cholecystitis. Another cause of nonvisualization of the gallbladder is imaging a patient who has been fasting for several days. This often occurs in patients who have been hospitalized for several days and have been given nothing by mouth. Other reported causes of nonvisualization of the gallbladder include a normal nonfasting state such as acute pancreatitis, alcoholism, total parenteral nutrition, and physiological gallbladder distention without fasting. In still other instances, the cystic duct may be occluded by intrinsic or extrinsic tumors without acute cholecystitis. Acalculous cholecystitis was reported by Weissman et al.[7–11] to produce nonvisualization of the gallbladder in 14 of 15 patients studied.

In conclusion, an abnormal sonogram is found in a high percentage of patients with acute cholecystitis. When the abnormalities consist only of the presence of gallstones, the specificity of the examination is not considered adequate enough to recommend surgery without additional studies. When a sonogram reveals associated signs such as edema of the wall, pericholecystic fluid collections, or the presence of a sonographic Murphy's sign, the accuracy of the diagnosis of acute cholecystitis is more certain; individual decisions must be made as to whether or not further diagnostic studies are required. In patients with normal gallbladder sonograms in whom there is a strong suspicion of acute cholecystitis, further evaluation with hepatobiliary scintigraphy is indicated. In our institution, the majority of patients with suspected acute cholecystitis have both studies performed. Scintigraphy alone, without ultrasound, is usually not done unless the scintigraphic study is normal. In instances where hepatobiliary imaging indicates cystic duct obstruction, ultrasound is valuable in providing ancillary information on whether the condition is urgent. Where ultrasound findings reveal hydrops of the gallbladder, marked edema of the gallbladder wall, and pericholecystic fluid collections, surgical intervention is usually indicated.

CHRONIC CHOLECYSTITIS

In chronic cholecystitis, ultrasound is superior to hepatobiliary scintigraphy; it demonstrates the presence of stones in the gallbladder with a greater than 95% accuracy. Scintigraphic studies, on the other hand, present variable findings; the range varies from a normal examination to delayed visualization to nonvisualization of the gallbladder suggesting cystic duct obstruction. The incidence of false-positive DISIDA studies in chronic cholecystitis is to a large extent dependent upon the time of termination of the study; delayed imaging decreases the number of false-positive studies. The excretion half-times of the differing ^{99m}Tc-labeled

IDA compounds range from 18.8 to 108 minutes; this causes an increase in the number of false-positive studies, especially when the more rapidly clearing agents are employed.

THE JAUNDICED PATIENT

In the diagnosis of jaundice, ultrasound is unquestionably superior to hepatobiliary scintigraphy in differentiating between surgical obstruction and medical jaundice. The ability of ultrasound to assess the presence of intra- or extrahepatic duct dilatation rapidly and noninvasively makes it an ideal modality in this situation. The recognition of dilated intrahepatic ducts is sometimes challenging when high-resolution, real-time scanners are utilized. Normal-size intrahepatic ducts are usually not visible, but the common hepatic duct should be viewed on all ultrasound examinations. Extrahepatic biliary obstruction causes the common duct and the common hepatic duct to be the first structures to show evidence of dilatation. With longstanding obstruction, dilatation of the intrahepatic biliary radicles take place. In early obstruction, there is no demonstrable dilatation of the common duct. In the latter instance, there is a role for hepatobiliary scintigraphy because a characteristic of good uptake by the liver with no excretion into the biliary ducts points to complete ductal obstruction. The latter can also be seen with normal-sized ducts. (Fig. 64).

Differentiation of dilated intrahepatic radicles from the other tubular structures within the liver, i.e., portal and hepatic veins, is not difficult with a real-time examination. The walls of the intrahepatic biliary radicles typically appear as irregular,

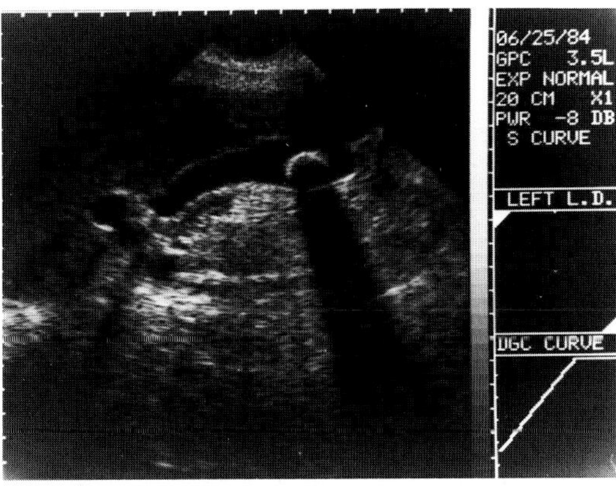

Figure 64. Longitudinal view of the gallbladder. Classic demonstration of a gallbladder stone. A semilunar echodensity within the lumen of the gallbladder (straight arrow) with associated posterior acoustic shadowing (curved arrow).

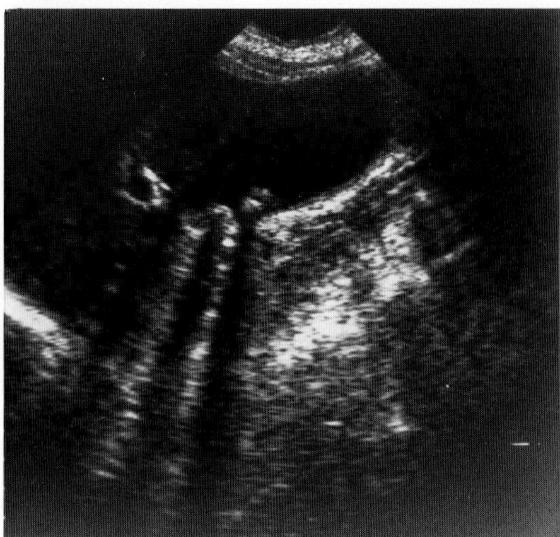

Figure 65. Longitudinal view of the gallbladder, which is somewhat distended and rounded in appearance (straight white arrows). Multiple echodensities with associated acoustic shadowing are demonstrated layering along the posterior wall of the gallbladder (open arrows).

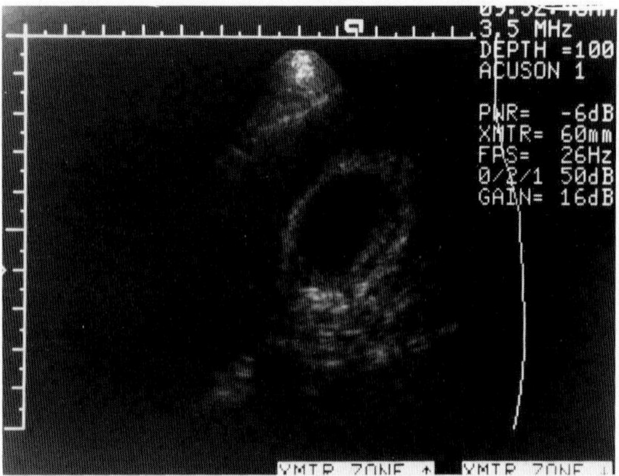

Figure 66. Transverse view of the gallbladder that reveals a rounded appearance to the gallbladder with a hypolucent, well-defined line seen within the wall of the gallbladder, an expression of edema (short white arrows).

undulating structures. In marked dilatation, finger-like projections of dilated bile ducts converging toward the left or right hepatic duct are frequently demonstrated. A subtle sign that is helpful in diagnosing dilated biliary radicles is enhanced transmission of the acoustic beam through the dilated ducts. This is not seen in either the portal or hepatic veins. The portal and hepatic venous systems can easily be differentiated under real-time examination by following the anatomical course of the vessels; the portal veins converge in the porta hepatis, and the hepatic veins are directed into the inferior vena cava. The walls of the portal veins are typically better demonstrated than the walls of the hepatic veins. The irregular-appearing walls of the biliary ducts allow better differentiation from the hepatic venous system. With marked dilatation of the intrahepatic biliary radicles, distended ducts are occasionally observed at the periphery of the liver, but it is most unusual to visualize portal veins.

The common hepatic duct should be visualized in all patients by locating it in relationship to the portal vein. The value chosen for the upper limits of normal for the diameter of the common hepatic duct will determine the sensitivity and specificity of the study. When a 4-mm internal diameter is used as the upper limit of normal, there is a sensitivity of 99% and a specificity of 87%. Using a larger value will improve the specificity at the expense of the sensitivity. The common bile duct must be carefully evaluated in every patient. It has

been demonstrated that the extrahepatic bile ducts may undergo rapid changes in caliber during radiological investigations. Rapid decreases in the size of the common duct can occur promptly with the passage of an impacted stone or the release of a ball-valve obstruction. There are abundant elastic fibers in the extrahepatic common bile duct walls

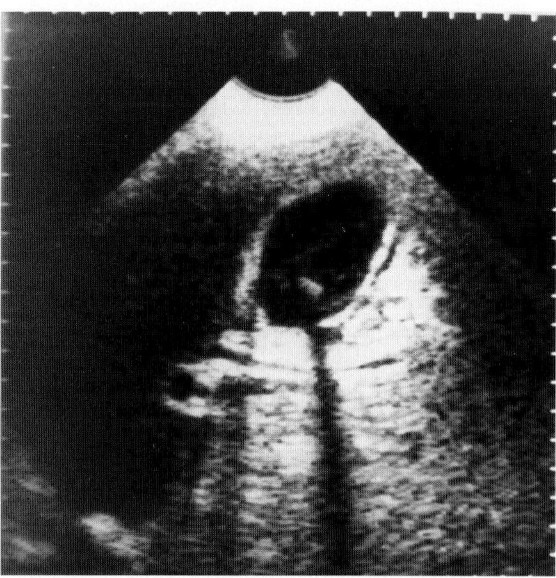

Figure 67. An oblique view of the gallbladder that demonstrates septations within the lumen of the gallbladder, which has a rounded appearance. In addition, a hypoacousant line (black arrowheads) is seen along the inferior wall of the gallbladder, an expression of edema of the wall. In addition, a high level echodensity with acoustic shadowing is seen floating within the lumen of the gallbladder (curved arrow). This is an example of empyema of the gallbladder.

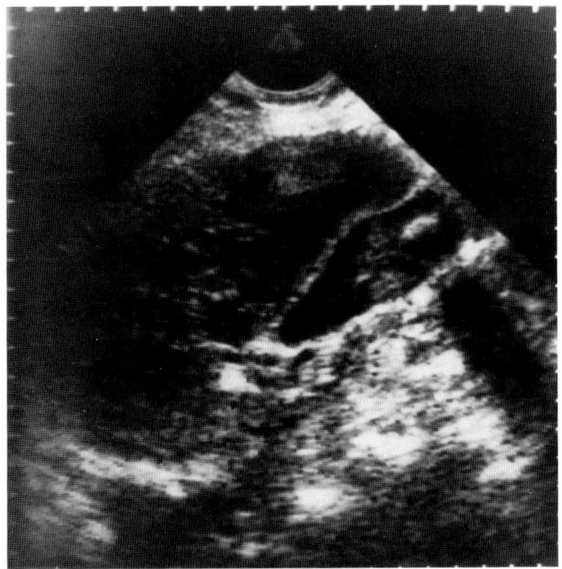

Figure 68. Sagittal view of the gallbladder demonstrated in Figure 67 showing the high level echo (straight white arrow) in the gallbladder lumen with associated septations and diffuse high level echoes within the gallbladder (small white arrows).

that allow for rapid duct expansion and recoil. Because there is little to no smooth muscle, active peristalsis does not occur.

It is difficult to compare duct measurements made ultrasonically with those made by endoscopic retrograde cholangiopancreatography (ERCP) or percutaneous transhepatic cholangiography; discrepancies which may result from several factors are invariably present. Changes in ductal size may be seen over short periods of time, and delay between different studies can easily account for differences. Another important factor is the magnification effect that takes place in radiographic examinations. Ultrasound measurements are made while the duct is in a physiological state, whereas measurements made during percutaneous cholangiography or ERCP are taken following the injection of contrast material at various introductal pressures and volumes.

The common bile duct should measure less than 7 mm in any patient who has not had a previous cholecystectomy; values in the range of 4–6 mm have been used as normal. In patients with an equivocal dilatation of the common duct, additional information can be obtained by administering a fatty meal and observing the changes that occur in the diameter of the duct. Under normal circumstances, a fatty meal will increase the flow of bile in the extrahepatic ducts while causing relaxation

of the sphincter of Oddi. In normal patients, a post–fatty meal sonogram shows a decrease in the diameter of the common duct in the range of 2–3 mm. Failure to see a decrease or increase in duct caliber is considered abnormal; it may be due to benign fibrosis, spasm of the sphincter of Oddi, or secondary choledocholithiasis. Use of the fatty meal demonstrates the dynamic nature of the common duct, with which sonographic techniques can further enhance diagnostic acuity.

The demonstration of stones within the common duct is a more difficult problem. They may be demonstrated as a typically appearing hyperechoic structure with distal acoustic shadowing. The absence of surrounding bile makes common duct stones difficult to differentiate from periductal structures, especially bowel. Most published series show a sensitivity in the range of 10–33% for the diagnosis of choledocholithiasis. A significant number of patients with choledocholithiasis will not manifest evidence of dilatation of the extrahepatic ductal system. In this group of patients, the diagnosis of choledocholithiasis cannot be made in 25–35%. When there is still a suspicion of common duct pathology, ERCP is recommended. This is also one of the few indications for an intravenous cholangiogram.

Hepatobiliary scintigraphy has very limited value in evaluating the common duct, except in postoperative patients. While massive dilatation of the duct can be conclusively demonstrated by scintigraphy, small degrees of enlargement cannot. Occasionally, it may be possible to demonstrate a large defect within the duct that represents a stone. He-

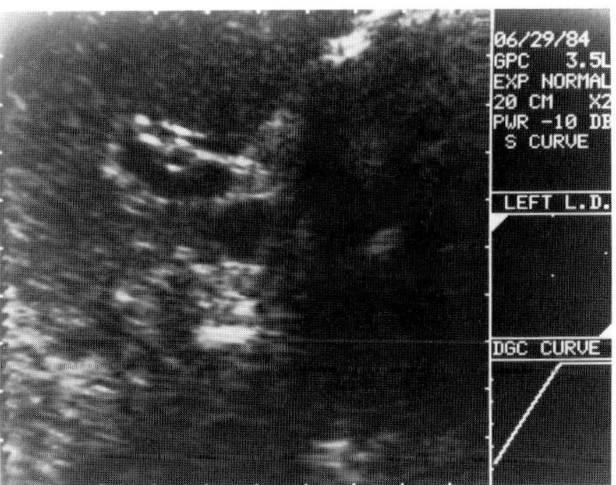

Figure 69. Sagittal view demonstrating the normal relationship of the common hepatic duct (straight white arrows), hepatic artery (curved short white arrow), and portal vein (straight large white arrows). The common hepatic duct measures no greater than 7 mm in anterior-posterior diameter.

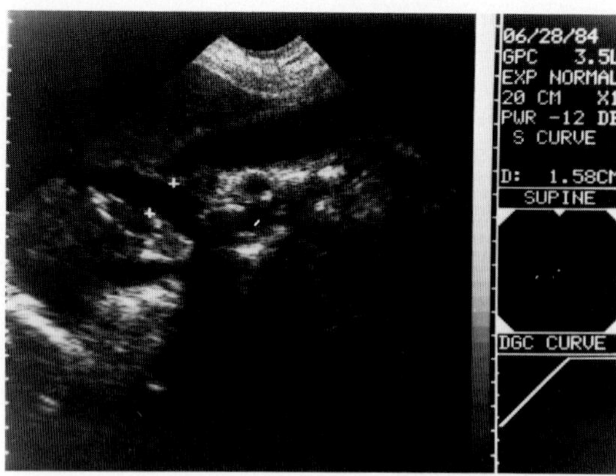

Figure 70.   Longitudinal view of the common hepatic duct, which measures 1.58 cm in anterior-posterior diameter. A curvilinear echodensity with associated acoustic shadowing is seen emanating from the lumen of the common duct. Impression: Choledocholithiasis. G.B. denotes the gallbladder. The anterior and posterior walls of the common duct are demarcated by the cross-hatched lines.

patobiliary scintigraphy is sometimes worthwhile in instances of common duct dilatation to demonstrate whether there is complete or partial obstruction. The demonstration of activity within the duodenum and the small bowel conclusively indicates incomplete obstruction.

THE POSTOPERATIVE PATIENT

Persistent or recurrent symptomatology following cholecystectomy or other biliary tract surgery is not uncommon. Following cholecystectomy, the reported range of symptomatic relief has been 50–88%. Even with a long symptom-free interval, however, it is not uncommon for signs and symptoms to reappear years after cholecystectomy. Ultrasound and hepatobiliary scintigraphy both offer useful and complementary information in the evaluation of postoperative patients. In these patients, despite numerous studies, there still remains some controversy concerning the so-called normal-sized common duct. The belief that the extrahepatic ducts may dilate postcholecystectomy was first proposed by Oddi in 1887. Numerous subsequent studies based on intravenous cholangiography have refuted this contention. In a study by Graham et al. employing ultrasound in 67 asymptomatic patients 4–16 months after cholecystectomy, 84% demonstrated common hepatic ducts with an internal diameter of 4 mm or less. Four patients had ducts measuring 5 mm, and seven patients had ducts measuring 6–10 mm. This study reveals that 16% of the asymptomatic group had hepatic ducts

ranging from 5 to 10 mm. In our experience with postcholecystectomy patients (with or without symptoms), we have encountered common hepatic duct enlargements as great as 10 mm without proven obstruction. This same observation has also been reported by other writers. The reasons for a dilated duct postoperatively without associated disease may be related to other factors, such as a combination of age, chronic inflammation of the duct wall, and previous dilatation that has not returned to normal. Other factors that still cannot be excluded on clinical or radiographic grounds are the recent passage of a ductal stone or low-grade ampullary stenosis. We recommend that whenever the duct size is in the range of 4–10 mm, a diligent search should be made to exclude pathology in or about the distal duct.

Ultrasound's difficulty in detecting retained stones in the common duct is one of its limitations. Hepatobiliary scintigraphy does offer additional information and can help to exclude pathology. In a study of 125 postcholecystectomy patients, Weissman et al. reported typical scintigraphic patterns (see Table 1). This group of patients had a larger variety of pathological conditions that ranged from biliary leaks to cystic duct remnants and retained ductal stones. There was a reported accuracy of 94.4% in detecting the associated pathology. The resolution of the hepatobiliary scintigraphy study does not identify the specific cause of obstruction; its ability to recognize biliary kinetics is a great diagnostic aid. The presence of ductal dilatation with functional patency, as shown by normal transit of the agent into the bowel, permits differentiation of patients with pathological conditions that show dilatation with an obstructive pattern. The ability to detect cystic duct remnants and biliary leakage with a high degree of certainty is a marked advantage of hepatobiliary scintigraphy. The evaluation of biliary kinetics with ^{99m}Tc-IDA compounds is not yet fully understood or utilized clinically. At present, we foresee that future development will undoubtedly add to its clinical usefulness.

In patients who present with signs and symptoms in the postcholecystectomy period, our examination consists first of an ultrasound scan, with careful attention paid to the biliary ducts and head of the pancreas. If the common hepatic duct measures less than 4 mm, retained stones or other obstructive pathology is unlikely. If the duct is in the range of 4–10 mm, hepatobiliary scintigraphy is of value in determining if normal biliary kinetics exist. Prolonged visualization of the ducts or delayed activity within the bowel suggests ductal pathology, and further evaluation by ERCP is recommended.

In those patients with ductal dilatation greater than 10 mm, hepatobiliary scintigraphy may be most useful in evaluating biliary kinetics. The presence of functional patency, without totally excluding the possibility of a retained common bile duct stone, should suggest the possibility of another diagnosis.

In patients with biliary enteroanastomoses, hepatobiliary scintigraphy also provides useful information concerning the patency of the anastomosis. In the latter group of patients, ultrasound examination is often difficult due to the distorted anatomy secondary to surgery. The frequent occurrence of air bubbles within the biliary system may mimic stones, and variable degrees of ductal dilatation may be seen following surgery. Scintigraphic patterns of complete or partial obstruction result in abnormal biliary kinetics similar to those seen in the postcholecystectomy patient. The degree of patency of an occlusion of the anastomosis can be demonstrated with a high degree of accuracy using hepatobiliary scintigraphy. The latter may probably be the procedure of choice.

CONCLUSIONS

It is clear that in a wide variety of pathological conditions affecting the biliary tract, ultrasound and hepatobiliary scintigraphy offer complementary information. *The high anatomical resolution of ultrasound, its high accuracy in detecting stones within the gallbladder, and its ability to evaluate other anatomical structures in the region of the gallbladder make ultrasound the procedure of first choice.* Hepatobiliary scintigraphy, on the other hand, provides information concerning biliary kinetics and the patency of the cystic and common ducts. *The latter cannot be deduced from the purely anatomical information attained by ultrasound. We believe that additional information, which improves the accuracy of diagnosis without risk to the patient, justifies the performance of a combined study in the majority of instances.*[*]

Recommended Reading

Bergman AB, Neiman HL, Draut B: Ultrasonographic evaluation of pericholecystic abscesses. *AJR* 132:201, 1979.

Berk RN, Ferrucci JT Jr, Fordtran JS, et al: The radiological diagnosis of gallbladder disease. *Radiology* 141:45, 1981.

Budvall B, Oevergaard B: Computer analysis of postch-

olecystectomy biliary tract systems. *Surg Gynecol Obstet* 124:723, 1967.

Brachman M, Levy R, Tanasescu D, et al: False-negative gallbladder scintigram in acute cholecystitis (letter to the editor). *J Nucl Med* 22:291, 1981.

Brown PH, Krishnamurthy Gt, Bobba VE, et al: Radiation dose calculation for five Tc-99m-IDA hepatobiliary agents. *J Nucl Med* 23:1030, 1982.

Callon PW, Filly RA: Ultrasonic localization of the gallbladder. *Radiology* 133:687, 1979.

Conrad MR, Janes JO, Dietchy J: Significance of low level echoes within the gallbladder. *AJR* 132:967, 1979.

Cooperberg PL, Pn MS, Wong P, et al: Real-time high-resolution ultrasound in the detection of biliary calculi. *Radiology* 131:789, 1979.

Cooperberg PL, Li D, Wong P, et al: Accuracy of common hepatic duct size in the evaluation of extrahepatic biliary obstruction. *Radiology* 135:141, 1980.

Crade M, Taylor KJW, Rosenfield AT, et al: Surgical and pathologic correlation of cholecystosonography and cholecystography. *Am J Roentgenol* 131:227, 1978.

Cronan JJ, Mueller PR, Simeone JF, et al: Prospective diagnosis of choledocholithiasis. *Radiology* 146:467, 1983.

Ferrucci JT Jr, Adson MA, Mueller PR, et al: Advances in the radiology of jaundice: A symposium and review. *AJR* 141:1, 1983.

Filly RA, Morse AA, Way LW: In vitro investigation of gallstone shadowing with ultrasound tomography. *J Clin Ultrasound* 7:255, 1979.

Fiske CE, Filly RA: Pseudo-sludge. *Radiology* 144:631, 1982.

Fiske CE, Laing FC, Brown TW: Ultrasonographic evidence of gallbladder wall thickening in association with hypoalbuminemia. *Radiology* 135:713, 1980.

Freitas JE: Cholescintigraphy in acute and chronic cholecystitis. *Semin Nucl Med* 12:18, 1982.

Freitas JE, Mirkes SH, Fink Bennett DM, et al: Suspected acute cholecystitis. Comparison of hepatobiliary scintigraphy versus ultrasonography. *Clin Nucl Med* 7:354, 1982.

Glazer GM, Filly RA, Laing FC: Rapid change in caliber of the nonobstructed common duct. *Radiology* 140:161, 1981.

Glenn F, McSherry C: Secondary abdominal operations for symptoms following biliary tract surgery. *Surg Gynecol Obstet* 121:979, 1965.

Graham MF, Cooperberg PL, Cohen MM, et al: The size of the normal common hepatic duct following cholecystectomy: An ultrasonographic study. *Radiology* 135:137, 1980.

Greenwald RA, Pereiras R, Morris SJ, et al: Jaundice, choledocholithiasis and a nondilated common duct. *JAMA* 240:1983, 1978.

Gross BH, Harter LP, Gore RM, et al: Ultrasonic evaluation of common bile duct stones: Prospective comparison with endoscopic retrograde cholangiopancreatography. *Radiology* 146:471, 1983.

Harbin WP, Ferrucci JT Jr, Wittenberg J, et al: Nonvisualized gallbladder by cholecystosonography. *AJR* 132:727, 1979.

Harvey E, Loberg M, Cooper M, et al: Tc-99m HIDA: A new radiopharmaceutical for hepatobiliary imaging (abstracted). *J Nucl Med* 16:533, 1975.

Hughes J, LoCurcio SB, Edmonds R, et al: The common bile duct after cholecystectomy. *JAMA* 197:247, 1966.

Jeffrey RB, Laing FC, Wong W, et al: Gangrenous cholecystitis: Diagnosis by ultrasound. *Radiology* 148:219, 1983.

---

[*]Author's note: The reader is referred to Chapter 8, "Chronic Cholelithiasis," in which the importance of a correct diagnosis is stressed.

Juttner HU, Ralls PW, Quin MF, et al: Thickening of the gallbladder wall in acute hepatitis: Ultrasound demonstration. *Radiology* 142:465, 1982.

Kalff V, Froelich JW, Lloyd R, et al: Predictive value of an abnormal hepatobiliary scan in patients with severe intercurrent illness. *Radiology* 146:191, 1983.

Kane RA: Ultrasonographic diagnosis of gangrenous cholecystitis and emphysema of the gallbladder. *Radiology* 134:191, 1980.

Klingensmith WC, Fritzberg AR, Spitzer VM, et al: Clinical comparison of diisoprophyl-IDA Tc 99m and diethyl-IDA Tc 99m for evaluation of the hepatobiliary system. *Radiology* 140:791, 1981.

Klingensmith WC, Spitzer VM, Fritzberg AR, et al: The normal fasting and postpradial diisopropyl-IDA Tc 99m hepatobiliary study. *Radiology* 141:771, 1981.

Krishnamurthy Gt, Turner FE: Letter to the editor, *SNM Newsline*, March 1984.

Krook PM, Allen RH, Bush WH Jr, et al: Comparison of real-time cholecystectosonography and oral cholecystography. *Radiology* 135:145, 1980.

Larsen MJ, Klingensmith WC, Kuni CC: Radionuclide hepatobiliary imaging: Non-visualization of the gallbladder secondary to prolonged fasting. *J Nucl Med* 23:1003, 1982.

Lecklitner ML, Rosen PR, Nusynowitz M: Cholescintigraphy: Gallbladder nonvisualization secondary to neoplasm. *J Nucl Med* 22:699, 1981.

LeQuesne LP, Whiteside CG, Hand BF: The common bile duct after cholecystectomy. *Br Med J* 5118:329, 1959.

Longo MF, Hodgson JR, Ferris DO: The size of the common bile duct following cholecystectomy. *Ann Surg* 165:250, 1967.

McIntosh DMF, Penney HF: Gray-scale ultrasonography as a screening procedure in the detection of gallbladder disease. *Radiology* 136:725, 1980.

Marchal FJF, Casaer M, Baert AL, et al: Gallbladder wall sonolucency in acute cholecystitis. *Radiology* 133:429, 1979.

Massie JD, Moinuddin M, Phillips JC: Acute calculous cholecystitis with patent cystic duct. *Am J Roentgenol* 141:39, 1983.

Maturo VG, Zusmer NR, Smoak WM III, et al: The role of biliary scintigraphy and ultrasonography in the diagnosis of cholecystitis. *Revista Interamericana Radiologia*, 6:47, 1981.

Mauro MA, McCarney WH, Melmed JR: Hepatobiliary scanning with ^{99m}Tc PIPIDA in acute cholecystitis. *Radiology* 142:193, 1982.

Mueller PR, Ferrucci JT Jr, Simeone JF, et al: Observations on the distensibility of the common bile duct. *Radiology* 142:467, 1982.

Oddi R: D'une disposition a sphincter speciale de l'ouverture du canal choledoque. *Arch Ital Biol* 8:317, 1887.

Raptopoulos V, D'Orsi C, Smith E, et al: Dynamic cholecystosonography of the contracted gallbladder: The double-arc-shadow sign. *AJR* 138:275, 1982.

Sample WF, Sarti DA, Goldstein LI, et al: Gray-scale ultrasonography of the jaundiced patient. *Radiology* 128:719, 1978.

Samuels BI, Freitas JE, Bree RL, et al: A comparison of radionuclide hepatobiliary imaging and real-time ultrasound for the detection of acute cholecystitis. *Radiology* 147:207, 1983.

Sanders RC: The significance of sonographic wall thickening. *J Clin Ultrasound* 8:143, 1980.

Schein CJ, Beneventano TC: Choledochal dynamics in man. *Surg Gynecol Obstet* 126:591, 1968.

Scheske GA, Cooperberg PL, Cohen MM, et al: Dynamic changes in the caliber of the major bile ducts related to obstruction. *Radiology* 135:215, 1980.

Shuman WP, Gibbs P, Rudd TG, et al: PIPIDA scintigraphy for cholecystitis: False positives in alcoholism and total parenteral nutrition. *Am J Roentgenol* 138:1, 1982.

Simeone JF, Mueller PR, Ferrucci JT Jr, et al: Sonography of the bile ducts after a fatty meal: An aid in the detection of obstruction. *Radiology* 143:211, 1982.

Sommer FG, Taylor KJW: Differentiation of acoustic shadowing due to calculi and gas collections. *Radiology* 135:399, 1980.

Sukov RJ, Sample WF, Sarti DA, et al: Cholecystosonography—the junctional fold. *Radiology* 133:435, 1979.

Sullivan RJ, Eaton SB Jr, Ferrucci JT Jr, et al: Cholangiographic manifestations of acute biliary colic. *N Engl J Med* 288:33, 1973.

Taavitsainen M, Jarvinen H, Tallroth K: Cholescintigraphy in the diagnosis of acute cholecystitis. *Ann Clin Res* 10:227, 1978.

Way LW: Diseases of the gallbladder and bile ducts, in Beeson PB, McDermott W, Wyngaarden JB (eds.): *Textbook of Medicine*. Philadelphia, WB Saunders Co, 1979.

Weill F, Eisencher A, Zeltner F: Ultrasonic study of the normal and dilated biliary tree. *Radiology* 127:221, 1978.

Wise RE: Current concepts of intravenous cholangiography. *Radiol Clin North Am* 4:521, 1966.

Worthen NJ, Uszler JM, Funamura JL: Cholecystitis: Prospective evaluation of sonography and 99m-Tc-HIDA cholescintigraphy. *AJR* 137:973, 1981.

Zeman RK, Segal HB, Caride VJ: Tc-99m HIDA cholescintigraphy: The distended photon-deficient gallbladder. *J Nucl Med* 22:39, 1981.

Zeman RK, Lee C, Stahl RS, et al: Ultrasound and hepatobiliary scintigraphy in the assessment of biliary-enteric anastomosis. *Radiology* 145:109, 1982.

Zeman RK, Burrell MI, Cahow Ce, et al: Diagnostic utility of cholescintigraphy and ultrasonography in acute cholecystitis. *Am J Surg* 141:446, 1981.

Zusmer NR, Janowitz WR: *Ultrasound and Scintigraphy of the Biliary Tree: Ultrasound Annual, 1984*. New York, Raven Press, 1984.

References

1. Leopold GR, Sokoloff J: Ultrasonic scanning in the diagnosis of biliary disease. *Surg Clin North Am* 53:1043, 1973.

2. Taplin GV, Meredith OM, Kade H: The radioactive 1–131 tagged rose bengal uptake excretion test for liver function using external gamma ray scintillation counting techniques, 1955.

3. Baker RJ, Bellen JC, Ronai PM: ^{99m}Tc-pyridoxylidene glutamate: A new rapid cholescintigraphic agent. *J Nucl Med* 15:476, 1974.

4. Chervu LR, Nunn AD, Loberg MD: Radiopharmaceuticals for hepatobiliary imaging. *Semin Nucl Med* 12:5, 1982

5. Laing FC, Federle MP, Jeffrey RB, et al: Ultrasonic evaluation of patients with acute right upper quadrant pain. *Radiology* 140:449, 1981.

6. Laing FC, Jeffrey RB: Choledocholithiasis and cystic duct obstruction: Difficult ultrasonographic diagnoses. *Radiology* 146:475, 1983.
7. Weissman HS, Sugarman LA, Freeman LM: The clinical role of technetium-99m iminodiacetic acid cholescintigraphy, in Freeman LM, Weissman HS (eds): *Nuclear Medicine Annual 1981.* New York, Raven Press, 1981.
8. Weissman HS, Frank MS, Bernstein LH, et al: Rapid and accurate diagnosis of acute cholecystitis with 99mTc-HIDA cholescintigraphy. *AJR* 132:523, 1979.
9. Weissman HS, Badia J, Sugarman LA, et al: Spectrum of 99m-Tc-IDA cholescintigraphic patterns in acute cholecystitis. *Radiology* 138:167, 1981.
10. Weissman HS, Berkowitz M, Fox MS, et al: The role of technetium-99m iminodiacetic acid (IDA) cholescintigraphy in acute acalculus cholecystitis. *Radiology* 146:177, 1983.
11. Weissman HS, Gludman ML, Wilk PJ, et al: Evaluation of the postoperative patient with Tc-99m-IDA cholescintigraphy. *Semin Nucl Med* 12:27, 1982.

Intraoperative Ultrasonography

W. Kirt Nichols, M.D., F.A.C.S.

Ultrasound (B-mode) imaging is an important diagnostic method used to detect biliary and pancreatic disease. In our institution, transcutaneous, real-time, B-mode ultrasound scanning is the procedure of choice to detect cholelithiasis. It is often used as the principal screening test in patients suspected of having chronic cholecystitis and/or cholelithiasis.

Ultrasound has been used intraoperatively during biliary surgery on a sporadic basis since the early 1960s. The earliest efforts used A-mode ultrasound, but more recent reports are limited to real-time, high-resolution, B-mode ultrasound imaging.

Two major factors appear to have limited more widespread use in the operating room. First, there has been the lack of an easy-to-use, truly portable scanner. Second, there seems to be a reluctance on the part of surgeons/clinicians to learn to use a large, complex, expensive piece of electronic equipment in an operating room setting. In addition, the information in an ultrasound image is not always intuitive; one must learn to interpret what the image represents. One observer notes that the images resemble the satellite weather maps seen on television newscasts.

This section briefly presents our preliminary experience in evaluating the biliary tract with a new, portable, "user-friendly," real-time, B-mode ultrasound scanner. The patients studied were undergoing either a gastric bypass procedure for

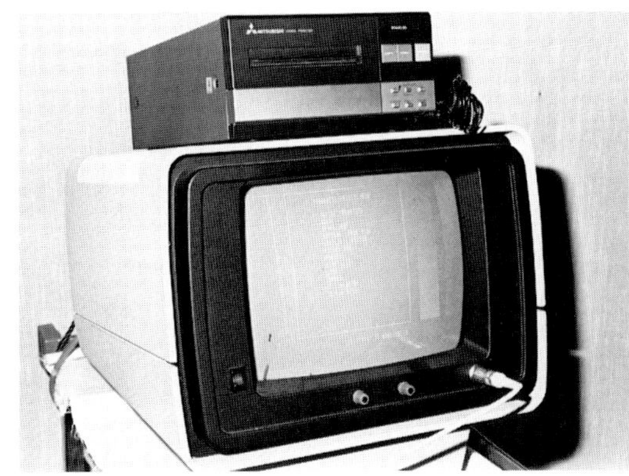

Figure 71. The Linscan™ Imaging System.

morbid obesity or a cholecystectomy, typically for recurrent attacks of cholecystitis.

METHOD

A Linscan Imaging System (Linscan Systems, Inc., Rolla, MO) real-time, B-mode, high-resolution ultrasound scanner was used (Fig. 71). The Linscan probe is shaped like a hockey stick and fitted or equipped with a 10-MHz transducer. It is mechanically driven to sweep a rectilinear scan 27 mm wide and 37 mm deep at a rate of 15 frames per second. The transducer has a focal zone between 10 and 15 mm.

The probe can be cold sterilized by soaking. However, we prefer a technique in which the probe and cord are placed inside a sterile plastic sleeve, which can then be used in the operative field (Fig. 72). This technique allows rapid, repetitive use of the same probe in different operations. A thin layer of acoustic coupling gel is placed between the probe and the inside of the plastic sheath.

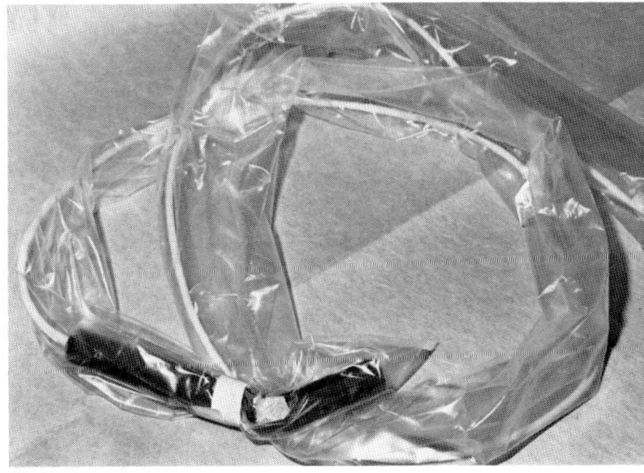

Figure 72. Probe and sterile plastic sheath for use in the operative field.

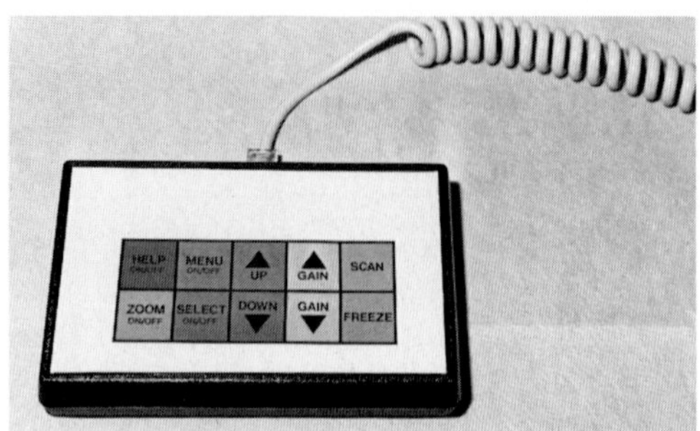

Figure 73. Membrane keypad used "off the table" to select functions or mode of operation.

The system's electronics are controlled by a state-of-the-art microprocessor. The functions are menu driven and controlled by a membrane key pad (Fig. 73) away from the operative field after the initial setup. This feature greatly simplifies the use of the machine during an operation. The real-time image may be recorded on a high-quality videotape recorder, or a hard copy of the video image for the patient's record can be obtained using either a Polaroid film camera or a video printer.

TECHNIQUE

The operative field is approached in a standard fashion. No special provisions are necessary. Visual and manual examinations of the abdominal organs are carried out as usual.

To scan the biliary tree fully, a Kocher maneuver should be performed before the ultrasound examination.

We usually scan the gallbladder first to confirm the presence and size of any calculi. Next, we methodically scan the extrahepatic bile ducts, beginning at the liver hilum with the hepatic ducts and progressing distally to the retroduodenal common bile duct (Fig. 74).

Sterile saline solution is maintained between the outside of the plastic sheath and the organ being scanned to provide a good acoustic window which permits imaging of the gallbladder or bile duct walls.

In this early evaluation, we still confirm our clinical and ultrasound scan impressions with conventional intraoperative cholangiography.

RESULTS

The gallbladder wall is typically echogenic and thin. Figure 75 is a sonogram of a normal gallbladder. The transducer in this and subsequent sonograms is at the top of the field. The transducer produces

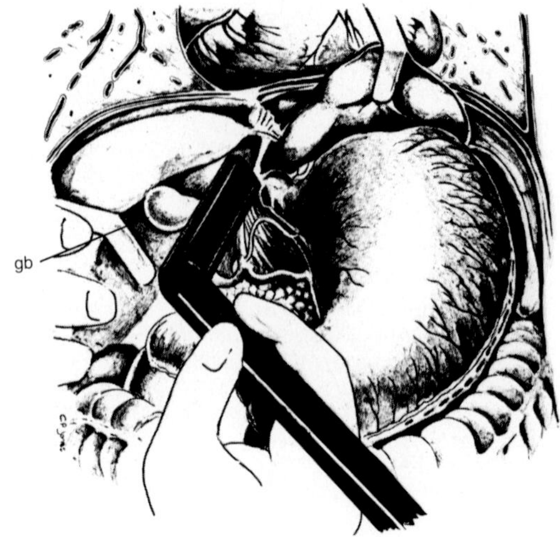

Figure 74. Schematic representation showing intraoperative scan of gallbladder (gb).

tissue "slices" that have approximately the size and configuration of a credit card. The top of the screen is superficial, and the bottom shows the deeper aspects of the organ. The location of the "heel" of the probe is variable, but is typically displayed at the left of the screen.

Calculi are seen as echoes represented in the image as an area of increased intensity (open arrows). Deep to or behind each calculus is an area known as an *acoustic shadow* (Fig. 76).

Figure 77 is a gallbladder viewed longitudinally. Its diameter can be accurately measured using the calibrated grid on the video monitor, which here shows a gallbladder 1.5–2.5 cm in diameter. Note the gallbladder polyp (arrow).

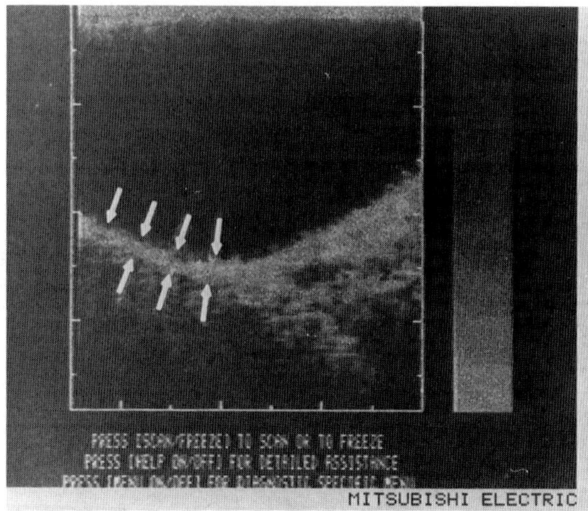

Figure 75. Normal gallbladder. Note the 3 mm echogenic wall (between arrows).

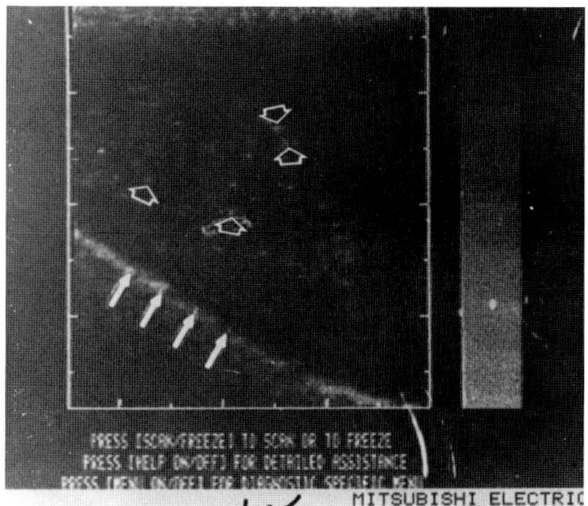

Figure 76. Gallbladder containing multiple calculi (open arrows). Note increased intensity of image representing echo. The gallbladder wall is the echogenic area shown by the solid arrows.

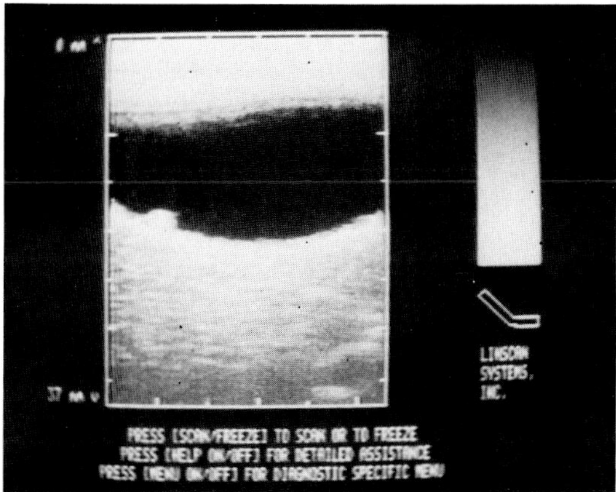

Figure 77. Gallbladder containing polyp (at arrow).

Figure 78 is a common bile duct view longitudinally. The caliber of the duct can be accurately measured using the calibrated grid on the video monitor, which here shows a duct 0.6–0.7 cm in diameter.

Figure 79 represents a dilated biliary ductal system in a patient with carcinoma of the head of the pancreas. Note the right and left hepatic ducts in transverse section. They measure approximately 1.5–2 cm in diameter.

COMMENT

Our preliminary experience with intraoperative ultrasonography has confirmed the ease of application of this diagnostic modality. The technique is relatively quick compared to that of intraoperative cholangiography, and although our numbers are quite small at present, the procedure seems accurate and reproducible.

Patients undergoing elective cholecystectomy for cholelithiasis generally have the presence of stones confirmed preoperatively. In other situations, when a surgeon is operating for another intra-abdominal condition, assessment of the gallbladder is routinely done. In certain instances, such as morbid obesity, the presence of calculi in the gallbladder may lead to cholecystectomy in addition to the planned gastric bypass procedure. Palpation of the gallbladder to detect calculi is usually reliable if the stones are large. However, the procedure is much

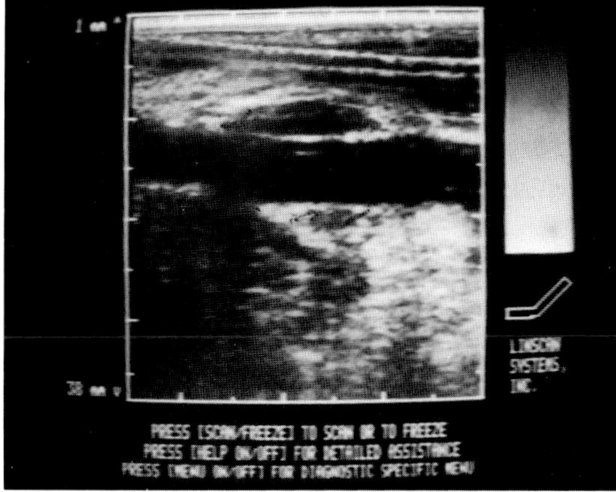

Figure 78. Normal common bile duct measuring 0.6–0.7 cm.

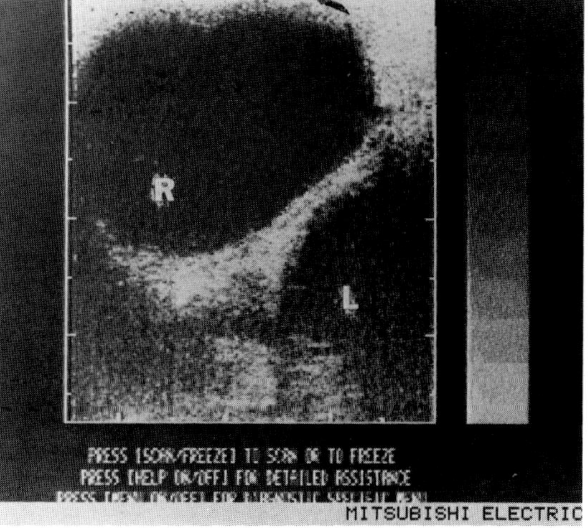

Figure 79. Dilated right and left hepatic ducts in a patient with obstructive jaundice secondary to an obstructing head of pancreas adenocarcinoma. The ducts measure approximately 1.5–2.0 cm in transverse diameter.

less reliable if the gallbladder is distended, has thickened walls, or is distorted by adhesions or inflammation. Operative sonography may provide valuable information about the presence of calculi in such instances.

Sigel et al. [1-4] indicate the most important applications of intraoperative ultrasonography which may be applied in the assessment of the extrahepatic bile ducts. An unanswered question is whether intraoperative ultrasound studies complement or replace intraoperative cholangiography or choledochoscopy. Certainly, operative cholangiography has reduced the number of unnecessary common bile duct explorations. Yet the cost effectiveness of this study has been questioned.[5] Sigel et al. have repeatedly shown that intraoperative ultrasound of the biliary tree provides results comparable to those of cholangiography.[1-4,6] They propose substituting intraoperative ultrasonography for intraoperative cholangiography in patients who, by their history and other examinations, are at low risk for having common duct stones.

Operative ultrasonography is a safe and quick procedure. It takes only about 5 minutes to scan the gallbladder and biliary ducts adequately, compared with an average of 30 minutes[7,8] for intraoperative cholangiography. A recent report concludes that intraoperative ultrasonography is safe and that there are no published reports of harm to patients caused by diagnostic ultrasound.[9]

Ultrasound studies provide dynamic information in real time, which intraoperative cholangiography cannot do. This is not apparent from a review of the static sonograms which accompany this chapter. A study in real time gives immediate feedback to the examiner which allows for rapid alterations or corrections in the technique of scanning. This is a difficult concept to convey, but the quality of the scans is operator dependent and the immediate feedback leads to a much better image with more information.

One disadvantage of ultrasound is its inability to display the anatomy of the entire ductal system at once. Intrahepatic radicles must be scanned one by one, if at all, and there is a potential danger of overlooking a stone in the intrahepatic biliary ducts. Nevertheless, I believe that the use of intraoperative ultrasound does have merit and promise.

THE FUTURE

The role of intraoperative ultrasonography in biliary tract disease is still to be determined. As more surgeons acquire and become familiar with its application, the significance of ultrasound will be de-

cided. It is a quick procedure and provides accurate information about some anatomical aspects of the biliary tract. It provides complementary information to intraoperative cholangiography and may replace that study in patients who are at low risk for choledocholithiasis.

To become popular, the equipment must be portable, must be easy to use, and must provide good, high-resolution images. Surgeons will need to learn to interpret the images and gain the expertise to operate the scanner. This has already been done with intraoperative Doppler ultrasound and can be done with intraoperative B-mode ultrasound in biliary surgery.

References

1. Sigel B, Coelho JC, Spigos DG, et al: Ultrasonic imaging during biliary and pancreatic surgery. *Am J Surg* 141:84, 1981.
2. Sigel B, Coelho JC, Nyhus LM, et al: Comparison of cholangiography and ultrasonography in the operative screening of the common bile duct. *World J Surg* 6:440, 1982.
3. Sigel B: Ultrasonography during biliary tract surgery, in *Operative Ultrasonography*. Philadelphia, Lea & Febiger, 1982.
4. Sigel B, Machi J, Anderson K III, et al: Operative sonography of the biliary tree and pancreas. *Semin Ultrasound, CT, MR* 6:2, 1985.
5. Skillings JC, Williams JS, Hinshaw JR: Cost-effectiveness of operative cholangiography. *Am J Surg* 137:26, 1979.
6. Sigel B, Coelho JC, Spigos DG, et al: Real-time ultrasonography during biliary surgery. *Radiology* 137:531, 1980.
7. Knight PR, Nevell JA: Operative use of ultrasonics in cholelithiasis. *Lancet* 1:1023, 1963.
8. Mogenstern L: Discussion. Digel B, Coelho JC, Spigos DG, Donahue PE, Wood DK, Nyhus LM: Ultrasonic imaging during biliary and pancreatic surgery. *Am J Surg* 141:89, 1981.
9. Diagnostic and therapeutic technology assessment. In Questions and Answers (DATTA). *JAMA* 254:285, 1985.

The Role of Radiation Therapy for Carcinoma of the Biliary Tract

Leonard M. Toonkel, M.D.

Because of the rich lymphatic network of the biliary submucosa and the relative proximity of the surrounding critical organs, primary tumors of the biliary tree tend at presentation to be in locally advanced or technically unresectable stages. These same factors account for the high local relapse rate following primary surgical extirpation of earlier resectable and presumed curable tumors. As biliary obstruction will cause progressive symptomatology and result in the death of the patient, effective palliative therapy can be expected to prolong the patient's survival. The role of radiation therapy is therefore twofold: firstly, as an adjunct to surgery for resectable lesions, and secondly, as a palliative modality for locally advanced, unresectable, or recurrent disease.

In a review of all surgical procedures for biliary tract cancer at the Massachusetts General Hospital, Kopelson et al.[1] reported that only 28 curative operations were performed on 82 patients. Local-regional failure occurred in 13 of 25 postoperative survivors, and 81% of all relapses had a component of local-regional failure. Despite these disappointing results with surgery alone, relatively few patients have been treated with postoperative radiation therapy.

Vaittinen[2] reported a median survival of 63 months for 7 patients receiving postoperative radiotherapy following curative resections for biliary cancer compared with 29 months for 24 patients treated by operation alone. The notion that tumors of the biliary tract are radioresistant probably accounts for the paucity of clinical data regarding adjunctive radiation therapy. While modern radiobiological principles base tumor radio resistance more on the quantity of malignant collagens (tumor burden) than on histological differences, it is likely that biliary tumors earned their reputation as radioresistant lesions due to the inability to deliver an adequate dosage of radiation because of the limited radio tolerance of surrounding normal tissues. Technical advances in radiation therapy over the last decade, including the development of high-energy linear accelerators (greater than 10 MeV), computed treatment planning interfaced with diagnostic computed tomograph scanning, and customized focus shielding, now permit the delivery of 4500–5500 cGy to the region of the porta hepatis with limited radiotoxicity, and postoperative radiation treatment is now recommended following most extirpative procedures for biliary tract cancer.

While significant palliation and occasional long-term survival can be seen with external beam radiation therapy used alone for locally advanced lesions, effective dose delivery requires precise tumor volume localization, optimally obtained by laparoscopy, and careful clipping of unresectable tumor. Biliary tract cancer provides an interesting model for two new radiation modalities that seek to increase the ability to deliver tumoricidal doses to the volume at risk while minimizing the exposure of sensitive surrounding structures. The first of these is transcatheter iridium-192 brachytherapy, in which the biliary drainage tubes are used to introduce small radioactive sources permitting the delivery of 4000–6000 cGy at a distance of 1.0 cm from the sources over 3–4 days. Several authors have reported encouraging short-term results using either transcatheter brachytherapy alone or as a "boost" technique combined with external treatment.[3-6]

Another promising modality is intraoperative electron beam therapy, in which a single massive fraction of electron beam irradiation (limited penetration) is delivered to unresected tumor under direct visualization under surgical control, with exclusion of normal tissues from the irradiated field. Intraoperative electron beam therapy has been employed as the sole palliative treatment in Japan but, like transcatheter iridium-192 therapy, is being investigated primarily as a boost technique in this country.[7]

Long-term preservation of the nonobstructed biliary system, preferably without permanent indwelling catheters which risk the development of ascending cholangitis, remains the major goal of palliative therapy of these most challenging tumors.

References

1. Kopelson G, Galdabini J, Warshaw A, et al: Patterns of failure after curative surgery for extrahepatic biliary tract carcinoma. *Int J Radiol Oncol Biol Phys* 7:413, 1981.
2. Vaittinen E: Carcinoma of the gallbladder. *Ann Chir Gynaecol* 168:1, 1970.
3. Herskovic A, Heaston D, Engler MJ, et al: Irradiation of biliary carcinoma. *Radiology* 139:219, 1981.
4. Chitwood WR Jr: Diagnosis and treatment of primary extrahepatic biliary duct tumors. *Am J Surg* 143:99, 1982.
5. Herskovic AM, Engler MJ, Noell KT: Radical radiotherapy for bile duct carcinoma. *Endocurie Hypertherm Oncol* 1:119, 1985.
6. Fletcher MS, Dowson JL, Wheeler PG, et al: Treatment of high bile duct carcinoma by internal radiotherapy with iridium-192 wire. *Lancet* 2:172, 1981.
7. Tepper JE: Intraoperative radiation therapy, in Perez C, Brady L (eds): *Principles and Practice of Radiation Oncology*. Philadelphia, JB Lippincott Co, 1987.

6

JAUNDICE

Introduction

Today, in undergraduate and postgraduate medical education, not enough stress is placed upon bedside diagnosis. The latter has become an accomplishment of the past; one rarely encounters a situation where the resident, internist, or surgeon makes an astute diagnosis at the bedside. Today one has merely to look at the size of the average hospital chart to see that a major portion of it is made up of laboratory data, blood tests, immunoassay studies, and more tests; often tests are costly and sophisticated studies are most expensive. When one opens the chart and looks for the history of the patient, one may or may not find it; if one does find the history, the chances are that it is brief, rather incomplete, or totally inadequate. Not infrequently, a good history is recorded; rarely, an exceptional one. A good history is still something to be hoped for.

My purpose in starting this complex chapter on jaundice with a plea for the return of the bedside diagnosis is to make an effort to simplify the differential diagnosis of jaundice. It is an attempt to show that a physician with a good knowledge of disease patterns can, by direct and knowledgeable questioning, come extremely close to differentiating a medical from a surgical jaundice. When additional assistance is required, more specific chemical and enzymatic blood studies are selected to elucidate further the underlying cause of the jaundice. There will, of course, be more difficult instances where the determination of the exact etiology, despite a good history and complete physical examination, will require additional sophisticated studies, such as blood studies, X-rays, percutaneous transhepatic cholangiography, needle biopsies, ultrasonic (sonographic) studies, computed tomography scans, and, ultimately, retrograde endoscopic choledochopancreatography and arteriography.

Jaundice, or the diffuse yellowing of the skin, may be caused by variable factors, both medical and surgical. Jaundice is not always due to a biliary obstruction; it may be due to infectious bacterial and viral causes; it may also be due to blood dyscrasias, such as hemolytic jaundice. Jaundice may be due to secondary viral involvement, as a result of direct blood transfusion, or viruses that cause hepatitis with jaundice. The commoner causes of jaundice are usually obstructive, and they ultimately become surgical problems. The causes, in order of their frequency, are stones in the common duct, with or without infection; benign or malignant neoplasms; and congenital atresias in the early phases of life. Jaundice is not an easy diagnosis to make in most instances; in many cases, it can be most perplexing.

Whenever possible, cases of jaundice should be dealt with jointly by the internist and the surgeon. Each can assist the other in making a more accurate definitive diagnosis, which can frequently be lifesaving. To enter in error into a surgical procedure for an infectious hepatitis that simulates an obstructive jaundice may result in a very sick or dead patient. It is also possible that a hepatitis, liver necrosis, or parenchymatous degeneration can be caused by faulty anesthesia. Hepatitis, liver necrosis, or liver degeneration, when operated upon needlessly, can result in serious postoperative complications and even death. To avoid such catastrophic errors, it is imperative that a diagnosis be made judiciously and without haste.

In making a differential diagnosis, one must utilize every diagnostic means at one's disposal in addition to a thorough physical examination. The diagnostic armamentarium should be up-to-date and should include all assistance possible from the departments of internal medicine, hematology, nuclear medicine, gastroenterology, and, of course, the general laboratory. Very often the laboratory will report equivocal results that further confuse and complicate the disease pattern. There are also studies that will require weeks before an answer can be attained, but these tests are of no consequence and no value in those cases in which a diagnosis must be made quickly. There should be enough time to get laboratory results in difficult cases where surgery is being contemplated. Not infrequently, the surgeon will keep the internist in abeyance because the latter may be too hasty in recommending surgery. The surgeon knows only too well that a postoperative death following an inaccurate diagnosis and premature exploratory laparotomy remains the surgeon's full responsibility, no matter how many consultants are on the case. This writer remembers various patients whose bilirubin level rose to 38–40 mg/100 ml with surgery appearing imminent, yet the evidence indicated that though the jaundice was deep and painless, there was no sign of weight loss, no significant change in appetite, and no liver changes, except elevated enzyme levels that, over time, fluctuated, dropped intermittently, and then rose again. Confusion persisted for weeks, yet surgery was delayed. Unexpectedly during the observation period, a sudden drop in bilirubin occurred, which, of course, may have been due to necrosis of a carcinoma of the ampulla that suddenly allowed the bile to pass; however, it may also have been a result of favorable changes in the liver, such as control of infection with reduction in edema. Regeneration allows an appreciable drop in bilirubin, or a ball-valve gallstone may have been present; in either case, one is encouraged to wait. If the waiting period does not allow the bilirubin to drop adequately and the enzymes, such as alkaline phosphatase, lactic dehydrogenase (LDH), and serum glutamic oxaloacetic transaminase (SGOT), remain elevated, it may become imperative to select a still more sophisticated study such as percutaneous transhepatic cholangiography as a last resort. Because of the serious nature of this test, and the need for immediate surgical intervention if sudden bleeding occurs, a surgical reservation should first be established with the operating room.

In cases of severe obstructive jaundice where the doctors, both medical and surgical, are undecided, transhepatic cholangiographic studies may reveal the exact site and cause of the obstruction. It may possibly rule out surgery, especially where obstruction cannot be demonstrated. An obstruction, if found, may be neoplastic, calculous, or neither. In cases where neoplasia is found to be the cause of obstruction, it may already be too late for surgery. To intervene surgically where no obstruction exists would be foolhardy. If stones are discovered, then, of course, surgery should be carried out at the propitious time. If jaundice continues to increase asymptomatically, it does not call for surgery unless there is evidence of associated pain, toxicity, leukocytosis, chills, and fever. These symptoms and signs indicate that a common duct stone is the most likely cause. Jaundice may increase without fever, chills, and pain, and may still be due to a calculous origin. The safest decision is to delay, because greater error and higher mortality will follow inadvertent, hasty surgical intervention. Given the risk of fatality, the surgeon must be conservative, but not too conservative, in the presence of certain facts that may indicate the need for urgent surgical intervention.

Laboratory tests will assist in determining whether the jaundice is due to parenchymatous liver destruction, as in hepatitis, cirrhosis, and varied forms of cholestasis. They will also help evaluate the type of obstruction, i.e., whether or not a virus infection or calculi are the cause, or whether the jaundice is due to a benign or malignant tumor. Table 1 is a list of tests in chart form to help differentiate the various types of jaundice.

Laboratory data correlated with X-ray studies, and the patient's clinical picture, will usually suffice to give the surgeon the necessary information for deciding whether surgery is indicated. There is no emergency in most cases. The investigational period will usually prevent needless laparotomy in those cases where intrahepatic pathology exists. The time utilized in evaluating the ultimate diagnosis will be well spent in better preparing the patient preoperatively for possible surgery. Despite all the studies and precautions taken, there will be instances where the diagnosis may be so complex that a tentative decision for surgery may have to be made even in the absence of proof of extrahepatic obstruction. Often the final diagnosis will be established after surgical exploration.

Welch[1] made reference to the anesthetic halothane as a causative factor in postoperative jaundice. In a study at the University of Oregon, 736 open heart operations were performed in which 63 patients developed postoperative jaundice, with two deaths developing from liver necrosis. There have been many anesthetists who have concluded that halothane and shock were the most relevant causal factors. The anesthetists believe that there appears to be a greater danger if the administration of halothane anesthesia has to be repeated. Kantrowitz et al.[2] reported four cases in which severe jaundice developed after surgery for the control of massive hemorrhage into body tissues. The jaundice was ascribed to the increased pigment load in the presence of decreased hepatic function, primarily because of shock. Low-grade jaundice may be due to idiopathic unconjugated hyperbilirubinemia; the latter was reported by Powell et al.[3]

Percutaneous transhepatic cholangiography using the skinny Chiba needle is considered a procedure of last resort in cases of jaundice where all available data are equivocal and therefore not sufficient to make a positive diagnosis. In most cases, the injected dye will pinpoint the exact site of obstruction and often the precise nature of the obstruction. If the liver problem is hepatocellular, little or no bile will be obtained and visualization of the biliary tract should no longer be attempted. A liver biopsy may be appropriate at this time. The surgeon must be aware of the possibility of complications that may follow transhepatic cholangiography. Perforation of the biliary tree can result in a retrograde escape of bile, especially when there is an extrahepatic obstruction. The operating room and the surgeon must stand by for immediate emergency surgery. The second complication may be hemorrhage; this will be due to inadvertent injury to a blood vessel. Regardless of the cause of the jaundice, the patient must be closely observed, especially in cases where surgery is contraindicated. Nevertheless, here too, the operating room and the surgeon must be ready to intervene at any time.

Table 1. Laboratory Studies in the Differential Diagnosis of Jaundice

	Extrahepatic Common Bile Duct Obstruction	Intrahepatic (Nonobstructive: Hepatitis-Viruses A, B; Toxic Hepatitis)	Neoplastic (Cancer of the Biliary Tree—Lymphomas; Cancer of the Ampulla; Cancer of the Head of the Pancreas)	Hemolytic
Alkaline phosphatase	High; increases with the duration of obstruction	Normal; increases later	Normal to high; depends if obstructive liver necrosis develops	Normal
LDH, SGOT	Early—normal to slightly elevated; later—elevated; as SGOT falls—LDH may rise	High; may fluctuate up and down	Normal to high; depends on degree of liver necrosis	Normal
Total bilirubin Van den Bergh—direct and indirect	High—Direct; increases with increasing obstruction; low—indirect—suggests intrahepatic cause	High—indirect; low—direct; occasionally, direct-indirect	High in obstructive type; elevation depends on degree of obstruction and involvement	Total—5–20 ml; direct—normal or increased; indirect—decreased
Urobilinogen (urinary and fecal)	Complete obstruction—incomplete obstruction—decreased; complete obstruction—absent	Normal to increased obstruction	Depends on degree of obstruction	Normal to increased
Australian antigen	Negative	Positive (+) in hepatitis caused by virus B	Negative	Negative
Albumin	Normal—early; lower—with liver necrosis	Low	Usually low; depends on degree of liver involvement	Decreased
Carcinogenic embryonic antigen	Normal findings	Normal findings	+ to + + + +—nonspecific	Normal findings
Prothrombin time	Increased early; greatly elevated later	Normal to greatly elevated	Early—elevated; late—very elevated	Normal
Stool (color)	Light brown-yellow to clay (acholic)	Brown to yellow	Brown to clay; depends on degree of CBD obstruction (acholic)	Urobilinogen—normal to increased
Urine	Bilirubin, normal; urobilinogen, decreased to absent	Bilirubin, increased; urobilinogen, increased	Bilirubin— 0; urobilinogen—normal or decreased to absent	Bilirubin—negative; urobilinogen—normal to increased

Recommended Reading

Berci G, Morgenstern L, Shore JM, et al: A direct approach to the differential diagnosis of jaundice. *Am J Surg* 126:372, 1973.

Block MA, Brush EE, Ponka JL, et al: Stenosis of sphincter of Oddi as a cause of jaundice. *Arch Surg* 76:88, 1958.

Cotton PB: Duodenoscopic placement of biliary prosthesis to relieve malignant obstructive jaundice. *Br J Surg* 69:501, 1982.

Ferrucci J Jr, Eaton SB: Advances in the radiology of jaundice; a symposium and review. *AJR* 141:1, 1983.

Ferrucci J Jr: Radiologic evaluation of obstructive jaundice. *Surg Clin North Am* 54:573, 1974.

Frey CF, Glenn F: Cholecystography in jaundiced patients with normal liver excretory function. *Ann Surg* 157:271, 1963.

Jordan GL Jr: *Curr Prob Surg* 19:No. 12. Chicago, Year Book Medical Publishers, 1982. pp. 338;511:742:744.

Longmire WP Jr: The diverse causes of biliary obstruction and their remedies. *Curr Prob Surg* 143:304, 1982.

Longmire FH Jr, Sanford MC: Intrahepatic cholangiojejunostomy for biliary obstruction. Report of 24 cases. *Ann Surg* 130:455, 1949.

Powell CS, Sawyer JR, Renolds VH, et al: Management of adult choledochocysts. *Ann Surg* 193:666, 1981.

Watkins DFL, Thomas GG: Jaundice in acute cholecystitis. *Br J Surg* 131:527, 1976.

References

1. Welch CE: Abdominal surgery. *N Engl J Med.*
2. Kantrowitz PA, Jones WA, Greenberger NJ, et al: Severe postoperative hyperbilirubinemia simulating obstructive jaundice. *N Engl J Med* 276:590, 1967.
3. Powell CS, Sawyer JR, Reynolds VH, et al: Low grade jaundice due to idiopathic unconjugated hyperbilirubinemia. *Ann Surg* 193:666, 1981.

Postcholecystectomy Jaundice

When jaundice occurs shortly after surgery, there are certain questions that must be answered: (1) Will the jaundice be life-threatening if allowed to continue? (2) Can the surgeon wait for a definitive diagnosis, allowing the patient to recover from the immediate surgery? (3) Will reoperation be required, and if so, how soon? (4) Is the patient at high risk? The first considerations are these: What was the condition of the patient immediately after surgery? What type of recovery did the patient have, and how soon did the icterus develop after surgery? Liver studies should, of course, be obtained and the results carefully evaluated. To reoperate very shortly after surgery is very serious and can well be life-threatening. It is very unwise and risky to place under anesthesia a patient with unexplained elevated liver studies, particularly elevated bilirubin, alkaline phosphatase, and unduly elevated prothrombin time. Jaundice after surgery is an unfortunate situation and may well lead to tragic consequences. The surgeon must ask the anesthetist whether halothane was given previously. If so, both must assume that there is existing liver damage; if surgery is to be carried out again, the anesthetist must ensure that halothane will not be used again.

In making the differential diagnosis, we must ask whether we are dealing with a medical toxic or viral hepatitis, or with an obstructing extrahepatic surgical jaundice (Table 1). A prothrombin time that is elevated and continues to rise unduly is a significant indication that the postoperative jaundice is becoming serious. When fever, chills, and leukocytosis develop, suppurative cholangitis must be considered. It is important to remember that if postoperative jaundice is not associated with an undue elevation of enzymes, prothrombin time, fever, chills, and leukocytosis, the situation is less urgent and additional time for an evaluation can be considered. In the routine study, one must include tests for viral hepatitis. Important studies include SGOT, LDH, alkaline phosphatase, total bilirubin and direct and indirect bilirubin studies, as well as a complete blood count (CBC) and a reticulocyte count. It should be kept in mind that a patient who has received multiple transfusions during past surgery, and subsequently reveals a palpable spleen, a reticulocytosis with further evidence of an indirect van den Bergh study, and a low hemoglobin reading, should suggest a hemolytic process.

Transient, low-grade, or mild postoperative hyperbilirubinemia is common in postoperative patients, particularly when they have been transfused. It needs no intensive investigation, but it should be carefully observed. If the serum bilirubin and SGOT and LDH levels continue to rise, if blood transfusions were given during the past surgery, and if a hepatitis B surface antigen (HBsAG) study is positive, the diagnosis of hepatitis is established. However, if the HBsAG remains negative, liver biopsy should be considered. In some cases, a needle biopsy of the liver may help differentiate a halothane induced hepatitis from a viral hepatitis. It should be noted that a postoperative liver biopsy is not unduly hazardous and can be useful in uncovering a rather obscure diagnosis such as alcoholic hepatitis. The surgeon can do a liver biopsy routinely at surgery, making needle biopsy unnecessary. If the stools become acholic and remain so for about 10 days or more, it may be necessary to consider a percutaneous transhepatic cholangiogram or transduodenal retrograde endoscopic (ERCP) study.

A transhepatic cholangiogram will usually exclude mechanical factors or obstruction in the major biliary ducts such as the hepatic and common bile ducts. If the cholangiogram is normal, a needle liver biopsy may then give clear-cut evidence of a specific parenchymatous liver disease. Biopsy and retrograde endoscopic cholangiopancreatography will, in most instances, differentiate between benign postoperative cholestasis, primary liver disease, and extrahepatic causes of jaundice. On occasion, a serious postoperative jaundice may be associated with bacteremia, sepsis, or endotoxic shock. The surgeon must constantly be on the alert whenever a postoperative jaundice develops to determine whether the jaundice is related to a prehepatic or posthepatic problem. Nonhepatic etiologies include the hemolytic anemias, transfusion reactions (especially when old stored blood had been utilized), reabsorption of blood as hematomas, blood in the gastrointestinal tract, and Gilbert's syndrome.

At times, there will be a low-flow syndrome related to the renal parenchyma. One should recognize that hepatic anoxia may develop as a precursor disease, and will be manifested by a peculiar clinical picture associated with jaundice. Jaundice may occur after any biliary tract or pancreatic surgery and, more often than not, is mechanical or obstructive in origin. Some refer to the latter causes as *iatrogenic*; this word has come to mean an inadvertent or careless accident that has occurred during surgery. Mechanical obstructive lesions following biliary and pancreatic surgery, or even gastric surgery, should be recognized and corrected as they occur, since their persistence will threaten possible liver failure and patient survival.

One must always keep in mind that there are preoperative precursor instances of jaundice, but with surgery and blood transfusions, jaundice is manifested more definitively in the postoperative period. Jaundice may be multifactorial, including such causes as benign cholestasis, unrecognized liver disease, and undue stress created by previous halothane anesthesia. The operation itself must be considered a factor, but transfusions during surgery must always be considered a strong contributing factor in postoperative jaundice. It is imperative that the anesthetist be constantly aware of good profusion of the liver parenchyma with good oxygenated blood, and be careful to avoid drug overload, drug sensitivity, and infection.

A history of the patient with a previous hepatitis, a history of alcoholism, or any sort of liver disease in the past contributes to a better evaluation of the postoperative period. Many times an overlooked fatty or congested liver fails to withstand surgery, and in most instances this preventable error can result in a jaundice that can be so perplexing as to require a detailed differential diagnosis. How does the jaundice develop? Does it intensify gradually or rapidly? Does it recede? Recurrent jaundice, worsening jaundice, or severe persistent jaundice demands strict attention from the surgeon as well as the internist. Retrograde endoscopic choledochopancreatography is an important contribution; selective visceral arteriography is a test of last resort and requires skilled personnel to evaluate the findings. This specialized talent is not always available, particularly in the average community hospital. In the last analysis, exploratory laparotomy may be necessary, but it carries high morbidity and mortality. The surgeon must also be aware that during anesthesia it is possible that hypotension with hypoxia before and during surgery can result in excessive amounts of blood accumulating in the extravascular tissues, resulting in the production of postoperative jaundice.

Whatever its cause, the surgeon must keep in mind that postoperative jaundice is linked with some form of preoperative impaired liver cell function; whether it is functional or mechanical is unimportant; the fact that the liver is functionally impaired is a constant reminder of the seriousness of the jaundice when the question of secondary surgery arises. However, one should not move too hastily to obtain exotic studies that evaluate postoperative jaundice, because in the period after biliary surgery, the most likely and significant cause of this condition is usually related to trauma in the biliary tree. Therefore, to seek a cause for the jaundice within the hour or within the first day after surgery is unnecessary and indicates undue concern. Primarily, one should know the patient, reevaluate what was done, and then carefully and calmly watch the patient's progress. One should order the studies that are necessary, and not resort unnecessarily to sophisticated and costly tests.

One must keep in mind that, depending upon whether the jaundice persists, appears intermittent, or declines and disappears, the behavior of the abnormality will determine when more diagnostic studies will be required. The employment of ERCP should be determined by the progress and course of the disease and by its absolute need as a diagnostic tool. It should be held in abeyance until all clinical evaluations have been made and all liver and function studies completed. Jaundice is usually recognized after the surgery, i.e., 1, 2, or 3 days postoperatively with increasing intensity. On occasion, it may be manifested by the development of an external biliary fistula. The surgery may have involved the biliary, pancreatic, gastric, or common duct, or any combination of these structures but, *most of all, postoperative jaundice must initially be considered traumatic (iatrogenic), and surgery must be kept in mind as a final means of offering relief.*

As previously stated, halothane-induced jaundice generally occurs only after the anesthetic has been used previously. The use of halothane should be discussed with the anesthetist. Inadvertent repeated exposure to halothane may prove fatal. Jaundice may be related to parenteral introduction of the virus either by a needle, a blood transfusion, or a viral carrier. Since jaundice due to viral hepatitis takes 5 weeks or more to develop, there should be no difficulty in recognizing jaundice related to viral infection. Any jaundice that occurs before 5 weeks after surgery is probably not related to B-virus hepatitis. Pancreatitis can be ruled out because even though postoperative jaundice related to pancreatitis may occur, it is rare. It is not uncommon after major abdominal surgery for a postoperative jaundice to develop, because a stone in the common duct or a tumor of the duct or the ampulla of Vater could have been overlooked at the time of previous surgery. In this situation, jaundice is usually manifested shortly after surgery.

If the causative factors were not recognized during the surgery, it may be necessary to perform further studies, and possibly ERCP should be considered. A transhepatic cholangiography is also a diagnostic possibility, but it is not as informative as retrograde cholangiography when the latter is successful. This writer feels that whatever the cause of postoperative jaundice, speed is not essential, though delay should be avoided. If reoperation is considered, it should not necessarily take place in the first, second, or third week unless the jaundice is so severe and progressive as to demand immediate interruption of the jaundice with its associated liver involvement.

Clinical Diagnosis of Jaundice

The most important single factor in making a correct diagnosis of jaundice is the *history* of the patient. A careful and guided evaluation of the sequence of events reported by the patient is most valuable.

ONSET

In taking the patient's history, one should pay strict attention to the mode and manner in which the jaundice developed. Did it develop gradually or appear suddenly? Was it painful or painless? Was there evidence of obstructive features such as darkening of the urine, or did the stool become paler until it turned gray? Has the jaundice fluctuated? Has it fluctuated over the past years or months, or even since birth? One must constantly be aware of whether the patient has ever been treated or diagnosed as having hemolytic anemia or cirrhosis that has been well compensated for by good management.

In making a clinical diagnosis, the surgeon must decide whether the jaundice is *medical* or *surgical.* One cannot proceed with surgery until the jaundice is classified into one of these two categories. The breakdown for the specific diagnosis comes later (see Differential Diagnosis of Jaundice). Obstructive jaundice, if medical, will be unfavorably influenced by surgical intervention. The mortality will invariably be increased by unnecessary or hasty laparotomy. The history of onset is especially important because hepatitis characteristically starts with a *gastrointestinal upset* which may or may not be preceded by *fever. Anorexia* is associated with *nausea* and sometimes *diarrhea* and may be very severe. Before the jaundice develops, a preliminary period of *erythematous or urticarial rash* may develop which is associated with *fever, malaise, weakness, fatigue,* and a generalized *abdominal discomfort* that cannot be localized. However, patients may state that after several days, they noticed that the *urine became darker* and the *stool paler,* and that *yellow skin* was first noticed by their friends and later by themselves. The *conjunctiva* and the underside of the *tongue* are often the first sites of *discoloration. Pruritis* is a common accompaniment. After several days, when the jaundice becomes quite intense, there may be a *strong history of contact with other hepatitis patients* or instances where *patients injured themselves* with a *needle or pin,* usually in the laboratory. The prodromal period may last for 2, 4, or 6 months with hepatitis B and 1 to 2 weeks with hepatitis A. Laboratory technicians should be carefully questioned about the possibility of even the slightest accident. This should be strongly suspected even if the patient cannot remember any accident. A *history of foreign travel* can be important because there are many *oriental forms of jaundice* caused by infestations and virus infections, as in yellow fever, *Clonorchis-sinensis, malaria, Ascaris lumbricoides,* and

Weil's disease (Leptospira icterohemorrhagiae). In the history of the onset of jaundice, the patient may be able to reveal that he or she was taking specific drugs for malaria, i.e., *quinacrine (Atabrine),* or phenothiazines such as *chlorpromazine.*

Patients may reveal that they have been on *steroids or arsphenamines.* A history of chronic *alcoholism* can be a causative factor in biliary cholestasis. There are patients who, because of a previously damaged liver, may be *sensitive or allergic* to one or more drugs, or perhaps any drug. There are patients with incipient jaundice who have not yet revealed their clinical jaundice, and who may be susceptible to a *toxic or nontoxic drug* or any combination of drugs. Patients are often told to bring in all the medications they are presently taking so that the physician can determine what the drugs are and how they concern this case of jaundice. Usually if a drug is considered the possible cause of the jaundice, its complete withdrawal may frequently be followed by complete relief. Recently, *halothane* anesthesia has been incriminated as the cause of postoperative jaundice, but there are presently two schools of thought on that possibility. It is important to remember that some patients have been in near shock or frank shock, and have been brought out of that state quickly and taken to surgery, where halothane was employed. In these instances, there has been a high percentage of postoperative jaundice. In cases where previously existing liver disease or damage existed, halothane or repeated surgery with halothane frequently led to postoperative jaundice and death. The greatest care must be given to such cases, and consultation with the anesthesiologist is mandatory before halothane is used.

Weil's disease (leptospira icterohemorrhagial) usually begins with a high fever and severe backaches and/or pain in the limbs. Headache is a common finding, and this disease can be mistaken for the common cold or flu. The occupation of the patient must always be considered because the inhalation diseases caused by various chemicals can produce jaundice, and this knowledge can be of help in ruling out Weil's disease. Disease onset that becomes deeper and deeper without causing pain or any preliminary symptoms is usually the way a gradual obstructive jaundice begins. In the absence of a history of suspected drug use, the absence of occupational factor, and the absence of viral contacts or an oriental trip, one should think of extrahepatic biliary obstruction in which cholelithiasis and choledocholithiasis are the commonest causes. The next most common obstructive causes are due to tumors of the ampulla of Vater and to carcinoma of the head of the pancreas. Other neoplastic causes are usually in the biliary tract, i.e., hepatic duct, cystic duct junction, common hepatic duct, or distal portion of the common duct close to the ampulla of Vater. A *long history of intermittent pruritis,* which has preceded the jaundice, may be a significant sign of primary biliary cirrhosis or lymphoma. Hodgkin's disease may sometimes present with pruritis as a forerunner of jaundice. One should be able to evaluate a history of colic attacks with or without jaundice and with or without referred pain to the back (interscapular area) and right shoulder. Often the patient is of a *specific habitus* that encourages consideration of cholecystitis and cholelithiasis, e.g., female, fat, flatulent, fair, and 40.

The history may reveal an acute onset of jaundice, fever, and chills, with intermittent *relief of fever and chills followed by the disappearance of jaundice and a return to normal-colored stool.* This syndrome may be pathognomonic of a ball valve type of cholangitis (Charcot's intermittent fever), cholelithiasis, and choledocholithiasis. The latter form of cholangitis almost never accompanies a primary biliary cirrhosis, or any other intrahepatic form of cholestasis, or even an ampullary obstruction of the head of the pancreas. A history of *alcoholism* may also reveal a background for the development of *cholestatic jaundice.* Of course, the patient may say that the onset *started shortly after surgery,* in which case the surgeon may have clamped and ligated the common duct. Inadvertent operative trauma may lead to stricture formation with obstruction. In the latter instance, an obstructive jaundice may develop with or without cholangitis. A *biliary fistula* developing after the surgery is significant and may reveal how the jaundice became first intense and then less intense with fistula development. Not infrequently, jaundice may develop as a primary sclerosing cholangitis or a sclerosing cholangitis secondary to a previous operative procedure, the causative factor being excessive instrumentation during exploration of the common duct. In either case, it is conceivable that the jaundice is associated with a diffuse form of sclerosing cholangitis.

The history may reveal that the patient had had previous surgery other than cholecystectomy (e.g., a hysterectomy) in which *multiple transfusions* were utilized. The latter procedure may have occurred 4 to 8 weeks (usually 6) before the posttransfusion jaundice developed. With a previous diagnosis of *carcinoma* of organs other than the liver and biliary tree, i.e., the *colon, ovary, or rectum,* subsequent jaundice is the foreteller of *secondary metastases* to the liver. This is also true of *lymphomatous diseases* such as Hodgkin's disease and lymphocytic leukemias. The onset of *jaundice shortly after birth* or in the pre-teenage period is highly suggestive of *congenital defects,* i.e., biliary atresias and choledochal cyst.

PHYSICAL EXAMINATION

During the physical examination, one should routinely evaluate the patient by inspection, palpation, percussion, and auscultation.

Inspection

On inspection the patient may appear slightly, moderately, or deeply jaundiced. The patient may speak of stool that is changing from dark brown to clay in color. Depending on the age of the person, i.e., infancy or the teenage period, slight jaundice may be recognized as a congenital form of hyperbilirubinemia or possibly atresia. One must always think of jaundice even in the early stages of life. When one suspects viral hepatitis, examination of a thin person may reveal a bulge in the right upper quadrant. This bulge is not often seen in the left upper quadrant, where the spleen may be a factor in producing a similar visual elevation. In the right upper quadrant, a mass may be an enlarged gallbladder of the Courvoisier type. The latter is seen especially when carcinoma of the head of the pancreas or ampulla may have existed for a long time. The patient's general condition may or may not reveal severe illness. There may be no special complaint in view of the fact that the jaundice is silent; here one sees a normal person with a deep jaundice who is totally unaware of the discoloration.

The physician may find that the jaundiced patient has drugs at the bedside, in which case an immediate search for the specific drug is made to determine whether or not chlorpromazine, quinacrine (Atabrine), arsphenamine, or any other toxic drug can be identified. Whether the patient has a rash may be important; some cases are preceded or accompanied by a skin rash, either macular or erythematous; the palms may show evidence of spider formations. Many cases of jaundice accompany infectious mononucleosis, and patients may show evidence of anemia and lymph node enlargement that will necessitate a search for lymphomatous diseases. Continued objective study may reveal petechiae of the upper palate, membranous pharyngitis, and possibly cervical lymphadenitis. One should look for plantar erythema, spider naevi, white nails, and occasionally clubbing, as noted in cirrhosis of the liver with jaundice. The last may be of the alcoholic variety. In some instances, mental confusion may be a factor that could be interpreted as a sign of pre-coma; this, of course, suggests severe failure of liver function with ammonia intoxication.

Palpation

On palpation of a jaundice patient, one feels for nodes in the neck, axilla, and groin; cervical nodes may suggest a form of lymphomatous disease or a remote carcinoma. On palpation of the abdomen, one will often recognize an enlarged, firm liver. This finding may be seen in the various forms of obstructive jaundice. Palpation of the liver may also reveal tenderness along with the enlargement, i.e., in viral hepatitis. Palpation of the upper left quadrant may reveal a slightly or markedly enlarged spleen, and this finding may go well with hemolytic jaundice; cirrhosis of the liver may also be associated with portal hypertension and hypersplenism. Hepatomegaly may accompany toxic hepatitis, though as a rule the enlargement is not marked. In hyperbilirubinemias associated with congenital factors, the spleen may not be palpable. In Gilbert's syndrome, there may or may not be a palpable liver with icterus, but in the Lawrence-Biedel-Bardet syndrome the liver is enlarged more frequently, and is associated with congenital anomalies, i.e., cystic changes and dilatation of the common duct. Tenderness with enlarged hepatomegaly, as in viral hepatitis, is especially noted during percussion. Macular or urticarial rashes that may occur in the prodromal period of jaundice can be palpated as well as seen. When the liver is rapidly reduced in size, the patient may pass into hepatic coma. This phenomenon can be seen in yellow atrophy of the liver that carries with it a high morbidity and mortality. One percusses out fluid in the abdomen (ascites). This occurs frequently when jaundice persists. When splenomegaly increases, it is a poor prognostic sign and may indicate that the causative factor of the jaundice is chronic cirrhosis associated with liver cell failure, hemorrhage, and esophageal varices.

As stated previously, the withdrawal of drugs in toxic jaundice will cause a rapid subsidence of the jaundice. In infectious mononucleosis, palpation of the glandular phenomena, i.e., glandular enlargement in the neck, axilla, and groin, is rather common and is usually accompanied by a palpable spleen. Often a conspicuous sign, especially in thinner individuals, is the enlarged collateral abdominal veins (inferior epigastric veins inosculating with superior epigastric veins); this may be associated with ascites. In the late stages of hepatic disease with jaundice, one finds visual objective findings of confusion, and pre-coma with hepatic failure; not infrequently, one also smells "hepatic fetor." The latter findings lead to complete hepatic failure, most often as a result of viral hepatitis. In a thin person, a large Courvoisier gallbladder may easily be palpated, but in the moderately obese individual it is more difficult to palpate. One must give credence to Courvoisier's law because obstruction in the distal biliary tree, i.e., ampulla of Vater, or head of the pancreas will almost invariably lead to distention of the gallbladder in all instances where no previous gallbladder disease existed. In the writer's opinion, the latter is a highly dependable diagnostic sign. In metastatic carcinoma, one must expect that any disease that has metastasized to the liver may give rise to a palpable nodular liver. One should search the neck, looking for a primary carcinoma. We also look for primary carcinoma in the breast or anywhere in the gastrointestinal tract.

Percussion

Masses in the abdomen are dull to percussion; they are primarily the liver, spleen, and any solid abdominal mass, or fluid. Percussion will determine that the liver is enlarged and subsequent percussion will enable the physician to determine its variable size. Over a period of time, one can determine the rate of growth or shrinkage of the liver. A recession or enlargement of the spleen can also be recognized by percussion. Palpation of a mass may suggest a lesion that has metastasized to the liver, and percussion may be helpful in locating and evaluating its extent. The kidneys can also be percussed, but some prefer the well-known *Murphy punch*. This has some significance where tenderness is rather obvious, but when tenderness is minimal or equivocal, this maneuver may have no significance. Percussion of the lungs may reveal consolidation, i.e., carcinoma, pneumonia, or fluid in the lungs; such findings suggest that there is metastasis from the liver, stomach, colon, or breast.

Auscultation

In listening to the abdomen with a stethoscope, one can recognize hyperperistalsis, hypoperistalsis, or absence of peristalsis; a bruit in an area of dullness may suggest abdominal aneurysm or an arteriovenous fistula anywhere in the abdomen. In relationship to jaundice, auscultation itself is of little value. Therefore, on the basis of the history and physical examination, we have demonstrated how our present knowledge of disease patterns can help to diagnose jaundice without the aid of excessive laboratory tests. It is remarkable that in a high percentage of cases the diagnosis can be made just from the history and onset of jaundice, even before the physical examination is performed. This writer is in no way advocating the abandonment of laboratory tests; he merely wishes to emphasize the fact that a great deal of vital knowledge can be gained from a careful objective study of the patient before any sophisticated studies are employed. We have discussed various important laboratory tests that may be employed in the diagnosis of jaundice. We have also included a classification of laboratory studies which differentiate obstructive from nonobstructive jaundice (see Table 1).

These laboratory studies include alkaline phosphatase, serum albumin transaminase, SGOT, LDH, urinary and fecal bilirubin, urobilinogen, quantitative studies of bilirubin, thymol turbidity, cholesterol, cephalin flocculation, Australian antigen, carcinogenic embryonic antigen, stool studies for blood and color, and other exotic studies by immunoelectrophoresis (see Table 1). The sophisticated laboratory studies so often required in the differential diagnosis of jaundice are carried out by special modalities: X-rays, nuclear isotope studies, liver biopsy, percutaneous transhepatic cholangiograms, angiograms, and the noninvasive ERCP and ultrasonography. Exotic tests will be discussed separately.

ABDOMINAL EXPLORATION AS A LAST RESORT FOR DIAGNOSIS AND TREATMENT OF JAUNDICE

Exploratory laparotomy may occasionally be necessary. If all the laboratory studies mentioned prove to be unrevealing or equivocal, exploratory laparotomy becomes the only measure left for diagnosis and possible treatment. When the patient is not improving or is getting worse, surgery becomes the only option. In obstructive jaundice the condition is never so emergent that a good workup, continued observation, and consultation cannot provide a better diagnosis, as well as an improved patient for possible surgery. When an ascending cholangitis is associated with pancreatitis, palliative decompression is attained only by surgery. If the obstructive jaundice is caused by stones, the prognosis will probably be good after surgery; delaying surgery while measures are taken to improve the patient is a good practice. If the obstructive jaundice proves to be carcinoma, nothing is lost by improving the patient during the waiting period for more major surgery. When the tumor is found to be inoperable, a palliative procedure is performed when feasible. It is possible that a curative Whipple procedure may be carried out because of the patient's improved state. An exploratory laparotomy does much to relieve the severe itching and uncomfortable back pressure; it also improves the ultimate survival rate. Too hasty surgery can prove detrimental to the patient; it can even be responsible for a postoperative death if the patient did not have obstructive jaundice, but instead had viral hepatitis.

So, it appears best and necessary to watch the patient for weeks, and possibly months, so long as no emergency situation arises that calls for immediate surgical intervention. Continued observation and repeat laboratory studies can give significant indications and clarification regarding the progress of the disease. As mentioned before, a percutaneous transhepatic cholangiography using the skinny Chiba needle is one of the final tests performed; but here too, the operating room and the surgeon must stand by for immediate surgery.

Emergency surgical intervention is reserved for biliary peritonitis, frank hemorrhage, or the definitive surgery that may be required. But if the disease is nonobstructive and suggestive of hepatitis, and the patient is not improving, but rather shows evidence of being stationary, then cortisone or prednisolone may be tried for a 5- to 7-day trial period. In a few instances there is a response, in which case a daily study of the bilirubin level may indicate a significant improvement both in the jaundice and the condition of the patient. In such a case, steroids are continued until the patient is completely well; failure to respond indicates that further studies have to be done and that the hepatitis is not related to steroid deficiency. When a patient responds to steroid treatment (30–40 mg daily for 5–7 days) and the bilirubin level falls, it may be wise to continue the treatment. However, a decreasing level of dosage is advised so that the treatment may last longer, i.e., 4–6 weeks. It is not uncommon to have recurrent jaundice when steroid treatment is discontinued. Nevertheless, the response to steroids strongly indicates that the jaundice is not obstructive. When a diagnostic problem develops up to the last stages of decision, it should be kept in mind that some surgeons prefer the information of the cholangiogram. If he is going to operate, the surgeon may prefer a cholangiographic study at surgery with minimal complications to the liver. After obtaining the necessary sonograms, and X-ray studies, the surgeon is prepared to proceed with any necessary definitive surgery. Surgeons who prefer a transhepatic cholangiogram through a mini-laparotomy incision approach the biliary tree via an infrahepatic or an anterior liver route.

Classification and Differential Diagnosis of Obstructive vs. Nonobstructive Jaundice

A. Obstructive Jaundice (Extrahepatic)
  1. Congenital
      a. Biliary atresias
      b. Choledochal cysts
  2. Acquired
      a. Cholecystitis and cholelithiasis
          (i) Single or multiple stones
      b. Sclerosing cholangitis
          (i) Differential diagnosis: cancer of the biliary tree
      c. Neoplasms
          (i) Benign
              (a) Extrinsic and intrinsic biliary growths
          (ii) Malignant
              (a) Cancer of the ampulla of Vater
              (b) Cancer of the head of the pancreas
              (c) Cancer of the biliary ductal system (any portion)
              (d) Extrinsic obstructive neoplasms, i.e., lymphomas, Hodgkin's disease, secondary metastasis
      d. Strictures of the biliary tree
          (i) *Postoperative trauma*, i.e., inadvertent tears, manipulations, or suturing
      e. Parasitic infestations
          (i) *Clonorchis sinensis*
          (ii) Weil's disease (leptospira icterohemorrhagiae)
          (iii) *Ascaris lumbricoides*
          (iv) Malaria
B. Nonobstructive Jaundice (Intrahepatic)
  1. Hepatitis (viral)
      a. Hepatitis A
          (i) Not related to the Australian antigen
          (ii) Short incubation period (1–3 weeks); short prodromal period and short onset
      b. Hepatitis B
          (i) Australian antigen—antibodies produced by virus B
          (ii) Longer incubation period (6–8 weeks)
          (iii) History: laboratory injury (minimal), transfusions, previous surgery
      c. Hepatitis—yellow fever (mosquito virus—*Aedis egypti*)

2. Hepatitis (bacterial)
   a. Bacterial infection with ascending cholangitis, pyelophlebitis (portal vein)
   b. Bacteremia, septicemia
3. Hepatitis (toxic)
   a. Drugs
      (i) Quinidine, arsephenamines, Thorazine (phenothiazines), benzine
      (ii) Any drug, based on sensitivity or an allergy, is capable of producing toxic hepatitis, especially if the liver is already in the prejaundice phase.
      (iii) Anesthetics
         (a) Chloroform
         (b) Halothane—in patients with preshock or repeated anesthesia with same agent
      (iv) Alcoholism
         (a) Liver biopsy—cholestasis
         (b) Late—cirrhosis of the liver
4. Hemolytic jaundice
   a. Congenital and acquired
   b. Posttransfusion
   c. Allergic—autoimmune reaction, idiopathic
5. Post–upper and lower gastrointestinal hemorrhage
   a. Absorption of blood components or breakdown products, causing fever and jaundice; especially repeated bleeding with blood transfusions
6. Gilbert's syndrome
   a. Jaundice of teenagers—associated with elevated bilirubin level caused by selective liver cell failure to conjugate bilirubin; a cholecystogram may provide good visualization of the gallbladder
7. Lawrence-Biedel-Bardet syndrome
   a. Dilated cystic and common bile ducts; associated with congenital anomalies
8. Primary biliary cirrhosis—idiopathic; unknown etiology; progressive

Laboratory Studies to Differentiate the Causes of Jaundice

A. Blood Studies
   1. CBC—anemia—abnormal platelet count, white blood cell count, and differential; spherocytosis and sperocytes; megaloblasts, hemoglobin, haptoglobin below normal suggest hemolytic jaundice
   2. Biochemical profile
      a. Enzymes
         (i) Elevated LDH; SGOT increased with obstructive jaundice; *early* elevation in parenchymatous jaundice, *later* in obstructive jaundice
         (ii) Elevated alkaline phosphatase—early in extrahepatic obstructive jaundice
      b. Tests
         (i) BSP (Bromsulphalein) retention of over 10% after 1 hour—malfunctioning liver
         (ii) Cephalin-flocculation—increased in late liver necrosis (intrahepatic jaundice)
         (iii) Thymol turbidity—same as cephalin-flocculation
         (iv) Total bilirubin—important guide to increase or decrease
            (a) Van den Bergh—direct: indicates obstructive cause; indirect: indicates parenchymatous cause
         (v) Australian antigen
            (a) When positive, indicates B virus antibodies; suggestive of transfusion reaction
            (b) Rule out laboratory injuries or contact with known viral hepatitis patient; virus A has a shorter incubation period (2 weeks) and is not related to the Australian antigen
         (vi) Albumin—decreased in parenchymatous necrosis
         (vii) Globulin—compensatory increase to sustain circulatory hemostasis
         (viii) Coombs' test—direct (+) indicates blood dyscrasia, acute immune bodies; autoagglutinins cover red blood cells; hemolytic changes occur
B. X-ray Studies
   1. Flat X-ray films—upright, lying down, and left lateral
      a. Intensifies calcifications, stones, masses, organ displacement, gas patterns, fluid (ascites), ileus, etc.
   2. Upper gastrointestinal tract study
      a. "Duodenal sweep," when increased, suggests an enlarged head of the pancreas; cancer of the papilla, or the duodenum; pancreatic or choledochal cyst; organ displacement; neoplasm of the stomach
   3. Lower gastrointestinal tract study—cancer of the colon; polyposis of the colon; organ displacement; may suggest hepatomegaly and/or splenomegaly

4. Chest X-ray—primary carcinoma or evidence of secondary metastasis, ascitic fluid; may suggest associated liver metastasis

5. Percutaneous transhepatic cholangiography—may indicate, by dye, site and possible cause of jaundice; the finding of a normal common duct is very significant. Japanese skinny needle is preferable; biopsy of the liver can also be done

C. Special Procedures

1. Ultrasonic (sonographic) studies (noninvasive)

 a. Evaluation of pancreas and biliary system more reliable than that provided by a nuclear scan

  (i) Intrinsic findings—gallstones and/or biliary stones

  (ii) Extrinsic findings

   (a) Cancer of the head of the pancreas (enlargement)

   (b) Lymphoma, Hodgkin's disease, leukosarcoma, glandular involvement of the porta hepatis

   (c) Hepatomegaly, splenomegaly, pancreatic cyst

   (d) Abdominal fluid

2. Percutaneous transhepatic cholangiography (see under "X-ray studies")

3. Endoscopic retrograde choledochopancreatogram (ERCP)—must be performed by an expert endoscopist. Complications are bacteremia, septicemia, infection, perforation, and retropharyngeal abscess with tracheal obstruction

4. Computed tomography scan (CT-Scan) accurate, often confirmative; occasionally produces surprising findings; reliable and expensive

5. Magnetic resonance imaging (MRI)

Surgical Errors Made in the Jaundiced and Nonjaundiced Patient

A disease process simulating acute cholecystitis without a history strong enough to substantiate the clinical appearance of the patient should contraindicate immediate surgery. However, if the condition is established as cholecystitis but the general condition of the patient is poor (e.g., coexisting cardiovascular-renal complications), surgery should be delayed until it is considered safe. In some instances, the acute process will be so threatening that all precautionary steps discussed earlier will come to mind, and yet surgery will have to be considered as urgent or emergent. In such instances, a cholecystectomy is performed as soon as possible. The various local pathological changes that can take place during the acute inflammatory process in cholecystitis may render surgery very difficult. Many physicians recommend immediate exploratory laparotomy and cholecystectomy. They seem to disregard the fact that an inflammatory process involves hot, "wet" tissues that do not hold a clamp or a suture well. This can easily lead to serious postoperative complications, especially if blood vessels fail to hold a ligature. In the author's opinion, it would be wiser to wait—not too long, but long enough for the inflammatory process to subside and the patient to improve.

In the presence of serious distortive changes, it is conceivable that a mistake in dissection can occur; also, failure to recognize anomalies is not unusual. As stated before, incomplete surgery on edematous, inflamed, and friable tissue is not safe and therefore not recommended. The pathological changes that occur at the time of surgery or after 24–48 hours are well established; it is suggested that 1–3 weeks (or preferably several months) should be allowed to pass before the effects of the inflammation are completely resolved.

A thorough and effective cholecystectomy and choledochotomy can best be carried out as an elective procedure. When the infection has subsided and the inflammatory changes have resolved, a careful and more detailed exploration and evaluation of the common duct can be carried out more easily. During an acute infectious process, everything in the abdomen looks red, inflamed, and edematous; a correct, astute evaluation can be most difficult. In other words, a serious error can readily be made at this time. This writer wishes to stress that gallbladder disease associated with colic is an emergency only in the presence of a progressive inflammatory process suggesting impending gangrene, obvious gangrene, or impending perforation of the gallbladder. A wait-and-watch policy is far more effective and safer than immediate intervention without the opportunity to improve the patient with fluids, electrolytes, blood, and antibiotics. If diabetic factors coexist, they should be dealt with first.

Another common error made in performing an emergency cholecystectomy during the acute phase is failure to recognize the coexistence of an unsuspected acute pancreatitis. In most instances, acute pancreatitis can be dealt with conservatively;

however, the surgeon must be on the alert in regard to the progressive nature of this acute process. The development of an acute hemorrhagic pancreatitis must be kept in mind, and the surgeon should be ready to interrupt and terminate this potential fulminating complication. In most instances, acute pancreatitis can be dealt with conservatively, but where coexisting hemorrhagic pancreatitis intervenes, mortality will rise sharply and therefore the patient must be dealt with differently. In this situation, cholecystectomy alone is inadequate. The surgeon must institute common duct T-tube drainage, as well as drainage with a Penrose or Jackson-Pratt drain. The site of the necrotic process must be drained to the exterior. The surgeon may have to decide in favor of cholecystostomy and removal as a second-stage procedure.

Antibiotics, antispasmodics, and anticholinergic drugs are important and useful, but as stated before, the morbidity and mortality will continue to rise. Whenever a common duct is found to be enlarged (over 10 mm in diameter), with a history of jaundice or the presence of jaundice, that patient requires a choledochotomy, with a common duct exploration for stones or foreign material. After such a pathological process, postoperative intensive care is required. Consultants for coexistent cardiovascular-renal-pulmonary pathology should be made available immediately.

It must be remembered that jaundice in itself is not an emergency. All jaundiced patients should have a complete medical workup, especially a liver profile. As mentioned elsewhere, laboratory data are important; enzyme studies can be of great significance. A history of hemolytic disease is of great significance; a recent transfusion, especially 4 to 6 weeks prior to the appearance of jaundice, is also of the utmost importance. A recent operation can also be an important clue and should be analyzed in great detail. Hepatitis is a constant specter in these cases, and if it is present, the patient should not be operated upon, because the mortality in such instances is too high. This tragedy can occur only when a patient with hepatitis undergoes emergency surgery without having given a good history or not having obtained an adequate preliminary medical workup. At present, we are fortunate to have laboratory studies that help us evaluate and differentiate the disease process as a precise pathological entity. With percutaneous transhepatic cholangiography and ERCP, we can now diagnose the exact underlying pathological process. The latter procedures can be of great significance by helping the surgeon avoid the abdominal approach.

IMPORTANT CONSIDERATIONS IN THE TECHNIQUE OF BILIARY SURGERY

Once surgery is decided upon, the procedure and technique must be correct and meticulous in order to avoid complications. The operation must be based upon the surgeon's intimate knowledge of the disease process, as well as the technical details of the surgical anatomy. Delicate and experienced handling of all anatomical structures is required. Adequate relaxation is very important, and here is where the anesthetist must cooperate with the surgeon. Delicate instrumentation with a minimum of traumatic handling is of the utmost importance, and the writer wishes to stress the use of noncrushing instruments wherever possible. It may be wiser if no instruments at all were used because of the friability of the inflamed and/or necrotic tissue. The cystic duct must invariably be carefully dissected out. There are many surgeons who recommend that the cholecystectomy be performed from above down. The writer believes that this is not a wise routine procedure; rather, the best routine technique is from below up. With the latter technique, no blood rolls down from the liver to mask the most important surgical anatomy, namely, the ligation of the cystic artery and cystic duct without incident. It also prevents technical accidents ranging from ligation of the common duct to severance of the right hepatic artery (Figs. 5, 6, 7, 8). When the anatomy appears to be obliterated, a careful technique from above down is best. (See Technique of cholecystectomy.)

This writer recommends that as a first step in cholecystectomy, the cystic duct should be carefully dissected out and identified clearly at its junction with the common duct. The cystic artery, no matter where it comes from and no matter where it lies, either on top of or underneath the hepatic or common bile duct, must be positively recognized as it enters into the gallbladder wall. When a short cystic artery is encountered, it should be either ligated or clipped within the wall of the gallbladder itself. The cystic artery stump should remain long and visible on the premise that an emergency second or even third ligature may be required. *It makes no difference where the cystic artery arises: The artery that clearly enters the gallbladder wall is the cystic artery.* A serious complication may occur when a small hepatic artery, because of previous contiguous inflammation, becomes adherent to the gallbladder wall and simulates a cystic artery. Here, a careful dissection will accurately identify the short hepatic artery; the surgeon should now carefully dissect it off and away from the gallbladder wall. The gallbladder wall must be carefully separated from the hepatic artery in order to fully visualize the short cystic artery during cholecystectomy. The cystic artery must be ligated close to the side or within the gallbladder wall. Sometimes the cystic artery may be so short (less than 1/8 inch in length) that it can be seriously compromised. Here is where speed must be substituted for a fastidious dissection and careful ligation or clipping.

This writer emphasizes that traction on the cystic duct should not be too forceful for fear of tenting the common duct. A cystic duct ligature inadvertently placed around the common duct will produce an immediate partial or complete obstruction of the duct which will be recognized shortly after surgery by a sudden jaundice. The latter must never be allowed to happen; it is completely avoidable (see "Operative Technique for Cholecystectomy" in Chapter 10).

When the gallbladder is removed from the abdomen, it should be opened and attention given to the inner surface and diameter of the cystic duct, as well as the size and type of gallstones. If the gallstones are too large to pass through a narrow cystic duct, it is unlikely that they will have passed into the common duct. If the common duct reveals no palpable stone and is of normal size (1 cm in diameter), with no history of past or present jaundice, normal color (slate blue), and normal thickness (thin-walled), there is no indication for opening and exploring the common duct nor for performing a routine cholangiogram via the cystic duct. If the cystic duct is found to have a large lumen and small gallstones, then regardless of the size of the common duct, a cystic duct cholangiogram and exploration are indicated. If stones are found, a thorough exploration should be carried out; a T-tube must be employed routinely whenever a common duct is opened and explored for gallstones. This step is most important in order to carry out postoperative cholangiographic studies and treatment: to irrigate if necessary; to employ local solvents, such as deoxycholic acid derivatives; or to utilize "fishing" procedures such as the postoperative Burhenne method. Burhenne has successfully removed overlooked common duct stones with a long-arm Dormia basket and balloon techniques. Finally, if a secondary operation is required, the T-tube or its fistulous tract will assist in accurately guiding the surgeon down to the choledochotomy site amid many difficult obliterative adhesions.

The surgeon must make every possible effort to remove the stone or stones from the common duct at the first attempt. To do so, he must have the proper instruments. Several sophisticated gallstone extractor instruments are now available, and the hospital is obligated to make them available to the surgeon. The Glassman Extractor instruments are used to remove stones from the common duct, either from above (choledochotomy), from below (duodenotomy), or by a combined choledochotomy and duodenotomy. The Storz rigid choledochoscope can be used alone or combined with the Glassman filiform, basket, or balloon instruments. There is also the Machida flexible choledochoscope, Fogerty's balloon catetege and the Mazzariello-Ciprini long stone grasping forceps. If the instrument can bypass the impacted stone in the common duct, the surgeon should be able to remove it. If the instrument cannot bypass the stone, the effort to remove it from above must end, and all attention must be given to removing it from below via duodenotomy. Here too, the Glassman Gallstone Extractor instruments are very helpful (see "Technique 4" in Chapter 11). A Kocher incision and maneuver will invariably assist the surgeon in removing the retained stone from the lower common duct. Straightening out the common duct by using downward traction makes it easier to manipulate the instruments designed for stone removal; this maneuver also permits the surgeon to see, palpate, and even incise the common duct at a level not possible without the Kocher maneuver (see "The Kocher Maneuver" in Chapter 11).

When the patient's blood pressure is falling and the pulse rate is increasing, the surgeon should discontinue the attempt to remove the stone. At this point, the surgeon has two options: (1) If the patient's condition has suddenly worsened, a T-tube should be inserted and the procedure terminated. (2) If the patient is not doing too well but can still tolerate the surgery, a choledochoduodenostomy (or -jejunostomy) should be performed as a last-resort procedure to allow the stone to pass. In the later postoperative period, in either instance, ERCP or Burhenne's long Dormia basket method may be attempted as a last noninvasive attempt to remove the stone. The latter maneuver is carried out via the fistulous tract left by the T-tube. The surgeon should try to use a long-arm T-tube (14 to 18 F).

When a stone is palpable, the common and hepatic ducts should definitely be explored. On rare occasions, a small common duct reveals a stone on the cholangiogram. Here too, an exploration of the common duct is mandatory (see "Technique for Choledochotomy and Common Duct Exploration" in Chapter 12). When exploring the hepatic ducts, the common duct should be plugged with a piece of gauze or tape so that a stone will not roll down inadvertantly into the distal common duct. The opposite precaution should be taken when the common duct is being irrigated; that is, the hepatic duct should be plugged to prevent a stone from rolling up into the proximal hepatic duct (see Glassman's technique for hepatic duct exploration and hepatic stone extraction).

To be sure that a probe has passed through the common duct into the duodenum, the tip of the probe should be recognized by its metallic appearance through the thin duodenal wall. Not infrequently, the probe may push up the mobile duodenal mucosa, giving the mistaken appearance that the instrument had successfully passed through the ampullary stoma. To avoid this misinterpretation, it is essential that the metallic tip of the probe be clearly seen through the wall before the surgeon decides that it has in fact passed through the ampullary stoma. If there have been recurrent bouts of jaundice, and the common duct is distended to 14 mm or more, and the probe still fails to pass through the ampullary stoma, it will be necessary to open the duodenum (duodenotomy) in order to evaluate carefully the appearance and patency of the ampulla of Vater.

A sphincterotomy should be performed when it becomes necessary to allow an impacted stone to fall out (see the discussion of Glassman's common bile duct operative techniques in Chapter 11). Not infrequently, it may be necessary to biopsy the ampulla. When this is carried out, it is important that all layers be in the bite of the biopsy forceps. Where sphincterotomy has been performed, the writer recommends a long arm Cattell T-tube modified by the author; that is, the distal portion of the long arm is multiply perforated so as not to obstruct the outlet of the pancreatic duct of Wirsung, thus obviating retrograde pancreatitis. The use of the long-arm Cattell T-tube is an excellent ancilliary maneuver in such instances because an uninterrupted drainage of bile from the liver is assured while it decompresses itself and recovers.

The Cattell T-tube may be shut-off earlier to ensure that valuable bile passes into the duodenum without effort. The postoperative cholangiogram has some value, but the long-arm Cattell T-tube offers even greater benefit in the postoperative period by preventing stricture formation after a sphincterotomy has been performed. This writer recommends that an adequate ampullary incision be made; it should be approximately 1 cm long, with the edges sewn together with a very fine catgut suture (0000) to assure patency and healing without stenosis (see "Technique of Sphincterotomy" in Chapter 17).

How long should a T-tube be kept in place? Too often we hear that the T-tube is routinely removed in the first week. Actually, there is no hurry and no precise time for removal. A T-tube serves many functions. First, it helps to drain the liver properly so that the organ has a chance for rapid and effective recovery. It is also possible to irrigate through a T-tube and to evaluate a suspicious swelling of the ampulla of Vater. In addition, the T-tube indicates when the edematous structure has receded. Several weeks may be required. There should be no hurry to remove a T-tube. Before it is removed, a cholangiogram must be obtained by a trained radiologist so that no complications, diagnostic equivocations, air bubbles, and so on complicate the picture. Whenever a T-tube cholangiogram is planned, this writer prophylactically starts the patient on an antibiotic the day before; the antibiotic must be able to enter and mix with the bile as it leaves the liver. Tetracyclines and cephalosporins have been useful for this purpose (see Chapter 15). There have been innumerable instances where faulty technique in the X-ray laboratory has allowed contaminants to enter the biliary ductal system, resulting in serious cholangitis with fever and chills.

After the cholangiogram had proved negative for stones, the tube should be clamped off intermittently. If the patient is asymptomatic, the tube is completely clamped off. Only if the patient meets all of the above criteria should the T-tube be finally removed. The time required for final T-tube removal depends entirely upon the time it takes to meet the following criteria:

1. There must be no pain after the T-tube is clamped off.
2. There must be no recurrent jaundice.
3. There must be no fever and/or chills.
4. The stool must be brown, not acholic or light yellow.

When all the above criteria are finally met, the T-tube is gently pulled out; this may take place in the doctor's office. It is remarkable how quickly the external drainage from the common duct ceases.

The hepatic and cystic arteries have been discussed elsewhere, but to reiterate, either one can be quite variable. The two arteries can be very small in diameter and can fool the most experienced surgeon; the right hepatic artery may appear as small as the cystic artery, and the cystic artery may appear large enough to simulate the right hepatic artery. Therefore, it is essential that the artery ligated be the cystic artery. The artery must enter the gallbladder wall. Because the hepatic artery may adhere to the gallbladder wall, it must be carefully dissected off the wall before the short cystic artery can be positively identified, ligated, and severed. It is true that ligating the right hepatic artery does not invariably produce necrosis of the liver and death, since there is always the possibility that collateral circulation above the site of ligation may exist; that in a percentage of the cases, in addition to portal and systemic intermixture, there is also an intrahepatic anastomosis between the right and left hepatic arteries. However, whatever vascular anastomosis may or may not be present intrahepatically, the surgeon must play it safe, assume that no anastomosis exists, and make every effort to avoid ligating the right hepatic artery.

If brisk bleeding occurs during surgery, the surgeon must never reach for a hemostat and start blind clamping. He must first use suction in order to clean and identify the exact site of the bleeding. If during surgery, when the cystic and common ducts are being dissected out, brisk bleeding suddenly occurs, the surgeon must immediately become aware of the complications that can develop from hasty and careless clamping. One thing is certain: *The surgeon must never apply a hemostat blindly!* He must first suction out and sponge the area, and, by digital compression of the entire porta hepatis (common duct, hepatic vein, and hepatic artery) between forefinger and thumb, temporarily compress the circulation until all of the blood is sucked out and the involved area is rendered clean and dry. Then, under good light, the surgeon releases his forefinger and thumb intermittently so that the exact site of bleeding can be positively identified. This site should then be carefully suture-ligated or clipped without infringing upon the hepatic artery, common duct, or portal vein. The hepatic artery, as mentioned previously, provides a most important blood supply to the right lobe of the liver, and must not be cut or ligated by blind, indiscriminate clamping or suturing. Exact pinpoint ligation of the bleeding site in a dry field, under direct vision, is the surest, most uncomplicated way to deal with cystic or hepatic artery bleeding. Ligating the right hepatic artery may conceivably cause death from necrosis of the right lobe of the liver; however, this is not a consistent occurrence. Few surgeons are aware of an intrahepatic collateral circulation that exists between the right and left hepatic arteries, or that portal and systemic blood also intermix intrahepatically. So long as these facts remain controversial, the surgeon must continue to treat every ligation of the cystic artery with "love and attention."

Because oozing is sometimes difficult to control in the deep liver bed, hot, wet lap pads with pressure under a Deavor retractor for several minutes will usually stop the oozing; Surgicel, Avitene (a collagenous hemostatic agent), or Gelfoam can be of value in controlling active oozing from the liver bed. Oversewing the liver with a continuous-lock (00) chromic catgut on an atraumatic needle can also be helpful when the hemostatic agents fail. Sometimes placing a bit of muscle cut away from the abdominal wall may serve as an effective hemostatic. Clips are preferable to ligation whenever there is oozing or minor bleeding sites deep in the liver bed. A fine coagulator is also an excellent means of controlling spot oozing or minor bleeding.

7

AVOIDABLE ERRORS IN DIAGNOSIS AND JUDGMENT IN THE MANAGEMENT OF BILIARY DISEASES

Complications of biliary tract surgery are primarily based upon the failure to diagnose correctly, which in turn is based upon the failure to initially obtain and evaluate the history of the case. The history plays the most important role in the making of a diagnosis, since a knowledge of the disease pattern and its pathogenetics are all found within a good history. Most of the complications of biliary tract surgery can be avoided by (1) the correct diagnosis, (2) the assurance of an experienced surgeon, (3) the correctness of the selected procedure, and (4) the postoperative management. If all these factors are carefully considered, the mortality should be less than 1% and the results should be excellent.

Diagnostic Errors

In order not to err diagnostically, the surgeon must have a complete knowledge of disease patterns and the pathogenetics that lead to the usual signs and symptoms characteristic of biliary tract disease. In general, the surgeon should operate on the patient with biliary tract disease because the existence of stones will ultimately cause multiple complications. Surgeons should operate with an awareness of the possibility of congenital anomalies; they must operate even though acquired infectious processes may complicate the biliary picture. The surgeon must know that he may have to operate on neoplastic diseases that are relatively uncommon to the biliary tree. X-ray diagnostic procedures such as sonograms, cholecystograms and IV cholangiograms are very important. When the latter demonstrate stones in the gallbladder or biliary tree and the clinical picture suggests gallbladder disease, surgical intervention should be considered without delay.

The surgeon must understand that pain is created in the biliary tract when gallstones attempt to enter the cystic duct. A stone may escape from the gallbladder, enter the cystic duct, and then be expelled into the common bile duct. Once in the common duct, the stone may remain there or pass into the duodenum. The pathogenesis of this process is invariably associated with colicky pain which can start suddenly and become very severe. The knowledge of how colicky pain differs from peritoneal pain is also very important. Colicky pain causes great restlessness; the patient cannot find a comfortable position to lie in. Peritoneal pain, in contrast, is sharp and causes the patient to become extremely quiescent; all bodily movements are avoided. The patient remains immobile, because

any movement can stimulate or stretch the peritoneum, producing "rebound tenderness." It is conceivable that a large stone may not be able to escape through the cystic duct, and may fall short of passing through the neck of the duct. By settling back into Hartmann's pouch, a large stone may still obstruct the cystic duct and produce all the signs and symptoms of acute cholecystitis. Therefore a large single stone is not necessarily a "silent stone." A stone that fails to pass through the cystic duct but instead falls away will cause the colicky pain to cease. The surgeon must carefully evaluate this ongoing process while observing the patient. It should be remembered that the position of the patient may sometimes help to relieve or aggravate the pain. A stone may roll within the gallbladder; if the patient stands up and leans to the right, the stone may fall by gravity toward the fundus away from the cystic duct. If the same patient lies down flat and turns to the left, the stone may roll toward the cystic duct and obstruct it. It is important to keep this hollow, viscus-stone relationship in mind as part of the pathogenesis of the gallbladder disease pattern.

The knowledge of pathogenesis teaches us that if the stone continues to obstruct the cystic duct while the gallbladder remains filled with bile, the water in the bile becomes absorbed. As the bile becomes concentrated to the point where bile acids, salts, and cholesterol precipitate out and irritate the mucosa of the gallbladder, a chemical inflammation or acute cholecystitis is produced. If the stone completely obstructs the cystic duct when the gallbladder is empty, the gallbladder mucosa will continue to secrete mucus and create a distended gallbladder full of white mucus. This process is referred to as *hydrops* of the gallbladder. We now know that obstructive hydrops can be followed by bacterial invasion and infection; this results in an acute infectious process known as *empyema* of the gallbladder. Empyema of the gallbladder is usually caused by the organisms common to the gastrointestinal tract, i.e., *Escherichia coli, Klebsiella, Aerobacter*, and *Clostridium*. It is imperative for the surgeon to know that a closed system, as in hydrops, is the forerunner of an abscess of the gallbladder or empyema that requires immediate decompression or drainage. The surgeon must understand that external drainage in this case is carried out as an emergency; in addition, if judged feasible, a cholecystectomy may be performed. The judgment and action will depend upon the surgeon's knowledge of biliary disease patterns.

The surgeon must be aware that the presence of peritoneal adhesions can make a difference; that is, with adhesions, a perforated empyema of the gallbladder can lead to a *pericholecystic abscess.* Without adhesions, a perforated empyema of the gallbladder can lead to a *generalized peritonitis.* This latter disease pattern can be predicted in advance, and therefore can be prevented by the informed surgeon. In either event, the operation must be carried out immediately, and the pus of the pericholecystic abscess must be drained. Drainage of empyema of the gallbladder is imperative, but, as stated previously, when possible and feasible, a cholecystectomy may be performed. Where a generalized peritonitis develops due to rupture or perforation, the gallbladder must be drained and the peritoneal cavity evacuated of all foreign contaminants. Antibiotics should be used before, during, and after surgery. A pericholecystic abscess may resolve spontaneously, but ultimately surgery may still be necessary, not as an emergency, but as an elective procedure.

Knowing the pathogenesis of the disease process and the patterns of gallbladder disease, one recalls that in the elderly, arteriosclerosis is ever present and that an acute inflammation with undue distention of the gallbladder wall can lead to occlusion of the cystic artery branches. Obliteration of the cystic artery branches and capillaries occurs by stretching, which ultimately leads to occlusion and thrombosis. In either event, gangrene of the gallbladder wall will take place, either locally or generally. And in either event, perforation produces peritonitis. The rate at which necrosis and gangrene develops indicates the seriousness of the disease. In one instance, such as a localized perforation, it may be wise to do an emergency cholecystostomy or possibly cholecystectomy; in another instance, such as extensive gangrene of the gallbladder, immediate surgery must be performed in order to remove the entire gangrenous gallbladder. It is important to know that when the gallbladder starts to enlarge, the diagnosis may be hydrops, empyema, or pericholecystic abscess.

A dilated gallbladder is often referred to as a *Courvoisier* gallbladder, but in either case, the surgeon must interrupt the progressive disease process. Most enlarged gallbladders are palpable, but when the gallbladder is not palpable, it must be assumed to be normal or less than normal in size. In regard to cholecystography of the gallbladder, the surgeon must believe that most cholecystograms, when carried out carefully, are accurate, and will usually reveal the gallbladder pathology whenever a negative test or nonvisualization results. There will be instances where failure to observe a nonfunctioning gallbladder (nonvisuali-

zation) may not necessarily imply gallbladder disease. Today it is more likely that sonography and scintigraphy will incriminate a nonvisualization with greater than 98% accuracy. A nonvisualization of the gallbladder implies an obstructed cystic duct. Most often, nonvisualization of the gallbladder implies the existence of mechanical obstruction, cholecystitis, or cholelithiasis; remotely, carcinoma of the gallbladder. An intimate knowledge of the patterns of gallbladder and biliary tract diseases will help the surgeon differentiate those nonsurgical diseases that ordinarily confuse the picture and lead to a nonindicated operation.

Right upper quadrant pain similar to gallbladder colic can be caused by hyperacidity, peptic ulcer, spastic bowel, right renal colic, lower right pulmonary pathology, arthritis of the thoracic spine, angina pectoris, coronary thrombosis, and porphyria. Patients with these conditions have, at one time or another, mistakenly had a cholecystectomy performed upon them. It is obligatory to first exclude these conditions by utilizing one's intimate knowledge of disease patterns and differentiating them, preferably at the patient's bedside. Of course, further assistance from the laboratory will be of definite benefit. It should be remembered that gallbladder colic is rarely an emergency, and surgery should be postponed until a definite diagnosis can be established. This precaution will lead to an elective surgical procedure without avoidable errors and complications. Surgeons must be aware that while observing a biliary disease process, they may procrastinate too long and allow the stone to enter into the common duct. If that happens, common duct obstruction and jaundice may ensue. The latter obstructive jaundice may be transient, silent, and intermittent, or may become more intense. The presence of jaundice with a history of biliary colic increases the positiveness of a diagnosis of choledocholithiasis and the need for urgent operative intervention. Jaundice without pain may also constitute an urgent indication for surgery.

Silent common duct stones may exist as well as symptomatic common duct stones, but they must be differentiated from other diseases that simulate silent jaundice. With an intimate knowledge of the disease patterns of biliary tract disease, one will be aware that jaundice may also be caused by viral hepatitis and hemolytic jaundice; either condition can be a serious contraindication to surgery. There may also be a carcinoma of the liver or an obstruction of the common duct due to pancreatic involvement, either inflammatory or neoplastic. It is conceivable that postoperative common duct strictures may also cause jaundice, and of course, carcinoma of any portion of the biliary tree may similarly produce a painless jaundice. Where jaundice appears and is soon associated with fever and chills, the surgeon who recognizes the disease patterns knows that secondary infection has set in and that a suppurative cholangitis must be suspected. The latter disease process, unless relieved immediately, can lead to multiple liver abscesses, bacteremia, and endotoxic shock. A suppurative cholangitis calls for immediate relief, as stated, and this relief must include drainage of the common duct. A simple operative procedure in which the gallbladder is removed or drained has little or no value in this disease process and should not be depended upon (see "Acute Suppurative Cholangitis" in Chapter 12). Drainage of the gallbladder would not only fail but would result in a progression of complications, just as if no surgery had been done. It is imperative, then, that in suppurative cholangitis the common duct be opened, evacuated, and drained; an emergency choledochotomy with T-tube drainage should be carried out. The postoperative care of the patient must include adequate fluids and electrolyte replacement, with proper antibiotics.

Management of Acute Cholecystitis (Conservative vs. Interventional)

When treating an acute cholecystitis conservatively, one should make sure that a definitive diagnosis is established. Acute cholecystitis means that emergency surgery is a possible consideration, and the differential diagnosis must be that of acute surgical abdomen. All acute surgical problems must be considered during this period. The differential diagnosis should first consider acute appendicitis, penetrating peptic ulcer, acute pancreatitis, and an acute pneumonic process of the right lower lobe. Conservative treatment should not deter the surgeon from constantly being aware of his plan of differential diagnosis. The surgeon should also be aware of the existence of a biliary colic that is not associated wtih an acute inflammatory process. This condition usually subsides spontaneously and does not call for immediate surgical intervention. Nevertheless, an acute inflammatory cholecystitis may develop at a later date. Because an acute cholecystitis may coexist with acute pancreatitis, one should not omit serum amylase and lipase studies. These tests usually show strong evidence of the coexistence of a primary pancreatitis in the acute

phase. One should also be aware that a cholecystectomy may not fulfill the entire requirement for the case associated with acute pancreatitis. Cholecystectomy alone will do little for the pancreatitis. In fact, the acute pancreatitis may exacerbate during the postoperative period. In an elective unhurried procedure the pancreas can be more carefully evaluated, whereas in a more hurried procedure it is usually overlooked or misjudged. Those who employ an intravenous cholecystographic study in making the differential diagnosis during the first 24 to 48 hours claim a high percentage of success. This writer feels that it is not so great an advantage. The results are far more accurate when ultrasonography is employed. The intravenous cholangiogram may show a good picture, yet the visualization of the gallbladder may or may not be good. The common duct and gallbladder will be more specifically outlined with sonography, and more information will be gained. Nonvisualization of the gallbladder is a common finding during an acute cholecystic process, but it is not a definitive diagnostic certainty. Failure to find an obstructed cystic duct or an obstructed biliary tree after the fifth to eighth day indicates that there is no need to consider a diagnosis of acute cholecystitis. Accurate information is more likely to be discovered after several days of waiting, and preoperative conservative management will often help to finalize the diagnosis as the patient improves. The writer wishes to emphasize that an unhurried workup and evaluation, including ultrasonography, intravenous pyelogram, and an upper gastrointestinal series to rule out a penetrating peptic ulcer can best be carried out by first improving the patient and then having these procedures carried out. Meanwhile, the patient can be prepared preoperatively for possible elective surgery.

Recommended Reading

Anderson RE, Priestly JT: Observations on the bacteriology of choledochal bile. *Ann Surg* 33:4786, 1951.

Becker WF, Powell JI, Turner RJ: A clinical study of 1060 patients with acute cholecystitis. *Surg Gynecol Obstet* 104:491, 1957.

Boey JH, Way LW: Acute cholecystitis. *Ann Surg* 191:264, 1980.

Bordley J, White TT: Causes for 340 reoperations on the extrahepatic bile ducts. *Ann Surg* 189:442, 1979.

Burnett W: Management of acute cholecystitis. *Aust NZ J Surg* 41:25, 1971.

Dunphy JE, Ross FP: Studies in acute cholecystitis. *Surgery* 26:539, 1949.

Flemma RJ, Flint LM, Osterhout S, et al: Bacteriologic studies of biliary tract infection. *Ann Surg* 166:563, 1967.

Hoerr SO, Hazard JB: Acute cholecystitis without gall-stones. *Am J Surg* 11:47, 1966.

Massie JR, Coxe JW III, Parker C, et al: Gallbladder perforations in acute cholecystitis. *Ann Surg* 145:825, 1957.

Schein CJ: *Acute Cholecystitis.* New York, Harper & Row, 1972.

Van der Linden W, Sunzel H: Early vs. delayed operation for acute cholecystitis; controlled clinical trial. *Am J Surg* 120:7, 1970.

Watkins DFL, Thomas GG: Jaundice in acute cholecystitis. *Br J Surg* 58:570, 1971.

Management of Incidental Cholecystitis and Cholelithiasis

How does one handle cholelithiasis when it is discovered at the time of another intra-abdominal surgical procedure? The surgeon must decide whether or not to perform a cholecystectomy. If it is delayed, will the patient develop a postoperative cholecystitis with obstruction and jaundice? The surgeon must also evaluate the risk. Will he add to the morbidity and mortality if concomitant cholecystectomy is performed? What does the vascular surgeon do when, in the midst of an aortic resection and a Dacron implant, he discovers an associated cholelithiasis? This writer's experience has shown that it is wiser by far to proceed with cholecystectomy if no obvious contraindications exist, such as in high-risk patients, the very ill, and aged patients to whom this added surgical burden may be enough to result in death. Thompson et al.,[1] of the University of Nebraska Medical Center, reported on 56 patients in whom incidental cholecystitis was discovered at the time of another abdominal procedure. This group comprised 33 women and 23 men with ages ranging from 18 to 85 years. Patients with preoperative signs and symptoms of cholecystitis were not included in this study. Of the 56 patients in whom coincidental cholelithiasis was found, 33 had concomitant cholecystectomy. The morbidity was 27% and the mortality was 3% (one case). Of these 25 patients who were not cholecystectomized, within 6 months 11 developed acute cholecystitis, 3 developed biliary colic, and 2 became jaundiced. Fifteen patients (65%) required cholecystectomy; 6 of this group required common bile duct exploration.

In patients in whom an unsuspected associated cholecystitis and cholelithiasis exists, a preoperative gallbladder workup should reveal its presence. Such preoperative biliary studies will benefit the surgeon, because it will give him advance information of coexistent cholelithiasis and will enable him to plan his procedure carefully.

Some surgeons believe that "a silent stone is as silent as a tombstone." That is, they believe that to allow a stone to remain after discovering it is to invite complications, either serious inflammatory disease, common duct obstruction, or, finally, incurable carcinoma. Other surgeons feel that the silent stone is indeed a myth. Gracie and Rausohoff[2] stated that few adult white males with gallstones go on to become symptomatic. This is not so in obese females. This writer is inclined to go along with the Mayo Clinic, whose surgeons generally believe that silent stones are no myth, but a reality to be dealt with. It should be mentioned at this point that there are patients, such as the aged, the very ill, and those at high-risk, in whom incidental cholelithiasis may be discovered. These patients in emergency situations will fare much better if a lesser procedure, i.e., cholecystostomy, is performed. In some, the latter procedure is all that will be required; in others, a secondary elective cholecystectomy will have to be performed. This writer believes that it is sometimes good judgment to think in terms of elective cholecystostomy.

The vascular surgeon who, during an aortic graft procedure, incidentally discovers cholelithiasis will find that concomitant cholecystectomy does not complicate the surgery. At the 1979 Southwestern Surgical Congress, McKroskey[3] reported on 521 aortoiliac constructions, during which 39 concomitant cholecystectomies were performed. No postoperative graft infection was reported.

References

1. Thompson JE Jr, Tompkins RK, Longmire WP Jr, et al: Factors in management of acute cholangitis. *Ann Surg* 195:137, 1982.
2. Gracie WA, Rausohoff DF: The natural history of silent gallstones. *N Engl J Med* 307:798, 1982.
3. McKroskey: Read before the Southwestern Surgical Congress, Kansas City, 1979.

The Differential Diagnosis Between Acute Cholecystitis, Angina Pectoris, and Acute Myocardial Infarction

Louis Lemberg, M.D.

Disease of the gallbladder, with or without stones, is very common in patients suffering from angina. Statistics indicate that diseases of the biliary tract are more common in patients who die of atherosclerotic heart disease than in control groups of patients. When upper gastrointestinal (GI) disease is present, the symptoms must and often can be differentiated from those resulting from heart disease.[1] Difficulties are encountered in some cases where common afferent pathways cause the referred pain in biliary disease to simulate that of angina pectoris and vice versa.[2] During an acute gallbladder attack, differentiation can be made more difficult by acute but transient changes in the electrocardiogram that resemble those of acute myocardial injury. Electrocardiographic injury patterns have been recorded in dogs during distention of the gallbladder, but only in those animals who had previous experimental coronary artery ligation. This would suggest that gallbladder-induced electrocardiographic changes can occur only in a background of atherosclerotic heart disease. A variety of cardiac arrhythmias that ordinarily accompany acute cardiac states can be induced while applying traction on or distending the gallbladder during surgery, e.g., ventricular and atrial premature beats, atrial tachycardia, atrial fibrillation, and cardiac arrest. Theodore Struhl describes a case in which excessive traction on the gallbladder repeatedly produced cardiac arrest requiring resuscitation. Local and intravenous novocaine solution permitted completion of the gallbladder surgery without further incidents.[3]

Right upper quadrant tenderness is a common finding in patients with congestive heart failure. Passive congestion of the liver causes stretching of Glisson's capsule, resulting in right upper quadrant tenderness, discomfort, or pain. It is apparent that the symptoms and signs, and at times the electrocardiographic findings, in both gallbladder and heart disease often overlap, frequently requiring careful reevaluation of the history, physical findings, and laboratory results (see Table 1).

MANAGEMENT OF ACUTE CHOLECYSTITIS

When gallbladder disease and angina pectoris coexist a cholecystectomy greatly ameliorates the cardiac symptoms. Angina pectoris is known to be aggravated or initiated by acute gallbladder disease. Removal of the gallbladder is thus indicated in patients who have an anginal syndrome due to atherosclerotic heart disease but who also show signs and symptoms of gallbladder disease. The management of acute gallbladder disease depends upon an accurate diagnosis and the patient's general health status. When the diagnosis of acute cholecystitis is definitely established, cholecystectomy may well be the treatment of choice. However, if cardiac disease presents a complicating factor, the cardiovascular state requires stabilization prior to any consideration of cholecystectomy; this will significantly reduce the risk of abdominal surgery.

GALLBLADDER WORKUP

1. A *complete history* is essential.
2. A *complete physical examination* establishes the site and degree of the pathological process. Signs of peritoneal inflammation and evidence of jaundice should be revealed by the examination. Rebound tenderness in the right upper quadrant is most significant. Abdominal auscultation for bowel sounds is mandatory.
3. *Laboratory tests*
   a. CBC—usually reveals a leukocytosis with a shift to the left.
   b. Biochemical profile.
   c. Urinalysis—positive for bile.
   d. Sonography (ultrasonic) is more accurate than oral cholecystography or an intravenous cholangiogram; it is noninvasive and preferred (see Chapter 5).
   e. Flat X-rays of the abdomen (anteroposterior and lateral views) may show a stone or stones. The bowel gas pattern can be helpful.
   f. Radiological examination of the chest (posteroanterior and lateral views) provides a convenient survey for the detection of unsuspected heart or lung disease.
   g. An electrocardiogram and (usually) serial electrocardiograms are needed to detect acute myocardial injury or infarction.
   h. A computed tomography scan may be an important adjunct to the workup.

PROGNOSIS

The operative mortality for cholecystectomy in patients with coexistent gallbladder and cardiac disease can approach zero, provided that the cardiac disease process is stabilized preoperatively and maintained throughout the postoperative course.

Recommended Reading

Babcock RH: Chronic cholecystitis as a cause of myocardial incompetence. *JAMA* 52:1904, 1909.

Table 1. Comparison of Acute Cholecystitis Angina Pectoris, and Acute Myocardial Infarction*

	Acute Cholecystitis	Angina Pectoris	Acute Myocardial Infarction
History	Recurrent attacks of right upper quadrant (RUQ) pain of varying severity; usually related to ingestion of fried or fatty foods	Transient precordial or substernal pain or pressure of varying severity, usually related to physical or emotional stress	Precordial or substernal pain or pressure lasting for 30 minutes or longer
Onset	May be spontaneous; usually related to ingestion of fried or fatty meals	Usually brought on by physical or emotional stress	Usually occurs without any precipitating cause, but may be related to physical or emotional stress
Type of pain	Sharp, often colicky; patient may have a sense of deep epigastric pressure	Substernal or precordial tightness or heaviness, with radiation to left upper extremity	Similar to angina but more severe, accompanied by diaphoresis
Duration	Often prolonged; lasts for hours	2–15 minutes	30 minutes or longer
Nitroglycerin	No relief	Relief within 3–5 minutes	No relief
Radiation of pain	RUQ pain radiating to the epigastrium, interscapular area, and right shoulder.	Radiation usually to the left, but may be to either or both upper extremities; lateral aspects of the neck, jaw, teeth, or face; pain may be confined to the referred areas	Similar to that of angina pectoris
Patient's response	Patient moves about, is restless, and may thrash about	Quiet, guarded, and apprehensive; sense of impending death	Similar to that of angina pectoris
Abdominal examination	RUQ tenderness; often rebound; varies (1 + − 4 +)	Negative	Negative

Laboratory tests	1. High white blood cell count with shift to the left
	2. Bile in urine; jaundice
	3. Flat films of abdomen may show stone in gallbladder
	4. Sonography (ultrasonic) shows calculi in gallbladder or common bile duct
	5. In rare cases, ECG may reveal inverted T waves which require several ECGs
		1. ECG findings
		  a. Acute injury pattern
		  b. Old myocardial infarction
		  c. Arrhythmias
		  d. Interventricular conduction abnormalities
			1. ECG findings
			  a. Acute injury pattern
			  b. Arrhythmias, e.g., ventricular premature beats, atrioventricular block, bradycardia
			2. Elevated cardiac enzyme levels

*When cardiac and hepatobiliary diseases coexist, diagnosis and management become more difficult. Cardiac disease management invariably precedes surgical intervention.

References

Birnbaum D, Braun K: Cholelithiasis and coronary artery disease. *Am J Med Sci* 235:45, 1962.

Cullen ML, Reese HL: Myocardial circulatory changes measured by clearance of Na-24. Effect of common duct distention on myocardial circulation. *Appl Physiol* 5:281, 1952.

Keys JR, Walters W, Gage RP: Sections of medicine, surgery and biometry and medical statistics. *Proc Staff Meet Mayo Clin*, vol 30, no 25, Dec 1955.

1. Tennant R, Zimmerman HM: Association between disease in the gallbladder and the heart as evidenced at autopsy. *Yale J Biol Med* 3:495, 1931.
2. Doran FSA: The sites to which pain is referred from common bile duct in man, and its implication for the theory of referred pain. *Br J Surg* 54:599, 1967.
3. Struhl T: Personal communication.

The Differential Diagnosis Between Renal Colic and Acute Cholecystitis

Oscar Kurzer, M.D.

To differentiate renal colic from acute cholecystitis may not always be an easy task. On occasion, it may demand all the diagnostic acumen of the surgeon and urologist working together. Most important is that acute cholecystitis is often accompanied by serious complications such as rupture, peritonitis, septic shock, and empyema, making early diagnosis and prompt surgical intervention imperative. On the other hand, from the standpoint of life and death, renal colic does not call for immediate surgical intervention. Rather, acute renal pain allows the surgeon and urologist sufficient time to localize the origin and decide whether or not the patient should be treated conservatively or surgically.

It is helpful to start this discussion by presenting a typical case.

A 58-year-old obese female came to the emergency room complaining of colicky pain for approximately 12 hours. The onset was sudden, following the ingestion of her evening meal. The pain was located over the right upper quadrant and was referred to the right costovertebral angle. She was nauseated and vomited four times. Prior to admission, the patient experienced fever and chills. She denied having any urinary symptoms.

Past history: Appendectomy at age 15. Three pregnancies, all uncomplicated deliveries. The patient had been treated on several occasions for nonspecific urinary infections.

Medications: None

Physical examination: Obese 58-year-old female, restless and obviously with acute distress. Rectal temperature was 101.5°F. Pulse, 110/m. Blood pressure, 130/90 mm Hg.

Lungs: Bilateral occasional coarse rales.

Abdomen: Palpation: Soft, with exquisite tenderness over the right upper quadrant. Rebound tenderness 2 plus. No masses noted.
Percussion: Murphy's punch was positive over the right costovertebral angle.
Auscultation: Hyperperistaltic bowel sounds.

Laboratory tests: Elevated white blood cell count (15,500/mm^3). Hemoglobin, 13.5 gm/100 ml. He-

matocrit, 46. Serum electrolytes within normal limits; urea nitrogen, 32 mg/100 ml; creatinine, 1.2 mg/100 ml. Urinalysis showed 50–55 white blood cells and 10–15 red blood cells. The chest X-ray showed no evidence of any acute cardiopulmonary process. The flat and erect abdominal films revealed nonspecific bowel gas distention; a 2-mm calcification was found on the right side of the abdomen consistent with a stone in the ureter.

The surgeon called for a urological consultation. The urologist ordered the placement of a Foley catheter to obtain a specimen of uncontaminated urine, for routine urinalysis, culture and sensitivity. The catheter was left in place to monitor urinary output. The catheterized urine specimen revealed 1–3 white blood cells, 0–2 red blood cells, and occult blood + +. An intravenous urogram demonstrated normal kidneys, and normal collecting systems were seen all the way down to the bladder, without any evidence of obstructive uropathy. The calcification noted on the scout film was outside of the urinary tract, most likely a phlebolith. With clearance by the urologist, a diagnosis of acute cholecystitis was pursued. *A gallbladder sonogram was taken, and a diagnosis of cholelithiasis was established.* The patient went to surgery and an acutely inflamed gallbladder with peri-cholecystic adhesions was found. A cholecystectomy was performed; postoperative recovery was uneventful.

DISCUSSION

Renal Pain

Renal pain may mimic a variety of gastrointestinal, musculoskeletal, and gynecological diseases, and therefore can be difficult to diagnose. There are three types of renal pain:

1. *Visceral pain* is often felt over the costovertebral angle but may occur subcostally below the 12th right rib. Pressure or stretching of the renal capsule produces visceral pain.
2. *Renal colic* is sudden, sharp, and acute, usually felt over the costovertebral angle and flank below the right 12th rib. Colicky pain is not related to ureteral hyperperistalsis or spasm, but rather to sudden distention of the renal pelvis. If obstruction is complete, the pain is more severe and colicky. If the obstruction is partial, renal tenderness may be absent.
3. *Referred renal pain* is manifested at a point away from the site of origin; this is due to common afferent nerve pathways. The kidney and ureter receive sensory innervation from the 11th thoracic to the 2nd lumbar spinal nerve roots (T-11

to L-2). Thus, pain from the proximal urinary tract may be referred, simulating the colicky pain of cholecystitis, appendicitis, and epididymitis. Nausea, vomiting, meteorism, and local or generalized paralytic ileus may also appear.

Causes of Acute Renal Pain

The renal conditions causing pain that may simulate acute cholecystitis are:

1. Acute ureteral obstruction; calculus, blood clot, and sloughed papilla.
2. Acute renal infection; pyelitis and pyelonephritis.
3. Acute renovascular obstruction (embolic or thrombotic).
4. Acute renal hemorrhage (intraparenchymal, subscapular, and perirenal).

It is important to know that signs and symptoms arising from urinary tract disease may so closely resemble those of acute gallbladder disease that even the most experienced urologist will have difficulty differentiating between the two.

Evaluation of Acute Renal Pain

Workup:

1. Complete history.
2. Complete physical examination.
3. Urinalysis
   a. *Hematuria:* Gross hematuria is frequently associated with acute renal disorders, but microscopic hematuria (microhematuria) is more common. Any patient with a urinalysis showing 2 red blood cells per high-power field *or more, without exception,* should receive a thorough urological survey. The presence of hematuria should be confirmed by a second urine specimen; a catheterized specimen is preferable, but a midstream specimen (clean catch) should be acceptable. If the second urinalysis shows hematuria, a urological consultation should be requested.
   b. *Pyuria:* Any acute or chronic inflammatory process of the urinary tract may result in an increased number of white blood cells in the *urinary sediment. Pyuria (or leukocyturia) is present when the urinary sediment shows more than 2 white blood cells per high-power field.*

A catheterized urine specimen eliminates the possibility of contamination of the urine specimen from the external genitalia and rectum. Pyuria indicates an inflammatory process in the bladder, ureters, or kidneys. One should discard a urine specimen from a catheter that has been in place for more than 72 hours; such a specimen is completely unreliable for an evaluation of hematuria, pyuria, or bacteruria.

Flat X-rays of the abdomen (kidneys, ureters, and bladder, KUB) consist of anteroposterior views of the abdomen in the recumbent and erect positions. These are obligatory studies in acute abdomen. Attention should be given to the areas corresponding to the kidneys, ureters, and bladder and to a search for calcific densities that overlap them.

The difficulty in diagnosing calculi arises when the stones are small, low in density, or obscured by gas; overlapping bony structures also create diagnostic problems. Most often, the transverse process of the lumbar vertebra will obscure visibility.

CHEMISTRY OF URINARY CALCULI

Approximately 80–85% of all kidney and ureteral calculi are composed (in decreasing order of opacity) of calcium phosphate, calcium oxalate, magnesium ammonium phosphate, and cystine. The incidence of complete radiolucent stones is 15–20%; they are made up of pure uric acid and urate crystals. They are the so-called soft stones composed of organic material with calcareous deposits. *The possibility of a nonopaque stone should be kept in mind* when evaluating the KUB in a patient complaining of acute abdominal pain with hematuria or pyuria. A diagnosis of urinary tract calculi based on an examination of the KUB film alone is *not* reliable, because there are too many extrabiliary opacities that can simulate urinary calculi.

Gallstones in the Gallbladder and Common Duct

Multiple calcifications or a solitary large calcification in the right upper quadrant may overlie the right renal shadow. Their roentgenographic appearance is almost pathognomonic for gallstones. They are recognized by their laminated structure and faceted appearance. On rare occasions, renal calculi may also be laminated and faceted, and can be misleading. An oblique film will ensure that the densities are not within the confines of the urinary tract. Often an intravenous urogram is necessary for further clarification. Stones in the common bile duct occasionally may calcify sufficiently to visualize.

Calcified Costal Cartilages

Calcifications closely follow the course of the cartilages; often cartilaginous shadows may be bilateral and involve several ribs.

Phleboliths (Calcified Venous Valves)

These calcifications are found within the pelvic veins and can be differentiated from ureteral calculi.

Calcification of the Blood Vessel Wall

Mistaken for calculi are fragmentary calcifications of the blood vessel wall. These calcifications are seen as a series of crescent-shaped opacities or pipe-like calcifications. They are seen more frequently in the iliac vessels. When they are not characteristic, an intravenous urogram may reveal the difference.

Calcified Mesenteric or Retroperitoneal Lymph Nodes

Calcified nodes are extremely common, but fortunately, their radiological appearance is so characteristic that they rarely cause difficulties.

Radiopaque Residual Material in the Abdomen

Undissolved pills within the bowel are frequent offenders. A lateral film reveals that the shadows have moved or disappeared. Residual barium in the bowel may also confuse the picture. If the patient requires an emergency workup, one should clear the bowel of barium.

Miscellaneous Calcific Shadows

Such shadows may be caused by metal clips and nonabsorbable sutures. Calcifications from previous inflammatory processes or trauma, i.e., pancreatic calcifications and adrenal calcifications, may also produce shadows. In the female, calcified fibromatous tumors of the uterus may assume unusual positions; when high as in pedunculated fibroids, they may be confused with gallstones or renal calculi.

Emergency Intravenous Pyelogram

An intravenous pyelogram (IVP) is the *fundamental X-ray study* of the urinary tract. It is an *obligatory study* in any patient with acute abdominal pain thought to arise from the urinary tract, especially when hematuria or pyuria is present.

Patients requiring emergency IVP are almost never prepared; there is no need for an enema, because it may result in increased intestinal gas and distention. A good IVP depends upon concentration of the urine, and since acutely ill patients are mildly dehydrated, they are in the proper physiological condition for this test.

There is no absolute contraindication for an IVP; all contraindications are relative.

Available evidence suggests an allergic reaction to the iodine. The chance of a second reaction occurring in the same patient is approximately 16:100. IVP should be avoided in patients with a strong history of allergic reaction to seafood and iodine.

The Presence of Preexisting Systemic Disease

IVP can be dangerous in such patients because of its potential renal toxicity; the iodine contrast medium may produce renal impairment. One such preexisting disease is diabetes mellitus, especially if diabetic nephropathy exists.

Pregnancy

If the indications for IVP are strong, there should be no hesitancy in performing this study. The X-ray exposure must be reduced to an absolute minimum.

Chronic Renal Failure

Renal toxicity due to the iodine contrast medium may exacerbate preexisting kidney insufficiency. Patients with a serum creatinine level of over 4.5 mg/100 ml should *not* have an IVP. About 3% of the patients with chronic renal failure whose creatinine level is 4.5 mg/ml will suffer *acute renal failure* following an IVP. The latter complication is non-oliguric and lasts for an average of 3 days. It is usually reversible, but in about 20–30% of these patients, this impairment can be permanent and will require dialysis.

Cystoscopy with Retrograde Pyelogram

This is a diagnostic procedure that should be done only at the urologist's discretion. It may be performed once the patient is asleep prior to the surgical exploration to either confirm or exclude an acute process of the urinary tract and possibly avoid unnecessary surgery.

Renal Ultrasonography

When delaying therapy will not jeopardize the patient's life, this procedure may be useful, but it will probably never replace IVP as a diagnostic tool. Renal ultrasound is primarily used to differentiate between solid and fluid renal masses. In the presence of acute renal pain, ultrasound may be most helpful.

Renal Radioisotopic Photoscanning (Renal Scan)

Renal scanning reveals the physiological configuration and function of the kidneys. Urinary tract dilatation can be assessed, but the renal scan is *not* able to differentiate between obstructive and non-obstructive nephrosis. The level of obstruction is also difficult to establish.

Computed Tomography (CT) Scan

The CT scan permits rapid and accurate differentiation between renal parenchymal disease and obstructive uropathy. An obstructed and dilated ureter can be followed through its retroperitoneal course, and the exact level of blockage (and possibly its etiology) can be determined. CT scanning can obviate the delay caused by follow-up films with IVP, thus leading to earlier surgery. The CT scan also requires an intravenous injection of iodine contrast dye, and the same contraindications that apply to IVP must be observed. The great disadvantage of CT scanning in a patient with acute abdominal pain is the constant diaphragmatic motion caused by the pain. This causes technical artifacts to appear, which make an accurate diagnosis almost impossible.

Recommended Reading

DeWolf WC, Fraley EE: Renal pain. *Urology* 6(4):403, 1975.

Emmett JL: *Emmett's Clinical Urography.* Philadelphia, WB Saunders Co, 1977.

Friedland GW: Urography, in Stamey TA (ed): *1984 Monographs in Urology,* vol 5, no 2. Princeton, NJ, Costum Publishers Service, 1984, p 26.

Friedland GW, Filly RA, Goris ML, et al (eds): *Uroradiology: An Integrated Approach.* New York, Churchill Livingstone, 1983.

Greene LF, Parsons CL: Urologic diagnosis, in Kendall AR, Karafin L (eds): *Urology,* vol 1. Philadelphia, Harper & Row, 1980.

McAfee JG, Donner MW: Differential diagnosis of calcifications encountered in abdominal radiographs. *Am. J Med Sci* 243:609, 1962.

Straffon RA, Higgins Ch C: Urinary lithiasis and foreign bodies, in Campbell MF, Harrison JH (eds): *Urology,* Vol. I. Philadelphia, WB Saunders Co, 1978, p 687.

8

CHRONIC CHOLECYSTITIS

Introduction

One cannot speak of chronic cholecystitis without mentioning that gallstones are usually present in the gallbladders of 25–35% of all people over 40 years of age. Cholelithiasis is about four to five times more common in women than in men, and the stones may be of many varieties. The different varieties of stones found in the gallbladder will be discussed in relation to chronic cholecystitis. Some stones are made of pure pigment and may develop as a result of blood dyscrasias. The stones of pure cholesterol may be of various sizes and are more likely to be caused by metabolic factors. They usually occur in the pure cholesterol form. *Cholesterol stones* are often seen shortly after pregnancy, and many times they occur in great numbers and frequently are of one size. This writer has seen young women of 19 to 25 after pregnancy with hundreds of small stones in their gallbladder, all of the same size—possibly formed at the same time in the pregnant or postpartum period. Cholesterol stones, when mixed with other chemical substances, are known as *mixed stones.* The type of stone one sees depends upon what elements are involved. Some stones possess calcium carbonate in their makeup, and they frequently show up readily on flat X-ray films. Therefore, it is mandatory to order routine initial flat films. Though we are not concerned at this point with the various types and causes of gallstones; they are fully discussed in Chapter 3. There seems to be no question that metabolic disorders such as those that occur during pregnancy and glandular diseases are associated with calcium or cholesterol dysfunction. Infection cannot be entirely excluded; it is certainly a secondary factor, but its role in the formation of acute and chronic cholecystitis is not fully known.

The gallstone certainly plays an etiological part in producing acute cholecystitis. Over a period of time, it becomes a factor in which a chronic process is likely to occur and lead to minor attacks of acute cholecystitis with varying degrees of severity. These minor attacks often pass as acute indigestion until the final episode becomes more definitely characterized, and ultimately diagnosed, as acute cholecystitis. Therefore, acute cholecystitis is usually nothing more than an acute exacerbation of a long preexiting chronic cholecystitis. How bacteria may get into the gallbladder is still a question. It may be by a direct ascending entrance into the cystic duct from the gastrointestinal tract; infection may enter along the lymphatics; it may be hematogenous in origin; or it may be secondary to ulceration of the mucosa associated with secondary bacterial invasion. Nevertheless, whenever the stone is large enough to obstruct the neck of the cystic duct, existing bacteria which may not be actively infecting the gallbladder can become activated in an obstructed gallbladder. There are forms of cholecystitis in which gravel, mud, or sand-like material is found without any evidence of stone formation. Yet, a clumping together of these materials at any given moment may produce an obstruction in the narrowest portion of the cystic duct. When such an obstruction occurs, the signs and symptoms of acute cholecystitis can be of the same severity as with a real stone.

The picture presented to the pathologist may show none of the characteristics common to chronic cholecystitis; why no typical chronic pathological picture develops at times is unexplained. On occasion, one may see a degenerative process in the mucosa of the gallbladder, but this may be attributed to secondary inflammatory changes caused by possible bacterial infection. In chronic cholecystic disease where no stones are recognized before surgery, one must think of cholesterosis or *strawberry gallbladder.* The author recommends that this form of gallbladder be operated on and removed; this includes adenomyomatosis, cholesterosis, and gallbladders with diverticula or Aschoff-Rokitansky bodies. One must consider the status of the entire biliary tract when searching for possible causes of cholecystitis. Malfunctions of the sphincter of Oddi may be a factor in producing a reflux of activated pancreatic digestive juices into the lumen of the gallbladder. A competent but spastic sphincter of Oddi may account for the back pressure of pancreatic juice that makes its way up into the biliary tract. Also, its spastic action can produce a symptom complex often referred to as *biliary dyskinesia.* Because the exact cause of the so-called biliary dyskinesia can be multiple, it may be difficult to pinpoint the exact diagnosis.

In noninflammatory chronic cholecystitis, routine bacterial studies will not always grow bacteria. However, when bacteria have been isolated in inflammatory processes, they have most often been *Escherichia coli,* streptococci, and staphylococci; on occasion, *Clostridium welchi,* and more uncommonly, *Bacillus typhosus.* Fifty or more years ago, not infrequently, typhoid and paratyphoid organisms were found. In those days, typhoid was a very serious disease. How do bacterial organisms make their way into the gallbladder lumen and produce an infectious inflammatory process? No information exists other than that an infection often takes place in an obstructed gallbladder, where, for some reason, inactivated preexisting organisms become activated. For the present, the means by which activated bacteria invade the gallbladder remains undetermined. One of the older theories, but still a pertinent one, states that bacteria usually originate in the gastrointestinal tract and make their way up from the duodenum through the common bile duct and into the gallbladder via the cystic duct. Another theory is that bacteria travel from the stomach, duodenum, and jejunum via the lymphatics of the porta hepatis that drain these organs into the liver. Bacterial dissemination through the hematogenous route must always be considered a factor, and theory of embolism to the gallbladder also remains a possibility. It is conceivable that bacterial organisms make their way through the hepatic duct system and are excreted in the bile, which finds its way into the gallbladder. Organisms from an existing bacteremia can spread via the portal venous system.

Early pathological tissue studies of chronic cholecystitis often do not reveal cellular changes that are pathognomic of chronic disease. There is evidence of a low-grade inflammatory reaction, round cell infiltration throughout, and deposits of fibrous tissue (desmoplasia); in addition, as previously stated, aspirates of early chronically involved gallbladders do not usually reveal infectious bacteria. The lymph gland of Calot, located at the cystic duct junction with the common duct, may be enlarged and show nonspecific inflammatory changes. On two occasions, lymphosarcoma was diagnosed by routine removal of this gland, and the early institution of chemotherapy allowed these patients to remain well for over 30 years. With time, a chronic cholecystic gallbladder becomes markedly thickened by increased desmoplasia and edema; the latter occurs primarily in the mucosa and submucosa, with lymphocytic cell infiltration in all layers of the gallbladder wall. On occasion, Aschoff-Rokitansky sinuses (or diverticuli) may be found; these gallbladders usually contain mucous or mucopurulent material which on culture may still remain sterile. Many times biliary mud, sand, gravel, or stones will be found. Over time, the muscle is replaced by fibrous tissue and the wall appears thicker, more rigid, and scarred; occasionally, the cystic duct lumen becomes occluded to the point where the gallbladder becomes one fibrous mass. Any gallbladder containing stones over a prolonged period of time is subject to the development of a secondary pathological entity namely, carcinoma.

Gallbladder problems possibly develop when the cystic duct is obstructed for any reason. Whether a cystic duct stone is impacted, or an inflammatory process produces a fibrotic obstruction, or a congenital kink in the cystic duct exists, a complete obstruction ultimately develops and the bile cannot be received from the liver. The bile that remains trapped in such a gallbladder is usually sterile; after the bile is absorbed, an excessive accumulation of mucous secretion produces what is known as *hydrops* of the gallbladder. This condition can be easily recognized at surgery when a needle inserted into the gallbladder lumen withdraws *white bile*. The latter indicates that no bile has come from the liver through the obstructed cystic duct, and if infection of the white bile occurs, an acute infectious cholecystic process develops called *empyema* of the gallbladder. Empyema of the gallbladder, as stated previously, requires emergency surgical intervention, namely evacuation and drainage, and possibly cholecystectomy [see "Management of Acute Cholecystitis (Conservative vs. Interventional)" in Chapter 7].

There are pathological changes that may take place in a gallbladder afflicted with chronic cholelithiasis (with or without infected bile) that can, through undue pressure and distention, produce eventual ischemia with necrosis. By causing undue intracholecystic pressure, an inflammatory reaction associated with a necrotic process may cause the gallbladder to become adherent to its surrounding contiguous structures. With adherence to the duodenum continued pressure may result in necrosis and fistula formation. A stone from the gallbladder may then pass into the duodenum and create a permanent cholecystoduodenal fistula. The stone may finally make its way down the gastrointestinal tract and ultimately lead to intestinal obstruction (gallstone ileus). A scout film will not only reveal an obstructive gas pattern, but will frequently indicate air throughout the biliary tree. Here, too, one may see an ascending cholangitis with all of its associated signs and symptoms. The sequelae of chronic cholecystitis with cholelithiasis are dealt with elsewhere (see "Avoidable Errors in Diagnosis and Judgment in the Management of Biliary Diseases" and "Diagnostic Errors" in Chapter 7). Let us once again enumerate the sequelae:

1. Obstruction of Hartmann's pouch or cystic duct.
2. Ulceration that may lead to:
    a. Perforation and pericholecystic disease.
    b. Emphysematous gallbladder.
    c. Peritonitis (local or generalized).
    d. Subhepatic and/or
    e. Subphrenic abscesses.
    f. Possibility of liver abscess and acute pancreatitis.

3. Ultimately, possible adenocarcinoma of the gallbladder with asymptomatic liver invasion.
4. Choledocholithiasis with jaundice often associated with an ascending cholangitis (pyrexia with chills). The latter is known as *Charcot's intermittent fever* and results from a *ball-valve action* of the gallstone that occludes the common bile duct intermittently and is associated with intermittent chills and fever.

Signs and Symptoms of Chronic Cholecystitis

Most cases of acute cholecystitis usually represent an exacerbation of a preexisting chronic cholecystitis that has developed insidiously over the years. Therefore, acute cholecystitis is usually an exacerbation of a chronic cholecystitis that has been preceded by many minor attacks of vague dyspepsia, i.e., pain and "gas." Sometimes the patient's history will reveal a colicky pain usually directed to the right upper quadrant and epigastrium, with referred pain down either arm or right shoulder; not infrequently pain is localized to the interscapular area. Often these attacks of pain are referrable to the substernal area and may strongly simulate an attack of angina pectoris. Not infrequently, the pain has been confused with a genuine heart attack; similarly, heart attacks have been mistaken for gallbladder disease (see "The Differential Diagnosis Between Acute Cholecystitis, Angina Pectoris, and Acute Myocardial Infraction" in Chapter 7). *Acute indigestion* is a diagnosis that was once often used in reference to either peptic ulcer disease or gallbladder colic. A coronary thrombosis has often resulted in death, and at autopsy the true diagnosis was revealed. What was once the so-called acute dyspepsia or acute indigestion was nothing more than an unrecognized coronary thrombosis with myocardial infarction. Dyspepsia or "stomach upset" may be a common symptom complex, but when the symptoms reach their height, anorexia and vomiting become concomitant complaints. Early attacks of acute cholecystitis may be stimulated by the same factors that excite a chronic cholecystitis, but apparently the severity of the attack is greater where a preexisting well-developed chronic cholecystitis pre-existed.

This writer maintains that only a surgical condition can be improved or cured by a surgical procedure. In other words, surgical conditions require surgical treatment, and only surgical conditions can truly improve with surgical intervention. If it is not a surgical condition, surgery cannot help; in fact, nonindicated surgical procedures can only complicate and add extra difficulties to the problem. For example, surgery for inaccurately diagnosed gallbladder disease may cause the patient to continue to complain of vague symptoms and signs that the surgeon will often diagnose as postcholecystectomy syndrome or biliary dyskinesia. Though the latter diagnosis has been used for years, this writer believes that in reality it is a myth, because no one has ever proven its existence. When one of these cases is evaluated at later surgery, with a more extensive workup, it is discovered that a cholecystectomy was not indicated in the first place; that another pathological condition existed or coexisted, such as hiatus hernia, diverticulitis, carcinoma of the colon, duodenal or gastric ulcer, and spastic bowel.

Not infrequently, a cholecystectomy is necessary but the surgeon fails to recognize the coexisting common duct problem. An unrecognized residual stone in the common bile duct is often diagnosed as postcholecystectomy syndrome. Biliary dyskinesia, if ever diagnosed correctly, will most likely turn out to be a physiological malfunction of the ampullary structure; in other words, a spastic sphincter of Oddi may be at fault. The writer has rarely utilized this diagnosis; in fact, he had found that surgical diseases are most often based not so much on malfunction of the biliary system as on coexisting unrecognized organic pathology. Postcholecystectomy syndrome may be diagnosed by the surgeon, but in reality the cause may be the fault of the operation itself. A hastily performed cholecystectomy may have left a large cystic duct stump that may have contained a calculus. The latter condition can produce colicky pains just as if the gallbladder had never been removed. Not infrequently, inadequate surgery is a strong iatrogenic factor that accounts for many of the complex problems called postcholecystectomy syndrome.

Recently, this writer examined a 75-year-old man who was diagnosed as having a postcholecystectomy syndrome. This patient stated that he had a cholecystectomy about 8 years ago. On examination his abdomen revealed a Kocher incision in the right upper quadrant. A routine cholecystogram showed an intact, full-sized, but poorly functioning gallbladder. Many sins of omission and commission are concealed by a diagnosis of postcholecystectomy syndrome or biliary dyskinesia. The patient was subsequently reoperated on and the usual chronically inflamed gallbladder was found and removed. Recovery was uneventful, and the patient never complained again.

Forms of Chronic Cholecystitis

CHOLESTEROSIS OF THE GALLBLADDER (STRAWBERRY GALLBLADDER)

Cholesterosis refers to a gallbladder disease that consists of small deposits of cholesterol in the mucosa, epithelial cells, and macrophages in the subepithelial layer of the gallbladder wall. On cholecystography the gallbladder may not show any evidence of existing pathology, and there is no impairment in the concentration of the dye by the gallbladder. Accumulation of cholesterol or lipid material is not necessarily associated with acute cholecystitis but is related to a high concentration of cholesterol in the bile of the gallbladder. The cholesterol deposits are found in the villi of the lining of the gallbladder mucosa, and they form polyp-like structures; these small polyps can be seen on a good cholecystogram as definite filling defects. Some believe that when these cholesterol-containing villi ultimately detach, they form a nucleus or nidus for subsequent stone formation; they certainly form a part of the debris that accumulates within the gallbladder. This debris can obstruct when it accumulates as a mass in the cystic duct and may cause symptoms of colic if the mass cannot pass further along the valves of Heister. Cholesterosis occurs equally as often in males and females, and the signs and symptoms often simulate those of acute cholecystitis. Occasionally, a sharp diagnosis based on good visual acuity may indicate the possibility of the existence of a strawberry gallbladder. During surgery, this gallbladder will present not as the chronically inflamed gallbladder, which is thick and lusterless, but as one whose wall is usually rather thin and still of a normal slate blue color.

Cholesterosis is best seen when the gallbladder is opened. It resembles the surface of a strawberry, with yellow flicks or spots on an inflamed, beefy red background. All signs and symptoms are most likely related to the strawberry gallbladder. Cholecystectomy usually gives complete relief. At times, there may be some localized cholesterol deposits that measure more than 2 or 3 mm in size, and in the differential diagnosis one must consider papillomatosis of the gallbladder. No one has yet clarified the relationship between papillomatosis of the gallbladder and carcinoma of the gallbladder, but this writer recommends cholecystectomy when signs and symptoms are attributed to the cholangiographic findings.

PORCELAIN GALLBLADDER

Porcelain gallbladder[1-10] is a condition in which calcification involves the wall of the gallbladder. The calcific process may be limited to the muscularis, the mucosa, or both. It occurs most frequently in patients over 65 years of age, predominantly in females; the female:male ratio is about 5:1.

This disease process may be relatively asymptomatic; the diagnosis is usually made on routine oral cholecystography and/or ultrasonography. The incidence of porcelain gallbladder at autopsy is 0.06–0.08%; by cholecystography, about 1 in 1500 cases; and at surgery, 0.4–0.8%.

The pathology depends upon which layer of the gallbladder wall is involved. It is believed that necrosis and fibrosis of the musculature precede the deposition of calcium (calcium carbonate). The mucosal lining develops a plaque-like formation, which is most likely the result of calcium deposits derived from mucus secretion.

It is believed that cystic duct obstruction is related to the abnormal pathological process, as well as to the frequency of gallstones. There is no evidence to suggest the coexistence of an abnormal calcium metabolism.

Microscopic studies of the gallbladder wall reveal varied pathological findings such as focal hemorrhage, necrosis, fibrosis, chronic inflammation, and metaplasia. A precancerous condition may also be seen. About 22% of the cases are associated with carcinoma (infiltrating and squamous cell carcinoma).

Complications occur in less than 10% of the cases.

References

1. Allison SS: Complete ossification of gallbladder. *London Med Gas* 137:35, 1844–1845.
2. Cornell CM, Clarke R: Vicarious calcification involving the gallbladder. *Ann Surg* 139:267, 1959.
3. Davis C, Galt RM: Porcelain gallbladder associated with carcinoma of the colon. *Am J Surg* 83:217, 1961.
4. Germain M, Martin E, Gremilet C: Vesicules porcelains and cancers. *Semain Hop Paris* 55:1629, 1979.
5. Kazmierski RH: Primary adenocarcinoma of the gallbladder with intramural calcification. *Am J Surg* 82:248, 1951.

6. Maingot R: *Abdominal Operations*, ed 7. New York, Appleton Century Crofts, 1980, p 999.

7. Naisons P: Presentaiton d'une vesicule biliare comletement certifice. *Bull Mem Soc Anat Paris* 84:15, 1909.

8. Ochsner SF, Carrera GM: Calcifications of the gallbladder—porcelain gallbladder. *Am J Roentgenol* 89:847, 1963.

9. Phemister DB, Rewbridge AG, Rudisill N: Calcium carbonate gallstones and calcification of the gallbladder following cystic duct obstruction. *Ann Surg* 94:493, 1931.

10. Polk HC: Carcinoma of the calcified gallbladder. *Gastroenterology* 50:582, 1966.

ACALCULOUS CHOLECYSTITIS

Acute acalculous cholecystitis is, in effect, an acute cholecystitis that develops without the formation of stones in the biliary tract. It is an uncommon disease entity with a diverse etiology. Acute acalculous cholecystitis has been known to follow severe trauma, burns, and extensive surgical procedures. Many other diseases, such as typhoid and brucillosis, have also been associated with this unusual disease process. It is believed that the gallbladder wall becomes primarily involved, followed secondarily by bacterial invasion. Acute acalculous cholecystitis has followed debilitating infectious disease in children and extensive trauma in the military. It is believed that the cystic duct is obstructed first, followed by bacterial invasion and inflammation. The physical signs are mainly tenderness and a possible mass in the right upper quadrant. Fever, leukocytosis, and elevated liver enzyme levels may also be present; jaundice too may appear. Ultrasonography may show a distended gallbladder with sludge and edema of the gallbladder wall. No stones can be found anywhere in the biliary tract, so that accompanying jaundice is most likely related to liver damage.

A published report by Munster et al.[1] states that acalculous cholecystitis is most often encountered in young patients with congenital biliary malformations. In middle-aged and elderly patients, coexistent diseases such as diabetes, vascular disorders, and pancreatitis are regarded as predisposing factors. In patients with extensive thermal injury, the incidence of acalculous cholecystitis was reviewed. The authors' study consisted of 2456 autopsies of patients who had suffered burns. Of this group, 10 patients were found with acalculous cholecystitis. The authors concluded that the surgeon should be aware of the existence of acalculous cholecystitis during the postburn period. In patients with jaundice, acalculous cholecystitis should be included in the differential diagnosis. The authors state that maintenance of adequate hydration is important during the postburn period. *They conclude that once the diagnosis of acute acalculous cholecystitis is established, a cholecystectomy should be carried out with a minimum of delay, since these patients are usually debilitated and easily prone to develop complications from sepsis. Nonoperative management may invite serious consequences.*

This form of acute cholecystitis was studied by Anderson et al.[2] They concluded that acute acalculous cholecystitis is an enigmatic condition and that different opinions exist regarding its cause and treatment. In approximately one-third of their cases, unsuccessful results followed surgical intervention. The complications and the mortality rate that followed surgery for acalculous cholecystitis were especially high. These writers studied acalculous gallbladders for over 8 years, and in their review paid special attention to the possible etiological factors and the results of their surgery.

This writer believes that the high mortality due to acute acalculous cholecystitis is related to delayed diagnosis, which predisposes to earlier perforation and gangrene of the gallbladder wall; and that preexisting debilitating conditions brought on by trauma, traumatic surgery, burns, and infectious diseases predispose the debilitated patient to this uncommon disease process. The treatment is surgical—either cholecystostomy in the very debilitated patient or cholecystectomy in the patient who appears strong enough to tolerate it. This writer concludes that there are numerous preexisting and exacerbating factors. In all cases of acute cholecystitis, acalculous cholecystitis should be considered in the differential diagnosis. Actually, the final diagnosis will be established by the pathologist's report. The preoperative diagnosis and treatment must be judged and carried out by the same criteria applied to acute cholecystitis.

Fox et al.,[3] in writing on acalculous cholecystitis, stated that this disease entity has the highest mortality of all so-called benign gallbladder diseases. He reported that this disease entity usually affects elderly patients with cardiovascular and metabolic diseases. The mortality rises whenever sepsis enters the picture. Of the cholecystectomies performed from 1969 to 1979, 2.3% were diagnosed as acalculous cholecystitis. Ages of the patients ranged from 26 to 82 years; 80% of these patients were over 60 years of age; 50% had cardiovascular disease; 25% had diabetes mellitus. Technetium-99 image display analysis (cholescintigraphy) proved most useful in diagnosing gallbladder dysfunction in 14 out of 15 patients. Failure of the gallbladder to contract is considered by Fox et al. to be pathognomonic for biliary tract disease. Fifty percent of the patients had gangrenous cholecystitis. Sepsis, dehydration, and starvation are often associated with acalculous cholecystitis. Children may also develop acute and chronic forms of acalculous disease.

Recommended Treatment

The greatest incidence of acalculous cholecystitis was reported in patients after trauma, such as after major surgical procedures in critically ill patients; the disease had no relationship to the surgery.

To demonstrate *the importance of early surgical intervention,* Johnson[4] divided his cases into two groups:

Group A patients underwent *cholecystectomy for acute cholecystitis in less than 48 hours;* 8% developed gangrene and perforation (see "Signs and Symptoms of Chronic Cholecystitis" in this chapter).

Group B patients went to surgery after 48 hours; 48% developed perforation of the gallbladder (a rate six times greater than in those operated on sooner).

Johnson encourages heightened awareness of making an early diagnosis and, more importantly, urges earlier surgical intervention.

Johnson stated that in 25% of the patients studied, unexplained fever was the first sign, followed by the more usual signs and symptons of cholecystitis. In the more difficult cases, ultrasound proved to be very reliable. In the absence of cholelithiasis, ultrasonography demonstrated (1) *thickening* of the gallbladder wall associated with (2) *a tender mass* and (3) *a pericholecystic collection.* In 90% of the patients studied, at least one of these three findings was present. In 75% of the patients who developed postoperative complications, further study revealed the existence of more advanced cholecystic disease.

The author's experience with acalculous cholecystitis is quite similar to Johnson's, and therefore the recommendations are the same, namely, *early surgical intervention.*

Recommended Reading

Becker CJ, Dubin T, Glenn F: Induction of acute cholecystitis by activation of factor XII. *J Exp Med* 151:81, 1980.

Deitch EA: Utility and accuracy of ultrasonically measured gallbladder wall as a diagnostic criteria in biliary tract disease. *Dig Dis Sci* 26:686, 1981.

Deitch EA, Engel JM: Acute acalculous cholecystitis: Ultrasonic diagnosis. *Am J Surg* 142:290, 1981.

Deitch EA, Engel JM: Ultrasonic detection of acute cholecystitis with pericholecystic abscess. *Am Surg* 42:211, 1981.

Duncan J: Femoral hernia: Gangrene of the gallbladder; extravasation of bile; peritonitis; death. *North J Med* 2:151, 1844.

DuPriest RW, Khaneja SC, Cowley RA: Acute cholecystitis complicating trauma. *Ann Surg* 189:84, 1979.

Glenn F: Acute cholecystitis following the surgical treatment of unrelated disease. *Ann Surg* 126:411, 1947.

Glenn F: Acute acalculous cholecystitis. *Ann Surg* 189:458, 1979.

Glenn F, Becker CG: Acute acalculous cholecystitis: An increasing entity. *Ann Surg* 195:131, 1982.

Greenberg M, Kangarloo H, Cochran ST, et al: The ultrasonographic diagnosis of cholecystitis and cholelithiasis in children. *Radiology* 137:745, 1980.

Herlin P, Ericsson M, Holmlin T, et al: Acute acalculous cholecystitis following trauma. *Br J Surg* 69:475, 1982.

Howard RJ: Acute acalculous cholecystitis. *Am J Surg* 141:194, 1981.

Lindberg EF, Grunnan GL, Smith L: Acalculous cholecystitis in Viet Nam casualties. *Ann Surg* 171:152, 1970.

Long TN, Heimbach DM, Carrico CJ: Acalculous cholecystitis in critically ill patients. *Am J Surg* 136:31, 1978.

Marchal G, Crolla D, Baurt AL, et al: Gallbladder wall thickening: A new sign of gallbladder disease visualized by gray scale cholecystosonography. *J Clin Ultrasound* 6:177, 1978.

Orlando R, Gleason E, Drezner AD: Acute acalculous cholecystitis in the critically ill patient. *Am J Surg* 145:472, 1983.

Ottinger LW: Acute cholecystitis as a postoperative complication. *Ann Surg* 184:162, 1976.

Peterson SF, Sheldon FG: Acute acalculous cholecystitis: A complication of hyperalimentation. *Am J Surg* 138:814, 1979.

Raghavendra BM, Feinder HD, Subramanyam BR, et al: Acute cholecystitis: Sonographic-pathologic analysis. *AJR* 137:327, 1981.

References

1. Munster AM, Goodwin JR, Pruit JR: US Army Institute of Surgical Research, Brooke Army Medical Center, Texas.

2. Anderson A, Bergdahl L, Boquist L, et al: Non-malignant gallbladder disease in the aged. *Acta Chir Scand* 140:242, 1974.

3. Fox TA, Block MA, LoGrippo GA: The importance of early diagnosis of acute acalculous cholecystitis. *Surg Gynecol Obstet* 1987.

4. Johnson AG: Cholecystectomy and gallstone dyspepsia. *Ann R Coll Surg Engl* 51:69, 1975.

EMPHYSEMATOUS CHOLECYSTITIS

Emphysematous cholecystitis is an uncommon form of inflammation of the gallbladder, characterized by the presence of gas in its lumen, wall, and surrounding spaces. Terms like *gaseous cholecystitis, pneumocholecystitis,* and *pyopneumocholecystitis* have also been employed to describe this condition. However, *emphysematous cholecystitis* appears to be most apt, as it denotes the characteristic swelling and inflation of the inflamed gallbladder due to the presence of air or gas.

The credit for making the first diagnosis of emphysematous cholecystitis preoperatively on the basis of roentgenograms goes to Hegner.[1] It was after his classical description of its radiological appearance, published in 1931, that this condition became better known and accepted. As recently as 1966, Sarmiento[2] was able to find only 105 cases reported in the world literature; this indicates the rarity of the entity.

The condition occurs most commonly in the sixth and seventh decades of life and is more frequent in males than in females. Its increased incidence in diabetics has been noted by other authors. The etiology appears to be due to invasion of the gallbladder by clostridia or other gas-forming organisms in a patient already afflicted with acute cholecystitis and an occluded cystic duct. The gas first appears in the gallbladder lumen and then dissects into the subserosa as the intraluminal pressure rises. The gas finally disseminates and perforates through the wall and into the pericholecystic tissue and subhepatic space. Twenty-four to 48 hours are required for sufficient gas to be produced for demonstration on a flat abdominal X-ray film.

Other sources of gas in the biliary tract must be ruled out, including that from an enterobiliary fistula or incompetent sphincter of Oddi. The differential diagnosis of right upper quadrant gas includes adjacent loops of bowel, subphrenic abscess with gas formation, and, rarely, a lipoma of the gallbladder.

Laboratory Findings in the Author's Patient

In a 70-year-old male Caucasian patient examined by the author, there was an infiltrate in the right lower lobe, with slight elevation of the right hemidiaphragm. The heart was increased in the cardiothoracic ratio. The initial abdominal X-rays (flat films, both upright and supine) revealed that the bowel gas pattern was unremarkable, with no evidence of air-fluid levels or free air under the diaphragm; otherwise, the films were essentially normal. A tentative diagnosis of acute cholecystitis was made, and the patient was managed by bed rest, nothing by mouth, continuous nasogastric suction, and antibiotics in the IV fluids. With this conservative management, the patient's previously elevated temperature began to drop, his vital signs

became more stable, and the patient started to feel better. His local abdominal signs, however, persisted. An oral cholecystogram failed to opacify the gallbladder, but in the region of the gallbladder a round air shadow (6 cm in diameter) with a peripheral ring of radiolucency was seen. On the basis of these findings, the X-ray diagnosis was revised to acute emphysematous cholecystitis. A barium enema was given, and an upper gastrointestinal series of X-rays was carried out in the following 2 days. The X-rays again confirmed the gaseous shadow to be extragastrointestinal. No fistulous communication could be demonstrated between the gallbladder and the gastrointestinal tract. Subsequent flat X-rays of the abdomen revealed a distinct horizontal air-fluid level in place of the previous round air shadow. Calculi were not demonstrable (Fig. 80).

Surgical Management

The patient was operated upon 3 weeks after the onset of the abdominal pain. The abdomen was opened, revealing a mass of adhesions in the right upper quadrant that consisted of the greater

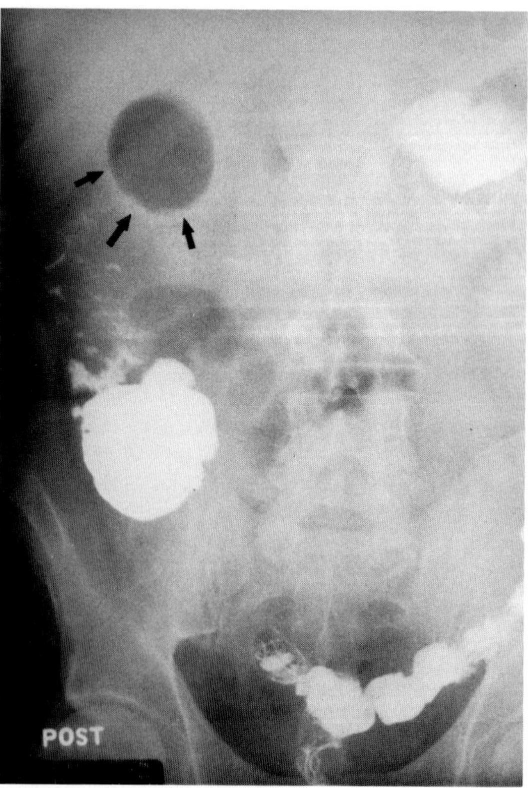

Figure 80. Postevacuation barium enema film demonstrating thickened wall of gallbladder with gas in the lumen.

omentum firmly adherent to, and completely obliterating, the inflamed gallbladder. Separation of the omentum by blunt and sharp dissection revealed a moderate amount of free pus in the subhepatic space (subhepatic abscess). Continued dissection revealed additional pus around the gallbladder (pericholecystic abscess). The gallbladder was markedly thickened and enlarged, fully distended, and severely inflamed. On introduction of a large trocar through the fundus (apparently the site of the original rupture), innumerable millet-sized stones, pus, and gas were released at once; the gas was under tremendous pressure, as seen by its explosive effect on the plunger of the trocar. The gas had no foul odor, but the mucosal lining of the gallbladder was completely necrotic and almost completely detached from the seromuscular wall. At no time was any bile encountered. There was gross distortion of the surrounding local anatomy, which was highly vascular and friable. The mucosal lining was circumferentially dissected from the seromuscular shell of the organ. The gallbladder shell was irrigated with normal saline, and a large Malecot catheter was introduced through the residual shell for drainage. The catheter was sewn in place to the shell wall. Morison's fossa and the subhepatic space were drained by Penrose drains brought out through a subcostal stab wound. The abdomen was then closed.

Postoperative Course

The Malecot catheter started to drain clear bile after 24 hours, but after 1 week, the bile drainage suddenly stopped. Culture of the gallbladder during surgery failed to grow any microorganisms. The negative culture was attributed to the intensive antibiotic therapy administered before the operation. The postoperative period was uneventful. Intravenous cholangiograms 6 weeks postoperatively outlined a normal biliary ductal system without any evidence of extrinsic obstruction or intraductal calculi. The gallbladder did not opacify, though there was a faint visualization of a short segment of the cystic duct. The Malecot catheter was removed, and the stoma in the abdominal wall closed spontaneously in 24 hours. When last seen 8 months after surgery, the patient was free of any biliary complaints.

Discussion

This writer managed the patient without surgery, but with antibiotics. Surgery was undertaken several days after the onset of the disease and after medical management. The flat films of the abdomen were taken at intervals; they gave us a better idea of the patient's pathological progress than did the clinical picture and laboratory data. A decision to operate 3 weeks after the onset of the disease process was influenced by the clinical picture, and more especially by the changing pattern of gas shadows seen in the flat X-ray films.

After the first postoperative day the bile drained freely, but it stopped soon thereafter. A retrograde study through the cholecystostomy tube revealed a normal biliary tree with no calculi. Six weeks later, an intravenous cholangiogram failed to opacify the gallbladder, showing that the patient had already achieved an effective "spontaneous cholecystectomy." The Malecot catheter was pulled out without any leakage, and the incision promptly closed without incident.

Summary

The author's case of emphysematous cholecystitis was presented.[3] The essential treatment consisted of draining the subhepatic abscess, excising the entire gangrenous lining (mucosa and submucosa) of the gallbladder, then doing an improvised cholecystostomy, utilizing the residual seromuscular gallbladder shell as the drainage site. The use of flat roentgenograms of the abdomen taken at intervals is advocated because it helps to reveal the progress of the pathogenesis of this disease process. Instead of the usual cholecystectomy or cholecystostomy, this writer believes that it may be better to excise only the gangrenous mucosal lining and drain the cored-out gallbladder shell, as was done in this case. This writer had a similar case about a month later in which the same treatment was carried out with success. After the mucosa and submucosa were excised, the gallbladder shell was drained; after the catheter was pulled out, spontaneous collapse of the gallbladder wall occurred, obliterating the gallbladder lumen—essentially a spontaneous cholecystectomy.

Recommended Reading

Bigler FC: Acute gaseous cholecystitis. *Am J Med* 29:181, 1960.

Blum I, Stagg A: Emphysematous cholecystitis. *Am J Roentgenol* 89:840, 1962.

Bockus HL: *Gastroenterology III*, ed 2. Philadelphia, WB Saunders Co, 1965, pp 713–715.

Boerema WJ, McWilliam RA: Emphysematous cholecystitis: An unusual form of presentation. *Aust NZ J Surg* 39:258, 1970.

Edinburgh A, Geffen A: Acute emphysematous cholecystitis. *Am J Surg* 96:66, 1958.

Ferguson HL: Emphysematous cholecystitis. *Am Surg* 37:431, 1971.

Friedman J, et al: Emphysematous cholecystitis. *Am J Roentgenol* 62:814, 1949.

Gordon-Taylor G, Whitby LEH: Incidence of anaerobic infections in the gall bladder. *Br J Surg* 19:619, 1932.

Gordon-Taylor G, Whitby LEH: Bacteriological study of 50 cases of cholecystectomy with special reference to anaerobic infection. *Br J Surg* 18:78, 1930.

Holgersen LO, White JJ: Emphysematous cholecystitis: A report of five cases. *Surgery* 69:102, 1971.

Marshall JF, Hartzog DC: Acute emphysematous cholecystitis. *Ann Surg* 159:1011, 1964.

McCorkle H, Fong EE: Clinical significance of gas in the gall bladder. *Surgery* 2:851, 1942.

McGregor JK: Surgical management of cholecystitis emphysematosa. *Can Med Assoc J* 85:863, 1961.

Rosoff L, Meyers H: Acute emphysematous cholecystitis. *Am J Surg* 111:410, 1966.

Sawyer RB, Lynch FP, Coppinger WR, et al: Infectious emphysema of the gastrointestinal tract in the adult. *Am J Surg* 120:579, 1970.

Schowengerdt CG, Wiot JF: Emphysematous cholecystitis following aortography. *Am Surg* 82:274, 1972.

Stevenson CA: Emphysematous cholecystitis. *Am J Roentgenol Radiol Ther* 51:53, 1944.

References

1. Hegner CF: Gaseous pericholecystitis with cholecystitis and cholelithiasis. *Arch Surg* 22:993, 1931.
2. Sarmiento RV: Emphysematous cholecystitis. *Arch Surg* 93:1009, 1966.
3. Glassman JA, Pieck C Jr, Bhuta V, et al: Emphysematous cholecystitis. *J Abdom Surg* vol 17, no 4, 1975.

ADENOMYOMATOSIS

It is believed that adenomyomatosis is a congenital anomaly and commonly involves the fundus of the gallbladder. It can be seen or palpated grossly and is normally covered by the serosa of the gallbladder. When cut, this tumor shows cystic spaces which, on occasion, may fill on X-ray study and can often be recognized. These spaces communicate with the gallbladder lumen at times; at other times, they do not. Here again, we have an equivocal problem. When this tumor is associated with signs and symptoms referable to the gallbladder, this writer recommends cholecystectomy as the best and safest course to follow.

Other names for adenomyomatosis are *cholecystitis cystica* and *adenomyoma.*

This lesion may be localized or diffuse; the localized form is usually found in the fundus of the gallbladder. Pathologically, adenomyoma exists as an admixture of smooth muscle, glands, and cystic stoma. Radiologically, its appearance may vary, depending upon the gallbladder involvement and the degree of distention.

POLYPS

Polyps of the gallbladder are lesions on a stalk and may be inflammatory or hyperplastic. Though they may undergo malignant change, they are not considered invasive. Cholecystography is the only means of diagnosing polyps of the gallbladder. When they are recognized, the safest procedure is cholecystectomy.

ASCHOFF-ROKITANSKY SINUSES

It is believed that Aschoff-Rokitansky sinuses are acquired. They are mostly seen in persons over 40 and, uncommonly in younger patients. This writer has had two cases of hourglass gallbladder; cholecystectomy revealed that the constriction of the body was caused by the inflamed Aschoff-Rokitansky bodies at the site of constriction. One patient was an 18-year-old female, and the other was a 60-year-old male. Aschoff-Rokitansky sinuses are outpouchings of the gallbladder mucosa that make their way out through the muscularis and force their way to the serosal surface, thus creating false diverticula which may be compared with the pharyngoesophagael diverticulum (Zenker's) of the esophagus. This should be considered an acquired pathological condition that is vividly revealed on radiological study. Aschoff-Rokitansky sinuses or diverticula project out from the lumen of the gallbladder and are often seen surrounding the gallbladder surface. Theoretically, the possible cause of Aschoff-Rokitansky sinuses or diverticula, though unknown, is believed to be related to occasional undue or excessive pressure that may develop within the gallbladder. This may occur, for example, when the gallbladder has difficulty in expressing bile through the cystic duct; the back pressure may act to create these protrusions. Many believe that stone formations develop in these diverticuli, which at a later date may lead to cholelithiasis. Whenever the writer recognizes that these findings are associated with symptoms and signs referable to the gallbladder disease, he recommends cholecystectomy.

HOURGLASS AND MULTISEPTATION OF THE GALLBLADDER

Multiseptation of the gallbladder is a rare congenital anomaly. The septa are believed to consist of a fibromuscular tissue lined with epithelium. The pathogenesis suggests that the gallbladder may have been "pushed" or "drawn" into the gallbladder vesicle. The author believes that in case 1 (Fig. 82), the Rokitansky sinuses within the gallbladder wall, by repeated inflammatory changes, may have constricted to create a septal formation with two communicating compartments—one compartment proximal and the other distal to the cystic duct. Cholangiographic studies revealed a septated gallbladder, with two compartments separated by a narrow lumen.

Clinically, all four reported patients complained of right upper quadrant pain and tenderness. Two of the patients had to be operated on as emergencies. Their ages ranged from the second to the fourth decade. The remaining two patients were operated on electively; they, too, suffered intermittently from the signs and symptoms of gallbladder dysfunction. One of the patients operated on as an emergency revealed a gallbladder that had to be dissected free from extensive pericholecystic adhesions. Otherwise, cholecystectomy was carried out in a routine manner. In case 1, the gallbladder was opened in the operating room. The septa were noted, and the Rokitansky-Aschoff sinuses (Fig. 81, arrow) were easily identified. The distal compartment appeared inflamed, but no stones were found (Figs. 81–83). Microscopically, the pathologist reported acute inflammation with thickening of the gallbladder wall. The patient made an uneventful recovery. In case 2, when the gallbladder was divided, multisepta were found, creating several compartments; stones were found in the distal and middle compartments. Microscopically, subacute recurrent cholecystitis with focal hemorrhages and ulcerations was reported (Figs. 81–83). This patient also made an uneventful recovery.

Multiseptation of the gallbladder was first described by Knetch[1] in 1952. Beilby[2] illustrated an infant's gallbladder with three locules separated by septa at the neck and fundus. Land et al.[3] reported a case of multiseptate gallbladder and suggested a hypothesis based upon embryogenesis.

The clinical pathogenesis of a characteristic gallbladder symptom complex may be due to the inability of the obstructed compartment to empty itself. Multiseptation creates a stenotic resistance to the outflow of thickened, viscid bile which results in stasis and ultimate cholecystitis. Figures 81, 82, and 83 illustrate the pathological picture that the author found at surgery. Based upon the marked bluish discoloration of the distal compartment, it is conceivable that gangrenous changes were in progress and that timely intervention prevented perforation and peritonitis.

References

1. Knetch: First description of multiseptation of the gallbladder, 77:587-89; Nov. 1952.
2. Beilby JO: Diverticulosis of the gallbladder. *Br J Pathol* 48:382, 1907.
3. Land AS, Bhagavan BS, Amin PB, et al: Multiseptate gallbladder: Embryonic hypothesis. *Arch Pathol* 89:382, 1970.

THE "SILENT" GALLSTONE

At times, gallstones will accidentally be found on routine X-ray study, and the patient will have no complaints in relation to them; these stones are silent. The patient may not be aware of having cholelithiasis for years. When doctors find a gallbladder full of stones, or just one large, symptomless stone, what should they recommend to their patient? Some doctors tell the patient, "If the 'silent' stone does not bother you, then don't bother it." This is a common statement, usually followed by: "If and when it bothers you, we will attend to it." This is the worst possible advice a physician can offer his patient. According to this writer, a "silent stone," as Charles Mayo once put it, "is as silent as a tombstone!" At times, a single stone will obstruct the gallbladder no matter how large it may be. A stone doesn't have to obstruct the cystic duct; it can obstruct the gallbladder at the ampulla or in Hartmann's pouch, yet the obstruction will be just as complete and just as dangerous. A stone that is silent may conceivably produce a silent carcinoma, or erode into the duodenum and roll down the intestine to produce intestinal obstruction, both of which do not give the patient the opportunity to receive the proper curative treatment, namely, elective cholecystectomy. This writer, despite opinions to the contrary, strongly urges the surgeon to recommend a cholecystectomy on every gallbladder that contains stones, silent or not. The surgeon must be a good diagnostician as well as a good salesman. He must sell the patient an operation because he has the opportunity to prevent a future serious complication, possibly an incurable one. There are surgeons (as well as internists) who recommend elective cholecystectomy only when the silent stone or stones provoke repeated attacks of pain, nausea, and vomiting. Some surgeons and internists wait for jaundice to develop before they recommend surgery. They do not understand that emergency surgery carries a higher mortality, especially in patients over 65.

Silent stones may not begin with a simple attack; rather, they may begin as a major inflammatory process which may be late in its pathogenesis. A

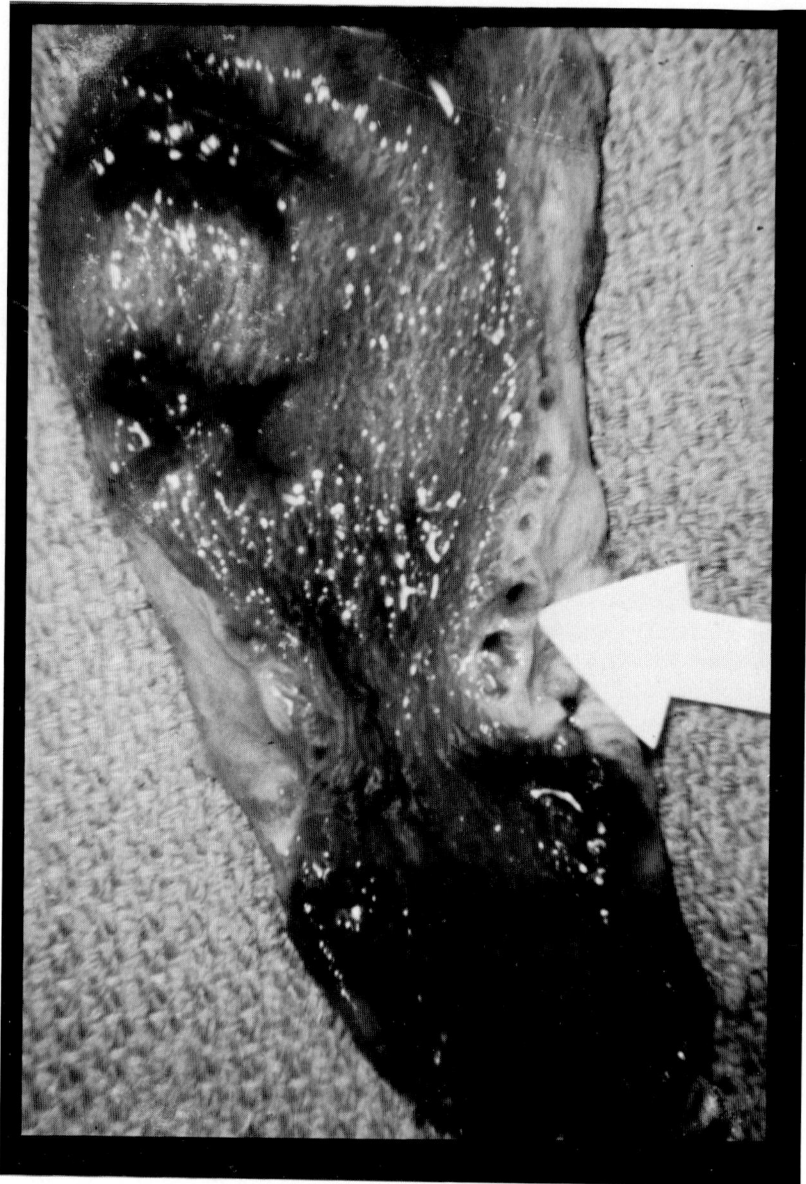

Figure 81. *This diagram of the cut gallbladder shows the constriction that leads to two compartments, known as the "hour-glass" gallbladder. See text for the pathogenesis of this entity; also the surgical treatment.*

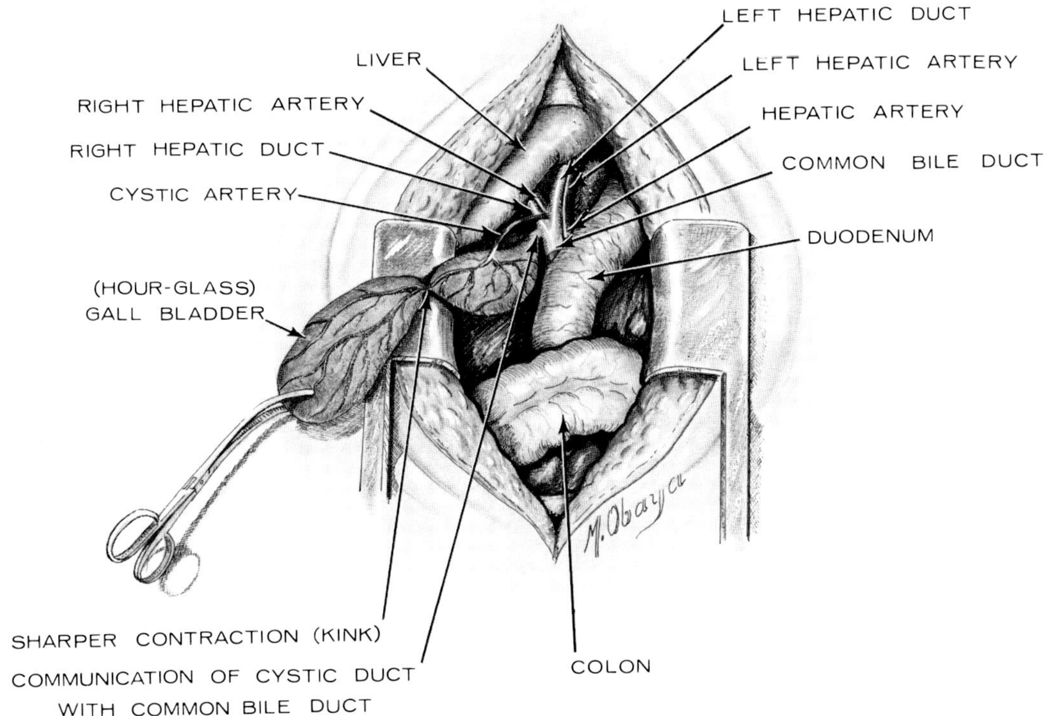

Figure 82. The "hour-glass" gallbladder is fully exposed. Cholecystectomy must be carried out carefully because of the adjacent inflammatory changes.

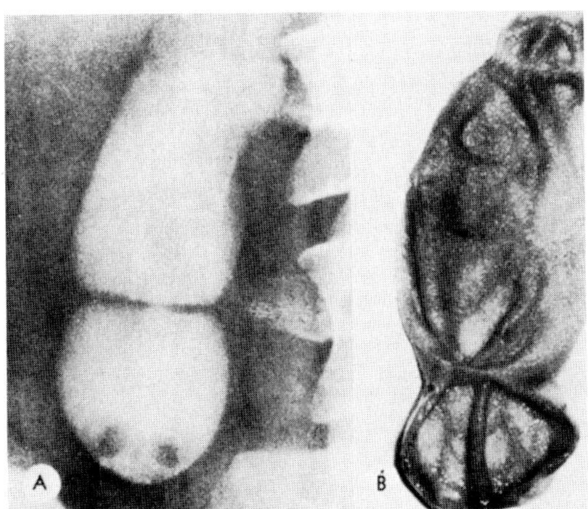

Figure 83. Adenomyomatosis, annular type, early stage. A. Phrygian cap; lithiasis beyond the septum. B. Surgical specimen. The gallbladder wall at the insertion of the septum appears slightly thickened, and the Rokitansky Aschoff sinuses are visible. (From The American Journal of Roentgenology, Radium Therapy and Nuclear Medicine Vol CVII, No. 1, September, 1969.)

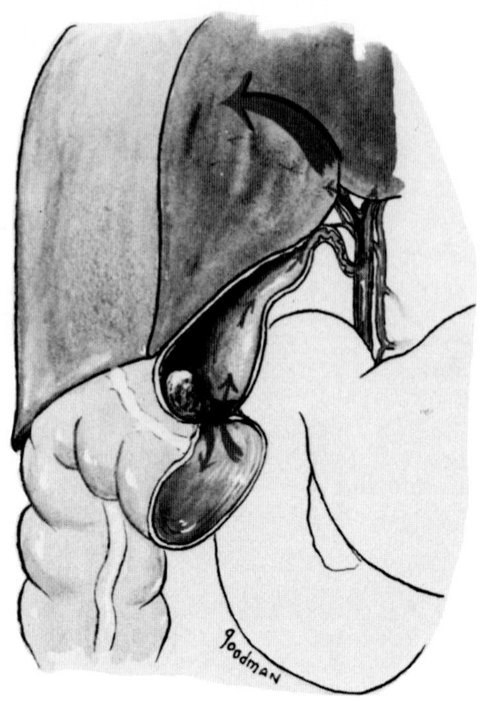

Figure 84. This diagram illustrates a more serious form of gallbladder erosion. When the gallstone erodes into the colon it usually passes out with the stool. Here the stone is shown eroding into the duodenum and beginning its passage down the gastrointestinal tract until it obstructs at the narrowest portion of the ileum or ileocecal junction. A "silent" gallstone obstructing the small bowel requires immediate surgery.

stone may make its way to the outlet of the gallbladder and obstruct it, causing an acute colicky attack, i.e., cholecystitis, hydrops, or empyema. A silent stone may, over a variable period of time, conceivably result in inoperable carcinoma. Silent stones may erode their way through the gallbladder wall into the duodenum, producing a fistula, and possibly, at a later date, a gallstone ileus. More often, a silent stone makes its way through the cystic duct into the common bile duct and produces obstructive jaundice and/or pancreatitis. All the associated concomitant problems, i.e., hepatitis, cholangitis, cholangiolitis, and cholestasis, may occur later in this progressive, silent disease process. Surgeons should not pacify their patients; rather, they should truthfully tell them what the future holds. Surgeons must take a stand and not play the passive role by giving in to the patient's procrastinating attitude (Figs. 84–86).

A silent stone, in the writer's opinion, presents a distinct surgical indication. The surgeon has every right to convince the patient that an operation at a time when no symptoms exist must still be carried out. Ideally, a silent stone, with all of its possible future consequences, should be removed by elective cholecystectomy as soon as the patient is properly prepared. The patient should be told about all the possible complications and should be made to understand that surgery at an early date

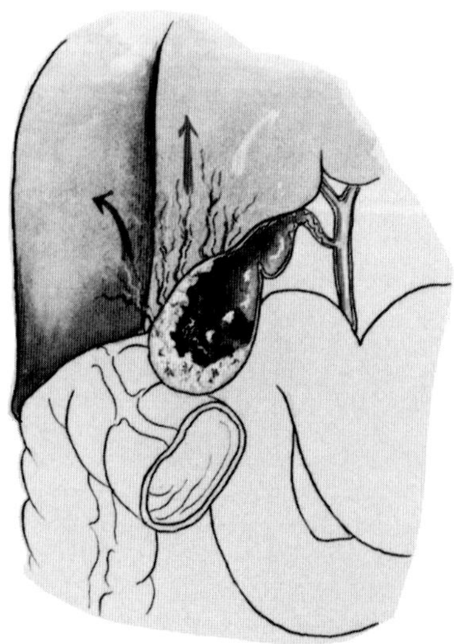

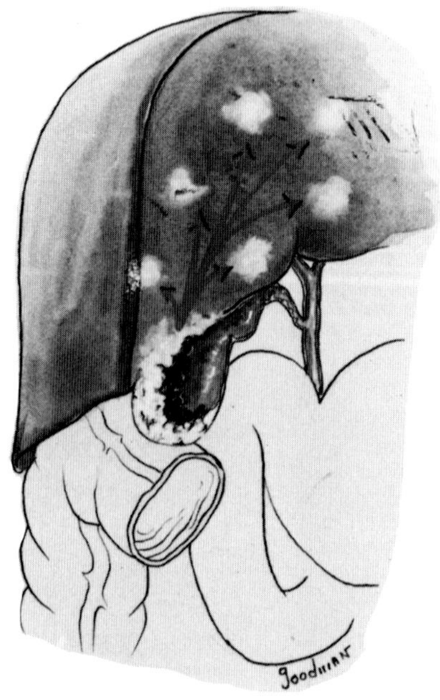

Figure 85. Carcinoma, not unlike a gallstone, may penetrate and perforate in the small or large bowel. Gallstones in the majority of cases are associated with carcinoma; therefore, whenever gallstone ileus is diagnosed, a search of the biliary tree should be made. If carcinoma of the gallbladder is suspected or recognized, it and a portion of bowel should be resected.

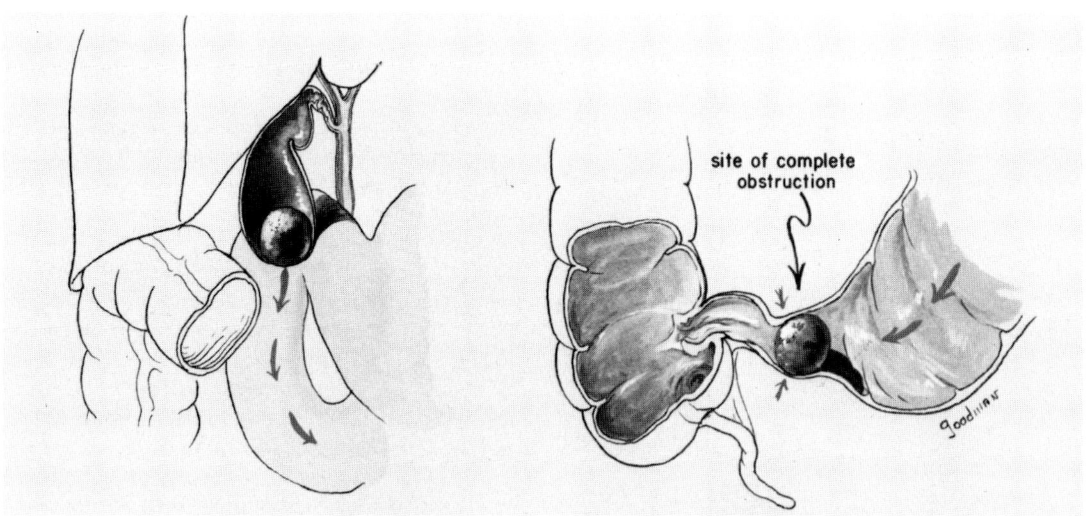

Figure 86. This diagram represents one of the most common complications that takes place in the course of chronic cholecystitis and cholelithiasis. The diagrams that follow will depict the pathological sequence of events when the gallstone exits the perforated gallbladder and proceeds down the gastrointestinal tract.

offers a minimum of risk and that surgery at a later date may possibly involve a higher risk and conceivably an incurable complication. The early-stage elective cholecystectomy is safer and more likely to be successful. An intelligent patient will listen and be convinced. Unfortunately, the patient makes the final decision, and the surgeon can only abide by it.

In this day of malpractice suits, the physician should fully inform the patient, the immediate relatives, close relatives, and friends. A full disclosure of the information given to the patient should preferably be recorded; the patient must fully understand the consequences of refusing surgery. It is imperative that everything said be recorded and dated. At a later date, it is quite common for the patient to claim, "The doctor did not fully explain it to me; he didn't tell me what the consequences would be. I was not fully informed!" *The physician should never put himself in a position to be judged.* To avoid this uncomfortable position, he must inform his patient fully and keep excellent records.

In a study by Sato and Matsushiro[1] from Tohoku University School of Medicine (Sendai, Japan), the authors reported on 784 patients with cholelithiasis operated on from 1961 to 1971. This study also included 3522 autopsies in which 152 patients (4.3%) had undiagnosed cholelithiasis. Of 51 selected patients with silent gallbladder stones, 29 had cholesterol stones, 16 had calcium bilirubinate stones, and 6 had pure pigment stones. These writers found that the incidence of silent gallstones was higher among the aged patients (60 years and over).

The development of symptoms in patients with silent gallstones occurred more suddenly, and in a severer form of acute cholecystitis; also, these cases carried a more unfavorable prognosis. The writers found that the incidence of cancer of the gallbladder increased progressively with age. The incidence was 3.8% in men and 9.3% in women; the patients were 60 years of age.

Histopathological studies revealed that where cholesterol stones were found, the gallbladder's mucosal lining developed prominent inflammatory changes; lesser changes developed with calcium bilirubinate and pigment stones. These changes were indistinguishable from those of symptomatic cholecystolithiasis. After reviewing the development of silent gallstone in younger patients (below 30 years of age), these authors concluded that this group, because of their youth, can be treated conservatively until the symptoms become aggravated and are associated with cholecystic complaints. They found that the younger patient rarely suffers a sudden onset of symptoms; complications are less frequent than in aged patients, and surgery carries less mortality. Conversely, surgery is recommended early for older patients (40 to more than 70 years of age). Early surgery in these patients is believed to avert serious complications such as empyema, toxic shock, and anaerobic bacterial septicemia. Late surgery in the latter forms of cholecystitis carries a high mortality.

The writers conclude that silent forms of cholecystolithiasis in older patients (40 to 70 years) require an elective cholecystectomy. In spite of this elective conclusion, however, they generally leave the decision to the patient.

Recommended Reading

Gracie WA, Ransohoff DF: The natural history of silent gallstones: The innocent stone is not a myth. *N Engl J Med* 307:798, 1982.
Method HL, Mehn WA, Frable WG: Silent gallstone. *Arch Surg* 85:338, 1962.
Strohl EL, Diffenbaugh WG, Anderson RE: Biliary tract surgery in the aged patient. *Geriatrics* 19:275, 1964.

References

1. Sato T, Matsushiro T: Surgical indications in patients with silent gallstones. *Am J Surg* 128:368, 1974.

GALLSTONE ILEUS

Gallstone ileus is a condition in which a gallstone or stones obstruct the lumen of the small intestine, usually causing a low intestinal obstruction with distention of the entire gastrointestinal tract. It is, as was mentioned in the discussion of biliary-intestinal fistula, common in patients over 65, especially when previous intermittent attacks of cholecystitis or cholelithiasis occurred, and more particularly in female patients (see "The 'Silent' Gallstone"). The mortality rate is high but varies with the alertness and diagnostic acuity of the surgeon. Early intervention with the proper surgical procedure, and proper pre- and postoperative care, can reduce the mortality rate significantly. This writer stresses the importance of early diagnosis, with detection of the triad of abdominal distention, X-ray evidence of a calculus in the small bowel, and the presence of air in the right upper quadrant (biliary tract). The obstruction may be caused by multiple stones or by a small stone that has "snowballed" down the intestinal tract, picking up layer after layer of fecal material and increasing in size to the point where it causes obstruction at the narrowest site of the intestinal lumen. Usually spasm and edema assist in further contracting the bowel wall down upon the stone, thereby fixing the stone and the site of intestinal obstruction. As stated, earlier cholecystointestinal fistula develop insidiously usually due to a silent gallstone that leads to gradual fistulous formation.

Therefore, it is incumbent upon the surgeon to know that there are different phases of this disease, and that early diagnosis implies that an elective operation for silent gallstones can be carried out successfully. A late diagnosis implies that immediate surgical intervention is required. It is therefore incumbent upon every surgeon to be alerted to this condition in its earliest stage. To review, it is imperative to know that routine studies of the gallbladder are important, since they may reveal an unsuspected or silent cholecystitis and cholelithiasis, and that the finding of air in the biliary tree during a routine upper gastrointestinal tract X-ray study may also reveal barium in the biliary tree. The latter are all early nonemergent findings that may be dealt with surgically on an early elective basis; and a more complete operation is possible. When a fistula forms, and the stones or stone have been released and intestinal obstruction develops, an emergency situation demands immediate surgery (Figs. 84–86).

Depending upon the size of the stone and the condition of the bowel, i.e., the degree of spasticity and the size of the lumen, the obstruction may take place at any level, starting as high as the pylorus, duodenum, jejunum, ileum, or ileocecal valve. While the patient is observed, the changing nature of a gallstone obstruction, due to the changing level of the obstruction, can prove to be pathognomonic for gallstone ileus. One should try to take repeated flat films to localize these changing levels of the stone. As the gallstone makes its way down the gastrointestinal tract, the signs and symptoms may vary. The earliest onset of symptoms and signs may be those produced by the cholecystitis and cholelithiasis, namely, nausea and vomiting. The presence of colic and vomitus may be of some help, depending upon its color (light or dark-stained bile); it may even be fecal in nature. The latter is not only symptomatic but actually diagnostic. Late signs and symptoms develop when the stone becomes impacted at a narrowed portion of the intestinal tract, usually the distal ileum or ileocecal site. Until complete obstruction occurs, the abdomen may not become distended, but with impaction of the stone, abdominal distention becomes a major feature, and this one important sign helps to make the diagnosis. This writer believes that the high mortality rate with this disease is due to neglect, late diagnosis, and too late surgical intervention, as well as the undue length of time of the surgical procedure. The mortality is usually greater in the aged patient who has concomitant degenerative and/or systemic diseases (see "The 'Silent' Gallstone").

Surgical Technique

After careful preparation of the patient, i.e., careful sterilization of the abdominal wall and sterile incise draping, a long right paramedian or midline incision is made from the xiphoid down to below the umbilicus, so that with the proper lateral retraction any portion of the abdomen may be reached. The gallbladder should immediately be evaluated to determine whether or not stones and/or a fistulous tract are present in any of its contiguous hollow structures. If the stone is found in the gallbladder or duodenum, it is imperative that the entire gastrointestinal tract be carefully searched for any other calculi that may be capable of producing possible intestinal obstruction. Typical episodes of intestinal obstruction resulting from stones that have been overlooked have been reported. Sooner or later (months or even years), when the stone is located, having been found at the site where the distention meets the collapsed portion of the bowel, the stone is palpated, recognized, and carefully milked back to a higher level in the intestinal tract, preferably in the portion of bowel that appears to be in a better nutritional state. A longitudinal incision is made on the antimesenteric border; the incision should be made small rather than large so that the stone can be squeezed through the smallest required opening to prevent the need to sew a larger defect. When the stone has been milked out of the lumen, the intestinal tract should be carefully palpated from the ligament of Treitz down to the ileocecal junction.

The intestinal contents should be aspirated as much as possible from the proximal loop before the closure is carried out. The closure should preferably be done in a transverse direction, particularly when dealing with a small ileal lumen. The closure should be sewn with chromic catgut (000), using a continuous-lock suture for the first row and a second row of interrupted (000) black silk on atraumatic intestinal needle. There will be times during the surgery when a stone will be so firmly fixed to the intestinal wall that it will not be possible to disimpact it or dislodge it without causing undue trauma. In those instances, rather than risk damaging the bowel at an unsuspected site, it is better to carry out a bowel resection of the involved portion. The stone impacted in the intestine should be resected as one and an end-to-end anastomosis performed. Though resection will usually not be required, there have been several reported instances where it was the procedure of choice.

As soon as the surgery is completed and the small bowel is completely evaluated, the surgeon should return to the gallbladder and evaluate it very carefully. If possible, a cholecystectomy should be performed and a common duct exploration carried out to exclude the existence of any other stones in this duct. Often the condition of the patient will not permit all of these procedures because of age and associated systemic problems. In such instances, it may be wiser to do a cholecystostomy and thoroughly cleanse the gallbladder of all calculi and debris. However, if the patient's condition is considered good and stable, the gallbladder should be removed and the common duct explored. A T-tube is inserted, and the gallbladder area (Morison's fossa) is drained with a Penrose-wick drain. The T-tube is brought out through the same lateral subcostal stab wound as the mushroom catheter that is draining the gallbladder.

In most elderly patients, it is customary to do a complete evacuation of all gallbladder contents, followed by irrigation and removal of all stones, as described in Chapter 10. A Malecot or cutout mushroom catheter is used to drain the cholecystostomy. The latter procedure seems to be very adequate in these special cases, especially where jaundice is absent, the common duct is 1 cm or less in diameter of slate blue color, and with no thickening of the duct wall. Cholecystostomy in the cases referred to will usually prove to be adequate. There are times when nothing can be done except to remove the stone from the intestinal tract, repair the opening in the small bowel, and leave the cholecystoduodenal fistula undisturbed. The patient will have to wait for subsequent signs and symptoms to indicate what has happened as a result of the fistulous opening. Cholecystographic studies in the future may indicate that there are no more stones. If in time cholecystitis, cholelithiasis, or choledocholithiasis is suspected, sonographic and X-ray studies should be carried out to indicate its presence or absence. Repeated attacks of gallbladder colic, with or without cholangitis, may mean that elective surgery will have to be carried out. If cholecystectomy is required, the fistulous opening in the small or large intestine should be closed. The common bile duct should be opened and explored, and all the tricks of irrigation and basket and balloon procedures should be carried out to be sure that no mud, gravel, or stones are left over. The dull-tipped flexible probe may be used to probe the common duct through the ampulla of Vater to check its patency. Bakes dilators may be utilized to dilate the ampullary stoma and, if required, to perform a sphincterotomy, depending, of course, upon what is found. This writer recommends that, because of age and poor nutrition, the abdominal closure in these cases should be reinforced with deep tension sutures. He prefers 2-0 nylon deep tension sutures for added security in questionable wound closures. Four to eight deep tension sutures may be employed, through and through the full thickness of the abdominal wall. Ti-chron (00) sutures on a swedged-on needle are placed interruptedly. Every precaution should be taken to avoid a postoperative evisceration. Postoperative preventive measures should be strictly adhered to, and continued gastric tube decompression is most important. Aftercare should emphasize the nutritional status of the patient, i.e., fluid, electrolytes, and blood requirements.

Recommended Reading

Kurt RJ: Patterns of treatment of gallstone ileus over a 45 year period. *Am J Gastroenterol* 80:95, 1985.
Pangam JC: Cholecystoduodenocolic fistula with recurrent gallstone ileus. *Arch Surg* 119:1201, 1984.
Svartholm E: Diagnosis and treatment of gallstone ileus. *Acta Chir Scand* 148:435, 1982.

BILIARY-ENTERIC FISTULA

Biliary fistulae may be external or internal. External fistulae include an enteric fistula and a cholecystic fistula created by cholecystostomy. Included are T-tube drainage of the common bile duct and the spontaneous external fistulae caused by stones that erode through the abdominal wall, like carcinoma of the gallbladder. Internal biliary fistulae are usually spontaneous or iatrogenic. They may be intentionally iatrogenic, used to create decompressive stomas between the common bile duct and the small bowel, i.e., between the gallbladder and jejunum. The latter fistulae are internal and represent procedures such as cholecystojejunostomy, choledochojejunostomy, and choledochoduodenostomy. In addition to these intentional iatrogenic procedures, there are the internal fistulae that occur spontaneously and are due to a gallstone eroding through the gallbladder wall into the duodenum, colon, or small intestine. Spontaneous external biliary fistulae represent neglected cases of cholecystitis and cholelithiasis. The latter complications occur particularly in the geriatric patient and usually are found in terminal states. Other fistulae extending outward are due to silent cancer of the gallbladder, as well as carcinomas of the liver and colon.

Pathogenesis

The majority of internal biliary fistulae are caused by long-standing cholelithiasis in which the chronically inflamed gallbladder wall becomes eroded from the pressure of one or more stones. In the inflammatory process that ensues, the gallbladder attaches itself to an adjacent viscus and perforates into it by continuous erosion due to pressure created by the stone. The biliary fistulae that extend into the duodenum are the commonest variety and are referred to as *cholecystoduodenal fistulae.* Other varieties include cholecystocholedochal and cholecystocolic fistulae. Biliary-intestinal fistula is most commonly associated with the ultimate intestinal obstruction caused by gallstone impaction, or gallstone ileus. The greatest number of patients fall into the geriatric group, where morbidity and mortality are highest (Figs. 84–86).

Patients with biliary-enteric fistula have other chronic systemic processes associated with their age group, namely, degenerative processes that involve the pulmonary, renal, and cardiac systems. This type of case, when recognized, is usually surgical and consists essentially of a triad of signs and symptoms: (1) distention of the gastrointestinal tract, (2) air in the biliary tract, and (3) a possible calcific stone shadow on flat film studies, frequently seen in the lower end of the ileum. In the majority of instances, these cases come under the heading of acute abdomen, and if this triad is kept in mind, the diagnosis may be readily made and surgery carried out at the earliest possible time. In the majority of cases of biliary-enteric fistula, the gallbladder is found to contain stones; this is also true in cases involving the common bile duct. The incidence of this disease in women is much greater than in men; therefore, gallstone ileus, being more common in the female, should be searched for especially in the elderly female patient when differentiating a diagnosis of acute surgical abdomen.

Although any part of the extrahepatic biliary system may communicate with the gastrointestinal tract by fistulous formation, the commonest site for this occurrence is between the gallbladder and duodenum. The next most common sites are where the common bile duct communicates with the stomach, duodenum, jejunum, or large intestine. A history of chronic cholelithiasis may be elicited in which there have been intermittent attacks; during these inflammatory periods, the gallbladder wall, by a process that is part of a defensive mechanism, becomes adherent to contiguous structures, as in the walling-off process that occurs in other organs. The adhesions that develop between both organs may remain until another attack occurs at the same site, and based upon the inflammatory process, edema, and pressure that exist within the gallbladder, a biliary-enteric fistulous tract gradually develops. The stone that makes its way through this cholecystoduodenal fistula has usually lain in the ampulla of the gallbladder for some time; it is the continuous pressure and erosive process that interfere with the blood supply of the gallbladder and intestinal walls. The increased intraluminal pressure, as well as the weakening of the wall associated with edema, inflammation, and reduced vascularity of the area, that creates a process that ultimately permits passage of the stone from one organ to another. The contiguous walls involved actually undergo an ischemic process that progresses to gangrene and fistulous formation. The opening, of course, grows larger over time because the continued pressure and decreased vascularity, together with the thrombosis that accompanies this process, results in progressive gangrene and further enlargement of the opening.

This increased enlargement of the opening allows a large stone to pass from the gallbladder into the duodenum or small bowel. One or more stones may make their way into the hollow viscus, and from that point on, by peristalsis, the stone or stones are carried down into the lower intestinal tract where the lumen gets progressively smaller. If the stone enlarges as it is carried down to the lower and narrower ileum, it reaches a point where obstruction takes place, with concomitant signs and symptoms, namely, abdominal distention, pain, and vomiting. Flat X-ray films of the abdomen may show calcific shadows in the small bowel; many times, obvious stone formations are seen in the terminal ileum associated with air in the right upper quadrant, which usually signifies gas or air in the biliary tree. Small stones, of course, may pass beyond the ileocecal junction and thence on, to be evacuated into the large intestine. *If the gallstones get larger as they descend in the intestinal tract or are large to begin with, they will obstruct at the narrowest point;* the most common site of the obstruction is the terminal ileum (Fig. 86).

The X-ray picture often confirms the site as low down because of the many dilated proximal loops of small bowel. Distention of the entire abdomen confirms a low intestinal obstruction. In those cases of intestinal fistula that do not create an acute surgical abdomen, the patient may merely present a history of chronic cholecystitis and cholelithiasis. It is possible that by doing a cholecystogram, in-

travenous cholangiogram, or upper and lower gastrointestinal studies, the diagnosis may finally be established. Not infrequently, a routine gastrointestinal study will show a fistula that has permitted the barium to pass up into the gallbladder and/or biliary system. Also, on occasion, only a barium enema may successfully demonstrate a communication between the biliary system and the colon; here, too, air will be discovered in the biliary tree. In cases of biliary-intestinal fistula, it is possible for the intestinal content to make its way into the biliary tree and produce an ascending cholangitis. The latter inflammation may lead to impairment of liver function and associated hepatitis.

It should be kept in mind that the presence of gas in the gallbladder area as seen on X-ray may result from either spontaneous rupture into or an iatrogenic communication between the biliary system and a hollow viscus. Gas in the biliary system may also be due to an incompetent sphincter of Oddi, resulting in regurgitation of intestinal air or gas into the common bile duct and its radicals. Within the gallbladder, bacterial growth may give rise to *emphysematous cholecystitis.* If an abdominal flat film fails to reveal stones and/or air in the biliary tract, the upper gastrointestinal study may show a cholecystoduodenal fistula, just as the barium enema reveals a cholecystocolic fistula.

Treatment

Surgery must be considered wherever a fistulous tract has been established between the two viscera. If, during the surgical exploration, a communication between the duodenum and gallbladder is found, a careful sharp and blunt dissection should separate the gallbladder from the site of penetration into the duodenum. The duodenum, as in any other duodenal defect or perforation, must be closed with permanent sutures—(000) black silk placed interruptedly, utilizing two layers in a manner that does not infringe upon the lumen. The gallbladder, of course, should be removed. Choledochotomy should be performed and a routine exploration of the common duct carried out to search for and remove any residual stones, mud, gravel, or sludge that may interfere with future drainage through the ampulla of Vater. A flexible metal dull-tipped probe may be used to establish the ampullary opening. If the sphincter is stenotic, Bakes dilators may be employed to enlarge the opening to approximately 5 mm. The common duct is drained with a T-tube, as described elsewhere. Following the placement and sewing in of the T-tube, a routine cholangiogram should be carried out before the final abdominal closure. Any additional new findings noted in the cholangiogram that were not known before should be dealt with by removing the T-tube and further exploring the common duct. When the T-tube is finally left in, the entire biliary system should be considered clean and in normal condition. Follow-up treatment should be no different than the routine postoperative treatment of cholecystitis and cholelithiasis. At surgery the Levin tube should be inserted and placed in the stomach with the aid of the anesthetist. The anesthetist should withdraw the tube until its tip is felt to be at the pylorus, with all kinks undone. An antibiotic is employed in the pre- and postoperative periods in all instances where a fistula existed.

Recommended Reading

Calonje MA, Ozenstark JL, Nice CM Jr: Internal biliary fistula. *JAMA* 179:112, 1962.

Constant E, Turcotte JG: Choledochoduodenal fistula: The natural history and management of an unusual complication of peptic ulcer disease. *Ann Surg* 167:220, 1968.

Feller ER, Warshaw AL, Schapiro RH: Observations on management of choledochoduodenal fistula due to penetrating peptic ulcer. *Gastroenterology* 78:126, 1980.

Fitchett CW: Spontaneous external biliary fistula. *Trans South Surg Assoc* 80:214, 1969.

Fox PF: Planning the operation for cholecystoenteric fistula with gallstone ileus. *Surg Clin North Am* 50:93, 1970.

Hicken NF, Coray QB: Spontaneous gastrointestinal biliary fistulas. *Surg Gynecol Obstet* 82:723, 1946.

Ikeda S, Okada Y: Classification of choledochoduodenal fistula diagnosed by duodenal fiberscopy and its etiological significance. *Gastroenterology* 69:130, 1975.

Kourias BG, Chouliaras A: Spontaneous gastrointestinal-biliary fistula complicating duodenal ulcer. *Surg Gynecol Obstet* 119:1013, 1964.

Norcross JW, Dadey JL: Medical complications of operative bile-duct injuries. *N Engl J Med* 257:1216, 1957.

Safaie-Shirzai S, Zike WL, Printen KJ: Spontaneous enterobiliary fistulas. *Surg Gynecol Obstet* 137:769, 1973.

Shocket E, Evans J, Jones S: Cholecysto-duodeno-colic fistula with gallstone ileus. *Arch Surg* 101:523, 1970.

Wagner GR, Passaro E: Choledochoduodenal fistula secondary to duodenal ulcer. *Arch Surg* 103:21, 1971.

9

DISSOLUTION OF GALLSTONES

Fifteen million Americans are believed to have gallstones, composed chiefly of cholesterol. Bile supersaturated with cholesterol is believed to be a prerequisite for cholesterol stone formation. Chenodeoxycholic acid (CDC) taken orally has been found to cause unsaturation of bile cholesterol.

The dissolution of gallstones is still in its experimental stages and cannot be compared in effectiveness and completeness with cholecystectomy and common bile duct exploration. Medical treatment for cholelithiasis utilizing chenodeoxycholic acid is an alternative treatment for patients in whom cholecytectomy is considered undesirable or contraindicated. This therapy should be reserved for high-risk patients with serious systemic diseases and those who have great fear of surgery.

One great disadvantage of medical dissolution of gallstones is that it fails to evaluate the entire biliary system, i.e., for cholelithiasis and choledocholithiasis, carcinoma of the papilla of Vater and the head of the pancreas, peptic ulcer, and hiatus hernia.

Patients with cholesterol gallstones have a reduced bile acid pool that is associated with a relative increase in bile cholesterol. Thistle and Schoenfield in 1971,[1] by administering chenodeoxycholic acid orally, were able to increase the bile acid pool and decrease the relative proportion of cholesterol in the bile. Studies by numerous researchers have confirmed these observations.

At the present time, there are two nonsurgical (noninvasive) treatments for cholelithiasis that originate from abnormal bile salt metabolism: oral chenodeoxycholic acid and lecithin feedings.

Gallstones have diminished in size or actually disappeared following the oral administration of chenodeoxycholic acid. The Mayo Clinic, in their experiences with chenotherapy, reported partial or complete dissolution of the gallstones in about 50% of their patients who were observed from 6 months to 3 years. Most of the reported statistics indicate that chenodeoxycholic acid dissolves about 50% of the radiolucent stones and that the response is usually slow. Unfortunately, discontinuance of the therapy is likely to result in recurrence of stones. This strongly suggests that a genetic metabolic abnormality in biliary physiology exists and accounts for the predetermination toward stone-forming diathesis. Therefore, it appears, that medical therapy will have to be continued for an indeterminate period of time. In such instances, an elective cholecystectomy is preferable and indeed indicated.

For some time, patients with gallstones have been suspected of having abnormal phospholipid metabolism; this observation has led to lecithin feedings. Lecithin administration has increased the phospholipid levels in the bile and in some cases has caused the disappearance of cholesterol crystals and gallstones. But thus far, lecithin feeding has not been as effective as chenodeoxycholic acid. In a number of cases with gallstones in the common bile duct (retained or impacted), perfusion with sodium cholate and/or heparin has resulted in dissolution of the stones over a period of several weeks.

Pribram[2] was the first to recommend and employ chemical dissolution of retained gallstones. He employed alcohol, ether, or ether and alcohol. His method is now obsolete.

In 1973, Thistle and Hoffmann,[3] at the Mayo Clinic, reported 50% of 53 patients with partial or complete dissolution of gallstones (6 months to 3 years) utilizing oral chendeoxycholic acid.

In 1973, Gardner[4] reported success with this therapy in 21 of 27 cases.

In 1978, Sali and Iser[5] established specific criteria for chenotherapy:

1. The patient must have a functioning gallbladder.
2. The gallstones must be radiolucent (cholesterol).
3. Cholesterol stones must be 22 mm or less; stones of this size respond best to chenotherapy.
4. Women who are capable of childbearing and who do not practice contraception should not be selected for treatment.
5. Patients with liver damage are unsuitable.
6. Pain must not be severe or too frequent; surgery is indicated if the patient suffers an attack during treatment.

It is important to know that not all stones will dissolve with lecithin, sodium cholate, and heparin; that the chemical composition of gallstones varies and, in fact, varies from person to person. Presently we must consider chemical dissolution of gallstones as an acceptable but limited medical therapy with specific indications for its use; at best, it is a limited adjunct to surgery.

Today there are many forms of treatment available for postoperative retained common duct stones:*

*All the ingenious tactics and techniques developed for gallstone dissolution or removal have proven to be most valuable: however, the prophylaxis against all of these methods still remains a complete first surgical procedure, good surgical judgment, and the patience to attempt every trick and tactic to remove the last remaining stone from the biliary tract. At the end of common duct exploration, it is mandatory to employ a T-tube of adequate size (if possible, not less than 14 F) and routinely perform T-tube cholangiography. If a stone is discovered, the T-tube must be removed and a renewed search made of the biliary tract. The author is aware that there will be instances where high-risk patients, prolonged operative time, undue traumatic manipulations, and prolonged anesthesia will mitigate against continuing a further search for the elusive gallstone. At this point, as a retreat procedure, choledochoduodenostomy is acceptable.

1. Oral administration of bile salts over a period of several months.
2. Saline irrigations, with the concomitant use of antispasmodics, amyl nitrite, and magnesium sulfate.
3. Exploration with a Dormia basket via the T-tube fistulous tract, utilizing a TV monitor.
4. Perfusion of the common duct with sodium cholate and/or heparin.
5. Retrograde endoscopic sphincterotomy, with or without the Dormia basket.
6. Surgical reexploration of the common bile duct; possible use of the Glassman Gallstone Extractor instruments, flexible lead probe, bipolar helix basket, and nylon brushes.
7. Failure to remove an impacted gallstone after every trick and tactic has been tried justifies a last-resort procedure, choledochoduodenostomy.

Johnson et al.,[6] at the Mayo Clinic, observed 90 patients with asymptomatic lucent gallstones. Of these patients, 52 received chenodeoxycholic acid for 2 years or longer, when necessary, to attain complete dissolution. The dose was as high as 25 mg/kg; in the presence of diarrhea, it was reduced. In 33 of the chenodeoxycholic acid–treated patients, 55% showed a definite decrease in the size and/or number of stones. In 17 patients treated with chenodeoxycholic acid, no change in the gallstones was noted, nor was there any change among the 18 placebo patients. In 10 of 12 patients who received 15 mg/kg (or more), 50% showed complete dissolution of the gallstones after 2 years. No complete stone dissolution was noted in 18 patients who were treated over a period of 1.5–3 years.

Diarrhea was a common and serious complication. Patients who received 15 mg/kg (or more) developed a mild increase in stool frequency. Liver changes were minimal; 3 of 15 patients had recurrent stone formation with discontinuance of therapy. In two, therapy was restarted and dissolution followed. Chenodeoxycholic acid can induce gallstone dissolution, with recurrence after 1–4 years. *It should be stressed that radiopaque stones (mixed and calcified) do not respond to chenotherapy.*

Instructions for Treatment

1. Acceptable criteria:
   a. The cholecystogram must show lucent gallstones no larger than 22 mm (2.2 cm). It must be repeated in 3–6 months.
   b. The bile aspirate must be analyzed before and after treatment. Bile must become unsaturated in cholesterol stone cases.
2. Dosage—15 mg per kilogram of body weight (more in obese patients).
3. Duration of treatment—smaller stones usually dissolve within 6 months; stones closer to 2.2 cm may require 2 years or longer.
4. Reactions—diarrhea; may stop spontaneously or the dosage may be reduced; alternatively, antidiarrheal medications may be tried.

Ursodeoxycholic acid is chemically related to chenodeoxycholic acid. It produces unsaturated bile, using a smaller dosage, and has reduced side effects, i.e., diarrhea and hypertransaminasemia. More extensive controlled studies are necessary.

Conclusion

It is conceivable and hoped for that medical treatment for radiolucent gallstones in selected patients who meet the criteria of Sali and Iser[5] may someday become a routine alternative to cholecystectomy.

Recommended Reading

Adler RD, Bennion LJ, Duane WC, et al: Effects of low dose chenodeoxycholic acid (chenodiol) feeding on biliary lipid metabolism. *Gastroenterology* 68:326, 1975.

Albers JJ, Grundy SM, Clary PA, et al: The National Cooperative Gallstone Study; the effects of chenodeoxycholic acid on lipoproteins and apoproteins. *Gastroenterology* 82:638, 1982.

Allen MJ, Borody TJ, Bugliosi TF, et al: Rapid dissolution of gallstones by methyl tert-butyl ether: Preliminary observations. *N Engl J Med* 312:217, 1985.

Angelin B, Einarsson K, Heilstrom K, et al: Effects of cholestyramine and chenodeoxycholic acid on the metabolism of endogenous triglyceride in hyperlipoproteinemia. *J Lipid Res* 19:101, 1976.

Beil U, Crouse JR, Einarsson K, et al: Effects of interruption of the enterohepatic circulation of bile acids on the transport of very low density lipoprotein triglycerides. *Metabolism* 31:438, 1982.

Bennion LJ, Grundy SM: Effects of obesity and caloric intake on biliary lipid metabolism in man. *J Clin Invest* 56:996, 1975.

Brown MS, Goldstein JL: Expression of the familial hypercholesterolemia gene in heterozygotes: Mechanism for a dominant disorder in man. *Science* 185:61, 1974.

Crouse JR, Grundy SM: Effects of sucrose polyester on cholesterol metabolism in man. *Metabolism* 28:994, 1979.

Einarsson KA, Grundy SM: Effects of feeding cholic acid and chenodeoxycholic acid on cholesterol absorption and hepatic secretion of biliary lipids in man. *J Lipid Res* 21:23, 1980.

Friedman GD, Kannel WB, Dawber TR: The epidemiology

of gallbladder disease: Observations in the Framingham Study. *J Chronic Dis* 19:273, 1966.

Grundy SM, Metzger AL, Alder RD: Mechanism of lithogenic bile formation in American Indian women with cholesterol gallstones. *J Clin Invest* 51:3026, 1972.

Hoffman NE, Hoffmann AF, Thistle JL: Effect of bile acid feeding on cholesterol metabolism in gallstone patients. *Mayo Clin Proc* 49:236, 1974.

Iserr JH, Maton PN, Murphy GM, et al: Resistance to chenodeoxycholic acid (CDA) treatment in obese patients with gallstones. *Br Med J* 1:1509, 1978.

Key PH, Bonorria GG, Coyne MJ, et al: Hepatic cholesterol synthesis: A determinant of cholesterol secretion in gallstone patients. *Gastroenterology* 72:A159, 1972.

Marinovic I, Guerra C, Larach G: Incidencia de Litiasis biliar en material de autopsias y analisis de composicion de los calculos. *Rev Med Chile* 100:1320, 1972.

Marks JW, Baum RA, Hanson RF, et al: Additional chenodiol therapy after partial dissolution of gallstones with two years of treatment. *Ann Intern Med* 100:382, 1984.

Metzger AL, Adler RA, Heymsfield S, et al: Diurnal variation in biliary lipid composition: Possible role in cholesterol gallstone formation. *N Engl J Med* 288:333, 1973.

Miller NE, Nestel PJ: Triglyceride-lowering effect of chenodeoxycholic acid in patients with endogenous hypertriglyceridemia. *Lancet* 2:929, 1974.

Mok HYI, von Bergmann K, Grouse JR, et al: Biliary lipid metabolism in obesity: Effects of bile acid feeding before and during weight reduction. *Gastroenterology* 76:556, 1979.

Mok HYI, von Bergmann K, Grundy SM: Regulation of proof size of bile acids in man. *Gastroenterology* 73:684, 1977.

Mok HYI, von Bergmann K, Grundy SM: Factors affecting bile saturation at low outputs of bile acids, in Paymgartner G, Stiehl A, Gerok W (eds): *Biological Effects of Bile Acids (5th Bile Acid Meeting)*. Freiburg, MPT Press 1978.

Nestel PJ, Schreibman PH, Ahrens Jr EH: Cholesterol metabolism in human obesity. *J Clin Invest* 52:2389, 1973.

Nestel PJ, Whyte HM, Goodman PS: Distribution and turnover of cholesterol in humans. *J Clin Invest* 48:982, 1969.

Northfield TC, Hoffmann AF: Biliary lipid output during three meals and an overnight fast: 1. Relationship to bile acid pool size and cholesterol saturation of bile in gallstone and control subjects. *Gut* 16:1, 1975.

Palmer RH: More on chenodiol: Continued treatment and prevention of recurrences. *Ann Intern Med* 100:450, 1984.

Pittman RC, Attie AD, Carew TE, et al: Tissue sites of degradation of low density lipoproteins: Application of a new method for determining the fate of plasma proteins. *Proc Natl Acad Sci USA* 76:5345, 1979.

Sampliner RE, Bennett PH, Comess LJ, et al: Gallbladder disease in Pima Indians. *N Engl J Med* 283:1538, 1970.

Schoenfield LJ, Lacgub M, and the Steering Committee, National Cooperative Gallstone Study: Chenodiol (chenodeoxycholic acid) for dissolution of gallstones; a controlled trial of efficacy and safety. *Ann Intern Med* 95:257, 1981.

Slater HR, Pckard CJ, Bicker S, et al: Effects of cholestyramine on reception-mediated plasma clearance and tissue uptake of human low density lipoproteins in the rabbit. *J Biol Chem* 255:10210, 1980.

References

1. Thistle JL, Schoenfield LJ: Induced alterations in composition of bile of persons having cholelithiasis. *Gastroenterology* 61:488, 1971.

2. Pribram BOC: The method for dissolving common duct stones remaining after surgery. *Surgery* 22:806, 1947.

3. Johnson AG, Thistle JL, Hoffmann AF, et al: Chemotherapy for gallstone dissolution. *JAMA* 239:1041, 1978.

4. Gardner B, Dennis CR, Patti J, et al: Current status of dissolution of gallstones. *Am J Surg* 130:293, 1975.

5. Sali A, Iser J: The non-operative management of gallstones. *Aust NZ J Surg* 48:484, 1978.

6. Thistle JL, Hoffmann AF, Ott BJ, et al: Chemotherapy for gallstone dissolution: Efficacy and safety. *JAMA* 239:1041, 1978.

Obesity, Gallstones, and Chenodiol

Scott M. Grundy, Ph.D.

The results of the National Cooperative Gallstone Study (NCGS)[1] confirmed that chenodiol has the potential to dissolve gallstones. Generally, treatment was not associated with major toxicity, and side effects alone do not proscribe the use of chenodiol in patients who are good candidates for dissolution therapy. The study revealed both a major and a minor problem with chenodiol therapy. The major problem is that a minority of patients had complete dissolution; the minor problem is that chenodiol caused an increase in plasma total cholesterol and low density lipoprotein (LDL)-cholesterol. I shall discuss the mechanisms responsible for these problems and how they might be overcome.

DISSOLUTION FAILURES IN THE NCGS

The NCGS was a double-masked trial including 196 patients who were divided into three equal-sized groups: high-dose chenodiol (750 mg/day), low-dose chenodiol (375 mg/day), and placebo. These groups were treated for 2 years. Confirmed complete dissolution occurred in 13.5% of patients on 750 mg/day, in 5.2% on 350 mg/day, and in 0.8% on placebo. Partial dissolution (over 50% reduction in stone size) is taken to indicate the potential for chenodiol to dissolve stones. Partial or complete dissolution occurred in 41% of the patients on high-dose chenodiol, in 24% of those on low-dose chenodiol, and in 11% of those on placebo. The major findings of this study were that dissolution occurred more frequently in women than in men, in thin rather than in obese patients, and with small gallstones rather than large ones.

In regard to the last observation—that dissolution occurred more commonly with small gallstones than with large ones—large gallstones may be inherently more difficult to dissolve. The large stones probably were older, more compact, and contained more calcium. Nevertheless, sometimes large stones dissolved, and it is possible that a longer treatment period (e.g., 3–4 years) may have resulted in greater success. To understand the basis of the observation that dissolution occurred less often in obese patients than in thin ones, the effect of obesity on sterol metabolism and its role in the pathogenesis of cholesterol gallstones must be considered.

EFFECTS OF OBESITY

It is a clinical fact, confirmed by epidemiological studies, that gallstones occur more commonly in obese than in nonobese subjects. The primary reason apparently is that overweight persons usually have bile that is supersaturated with cholesterol. Supersaturation, in turn, is usually the result of overproduction of cholesterol. Excess synthesis of cholesterol in obese patients has been demonstrated repeatedly by cholesterol balance and isotopic studies. The activity of reductase, the rate-limiting enzyme in cholesterol synthesis, is responsive to total caloric intake and plasma insulin, both of which are increased in obesity. In the obese person there is a high correlation between the degree of excess synthesis of cholesterol (as determined by cholesterol balance) and biliary cholesterol secretion. Recently, the activity of reductase has been shown to correlate with the rate of biliary cholesterol secretion.

Although hypersecretion of biliary cholesterol with obesity is probably a prime factor in cholesterol gallstone patients, certain obese patients are probably protected from gallstones by an increased synthesis of bile acids. Obese persons frequently have high production rates, high biliary secretion rates, and large pools of bile acids. Also, the synthesis of biliary lecithin is usually increased in obese patients. The excess of bile acids and lecithin in bile provides a buffer against increased biliary cholesterol; this may explain why a significant number of obese patients do not develop cholelithiasis. The importance of a compensatory increase in the synthesis of cholesterol and bile acids for protection against gallstones is revealed by studies in obese American Indians. In this population, obesity clearly enhances cholesterol production and biliary secretion, but because an increased synthesis of bile acids and lecithin does not occur, most obese Indians develop gallstones.

Some obese patients appear to be protected from gallstones by high secretion rates of bile acids and phospholipids. This protection may be limited by events occurring in a fasting state. At high biliary output of bile acids, secretion rates of cholesterol and phospholipids are usually linked. Biliary cholesterol is coupled closely with lecithin, and cholesterol output is linked to the level of lecithin creation; the latter, in turn, is coupled to the output of bile acids. On the other hand, when bile acid secretion falls, as occurs in the fasting state, cholesterol secretion becomes partially "uncoupled" from lecithin; that is, cholesterol output is maintained at a relatively higher level than lecithin and bile acid output. This leads to supersaturation of bile with cholesterol in the fasting state and produces the "diurnal variation" in biliary lipid composition. This diurnal variation seems to be enhanced in obese patients; that is, biliary cholesterol secretion during fasting tends to be markedly uncoupled from lecithin and remains much higher than normal; this leads to an accentuated supersaturation of bile. Despite an increased synthesis of both bile acids and lecithin, obese patients are still prone to develop highly supersaturated bile in the fasting state.

EFFECTS OF CALORIC RESTRICTION

The above discussion provides the theoretical framework of why chenodiol therapy is not highly effective in obese patients with cholesterol gallstones. Since the bile acid pool is relatively large in obese subjects, the addition of exogenous chenodiol to the extrahepatic circulation does not greatly expand the total bile acid pool. The capacity of the intestine to reabsorb bile acids is large but limited; therefore, overloading the bile acid pool in the presence of an already expanded pool provides little benefit.

Previous studies have shown that chenodiol not only expands the bile acid pool in normal subjects but also reduces hepatic secretion of cholesterol. Both alterations apparently contribute to the decrease in bile saturation associated with chenodiol therapy. It is not known whether chenodiol decreases cholesterol output in obese patients. If so, this might explain reports that very large doses of chenodiol (greater than 15 mg/kg/day) can dissolve gallstones in obese patients. Unfortunately, the NCGS did not use a very large dose of chenodiol;

with the moderate doses employed, it is doubtful that chenodiol can successfully desaturate bile in obese patients. Other workers have recommended that higher doses of chenodiol (up to 1.5 gm/day, if necessary) be used in obese patients to overcome the effects of increased secretion of biliary cholesterol and to affect gallstone dissolution in a good number of cases.

The results of the NCGS indicated that toxicity of chenodiol is dose related, and there has been concern that very high doses of chenodiol may be associated with significant hepatotoxicity.

Recent studies from our laboratory suggest another approach to gallstone dissolution in obese patients. This approach is based on our observation that caloric restriction can cause a normalization of biliary lipid metabolism. With reduced caloric intake, the synthesis of both cholesterol and bile acids returns to normal, as do their hepatic secretion rates during the fed state. Unfortunately, this normalization of biliary lipids does not extend to the fasting state, because many obese subjects actually have increased saturation with fasting. Therefore, caloric restriction alone will not bring about dissolution of gallstones in most obese patients.

Despite the frequent increase in bile saturation during fasting in many obese patients, our studies have shown that desaturation of bile can be achieved in most cases if only moderate doses (750 mg/day) of chenodiol are given simultaneously with caloric restriction. In this circumstance, the bile acid pool and hepatic secretion of bile acids can be enhanced at the same time that biliary output of cholesterol remains in the normal range. It is interesting to note that expansion of the bile acid pool alone is not sufficient to desaturate bile in obese patients undergoing weight reduction. In our study, when cholic acid was given, gallbladder bile did not desaturate despite marked expansion of the bile acid pool; in contrast, desaturation was achieved with chenodiol. The explanation of this difference is that chenodiol both expanded the bile acid pool and reduced biliary output of cholesterol, while cholic acid merely expanded the bile acid pool. We have reported recently that chenodiol represses the uncoupling of cholesterol and lecithin in the fasting state, while cholic acid does not.

The failure of chenodiol therapy in obese patients can probably be overcome by simultaneous reduction of caloric intake. The latter approach seems to have two definite advantages over markedly increasing the dosage of the drug. First, the potential hepatotoxicity of very large doses of chenodiol can be avoided; second, the problem of gallstone re-

currence following dissolution may be prevented. Since obesity is a major precursor of gallstone formation, little may be achieved by dissolving stones in patients who remain obese. It is probable that most patients will have a recurrence shortly after the termination of therapy. However, if a normal weight can be achieved and maintained simultaneously with gallstone dissolution, there is a possibility that gallstones may not occur.

Any future advances in the treatment of obesity should have a profound effect on the success of gallstone therapy. One such advantage may be the development of a new nonabsorbable fat, sucrose polyester. This material can be used as a substitute for fat, and because it is not digested and absorbed, it does not provide calories and thereby can lead to weight loss. Conceivably, the use of sucrose polyester in combination with chenodiol might prove effective for obese patients with gallstones.

CHOLESTEROL CRYSTALS AND GALLSTONES

Another factor leading to the relatively low rate of gallstone dissolution in the NCGS was that many of the patients had noncholesterol stones. One reason why women showed a higher dissolution rate than men was that they may have had a greater proportion of cholesterol stones. Our preliminary studies at the Veterans Administration Hospital in San Diego showed that men have a relatively high fraction of noncholesterol stones. Dissolution with chenodiol might be enhanced if gallstones containing little or no cholesterol could be identified and removed from treatment.

We have shown that there is a correlation between the presence of cholesterol crystals in bile and gallstone formation. Of interest was the finding that many patients with supersaturated bile did not have cholesterol crystals. These patients almost never developed cholesterol gallstones. Thus, development of cholesterol crystals may be a prerequisite for gallstone formation. The reason why some patients with supersaturated bile develop cholesterol crystals while others do not has not been determined, but the mechanism could represent a crucial link in the pathogenesis of cholesterol stones.

Since patients without detectable cholesterol crystals in bile usually do not have cholesterol gallstones, an examination of bile for crystals could provide a means to differentiate those with and without cholesterol stones. It might prove beneficial to intubate the duodenum, collect gallbladder bile, and examine it for crystals before selecting a patient for prolonged chenodiol therapy. If crystals are not found, the chances of a patient having cholesterol stones are lessened; it may be assumed that the stones do not contain cholesterol, and thus the patient would be rejected as a suitable subject for dissolution therapy. Our preliminary studies suggest that dissolution results might be improved by identifying patients with cholesterol stones.

CHENODIOL AND LIPOPROTEIN METABOLISM

Past studies suggested that chenodiol had no effect on total plasma cholesterol, but after a large number of patients were studied in the NCGS, a significant effect was observed. Small but definite increases in total cholesterol were observed in both the low- and high-dose groups; the increases, as compared to the placebo group, averaged about 5% (or 10 mg/day). In contrast, chenodiol caused a reduction in plasma triglycerides, as had been reported by earlier workers.

The rise in plasma cholesterol during chenodiol treatment was examined and was found to be confined to LDL. Most LDL is derived from degradation of VLDL (triglycerides); LDL can be catabolized by either the liver or extrahepatic tissue, although the distributions of these two pathways are not known. Data in animals indicate that approximately 40% goes to the liver and 60% to extrahepatic tissues.

During chenodiol therapy, the presumed rise in LDL is the reverse of that during treatment with bile acids sequestrants. Hepatic synthesis of receptors is likely inhibited, and less LDL is cleared by the liver. One result is a small rise in plasma LDL levels, but, more important, an increased amount of LDL may be directed to peripheral tissues for degradation. If so, this could lead to an increase in tissue cholesterol levels. The danger of expansion of tissue pools of cholesterol is that the increase might be extended to the arterial wall and thereby promote the development of atherosclerosis. Admittedly, this is only a theoretical concept.

Reference

1. Schoenfield LJ, Grundy SM, Hoffmann AF, et al: National Cooperative Gallstone Study (NCGS). *Gastroenterology* 84:644, 1983.

Chenodeoxycholic Acid Dissolution Studies in Sweden

The surgeons of the Karolinska Hospital in Sweden studied 342 patients who had indications for cholecystectomy but could be considered good subjects for dissolution with chenodeoxycholic acid.[1] Of this group, 136 patients (42.2%) had nonfunctioning gallbladders and were excluded; 100 patients (31.1%) with gallstones larger than 2 cm were rejected; 86 patients were excluded because of radiopaque calculi; and 7 were excluded because of hepatic disease. Of 342 patients requiring elective cholecystectomy, 49 were eligible for the dissolution treatment. Of the remaining 49 patients, 10 fertile women with inadequate contraception were eliminated; 6 patients with severe symptoms were unsatisfactory because dissolution therapy could not be considered the proper therapy. Three patients required laparotomy, and eight patients were ruled out for psychiatric and social reasons. Twenty-two patients were left out; 10 patients decided against the treatment. Finally, only 5 of the 342 patients actually completed the 2-year program. The result was disappointing; the gallstones remained in four patients, and only one patient (20%) had a successful result.

Reference

1. Karolinska Hospital, Dept. of Surgery: Stockholm, Sweden.

Monooctanoin

Monooctanoin is a semisynthetic esterified glycerol. It is used as a solubilizing agent for cholesterol gallstones retained in the biliary tract following cholecystectomy and choledochotomy and where reoperation is contraindicated. It is generally believed that in about one-third of the patients treated with monooctanoin, complete dissolution will occur, and that in about another one-third, partial dissolution will occur (reduction in size). Monooctanoin may be administered directly into the bile duct via a T-tube or an endoscopically placed into a naso-cholangio-catheter. Dissolution or reduction in stone size is reported to occur after 2–10 days of continuous perfusion.

Monooctanoin must never be employed in patients with clinical jaundice or infections, or in patients who have a history of duodenal ulcer or bowel inflammation.

The author cautions the reader that only those with experience in perfusion therapy should be entrusted with this form of therapy. A trademarked monooctanoin, Moctanin, is accompanied by a complete brochure of instructions; anyone who undertakes this form of therapy must read these instructions carefully.

Recommended Reading

Gadacz TR, Sharp K: Monooctanoin therapy for retained gallstones. *Surg News*, May 1983.
Thistle JL, Carlson GL, Hoffmann AF: Monooctanoin, a dissolution agent for retained cholesterol duct stones: Clinical application. *Gastroenterology* 78:1016, 1980.

Dissolution of Cholesterol Gallstones by Methyl Tert-Butyl Ether (MTBE)

MTBE has been tried by several endoscopists, who have reported both successes and failures. This new, powerful solvent, involving a tricky technique, has provoked differences of opinion regarding its use, safety, and effectiveness. Though MTBE is considered an acceptable alternative to chenodeoxycholic acid and ursodeoxycholic acid, it is certainly not an alternative to cholecystectomy with biopsy and abdominal exploration. The endoscopist must not forget that chemotherapy is not a cure for cholelithiasis; at best, it is a temporary means of improving gallbladder symptoms. To remove the stones and leave the diseased gallbladder is a temporizing procedure that has serious drawbacks.

Essentially, the MTBE procedure is performed as follows: Endoscopic retrograde pancreatography makes use of the endoscope, through which a nasobiliary catheter is passed through the ampulla of Vater into the common duct and further on through the cystic duct and into the gallbladder lumen. The bile is withdrawn, and 5 ml MTBE containing 10% fat-soluble X-ray contrast medium is instilled. X-rays reveal the gallstones bathed in MTBE. This combination is withdrawn, and 5 ml pure MTBE is instilled. Repeated aspirations and reinfusions are carried out to mix and stir up the combination more effectively. Every 15 minutes, 5 ml is aspirated and replaced 20 times on day 1, 10 times on day 2, and 7 times on day 6. During the days of irrigation and instillation, the nasobiliary catheter remains in place.

Sauerbruch et al.[1] described their technique as stated above; their experience was as follows: The first 10 aspirates revealed a thick layer of cholesterol crystals, as proved by light microscopy. On day 6 no more cholesterol crystals were noted, but evidence of residual stone material was present, confirmed by ultrasound. Two months later, the patient remained asymptomatic. Sauerbruch et al. concluded that cholesterol stones can be dissolved rapidly by instillations of MTBE solvent via nasobiliary catheter. There was leftover gallbladder residue that may have been noncholesterol material. At present, MTBE presents problems, especially when multiple mixed stones are present.

Even if MTBE treatment were successful (and it is not), follow-up treatments are still required. The underlying pathogenesis (etiological factors) has not been considered in this form of chemotherapy, and that is why the gallstones re-form, as before. The original gallbladder disease process remains; in no way has it been altered.

Sauerbruch now concerns himself exclusively with extracorporeal shock wave therapy for the fragmentation of cholesterol gallstones.

Recommended Reading

Allen MJ, Borody TJ, Bugliosi TF, et al: Rapid dissolution of gallstones by methyl-tert-butyl-ether (MTBE). *N Engl J Med* vol 312, no 4, 1985.

Reference

1. Sauerbruch T, Delius M, Paumgartner G, et al: Fragmentation of stones by extracorporeal shock waves. *N Engl J Med* 314:818, 1986.

Hyodeoxycholic Acid

McSherry et al.[1,2] reported their experiments with hyodeoxycholic acid and its isomer, 6^B-hyodeoxycholic acid, on prairie dogs and found that it prevented the formation of cholesterol gallstones and crystals. These workers have shown that the beneficial results take place in the presence of bile that is saturated with cholesterol. They found that when these animals were fed with hyodeoxycholic acid and 6^B-hyodeoxycholic acid, their bile contained abundant liquid crystals, which suggests that these new bile acids prevented the transition of cholesterol from its liquid crystalline phase to solid crystals and stones. McSherry et al. theorized that activity of reductase, the rate-limiting enzyme of cholesterol synthesis, prevented elevation of serum and liver cholesterol in the prairie dog fed a 0.4% cholesterol diet.

This writer believes that McSherry and his coworkers have made a definite advance in their search for the prevention and dissolution of the cholesterol gallstone. They are now studying the toxicity of hyodeoxycholic acid and 6^B-hyodeoxycholic acid, as well as their ability to dissolve the cholesterol stone.

References

1. McSherry AK, Mosbach EH, Cohen B, et al: Prevention of cholesterol induced gallstones by hyodeoxycholic acid in the prairie dog. *J Lipid Res* 25:539, 1984.
2. McSherry AK, Cohen BI, Mosbach EH, et al: Prevention of cholesterol induced gallstones by hyodeoxycholic acid in the prairie dog. *J Lipid Res* 25:539, 1984.

Ursodeoxycholic Acid

Ursodeoxycholic acid, (Ursodiol), in the U.S.A., and soon to be marketed as Actigall by Ciba-Geigy. Ursodeoxycholic acid is a naturally occurring bile acid and is being used for dissolution of radiolucent non-calcific cholesterol gallstones. The stones must not exceed 2 cm. in diameter.

The mechanism of Ursodeoxycholic acid action is believed to be that it lowers the cholesterol in the bile and alters the cholesterol-phospholipid ratio of lipid vesicles secreted into the bile. It also decreases the absorption of dietary and biliary cholesterol. About 90 percent of ursodeoxycholic acid is absorbed from the gastrointestinal tract and is extracted by the liver where it is conjugated with glycine and taurine.

CLINICAL RESULTS

Cholesterol stones have been completely dissolved in about 30 percent of the cases. It took 1–2 years; smaller stones dissolved more rapidly.

MONITORING AND RECURRENCE

For a period of one year a sonogram every 6 months. Cholecystography may not detect all stones.

If all stones disappear, the treatment should be discontinued for 1 to 3 months. Within 5 years 50 percent recur; a second course may be effective—and even then there are recurrences. Cholecystectomy is recommended after 2 failures. Where lithotripsy has failed to completely pulverize the stone, ursodeoxycholic acid has been successful in dissolving the residual.

Prophylactic use of ursodeoxycholic acid has been employed in cases of obese women who were undergoing rapid weight loss.

Ursodeoxycholic acid is *Contraindicated* in cases of liver cirrhosis. It does not produce hepato-toxicity and seldom causes diarrhea. Ursodeoxycholic acid has no effect on serum cholesterol or triglycerides. Concurrent use of cholestyramine, cholestipol, or aluminum antacids may interfere with the absorption of ursodeoxycholic acid. Its effectiveness is reduced by estrogens, contraceptives, and clofibrate.

DOSAGE

Optimum dosage: 8–10 mg./kgm./day; 2 or 3 divided doses.

Conclusion

Ursodeoxycholic acid is safe and can dissolve small cholesterol stones in 50 percent of the patients; its long time safety has not yet been established. Recurrences are common; *50-percent within a 5 year period.*

10

SURGICAL PROCEDURES FOR ACUTE AND CHRONIC CHOLECYSTITIS

Cholecystostomy

It is unfortunate that certain articles and textbooks still refer to cholecystostomy as a rather minor procedure. This writer wishes to contradict this view because cholecystostomy can be a very serious and difficult operation, especially in the extremely ill, obese patient in whom the gallbladder is small, deep-seated, shrunken, and thick, or completely covered with omentum and adherent to adjacent organs. At times, the gallbladder may be extremely difficult or impossible to recognize and isolate. Many surgeons still recommend a small incision because cholecystostomy is considered such a simple operation; *this is a fallacy.* The surgeon must make an adequate incision, since no one can predict what will be encountered or the difficulty in locating a portion of the gallbladder. "Buttonhole" incisions must be avoided at all times. Another common fallacy is that many surgeons believe that local anesthesia is good for a high-risk patient such as one who is sick, aged, and unprepared. This is unrealistic; if one is in a hurry to do emergency surgery without preparing the patient, local anesthesia may seem correct but is not necessarily so. A better-prepared patient in whom some time is allotted for conservative preoperative treatment is a better risk. The administration of antibiotics, and intravenous fluids with electrolytes to correct fluid and electrolyte imbalances, will do much to lower the operative mortality. If the surgery can be delayed, this will lessen the risk of administering a mild general anesthetic, allow a larger incision to be made, and permit an easier and faster operation to be carried out.

Where the abdomen has been opened and the gallbladder and common duct reveal no inflammation, distortions, or anomalies, it is unwise not to take advantage of the situation and do a cholecystectomy. However, since existing inflammatory distortion may lead to complications and possible dire consequences, it is safer and more prudent to choose the alternative course of cholecystostomy. This procedure offers several options in the months that follow. In a patient 65 years or over, with varied associated systemic problems and a severe case of acute cholecystitis, it may be wiser to do a cholecystostomy as a primary operation because the patient is so toxic and gravely ill that any other surgery would be unwise. Continuing to treat the patient postoperatively prevents endotoxic shock from developing. It is necessary to hydrate the patient properly and replace electrolytes. The electrolyte imbalance must be improved and the necessary antibiotic or antibiotics given to control a mixed infection (from aerobic and anaerobic organisms). The results of this program have been so gratifying that the writer urges every surgeon to consider cholecystostomy not just as an alternative or backdown procedure but as a primary lifesaving operation. In one instance, a 92-year-old patient suffered on-and-off attacks of acute cholecystitis, which the internist felt was related to intermittent cardiac complaints; it was finally decided that this man should have his gallbladder removed. His general condition was brought up to optimum levels, and at surgery the gallbladder was found to contain stones, which were easily removed. Because the operation was easily performed, it took only about 10 minutes to remove the gallbladder and close the abdomen. Unfortunately, though this patient was well controlled with cardiac medication, the procedure was too much for him; he never recovered from the pulmonary and cardiac complications that followed. The patient finally developed intractable pulmonary problems and died. This is another instance in which, even with good medical preparation and normal anatomy, but in an aged patient well prepared and supported by cardiac drugs, definitive surgery (cholecystectomy) proved too much of a strain. In retrospect, the best procedure would have been to evacuate the gallbladder of stones and débris, establish continuity with the biliary tree with a cholecystostomy, and bow out.

The underlying pathology in acute cholecystitis is usually an inflamed and very distended gallbladder which cannot empty itself because of an obstructed, edematous cystic duct. The stagnant, concentrated, or inspissated bile may become secondarily infected, and in patients over 65 with advancing arteriosclerosis, this marked distention adds a further burden to the vasculature of the gallbladder wall. These vessels stretch and narrow to the point where necrosis sets in focally, multifocally, or over a large area, ultimately to involve the entire gallbladder. Almost invariably infection accompanies the pathological changes that exist with mechanical obstruction of the gallbladder; when the gallbladder becomes infected more often than not, *E. coli,* aerobic, and anaerobic mixed intestinal organisms are present, and unless the toxicity is immediately treated, the infection may spread through the blood and lymphatics, creating a picture of bacteremia and endotoxic shock.

After rupture of one of the focal necrotic areas, a localized or generalized peritonitis may develop as a result of both the chemical action of the bile and bacterial contamination throughout the peritoneal cavity. Much depends upon the surgeon, who must make a final decision; many decisions can be made preoperatively, but the final decision must be made in the operating room after the abdomen is opened and the area evaluated. When the patient's general condition is poor and is associated with systemic problems requiring strong medications, or when the patient is critically ill and the condition shows signs of increasing severity, it may be wise, even in the presence of apparent normal anatomy, to proceed with a staged procedure such as a cholecystostomy. Thorough cleansing and irrigation of the gallbladder lumen, biopsy of the wall, culture of the bile, and drainage with a large mushroom catheter through a subcostal stab wound is all that is required. Even when one plans an elective cholecystectomy in a controlled poor-risk patient, if the open abdomen reveals distention, inflammation and anomalous-looking anatomy, one should readily recognize a possible catastrophe with a primary cholecystectomy. Here too, it would be best for the acute process to subside after a first-stage cholecystostomy. At a later date, i.e., several months later, and after careful evaluation via tube cholangiography, a more definitive second-stage procedure may be performed on the patient who is now in optimum condition.

Empyema of the gallbladder has almost always been treated by cholecystostomy, employing a large mushroom catheter that is brought out through a subcostal stab wound. At times there will be evidence of necrosis in the fundus of the gallbladder, in which case it is best to debride whatever gangrenous tissue exists, and do a cholecystostomy on the residual normal gallbladder (see Fig. 1-87). Failing to remove the gangrenous portion of gallbladder can only lead to peritonitis and possible endotoxic shock. The drainage tube will require additional protection; omentum, if available, is wrapped around it so that the tube reaches the subcostal stab wound. Thus, the tube is completely covered and is protected against leakage into the peritoneal cavity.

There will be times, when on entering the abdomen, not only will the fundus of the gallbladder be found to be necrotic, but the entire gallbladder and cystic duct will reveal gangrene. Regardless of the patient's condition, the surgeon has no choice but to proceed and cut away all existing gangrenous tissue and, if deemed necessary, to perform a choledochotomy, insert a T-tube, and drain the common duct. It is hoped that subsequent T-tube cholangiography will indicate the need for future surgery to remove residual gallstones that may become obstructive. There always will be situations where surgeons will find that their own clinical judgment cannot always be acted upon; that the pathology itself will dictate the choice of surgery and thus decide the ultimate prognosis.

In my own cases, the majority of patients were 75 years and over; *there was some morbidity, but no mortality.* Every patient who had a cholecystostomy improved, starting with the first postoperative day, and none of the biopsies ever revealed carcinoma. After a drainage period of 1 month, common duct studies with tube cholangiography indicated that there was no evidence of leftover stones in the gallbladder or biliary tree. In cases that had serious associated pathological conditions, i.e., cardiac and pulmonary problems, diabetes mellitus, or blood dyscrasias, fortunately no further surgery was required.

After a second study with tube cholangiography 2 months after surgery, similar negative findings corroborated the finding of no stones in the biliary tree. The mushroom (or Malecot) catheter was withdrawn, and the residual pathological gallbladder was left in. No further surgery was contemplated. All of these cases were followed for several years, with no evidence (signs or symptoms) of cholecystic disease. Given the advanced ages of these patients, it is conceivable that no further gallbladder disease will develop and that death will result most likely from causes other than gallbladder. It should be mentioned here that during an abdominal procedure in the extremely aged patient for reasons other than gallbladder disease, should asymptomatic cholelithiasis coexist, it is considered good judgment to do a prophylactic cholecystostomy, empty the gallbladder of its content, and perform a secondary definitive operation later—if justified. This prevents a possible serious acute attack in the postoperative period that may require immediate surgical intervention.

The subject of cholecystostomy is usually associated with the geriatric patient. The question of whether or not acute biliary tract disease should be treated by immediate definitive or delayed surgery must be decided. At present there are two schools of thought; one is to operate as soon as possible; the other is to wait until the infectious process and the acute symptoms subside, and then perform an elective procedure. Both schools of thought have their advocates; however, in the geriatric population, *each patient must be evaluated individually,* and there should be no waste of time in either instance other than close observation of the patient. This writer believes that neither early nor delayed surgery alone is the answer; both have merit, depending upon the patient and the associated diseases. Timing is the critical factor, in-

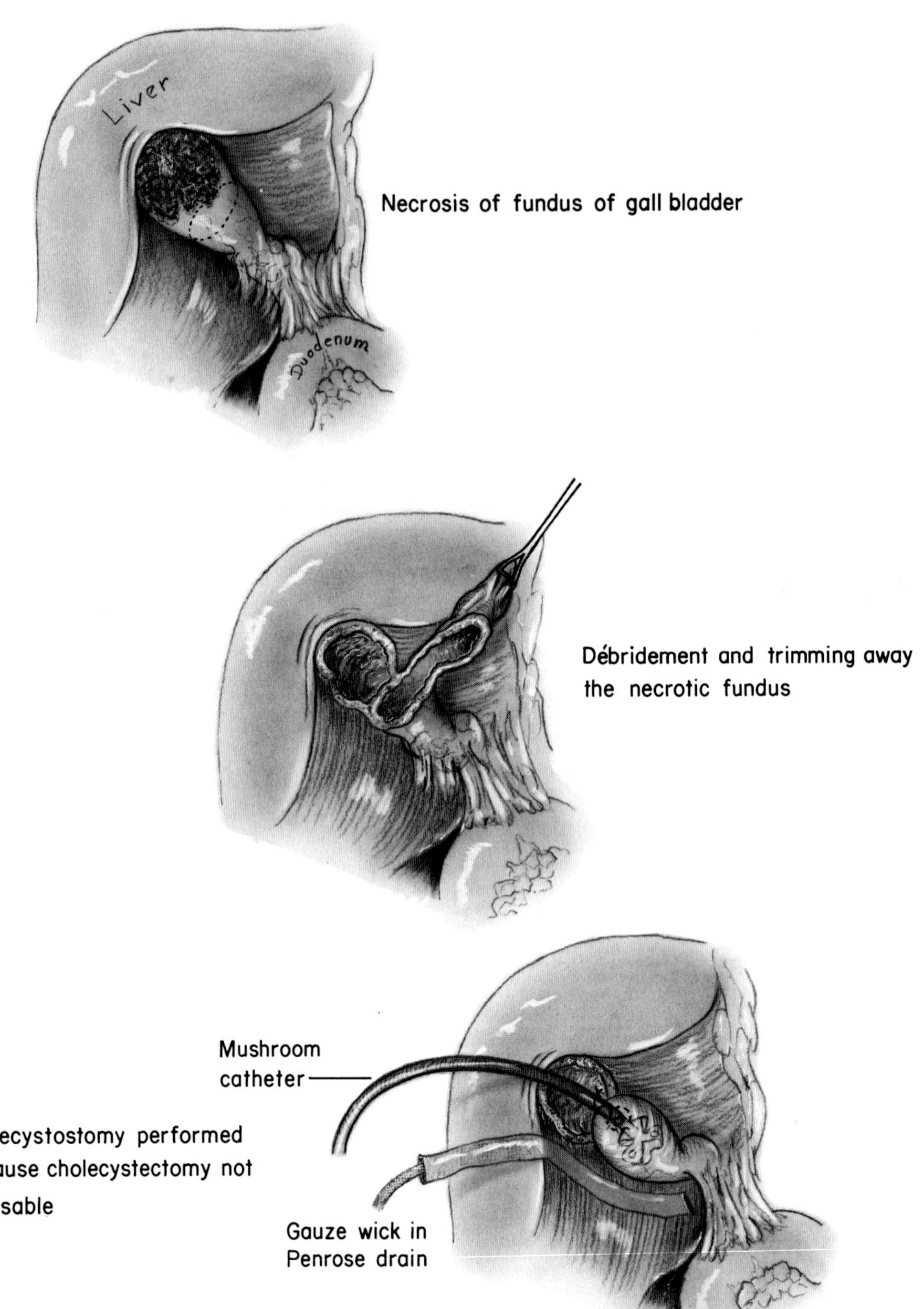

Figure 87. Cholecystostomy performed because cholecystectomy is not advisable. These diagrams illustrate the emergency measures that may be undertaken when existing conditions contraindicate complete cholecystectomy and exploration. In an inflamed necrotic gallbladder only the gangrenous portion need be carefully excised, and a cholecystostomy performed. After an acceptable period of time either an elective cholecystectomy may be performed, or in the very aged and debilitated, the tube may be withdrawn, provided that healing was uneventful and the cholangiogram shows no residual stones present.

cluding the preparation of the patient, i.e., preoperative management before any surgery is carried out. An attempt to make each case elective, if possible, should be the surgeon's goal; and only in the presence of evidence indicating that the patient is not responding should one consider emergency surgical intervention. *The surgeon's surgical judgment should always be individualized, rather than based upon a formula or rule.* The surgeon who cannot wait to operate will most often run into difficult or disastrous problems. The reason is, he has not given himself or the patient the opportunity to attain optimum preoperative conditions before deciding on surgery.

It is most important for the geriatric patient to be treated immediately, i.e., whenever the disease is discovered. The treatment should be aimed at stopping the progression of the disease process by conservative medical management unless surgical intervention becomes mandatory. The surgeon should stand ready at all times to interrupt any conservative approach when he sees incipient toxicity developing toward full blown-endotoxic shock, which elderly patients cannot easily overcome. In 1970, a report in the *Southern Medical Journal* by Field and Jones[1] cited 30 geriatric patients in whom the authors had performed a cholecystostomy not as an emergency last-resort procedure, but as a definitive primary procedure. They stated that their 20% mortality was acceptable to them, since the procedure they carried out was considered lifesaving. This opinion has been shared by many, including this writer, namely, that mortality is greatest in the oldest and sickest patients for whom only cholecystostomy is reserved. Those who survive that surgery represent pure salvage. Prophylactic cholecystostomy for gallbladder disease in the geriatric patient is the only real means of early diagnosis and treatment of carcinoma of the gallbladder. Among many surgeons, there is a tendency to feel defeated when the original intent was to perform a cholecystectomy, and then to back down or compromise, so to speak, and perform a cholecystostomy. *Glenn[2] felt that since cholecystostomy is a lifesaving operation, the surgeon should not feel apologetic about it* in cases where cholecystectomy is contemplated but not attempted because of inflammatory distortion, alteration of the anatomical relationship, and difficulty of structure identification. *Glenn also felt that since the primary problem in such instances was drainage of the bile, a cholecystostomy becomes the only consideration and the ideal procedure to perform.*

An infected gallbladder that progresses to generalized toxicity requires additional special therapy, namely, combination therapy. Large doses of corticosteroids, as well as vasodilators, should be given when indicated; the best broad-spectrum antibiotics, singly or in combination, should be administered, including tetracyclines, chloramphenicol (Chloromycetin with the consent of the family), and cephalosporins such as Mandol (Lilly) and Cefoxitin (S K and F), with or without an aminoglycoside (e.g., gentamicin).

INDICATIONS

1. Acute cholecystitis with right upper quadrant (RUQ) tenderness; RUQ mass increasing in size; or just a palpable mass associated with temperature and possible chills. A pathological process that fails to respond to conservative management, in the aged and/or poor-risk patient.
2. During surgery, when the surgeon recognizes a severe, acute inflammatory process associated with distorted anatomy, swelling, and edema. Friability of the tissue indicates a great risk of irreparably damaging important contiguous anatomical structures.
3. In patients who are poor risks and in those who appear toxic, suggesting incipient anaerobic infection with endotoxic shock; in patients with jaundice of varying intensity; and in those with associated cardiovascular-renal problems that would contraindicate a prolonged, definitive procedure.
4. Whenever acute suppurative cholangitis or empyema of the gallbladder is suspected, especially when associated with common duct obstruction, in the aged patient.
5. When the operating surgeon is working alone and is too inexperienced to tackle a difficult surgical procedure in a high-risk patient.
6. As a first-stage drainage procedure for carcinoma of the head of the pancreas, or to relieve the intense intrabiliary pressure and jaundice caused by obstruction (cholecystojejunostomy).
7. In acute pancreatitis caused by common duct obstruction at the level of the ampullary area, where there is a reflux of bile into the duct of Wirsung, causing an acute pancreatitis with jaundice. Cholecystostomy may serve as a vital decompressive form of therapy and may be lifesaving.
8. It may be contemplated as an elective procedure in patients aged 65 to 95 when the problem is associated with advanced pulmonary-cardiovascular-renal disease; in those patients who are under medication and management and are delicately balanced.

ADVANTAGES

1. This is a surgical procedure of minimal undertaking; that is, it is rapid, requiring a minimum of anesthesia, with a minimum insult to the patient; it usually assures a more rapid recovery.
2. The principle of gallbladder drainage is that of removing the infected content from a closed cavity. In an inflamed gallbladder obstructed at the cystic duct, drainage also serves to decompress the organ. Cholecystostomy is a preventive measure against empyema of gallbladder that usually progresses to rupture and peritonitis. It is also used when a severe toxemia develops that cannot be easily controlled and where there may be a gram-negative sepsis with impending endotoxic shock.
3. By performing a rapid temporizing procedure such as cholecystostomy, one allows drainage, with removal of the bile and pus to the outside, as well as decompression of the entire hepatic system. Liver function is improved, jaundice is reduced, existing infection is controlled, and the chances of toxemia are reduced. Finally, cholecystostomy allows subsequent study of the biliary tree with cholangiography and future safe secondary surgery.
4. Another advantage is that a second-stage operation may be planned at any elective period found necessary or desirable. A postcholecystostomy patient who has potential longevity should be allowed the risk of a second-stage elective cholecystectomy.
5. If after a cholecystographic study through a draining Foley or mushroom catheter no stones in the biliary tree are found, then the tube or catheter may be withdrawn and no cholecystectomy undertaken.
6. If a secondary elective procedure is planned, ideally the patient should be prepared so that the surgery and anesthesia will be better tolerated, over a longer period of operative time.

MANAGEMENT OF THE CHOLECYSTOSTOMY TUBE

1. Bile should be passed from the drainage tube into a collecting bag (usually a leg urinal collecting bag).
2. Precautions should be taken to secure the tube around its skin exit site to prevent its being pulled out.
3. The bile should be inspected from time to time, described carefully, cultured if necessary, measured twice daily, and a daily output chart kept. It is possible that on the first, second, or even third day, bile may not begin to flow. In due time, however, after tissue inflammation and edema have subsided and the biliary intraductal pressure has built up, bile will eventually begin to flow. At about 3–4 weeks, cholecystography may be carried out through the mushroom catheter. Enzymatic studies should indicate how the liver has improved during the period of drainage. The tube should be removed at the propitious moment. When no calculi can be found in the biliary tree, the tube may be withdrawn, with the expectation that no future exacerbation of cholecystitis will occur. However, in patients 70 years or less with a good chance of living for another 10 or more years, a second-stage procedure may be planned; the drainage tube should then be left in because it is a good guide to the common bile duct at later surgery.

In patients over 65 with associated systemic disease, and in whom the cholecystographic studies show a retained stone in the gallbladder, it is possible to do a secondary procedure to remove the offending stone without doing a cholecystectomy. These high-risk patients may be carefully prepared for a second-stage operation, in which case the common duct stone is removed and drained with a T-tube. *Before a second-stage operation is resorted to every noninvasive technique should be attempted* (see Casal's description of Burhenne's Techniques in Chapter 5). However, if the stone is not removable or dissolvable in its fixed position within the ampulla, a *duodenotomy* and *sphincterotomy* may have to be performed. Here too, *endoscopic retrograde pancreatography (ERCP)* should be tried before secondary surgery is considered. Other means, depending upon the condition of the patient, may be considered, i.e., *choledochoduodenostomy*, which works very well and may provide the ultimate surgical cure. As stated before, if the patient has associated diseases such as diabetes, arteriosclerosis, or cardiovascular-renal disease, it may be better to avoid surgery. However, in patients with a retained common duct stone, it may be *wiser to resort to the various noninvasive techniques* devised specifically to remove impacted stones before resorting to definitive secondary surgery (see "Common Duct Surgery," "Choledochoduodenostomy," "Sphincterotomy," "Sphincteroplasty," and "Cholecystectomy" in Chapter 17).

OPERATIVE TECHNIQUES

1. The *patient's condition* should be built up to the optimal level. The patient should be properly

hydrated (fluids, electrolytes, and vitamins), blood reserved in the blood bank, and appropriate preoperative antibiotics administered.

2. The ideal *anesthesia* for the patient should be chosen, preferably a nontoxic general anesthesia. Intubate the poor-risk patient, if possible. In special high-risk patients in whom any form of anesthesia is contraindicated, it may be necessary to consider local anesthesia.

3. The *incision* must be designed for the individual patient. Patients with a short, squatty, or transverse body type should receive a right transverse or oblique (Kocher) incision. Those with a long, phthisical body type should receive a midline or paramedian (longitudinal) incision. In either case, the incision must ideally be over the site of pathology. The moderate or medium-type patient will probably do best with a modified paramedian, midline or subcostal Kocher incision (see Figs. 92, 93, and 94).

When the abdominal cavity is exposed, the gallbladder is sought and inspected for color, fullness, and tension. One must look for gangrenous spots and for evidence of perforation. The surgeon must recognize any distortions, as well as associated diseases, (i.e.) jaundice. Whether the common duct is available with minimal manipulation is significant. A large trocar is attached to a suction device.

It enters the gallbladder fundus and immediately decompresses the tense, swollen gallbladder by removing its stagnant bile, or "white bile" (hydrops), or pus (empyema).

The entire gallbladder area is walled off, and the trocar opening is enlarged. This should be carried out in the direction of the gangrenous spot that has to be debrided. After the gallbladder stoma is enlarged, spatulas, spoons, or whatever stone-grasping forceps are available are used to pick up and remove all debris, stones, mud, and gravel from the gallbladder lumen. It may be necessary to finger-palpate the lumen for any possible residual stones that are not readily recognized. One should immediately remove the used glove and replace it with a new sterile glove (Fig. 88). A finger maneuver or tactic to dislodge an impacted stone near the cystic duct or in Hartmann's pouch is considered good technique. The stone can be better manipulated between the outside and inside fingers (see Fig. 88). Packing the gallbladder cavity with a moist gauze sponge often traps resistant debris and small stones that may still be present. The moist piece of gauze effectively picks up gravel and mud within its interstices as it is scraped mildly along the mucosa of the gallbladder.

When the gallbladder lumen is thoroughly cleansed of all its content, a biopsy is taken of the

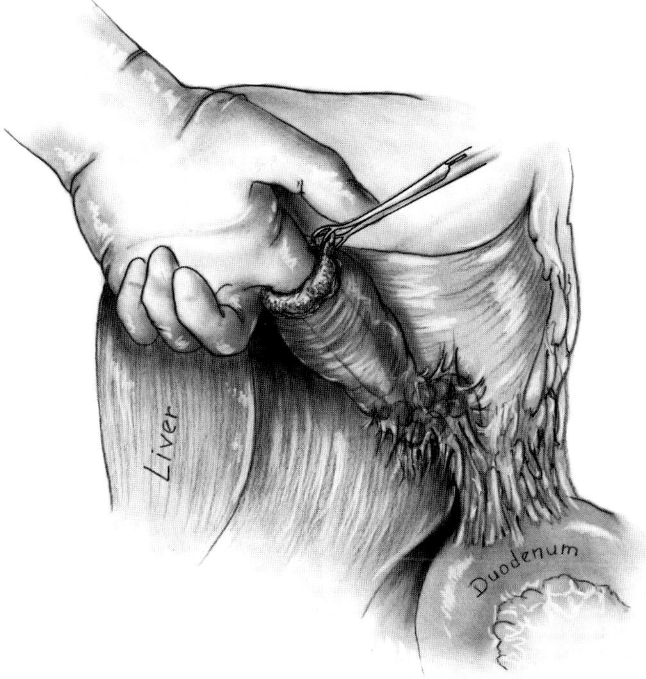

Figure 88. The McNealy-Glassman finger maneuver. The forefinger of left hand inserted into gallbladder helps to palpate residual stones, polyps, and tumors and safely guides external dissection to identify attached structures. Change glove after exploration.

gallbladder wall, as well as a swab of the lumen for culture and sensitivity. A No. 20–24 tube is employed; a Fogerty balloon catheter, a Malecot catheter, or even an ordinary mushroom catheter is acceptable. The writer prefers an ordinary mushroom catheter with cut-out openings to allow debris and small stones to pass through (Fig. 89). The tip is cut off before inserting and fixing it to the gallbladder wall. The surgeon should inspect the rest of the gallbladder without disturbing the adherent omentum and adjacent organs to see if further debridement is necessary. It is wise to leave the inflammatory adhesions alone; they should be disturbed as little as possible because they serve as a useful walling-off purpose.

With the forefinger and thumb, the surgeon should palpate along the common duct; it may be possible to determine whether there are any tumors, involved lymph nodes, or stones that may have been missed. The same two fingers can be used along the cystic duct level to milk a palpable stone back into the gallbladder lumen so that it can be removed with forceps. Caution should be observed at this time; if the operator finds more gangrenous spots in the gallbladder wall, it may be necessary to do a partial (subtotal) cholecystectomy, removing all the necrotic tissue and still carrying out the planned cholecystostomy (see Fig. 87). However, if the entire gallbladder is gangrenous, it is imperative, regardless of the patient's condition, to remove all available necrotic tissue and do a procedure as close to a complete cholecystectomy as possible. When it is discovered that the gallbladder is perforated at a point too low to do a safe cholecystostomy, it becomes necessary to persist and risk taking additional operative time to complete a cholecystectomy. After the drainage tube has been inserted into the gallbladder, it is sewn to the gallbladder wall, using a circumferential suture of (00) chromic catgut; several interrupted sutures are placed circumferentially around the gallbladder stoma, closing it watertight around the tube. The catgut suture that encircles the stoma is also tied to the tube so as to anchor it more effectively to the gallbladder; the latter will help prevent the accidental pulling out of the tube (see Fig. 89).

A subcostal stab wound is established just below the rib margin, and a curved Pean forceps is forced through to the peritoneum to grasp the drainage tube and bring it out through the stab wound. The tube is adjusted with a minimum of traction sufficient to bring the gallbladder wall in touch with the parietal peritoneum. It is preferable to have the gallbladder touch the parietal peritoneum because adhesions are created between the gallbladder and peritoneum to prevent leakage. Hurwitz[3] has recommended that a portion of the gallbladder fundus be exteriorized beyond the peritoneal surface. This writer feels that this maneuver is not essential; those who feel that it contributes to their results may use it. The omentum may be used to encircle the tube wherever there may be a short or fixed gallbladder that allows a space to exist between the fundus of the gallbladder and the parietal peritoneum. The omentum that encircles the tube helps to form a sort of canal that also prevents leakage into the peritoneal cavity. The Penrose or Jackson-Pratt drain is placed as far down along the body of the gallbladder as possible and out through the same stab wound. A word of caution here: When placing a suture circumferentially around the tube to make the gallbladder watertight, it is important to remember that an inflamed gallbladder wall is usually thick, fibrotic, and edematous, and that superficial stitching is inadequate. Either interrupted or circumferential through-and-through sutures should be made to be sure that maximum strength has been attained in snugging up the gallbladder wall around the tube.

The original abdominal incision is now closed in layers. If a midline incision was made, the peritoneum and linea alba are closed with interrupted Ti-chron (00) sutures. The skin and subcutaneous tissue are closed with interrupted (000) black silk or metal clips. Provided that carcinoma was not recognized, and provided that the patient is not debilitated, malnourished or obese, with no associated respiratory problems, deep nylon or wire tension sutures are not required. However, if any of the conditions mentioned do exist, the use of deep through-and-through tension sutures of either Ti-chron (0) or nylon (0) are justified.

Bile may not appear for as long as 24–48 or 72 hours. The only drainage that one may see at times is serosanguinous material. The Penrose drain is usually allowed to remain in place for about 3–7 days, depending upon the amount of bile drainage. If the Penrose drain shows no evidence of bile drainage after the third day, it may be carefully removed. There is no exact time limit for removing the Malecot, Foley, or mushroom catheter, because each case must be evaluated on its own merits; the best time to begin cholecystography is after about 3–4 weeks, when it is safe to traumatize the patient's biliary tree with a dye injection. There should be no hurry; the patient is usually improving, and the liver is being decompressed. This

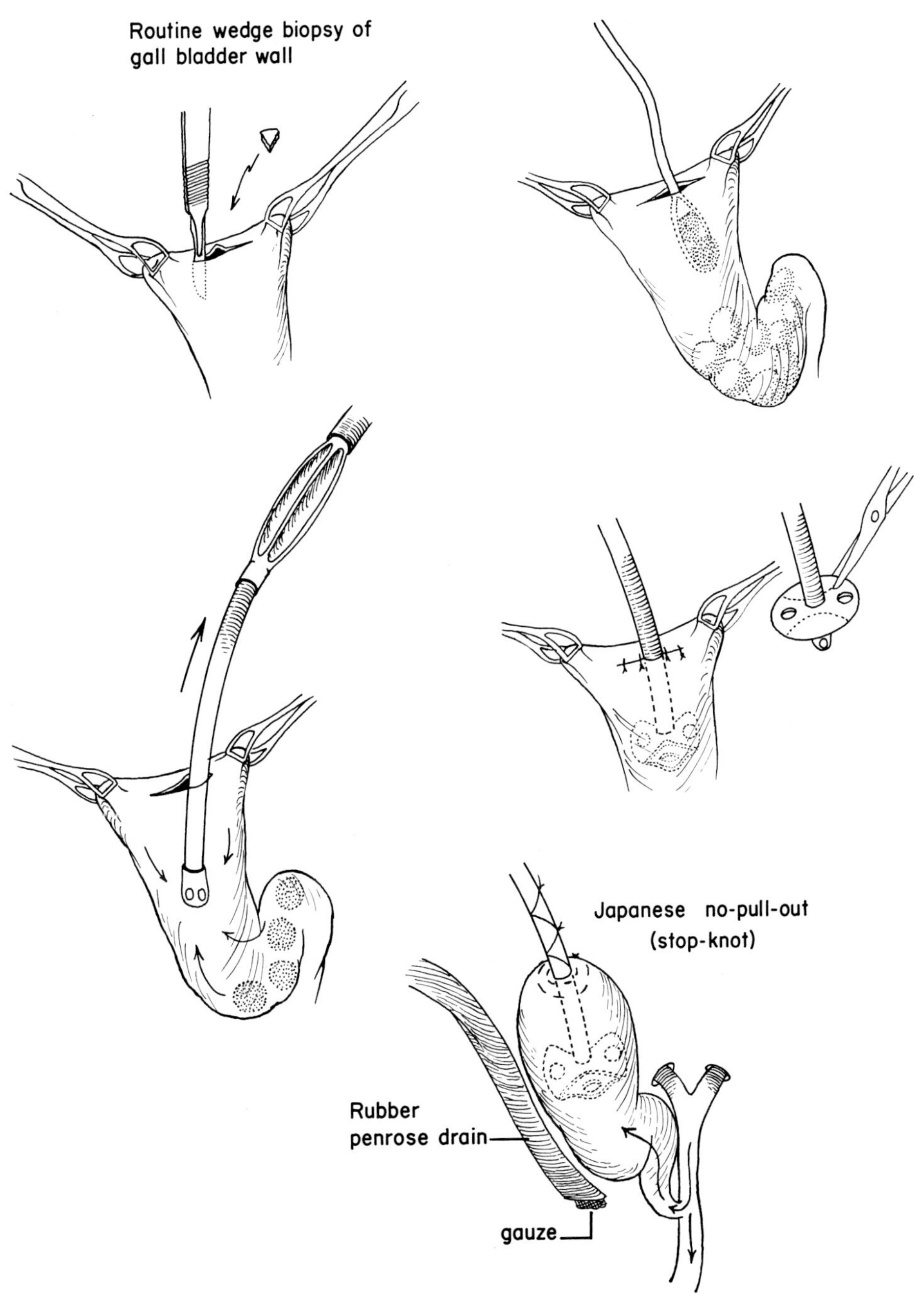

Figure 89.   Steps in cholecystostomy. Empty gallbladder completely; irrigate with saline; finger palpate inside of gallbladder for residual stones; dry gauze helps to enmesh small stones. If no stones obstruct the cystic and common bile duct, the tube may be removed in the aged poor-risk patient.

writer likes to continue antibiotics in decreasing dosage until the draining bile turns golden; then the antibiotic is discontinued.

If cholecystography indicates that there is a residual stone in the gallbladder, then through the original stab wound incision a secondary operative procedure can be carried out that allows the surgeon to follow the tube as he enlarges the incision. After the tube is followed into the gallbladder cavity, the stone can be removed by a stone-grasping forceps. Draining the gallbladder with the Malecot, mushroom, or Foley catheter should be continued for a few weeks longer. After cholecystography indicates no residual stones in the biliary tree, the drainage tube can be pulled out. Another option in patients 65 years old or more who have at least a 10-year survival period is a secondary cholecystectomy. In this operation, if a stone is discovered in the common bile duct, it can be opened and explored. If the common bile duct stone cannot be removed by other known techniques, it may be necessary to do a palliative bypass procedure as a last resort. The common duct is anastomosed to the duonenum; Choledochoduodenostomy (see Fig. 90). Secondary operation is undertaken only after the patient is brought up to his or her peak condition. When the second operation is performed, the drainage tube helps to guide the surgeon down to the cystic duct and then onto the common duct. The common duct is then opened, and if the stone cannot be removed immediately and with dispatch, a palliative choledochoduodenostomy is performed. These elderly patients, as a rule, do very well for the remainder of their life. They are watched closely in the hospital and subsequently are followed closely at the office. An important factor often overlooked in the postcholecystostomy period is that these patients with intact gallbladders and with a negative cholecystogram must still be watched carefully. They are not allowed to live and eat in any fashion they desire. They must be managed as a medical gallbladder problem; that is, they must be on a rigid gallbladder diet as a prophylactic measure to prevent recurrent cholecystitis and cholelithiasis. In the writer's experience in the past 35 years, only a few patients had to be reoperated on for recurrent cholelithiasis.

CLINICAL REPORTS

Ficarra[4] performed 75 cholecystostomy procedures in patients with acute cholecystitis, with or without perforation. He reported no postoperative morbidity or mortality.[4] He stressed that an acute inflammatory edema around the cystic duct and Hartmann's pouch prevents dissection and identification for ligation of the cystic duct and cystic artery. He noted that the gallbladder becomes more distended and that the cystic duct and artery become shorter. He further stated that the brevity of the vital structures makes it difficult to perform double ligations on the cystic duct and artery. Improper ligation of these structures is surgically perilous, and invites the possibility of biliary fistula, hemorrhage, or both. He stressed that whenever the cystic duct and cystic artery cannot be properly identified and ligated, the surgeon should be aware of the possibility of injury to the common duct and the cystic artery.

The temerity which favors cholecystostomy may be the price one pays for safety. Based upon their experience of the past two decades, Ficarra believes that cholecystostomy in the elderly patient allows 10 to 20 years of freedom from recurrence of cholelithiasis; this is especially true if the patient adheres to the recommended dietary regimen. The author concludes that cholecystostomy is safe and has a place in the management of acute fulminating obstructive cholelithiasis in the geriatric patient. This writer agrees wholeheartedly with him.

Field and Jones,[1] in their article in the *Southern Medical Journal*, speak of their experience with 30 seriously ill elderly patients whose average age was 76 and whose average postoperative follow-up period was 3 years. The existing contraindications to surgery were mainly cardiovascular-renal, yet they performed cholecystostomy on all 30 patients. They stated that wherever the biliary tree is free of stones, as recognized in the postoperative period by cholecystographic studies, no additional surgery should be performed. Further, wherever cholecystographic studies in the postoperative period indicate that a stone or stones are impacted in the cystic or common duct, they recommend cholecystostomy and exploration of the common bile duct. In their 3-year follow-up studies they reported eight postoperative deaths—two from pulmonary emboli, two from coronary occlusion, and one from a cardiovascular accident and mesenteric thrombosis. Of the remaining patients, one died 2 years after surgery from emphysema and pneumonia; two died from congestive heart failure, and arteriosclerosis after that period of time. Twenty patients are still alive and asymptomatic, with no cholecystographic evidence of stone recurrence; they still show normal cholecystograms.

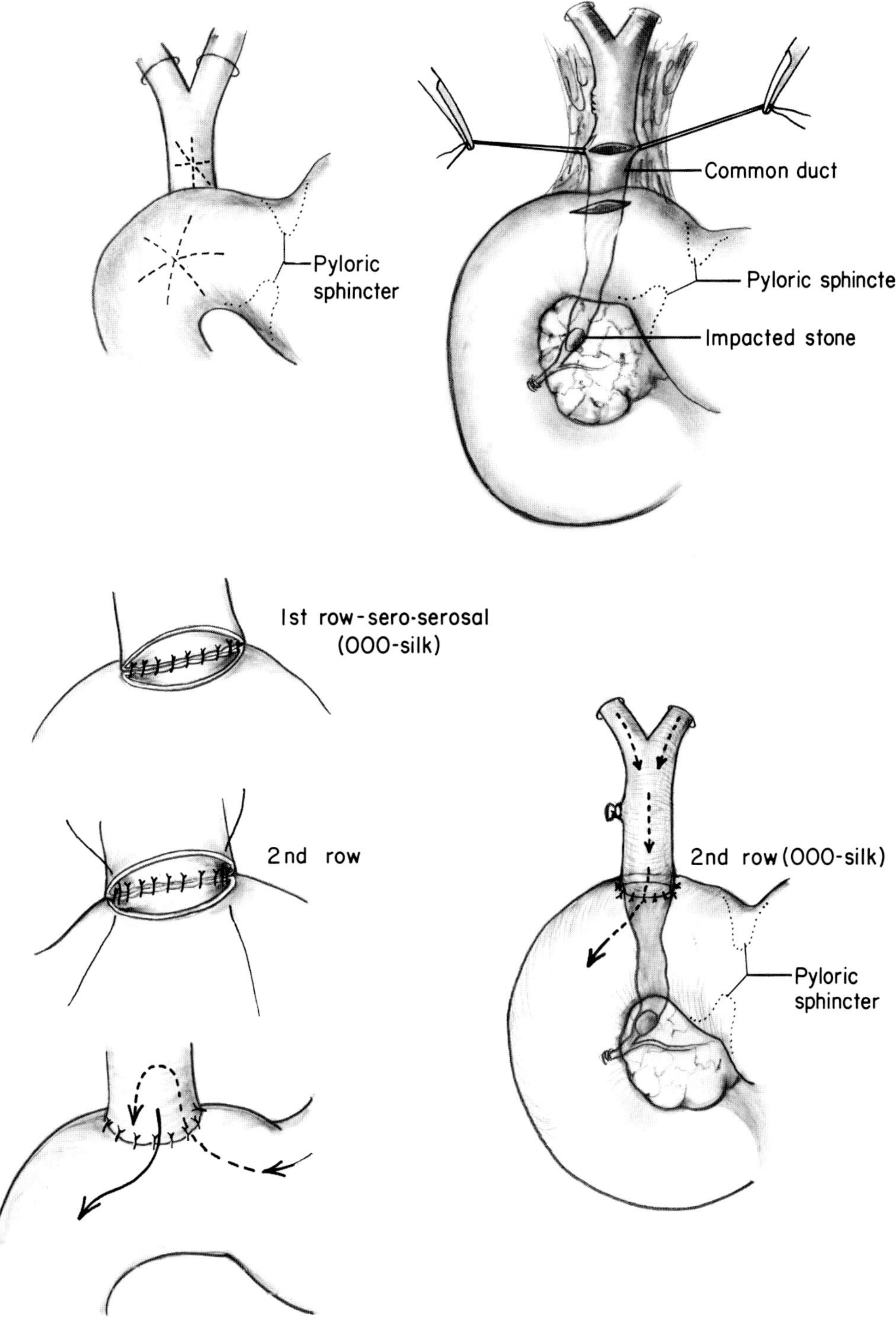

Figure 90.   The techniques for choledochoduodenostomy (side-to-side and end-to-side) are shown here. The surgeon is urged to employ this last resort procedure when absolutely indicated. When all available efforts have been attempted in removing a stone or stones from the common or hepatic ducts without success, then as a last resort procedure a choledochoduodenostomy or choledochojejunostomy, should be performed.

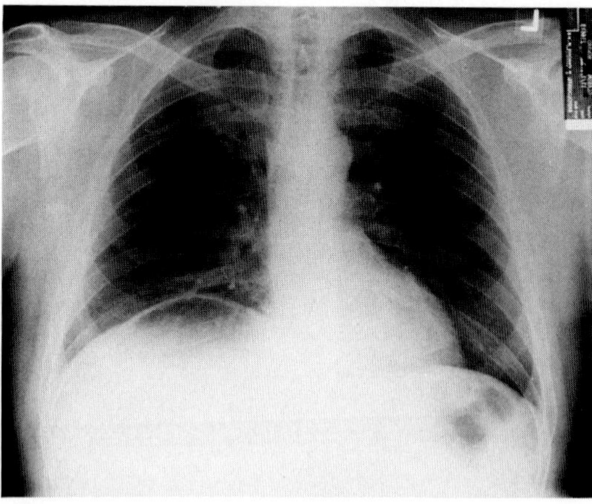

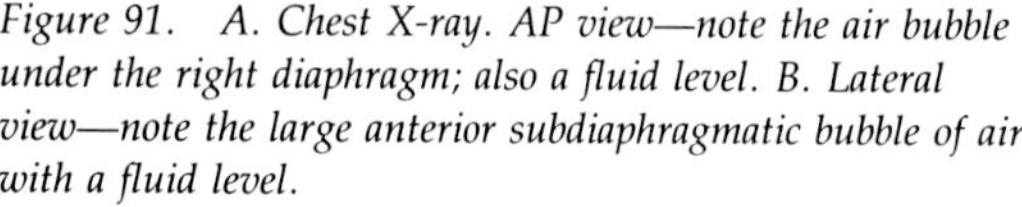

Figure 91. A. Chest X-ray. AP view—note the air bubble under the right diaphragm; also a fluid level. B. Lateral view—note the large anterior subdiaphragmatic bubble of air with a fluid level.

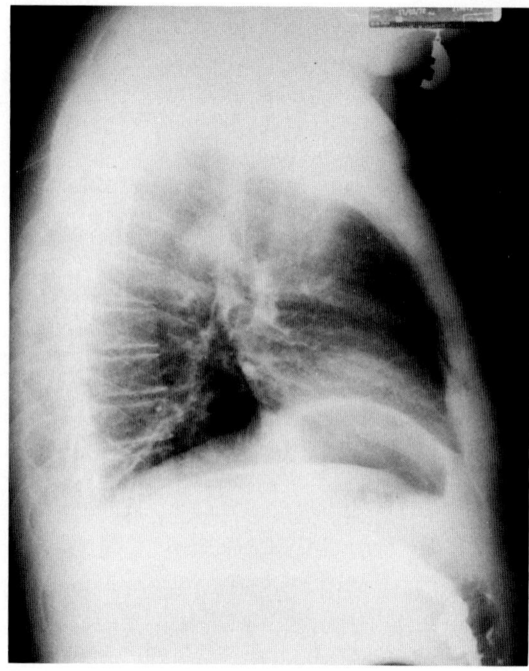

B

Recommended Reading

Pearse DM, Hawkins IF: Percutaneous cholecystostomy in acute cholecystitis and common duct obstruction. *Radiology* 152:365, 1984.

Skillings JC, Kumai C, Hinshaw JR Jr, et al: Cholecystostomy—a place in modern biliary surgery? *Am J Surg* 139:865, 1980.

References

1. Field Jones: Cholecystostomy, a safe operation in emergencies of the aged. *South Med J* 18:832, 1970.
2. Glenn F: Surgical management in patients 65 years of age and older. *Ann Surg* 193:56, 1981.
3. Hurwitz A: Personal communication.
4. Ficarra BJ: Cholecystostomy in the aged patients. *J Am Geriatr Soc* 1970.

Techniques for Cholecystectomy (McNealy-Glassman)

Two techniques are commonly employed for cholecystectomy. There are also many variations, depending upon the specific problems encountered.

When should one employ the *bottom-up* versus the *top-bottom* method? This writer prefers the bottom-up technique because it permits the surgeon to start his dissection in a clean, dry field without being distracted by the constant dripping and rolling down of blood from the raw liver bed above. The actual surgical field is no larger than the size of a silver dollar (see Fig. 93). It is in this limited area that the critical surgery is carried out, namely, the dissection and ligation of the cystic duct and cystic artery. It is here that most serious or fatal errors are committed. The surgeon needs all the help he can get, and should avoid all complicating factors such as the constant dripping of blood into the surgical field.

BOTTOM-UP TECHNIQUE

1. Incisions (Fig. 94)
    a. Long midline incision
    b. Long paramedian incision
    c. Subcostal-oblique (Kocher)
    d. Bilateral (joined) Kocher
    e. Transverse (unilateral)
    f. Transverse (joined) bilateral

The choice of incision will depend upon the type or habitus of the patient (see "Comments on Incisions").

2. A Pean forceps grasps the falciform ligament (ligamentum teres), and with gentle, steady traction, the liver and gallbladder are elevated and brought out of the wound. Another Pean forceps grasps the fundus of the gallbladder, and, with steady, gentle lateral traction, the surgeon straightens out that portion of the gallbladder. Another Pean forceps is applied to the body of the gallbladder, and more lateral traction is used. A fourth Pean forceps now grasps the infundibulum (or ampulla, or Hartmann's pouch), and here further lateral traction usually straightens out the cystic duct and contributes to better visualization of its junction with the common bile duct. The cholecystoduodenal ligament covers this area; that is, it covers the cystic duct as it joins the common duct and the cystic artery as it arises from the right hepatic artery. It is this peritoneal reflection that must be stripped off before the cystic duct and artery can be adequately dealt with.

Physical types are shown:

<u>PHYSICAL, OR LONGITUDINAL HABITUS</u> requires a long longitudinal incision; mid-line or paramedian.

<u>MEDIUM HABITUS,</u> between lean and obese types. · A longitudinal or a slightly oblique type of incision is usually adequate (Kocher).

<u>OBESE HABITUS</u> - requires an oblique or transverse incision; in the very wide-obese-type, a bi-lateral transverse or 'fish mouth' incision may be required.   A good incision is one large enough, over the site of the pathology and preferably a little larger than a little smaller.

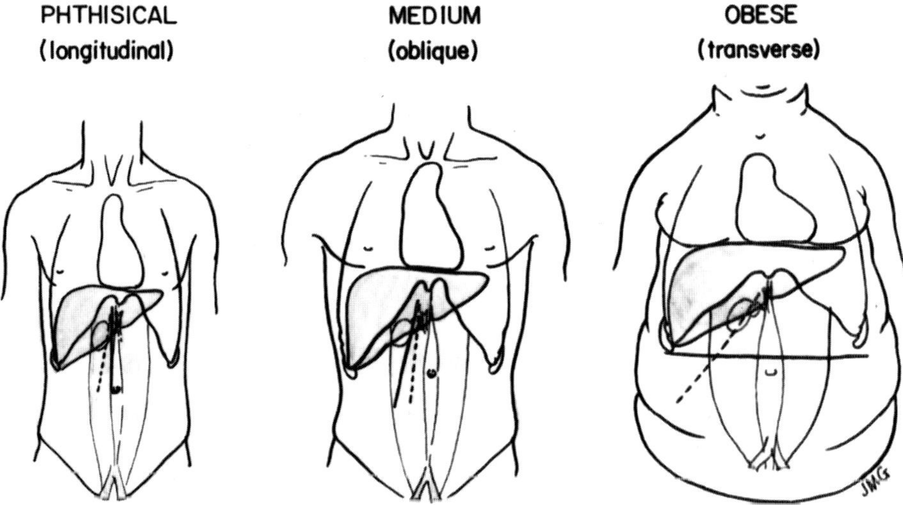

Figure 92.   Incisions must be individualized or made to order for various physical types as shown.

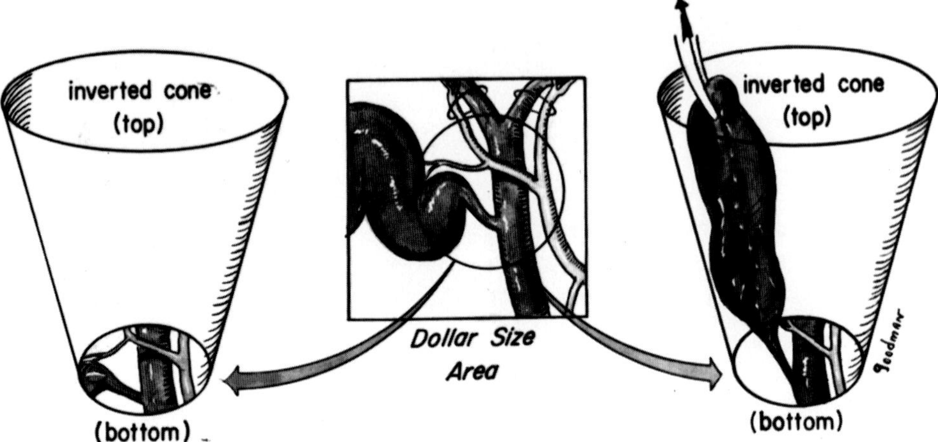

Figure 93. *Diagrammatic drawings showing how the critical site (cystic duct and cystic artery) is no larger than a silver dollar, and that looking down through the wide incision creates an inverted conelike structure. When a small amount of blood rolls down into this critical dollar-sized area, the entire field is quickly obliterated. If at all possible, cholecystectomy should be started from below, in a perfectly dry field, without even a fine film of blood to cloud the surgeon's visit.*

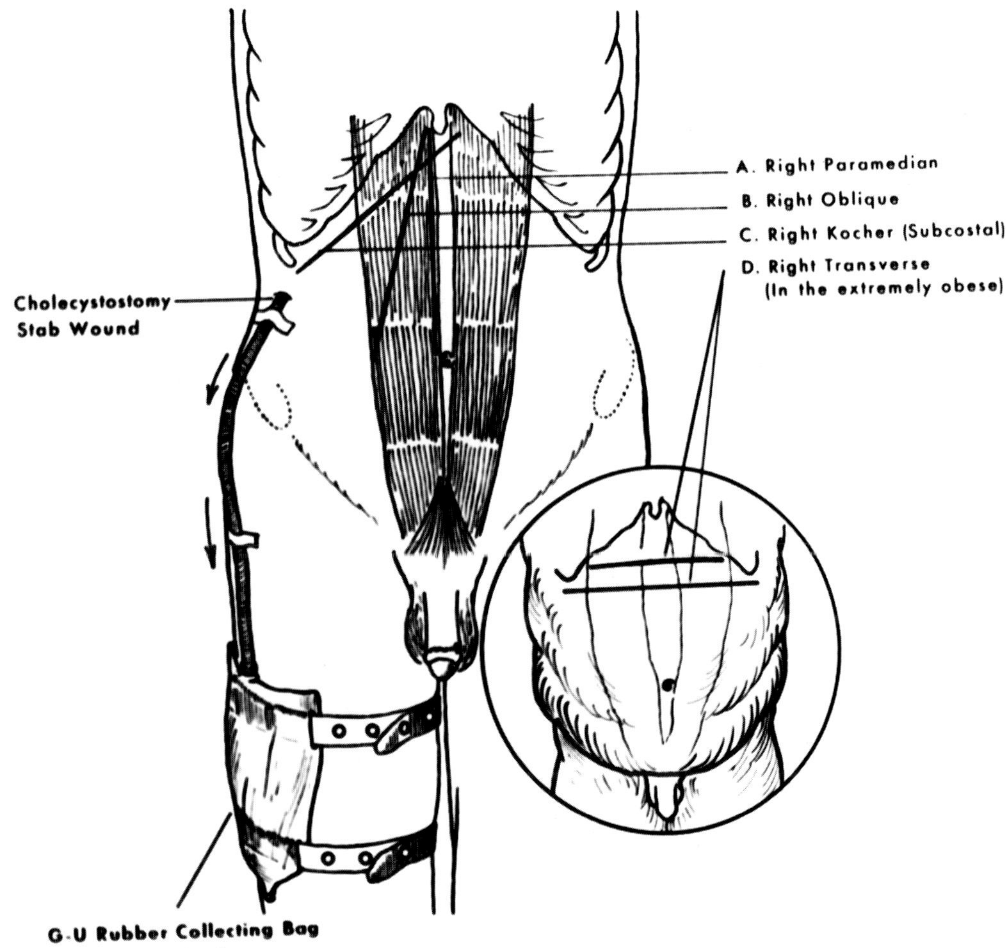

Figure 94.   *Illustrated here are various gallbladder incisions, each to be employed in specific instances. The longer the abdomen (acute costal angle), the more linear the incision. The broader the abdomen (obtuse costal angle), the more transverse is the incision. Also shown is a method for directing the bile in the long arm of the T-tube into a urinary bag that is strapped to the thigh.*

Figure 95. Dissection of gallbladder (bottom-up technique). Illustrated in this diagram is a simple technique for the removal of an uncomplicated gallbladder with chronic cholecystitis. After putting the gallbladder on stretch in order to straighten out the cystic duct at its junction with the common duct, the first maneuver is to clear the cystic duct and expose the cystic artery. This relationship must be carefully evaluated before the actual surgery is begun. This procedure is recommended because the field is still clear and untainted by blood running or oozing down from above. Since the destiny of success or failure is made at this time, it is safest for the surgeon to begin the operation when the field is cleanest and unencumbered by blood trickling down from above. When it is definitely established that the cystic duct and cystic artery are positively identified, then the irrevocable steps are taken; namely, the cystic duct is ligated, cut, and the gallbladder is reflected. This step usually exposes the extent of the cystic artery. When assured of the anatomy, the cystic artery is doubly ligated and cut. The final illustration shows how Morison's Fossa is drained. A Penrose drain with wick, or a Jackson-Pratt suction drain for continuous suction. The author strongly recommends drainage in all cases; *it is a pure gamble to close the abdomen without draining Morison's Fossa. (Refer to the author's text on this cholecystectomy in Chapter 10.)*

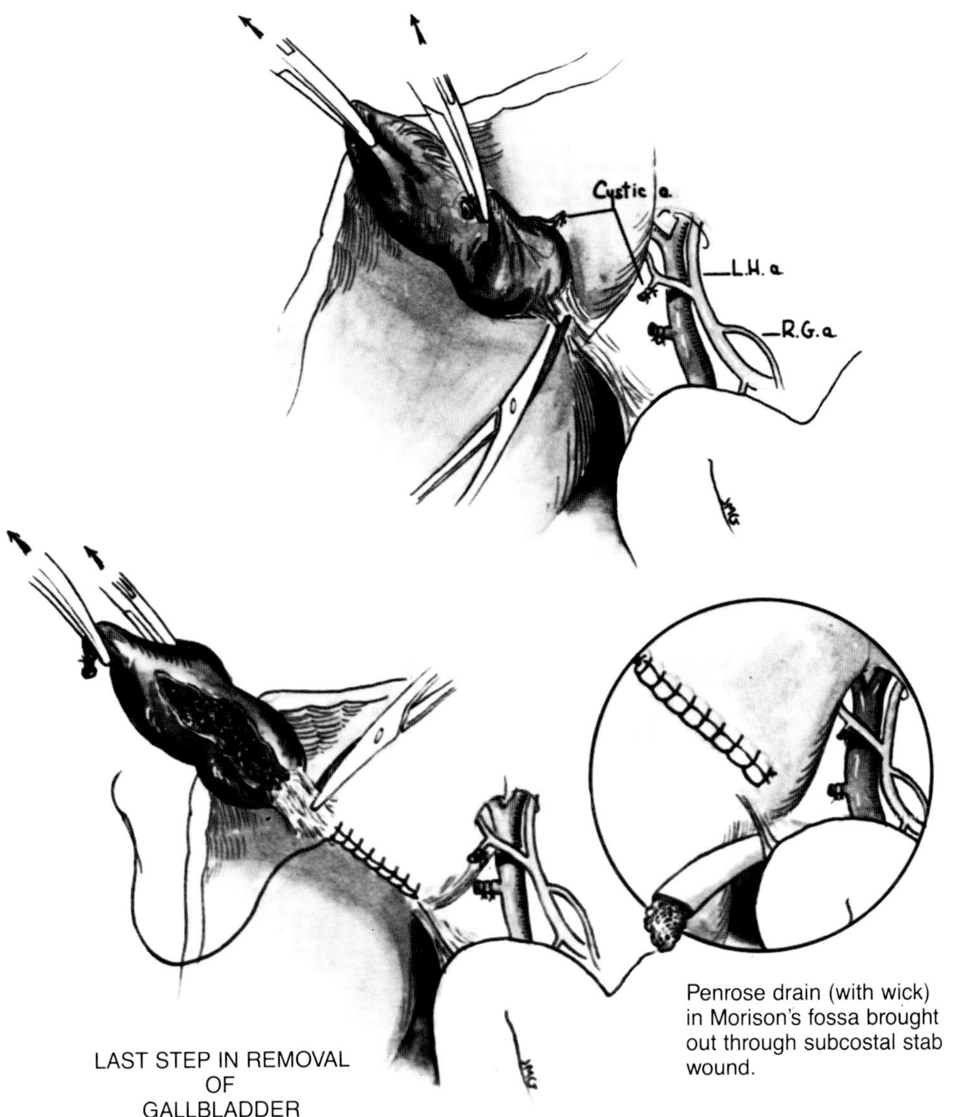

Penrose drain (with wick) in Morison's fossa brought out through subcostal stab wound.

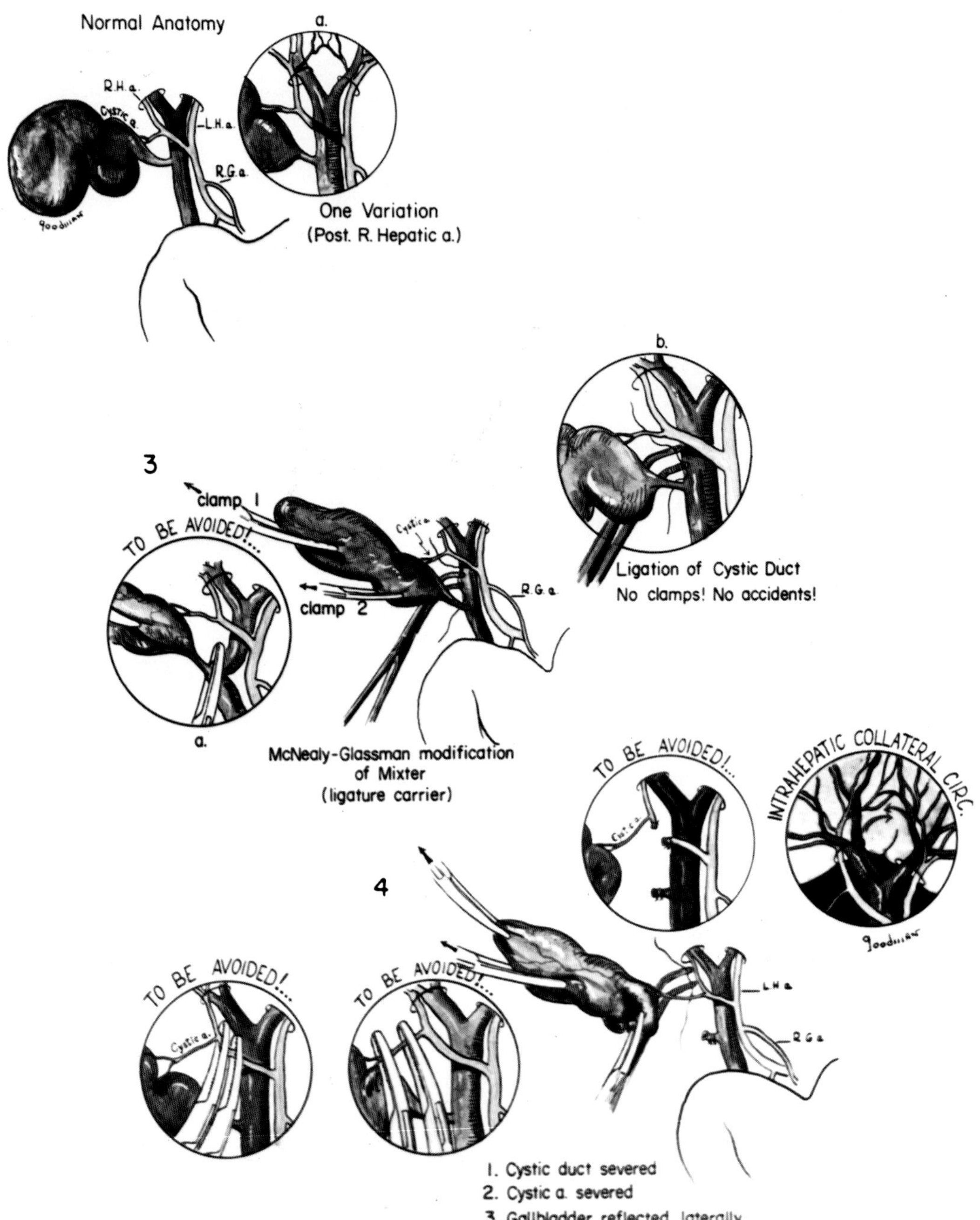

Figure 96.   The McNealy-Glassman technique for cholecys-   tectomy from bottom up.

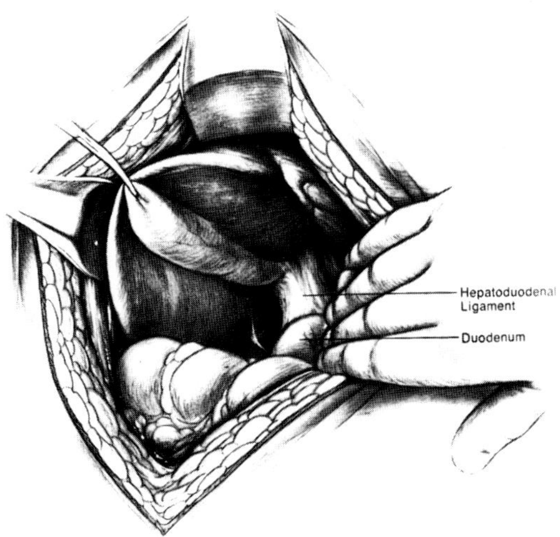

Figure 97. Bottom-up technique. *Gallbladder fundus is grasped with a Pean forceps and upward, outward traction is applied. If the gland is large and redundant, a second and third Pean forceps are employed; upward and outward traction should be maintained. Review the anatomy; then pack off stomach, colon, and liver to better expose the operational field.*

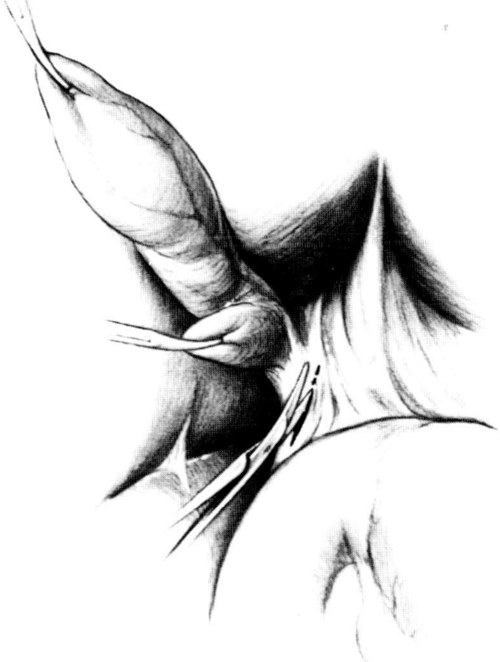

Figure 98. Bottom-up technique continued. *The last Pean forceps is applied to Hartmann's pouch and again upward and outward traction is applied. This traction puts the cystic duct and cystic artery on the stretch. At this point carefully dissect out the structure covered by the hepatoduodenal ligament. Blunt dissection using either a mixter clamp or as illustrated, a Metzenbaum scissors.*

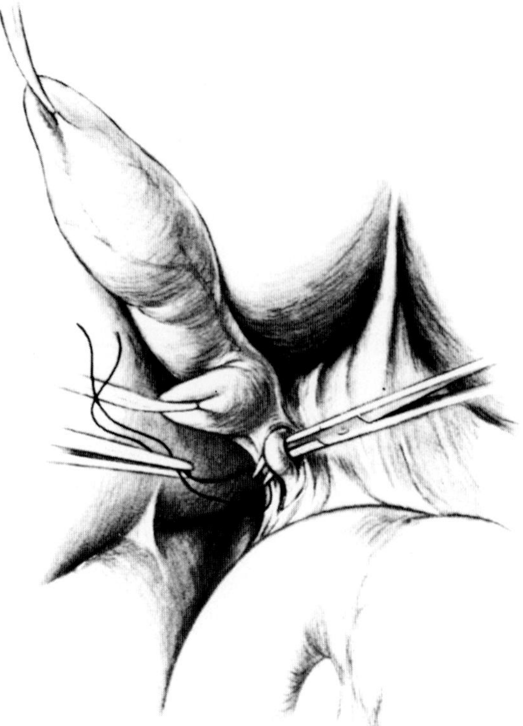

Figure 99. Bottom-up technique continued. *The cystic duct is usually the first structure exposed and isolated. At times, the cystic artery may be the first structure to be seen. Dissect both structures cleanly and adequately. Dissect the cystic duct toward its junction with the common bile duct. Then completely evaluate the cystic artery. Try to identify the cystic artery toward its source, (the right hepatic artery); if too difficult, trace the cystic artery to the gallbladder wall and observe its entrance into the gallbladder wall. If the cystic artery is easily identified, then its ligation may be close to the gallbladder. If it is not too easily substantiated, dissect it out from the gallbladder wall and ligate it there by (suture ligature). The artery that clearly terminates into the gallbladder wall is the cystic artery.*

3. With the tip of a mixter forceps (or with a Metzenbaum scissors), the peritoneum is gently stripped off piecemeal until the cystic duct is clearly exposed, and isolated. It is then encircled with a holding suture. Figure 99 shows the stripping and clearing process. The writer proceeds to doubly ligate the cystic duct distally about 1/4 of an inch from its junction with the common duct. A mixter forceps is applied to the cystic duct distal to the ligatures before it is divided (Figs. 101, 102). The clamped cystic duct is now reflected upward and to the right. This exposes the underside of the duct and usually reveals the cystic artery. The cystic artery is

bluntly dissected out, encircled with a ligature, and held as traction (Fig. 100).

Before doubly ligating the cystic artery, we evaluate its location and its direction of termination. We do not really know its name until we trace the artery directly into the gallbladder wall. If in fact the artery ends in the gallbladder wall, we name it the *cystic artery;* it is doubly ligated and divided. The cystic artery is the anchor of the gallbladder, and being severed, it now permits the gallbladder to be completely excised from its liver bed (Figs. 101, 102).

4. The mixter clamp on the cut cystic duct and the three Pean forceps on the gallbladder body are now held together in order to apply stronger upward traction. Sharp dissection will finally remove the gallbladder from its liver bed; when feasible, we preserve a flap of peritoneum on either side to peritonealize the raw liver bed later (Fig. 103). If this cannot be accomplished, an absolutely dry liver bed is sought. To this end we ligate, clip, or coagulate all bleeding and oozing points.

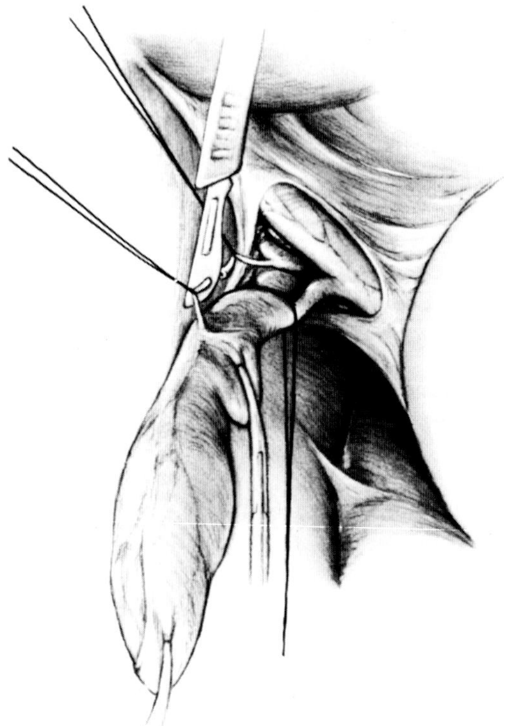

Figure 100. Bottom-up technique continued. *Here, both the cystic duct and cystic artery have been identified, and the cystic duct still remains encircled by a suture for traction.*

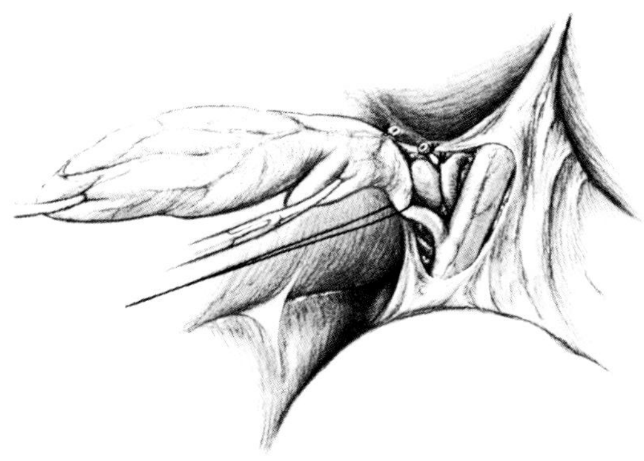

Figure 101.   Bottom-up technique continued. *Note that two cystic arteries had to be ligated instead of the usual one. This is not unusual. The ligatures are cut, but the gallblad-* *der is still under suture-traction. Note also the traction by Pean forceps at the fundus.*

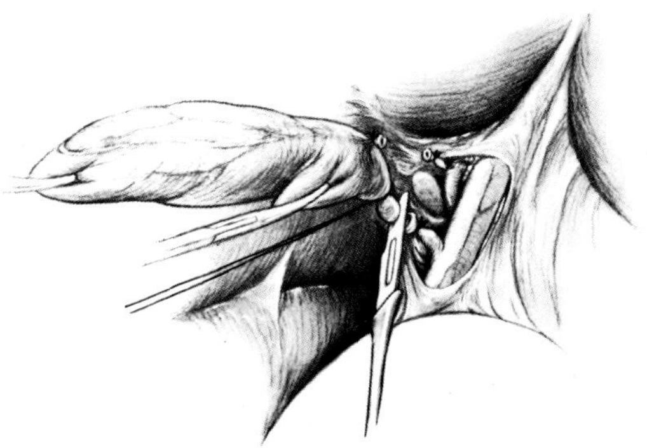

Figure 102.   Bottom-up technique continued. *The cystic arteries are ligated and cut. The cystic duct is doubly ligated and cut between ligatures; this writer uses 3-0 black silk. The field appears clean (bloodless), and all structures are re-identified.*

5. This writer uses a drain routinely. Either a Penrose-wick drain or a Jackson-Pratt suction drain may be employed. The drain is placed in Morison's fossa and brought out through a lateral stab wound (Figs. 103, 104). If a T-tube was used, it too is brought out through the same stab wound. Drains are anchored to the skin. This writer is aware of the advocates of no drainage. He is aware that this fad has appeared and died with each new generation of surgeons. There are no antibiotics that can overcome biliary peritonitis that results from unrecognized cut biliary canaliculi in the liver bed. "Clean" cholecystectomy pertains to no contamination or bleeding. *Bile leakage* is another story (see "Biliary Peritonitis").

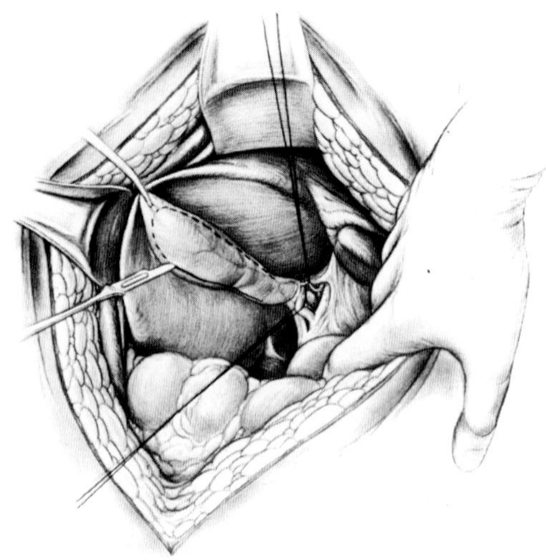

Figure 104.   Top-down technique. *The body of the gallbladder is marked out and a sharp, but superficial, incision is made. There will be instances where adhesions from previous inflammations will distort and render the site of cystic artery and cystic duct ligations difficult or treacherous to dissect from known anatomy toward the unknown. This dissection is slower because of adhesions and fibrinous covering; but slow, careful dissection will lead the surgeon to the cystic duct.*

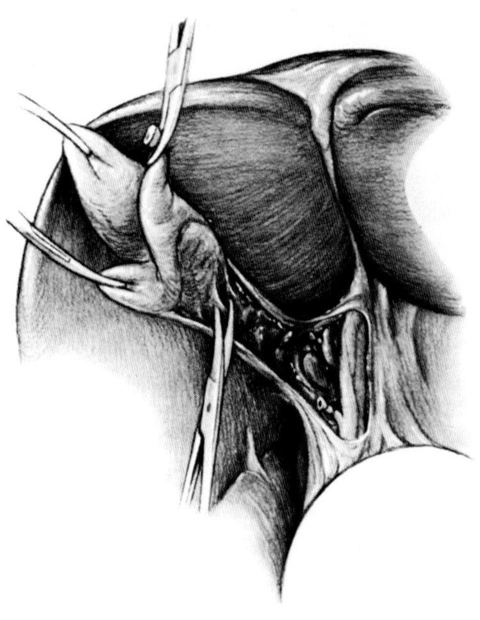

Figure 103.   Bottom-up technique continued. *With upward traction on the freed gallbladder, its underside is carefully dissected with a Metzenbaum scissors. Try to stay close to the gallbladder wall to preserve as much peritoneum as possible to use as flaps to cover the denuded gallbladder bed. Hemostasis is secured as you dissect; either coagulate or ligate oozers and clip active bleeders. At this time, this writer (despite claims to the contrary), strongly recommends drainage of Morison's space (infrahepatic). Either a Penrose drain, or a Jackson-Pratt continuous suction drain may be employed. (See Chapter 10.) Here, a Penrose-wick drain is placed in Morison's fossa; the drain should not touch the ligated structures because it may drain away some serofibrinous secretions, which are necessary for properly sealing of the sewn structures. Note that the deperitonealized gallbladder bed has been serosalized, but only after complete hemostasis and biliary canaliculi have been attended to.*

6. The incisional wound is closed as follows:

    a. The linea alba is approximated with interrupted Ti-chron sutures, (00).

    b. The skin is approximated with metallic clips.

Should the patient give a history of previous inflammation or multiple past abdominal surgeries, it would be best to plan a top-bottom cholecystectomy. Adhesions and possible anatomical distortions are a real possibility, and can better be dealt with by a procedure that starts from the top and slowly works down. There is an old rule in surgery: Start from the known or normal, and work toward the unknown or abnormal. This rule is certainly germane here.

If at surgery the operator sees problems that were not contemplated preoperatively, he should definitely switch to the safer top-bottom technique. If the operator identifies unexplained adhesions, an edematous cystic duct, or enlarged and thickened gallbladder walls that reduce the size of the operative field, he must alter his original plan of surgery from the bottom-up to the top-down technique.

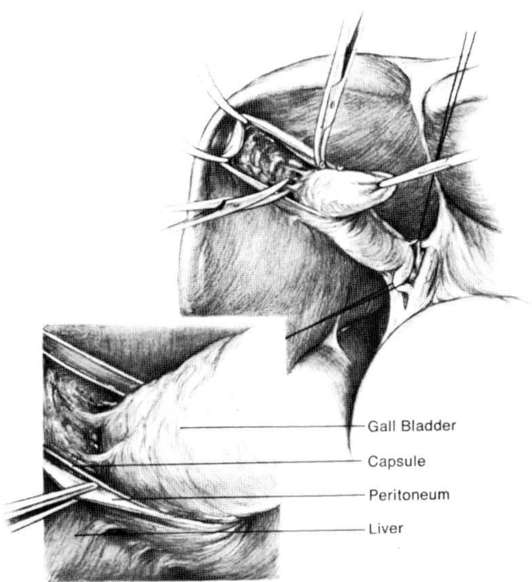

Figure 105. Top-down technique continued. *This illustration depicts small arteries being cut, coagulated, clamped, or ligated as the dissection progresses downwardly. Upward traction is most important to avoid doubling on itself, and thus avoiding an inadvertant cut with bile leakage. The cystic duct has been identified and isolated; it is put on suture traction while searching for the cystic artery. A cystic arterial branch has been found and will be ligated. After complete hemostasis the same surgical technique is carried out. The denuded liver bed is peritonealized, and a drain is placed in Morison's fossa. (See Figure 103 and Chapter 10 for 'drain or no drain' discussion.)*

TOP-DOWN TECHNIQUE

1. The incision is the same as that described for the bottom-up technique.
2. A Pean clamp grasps the fundus of the gallbladder and applies upward traction (Fig. 104).
3. Inject sterile saline subperitoneally around the periphery of the gallbladder. Using a small blade, incise the peritoneal covering, and by blunt and sharp dissection, separate the body of the gallbladder, preferably along the lines of cleavage. The gallbladder dissection from the top of the liver bed is continued downward until the cystic duct is reached (Fig. 105). Then, with more gentle dissection, expose the junction of the cystic duct with the common bile duct; check the location and direction of the cystic artery. Carefully check for anomalous accessory bile duct and other abnormal variations of the hepatic and cystic arteries (Fig. 106). Often in the downward dissection of the gallbladder, the smaller branches of the cystic artery are cut and ligated;

this should alert the surgeon that the main cystic artery is nearby. After the cystic artery is definitely identified and doubly ligated, other correctable anomalies, i.e., accessory biliary ducts, should be ligated. The last step is to doubly ligate the cystic duct about 1/4 of an inch from its junction with the common duct. Do not exert too much traction on the cystic duct where it joins the common duct before applying the ligatures.

4. Place a Penrose-wick drain or a Jackson-Pratt suction drain in Morison's fossa and bring the end out through a later subcostal stab wound. Suture the drain to the skin (Fig. 107).

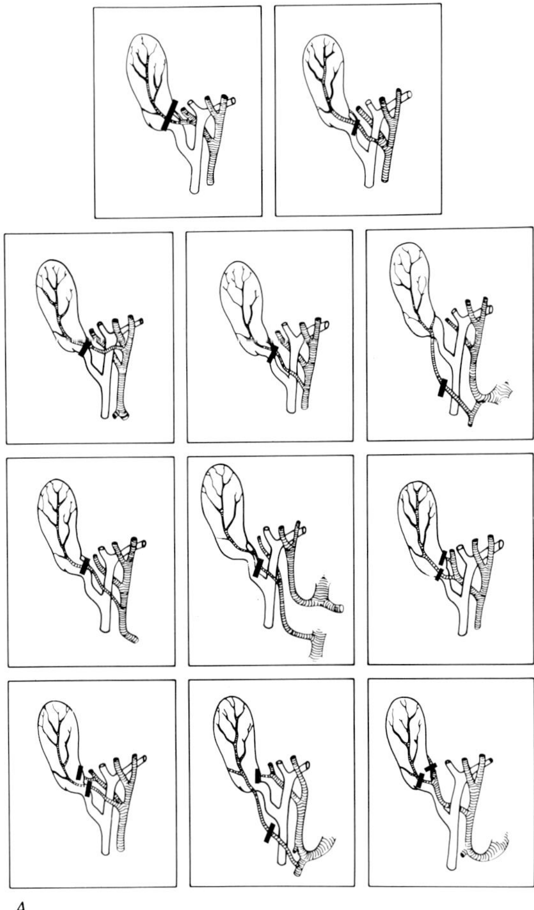

A

Figure 106. A. *Cystic artery anomalies are shown here. Note that the importance is not from where the cystic artery originates, but where it terminates. All ligations must be carried out where the artery terminates, namely, very close to the gallbladder wall or in the gallbladder wall. Note that all ligations are very distally placed; it is an extra assurance and precaution that the ligature is as far away from the right hepatic artery as possible. It is also a safe measure in case a cystic artery has to be reclamped.*

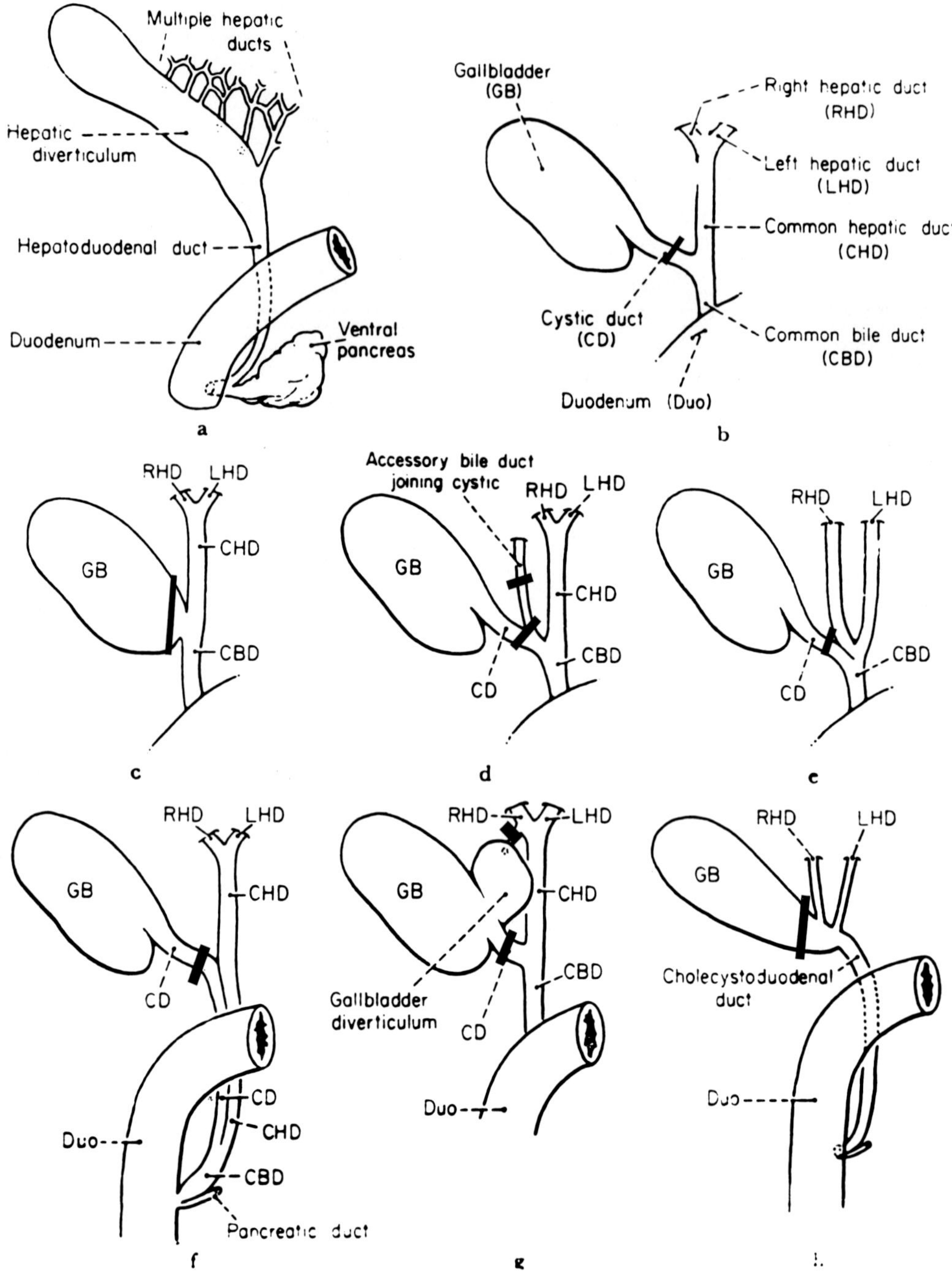

Figure 106 (continued) B. This illustration stresses variations of the cystic and common bile ducts. The ligatures show the important selected sites for ligations. The ligature must not in any way disturb or obstruct the natural flow of bile from the liver. The surgeon must at times allow a part of the gallbladder wall to be sacrificed because there is no cystic duct. If a long cystic duct has adhered to the common duct, (frozen), dissect the cystic duct to its safest farthest point on the common duct, and there apply the ligature.

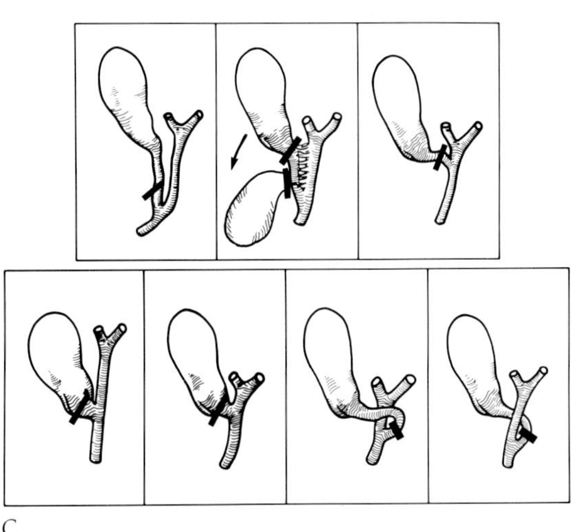

C

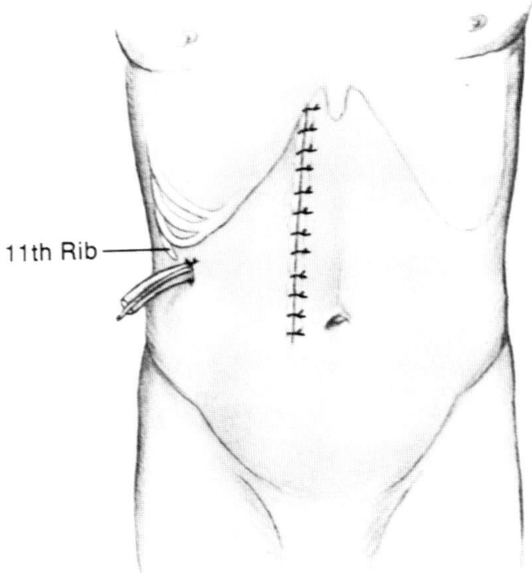

Figure 106 (continued)   C. Common variations of the cystic duct. Here the common duct is normal, but the cystic duct complicates the picture. The ligatures are so applied as not to interfere with the flow of the bile from the liver to the duodenum. At times a short cystic duct can, if improperly ligated (too close to the common duct), cause an immediate or late common duct stricture. If the long cystic duct is ligated too far from its common duct origin, a long cystic duct stump will most likely produce postoperative pain. The proper sites for cystic duct ligations are shown here.

Figure 108.   The final picture shows the paramedian incision closed by interrupted Ti-chron sutures, (3-0). The peritoneum and posterior rectus sheath also were approximately interrupted (3-0) Ti-chron sutures. The anterior rectus sheath was similarly sewn with the same interrupted sutures. Lately we have been using a midline incision, and the closure is completed with one row of interrupted (2-0) Ti-chron sutures. At times, a continuous-lock suture will be employed in a lean person. Skin is closed with 3-0 black silk. The Penrose drain is brought out through a subcostal incision below the 11th rib. One deep epidermal stitch may be placed to fix the drain in place.

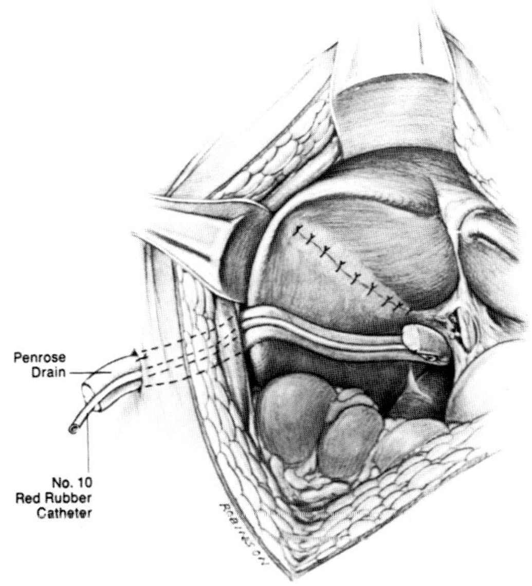

Figure 107.   This illustration shows the end of the cholecystectomy procedure. A Penrose drain with a wick has been placed in Morison's fossa and will be brought out laterally through a subcostal stab wound. The liver bed is secured by complete hemostasis followed by peritonealization of the denuded gallbladder bed. The abdomen is closed.

5. Close the incisional wound as for the bottom-up technique (Fig. 108).

Indications for common bile duct exploration, and techniques employed for stone removal, are discussed elsewhere. (See Chapter 10 on Common Duct Exploration; Indications; Criteria for Exploration of Common Duct; Routine Cystic Duct Cholangiography).

COMMENTS ON INCISIONS

Why is a longer incision superior to a smaller incision in biliary surgery?

1. A longer incision offers greater exposure and far better visualization. It allows for easier and faster surgery while reducing the number of iatrogenic accidents.

2. A longer incision, when made and properly closed, is less likely to result in dehiscence and herniation than a small incision made inade-

quately and closed improperly. The overall time gained by the ease of safer surgery more than compensates for the few extra minutes it may take to close a longer incision properly.

3. Preoperative X-rays will often assist the surgeon in selecting the ideal incision by identifying a high- or low-lying liver. A transverse-positioned gallbladder or a low-lying redundant gallbladder, when visualized preoperatively can significantly contribute to the selection of an ideal incision.

COMMENTS ON THE CYSTIC ARTERY

One of the common booby traps encountered in biliary surgery concerns the unpredictable cystic artery. Its varied locations, sizes, origins, and terminations often create difficulties in localizing, recognizing, and avoiding iatrogenic accidents (Fig. 106 a, b, c). The cystic artery most often lies behind the cystic duct; less often, superiorly or inferiorly. On occasion, the cystic artery will rest on top of the cystic duct. Less commonly, the cystic artery is inseparably fused to the undersurface of the cystic duct—a feature that is recognized only after the cystic duct and artery have already been ligated as one.

The cystic artery most often arises from the right hepatic artery (Fig. 106 a, b, c). The right hepatic artery most often passes over or under the common duct and then gives off the cystic artery. An artery, whether small or large, found passing across the common bile duct (either over or under it) *must never be ligated on the presumption* that it is the cystic artery. Such an artery must be considered to be the right hepatic artery until futher examination proves it to be so—or not. On occasion, a long cystic artery (small or large) will be found crossing the common bile duct, but before it can be considered to be the cystic artery, two criteria must be satisfied: (1) the right hepatic must be seen intact on its way to the liver, and (2) the terminal branches of the cystic artery must unmistakingly be seen entering the gallbladder wall.

If the cystic artery is found to be very short, with a very small distance existing between its hepatic artery origin and the gallbladder wall, the surgeon must not jeopardize the right hepatic artery by attempting to place a ligature too close to it. The cystic artery dissection should be extended farther into the gallbladder wall. When the artery is long enough, it can be ligated a safe distance away from its right hepatic origin.

When the cystic artery is doubly ligated, severed, and reflected, it may be discovered that because of previous inflammation, it has fused inseparably with the underside of the cystic duct, and the ligature had already encompassed both of the cystic structures. In such a situation, proceed with the removal of the gallbladder; the cholecystectomy has been completed.

COMMENTS ON THE CYSTIC DUCT

The cystic duct's anatomy is usually not too difficult to identify at first sight, but should the slightest suspicion arise during the surgery regarding any irregularity, stop and check it out. Figure 106(c) illustrates various biliary anomalies that may be encountered. The only way to rule in or out any serious biliary anomaly is to inject (using a fine needle) 50% Hypaque solution into the common bile duct. X-ray visualization should reveal any obvious biliary anomaly. A cystic duct injection with Hypaque (50%) may also assist in recognizing biliary tract anomalies.

Figure 106(c) shows the various biliary anomalies, with a black line located at the exact site where the proper ligature is to be applied. The consequences of improperly applied ligatures are self-evident. Any ligature that interferes with the normal flow of bile from the liver to the duodenum jeopardizes the patient's life. Therefore, ligatures to normal and abnormal biliary tract anatomy must be applied meticulously, preferably with the benefit of preliminary X-ray visualization when in doubt.

Recommended Reading

Colcock BP, Killeen RB, Leach NG: The asymptomatic patient with gallstones. *Am J Surg* 133:44, 1967.

Colcock BP, Perey B: The treatment of cholelithiasis. *Surg Gynecol Obstet* 117:529, 1963.

Comfort MW, Gray HK, Wilson JM: Silent gallstones: 10–20 year follow-up of 112 cases. *Ann Surg* 128:931, 1948.

Crump C: Incidence of gallstones and gallbladder disease. *Surg Gynecol Obstet* 53:447, 1931.

Edholm P, Jonsson G: Bile duct stones related to age and duct width. *Acta Chir Scand* 124:75, 1962.

Glenn F, Hays DM: The age factor in the mortality rate of patients undergoing surgery of the biliary tract. *Surg Gynecol Obstet* 100:11, 1955.

Gracie WA, Ransohoff DF: The natural history of silent gallstones: The innocent gallstone is not a myth. *N Engl J Med* 307:798, 1982.

Hays DM, Glenn F: A report on the fate of the cholecystectomy in acute cholecystitis. *Arch Surg* 92:689, 1966.

Hinderleider C, Saperstein L: A review of 814 cases of biliary tract surgery from 1957–1977. *Mt Sinai J Med* 46:243, 1979.

Ibach JR, Hume HA, Erb WH: Cholecystectomy in the aged. *Surg Gynecol Obstet* 126:523, 1968.

Lieber MM: Incidence of gallstones and their correlation with other diseases. *Ann Surg* 135:394 1952.

Lund J: Surgical indications in cholelithiasis. Prophylactic cholelithiasis: Prophylactic cholecystectomy elucidated on the basis of long-term follow-up. *Ann Surg* 151:153, 1960.

Meyer K, Capas ND, Mittlepunkt AI: Personal experience with 1261 cases of acute and chronic cholecystitis and cholelithaisis. *Surgery* 61:661, 1967.

Morrow DJ, Thompson J, Wilson SE: Acute cholecystitis in the elderly. *Arch Surg* 113:1149, 1978.

Schoenfield LJ, Lachin JM, Baum RA, et al: The National Cooperative Gallstone Study. *Ann Intern Med* 95:257, 1981.

Sullilvan DM, Hood TR, Griffen WO Jr: Biliary tract surgery in the elderly. *Am J Surg* 143:218, 1982.

Tangedahl TN: Who gets gallstones and why. *Postgrad Med* 66:175, 1979.

Wenckert A, Robertson B: The natural course of gallbladder disease: 11 year review of 781 non-operative cases. *Gastroenterology* 50:376, 1966.

Wright HK, Holden WD, Clark JH: Age as a factor in the mortality rate for biliary tract operations. *J Am Geriatr Soc* 11:422, 1963.

The McNealy-Glassman Round-The-Clock Abdominal Exploration

1. The round ligament is caught by a Pean forceps and turned toward the left shoulder.
2. The duodenum is brought into view and explored carefully for any sign of ulcer.
3. The lesser curvature is now followed up to the esophagus; a search is made for ulcers. The esophageal hiatus is examined to see if it is unusually large or if any herniation into the chest exists.
4. The spleen is palpated and checked for size, contour, and consistency.
5. The hand is brought back along the greater curvature of the stomach, feeling for any neoplastic lesion. The omentum is picked up and, when turned up, the transverse mesocolon is observed and examined. The transverse colon is examined from the splenic flexure across to the hepatic flexure, and carefully palpated for carcinoma and polyps.
6. The omentum is now folded inward into the palm of the left hand; the hand is thrust down toward the left anterior superior spine, where the omentum is turned loose. Check the descending colon, sigmoid, and rectosigmoid, and palpate carefully for neoplastic lesions.
7. The hand now drops into the cul-de-sac, and the uterus, tubes, and ovaries are palpated; check for endometriosis, cysts, and solid tumors.
8. The hand now sweeps toward the right iliac fossa, and the cecum is grasped and pulled up. An attempt is made to exteriorize the cecum in order to examine the appendix and to determine whether a cecal mass exists.
9. The left hand is now passed into Morison's fossa, and the index and middle fingers are inserted into the foramen of Winslow. The thumb is pressed toward the index finger to palpate first the pulsating hepatic artery and then the common bile duct for stones and lymph glands.
10. The common duct is palpated up toward the liver, including both hepatic ducts, and then down toward the duodenum for any existing stones, neoplasms, or any abnormality.
11. The forefinger and middle finger are now passed into the foramen of Winslow and, with the thumb topside, are used to palpate the head and body of the pancreas.
12. The gallbladder, liver, and convex borders of the duodenum should now be thoroughly investigated. Search for inflammatory changes, neoplastic growths, and stones in the common duct and ampulla of Vater.

Recognizing Immediate Postoperative Complications

BILIARY PERITONITIS

Biliary peritonitis may develop very early in the postoperative period and may be associated with the early development of jaundice, distention, fever, rapid pulse, hiccups, rebound tenderness, and a spreading type of severe pain. All of these signs and symptoms after surgery indicate that peritonitis is developing and is most likely due to bile leakage somewhere in the biliary tract. Since every patient with cholecystectomy or choledochotomy and common duct exploration is routinely drained, the dressings should be removed at once and checked. Bile may be oozing actively and in great amount around the Penrose drain. Profuse bile drainage may mean that bile is accumulating within the peritoneal cavity. An attempt to separate the wound may reveal a more copious escape of bile from the drain site. It should be apparent to the surgeon that a greater amount of bile is escaping around the drain than is expected. If bile is escaping from the biliary tree, it must also be escaping into the abdominal cavity. The immediate conclusion should be that bile leakage exists within the abdominal cavity, and an emergency laparotomy is indicated. Escaping bile sets up a chemical irritation that results in a loss of plasma into the peritoneal cavity. Plasma protein must be replaced, either by transfusion or the administration of plasma substitutes. (see "Cholecystectomy—Drain or No Drain?") Chapters 10 and 12.

When the abdomen is opened, the peritoneal cavity may be found to be full of bile that has walled itself off into multiple pockets. All synechiae must be broken down at surgery so that all of the bile can be aspirated from one major pocket. The source of the leakage must be found; the first place to look is the site of the cystic duct ligature, which may have slipped or been forced off. Many surgeons tie off the cystic duct too loosely when it should be tightly ligated, doubly ligated, or even suture-ligated to prevent cystic duct leakage. Exploration may reveal that bile is leaking from the fine ductules in the gallbladder liver bed. This should have been observed at the time of the cholecystectomy and dealt with properly. Penrose-wick drains, or Jackson-Pratt suction drainage should routinely be left in place to drain the bile out through a right subcostal stab wound. This latter routine precaution makes it possible to avoid the development of peritonitis. On occasion, a leak will occur from the common bile duct, which may have been inadvertently traumatized or nicked by a knife, clamp, or tear. This is less likely to occur, but it can happen and may not be recognized at the time. If it is recognized at surgery, it must be repaired on the spot. *The ideal time to repair any accidental cut, crush, or tear of the biliary tree is immediately.*

If the patient is at high risk and is not doing well, a tear or cut of the common duct is best treated by introducing a 14 or 16 French catheter through the tear and sewing it to the duct with a chromic catgut suture; the catheter is brought out through the subcostal stab wound. This emergency treatment creates a biliary fistula and prevents bile leakage into the peritoneal cavity. At a later date, after the patient has recovered, further surgery may not be necessary. If surgery does become necessary, the patient will at least be in better shape for a definitive operation. Reconstruction of the common bile and hepatic ducts is dealt with elsewhere by Drs. John Braasch and Ken Warren of the Lahey Clinic. The techniques employed in the reconstruction of the common and hepatic duct radicles are described by these surgeons, who have spent much of their careers attaining broad experience in this highly specialized field (see Chapter 13).

POSTOPERATIVE TECHNICAL CONSIDERATIONS

When patient develops signs of sepsis after biliary tract surgery, the surgeon must look for wound infection, common duct infection with or without suppuration, or sepsis possibly related to a leftover sponge or foreign body. Wound infection is usually suspected first, and should immediately be evaluated by removing the dressing and culturing whatever secretions or pus is present. Wound infections will also be discussed in connection with antibiotics, particularly in relationship to the prevention of wound infections or infections anywhere in the abdominal cavity, especially the biliary tract (see Chapter 15). The wound should be carefully evaluated for redness, edema, and separation, as well as drainage. Bacterial smears for culture and sensitivity studies should be done routinely. Anaerobic organisms should also be sought; this requires special culture tubes and immediate culturing. If there is evidence of gas within the wound, it should be immediately suspected of being *Bacillus welchii (Clostridium perfringens)* or another "gas" infection. If a common bile duct was explored and primarily closed without T-tube drainage, fever may well be due to cholangitis; alternatively, a stone may have been left, causing Charcot's intermittent chills and fever. If the latter does not subside and keeps mounting, reoperation may have to be undertaken. A choledochostomy should be performed to search for and remove any leftover stone, and especially to insert a T-tube to drain the common duct.

In the postoperative period, a careful study of the biliary tree should be carried out before the T-tube is removed. *Here again, the writer wishes to reemphasize the importance of routine use of the T-tube whenever a common duct is opened.* The common duct, contrary to recent publications, should never be primarily closed. The T-tube is the last bridge between the patient's disease process and the surgeon's judgment. To primarily close the common duct is to gamble with the patient's life. When a postoperative fever is undiagnosed and persists with undiagnosed pain, the patient's abdomen should be X-rayed routinely to search for the presence of any foreign body, i.e., a gauze sponge, lap pad, or instrument. Hemorrhage, whenever it occurs, is always serious and urgent. When the surgeon recognizes an escape of undue amount of bright red blood from the site of the drain, serious consideration must be given to possible emergency reoperation. Postoperative slight oozing or bleeding will most often stop, and there is no further problem; when serious internal bleeding occurs, the cystic artery must suspected first, but it may not be the only source of bleeding. It is possible that an anomalous blood vessel unrecognized during the surgery, may be actively bleeding. *The cystic artery still remains the commonest cause of postoperative hemorrhage in gallbladder surgery.*

If the postoperative patient has no fever, bleeding, or drainage problem, but is going into shock, the surgeon and certainly the internist must be alerted to the fact that in an elderly patient, coronary thrombosis may be taking place. Immediate electrocardiographic studies should be made, and the patient closely monitored. The assistance of the cardiologist will help, since a review and comparison of the pre- and postoperative electrocardiograms can help identify any new cardiac abnormality. A patient may also be suffering from acute hemorrhage, and a rapid diagnosis and decision must be made before it is too late. One precaution should always be exercised by the surgeon: *The abdomen must never be closed until he is confident that complete hemostasis has been secured.* When this precaution is taken, the surgeon can be more confident and can attribute shock to cardiovascular causes rather than to abdominal hemorrhage.

Preventable Late Complications

PERSISTENCE OF RUQ PAIN

When the same pain for which the patient was originally operated on persists or recurs and the patient appears to be suffering, it is conceivable that the surgery was needless and that the pain may be due to recurrent acute pancreatitis. The diagnostic error was committed before the surgery, and the disease that originally caused the pain still exists. There are other diseases, such as porphyria, that can produce the same pain that led to the surgery. This could have been recognized by testing for porphobilinogen and uroporphyrin in the urine. There are other rare cases that should also be kept in mind.

A stone left in the cystic duct can produce a similar recurrent postoperative pain. If it is left unrecognized for a long time, the cystic duct can stretch and dilate into an equivalent gallbladder sac. The colicky pain of an obstructed residual cystic duct stump can be identical to gallbladder colic. Reoperation and removal of the leftover stump

(which often includes a stone) usually relieves the pain. The writer recalls having to cut 2 inches into the liver substance in order to follow a long cystic duct containing a stone at its end that produced bizarre recurrent colicky pains. During cholecystectomy, the patient apparently had his cystic duct oversewn into a deep liver fossa. The cystic duct and the stone appeared as a base drumstick and were located deep in the center of the right lobe of the liver. The stone was clearly visualized on the X-ray, and its removal produced an immediate cure. The patient was originally diagnosed and treated for angina pectoris until the cystic duct and stone were excised. All cardiac medicaments were discarded. A long cystic duct stump that develops a neuroma at its end may also be a cause of persistent RUQ pain.

Finding a long cystic duct stump with a contained stone does not necessarily exclude the presence of a neuroma and/or the possibility of a coexisting chronic pancreatitis. Chronic pancreatitis, especially if recurrent, may ultimately have to come to surgery, though it is perferably controlled medically. However, when there is evidence of shock and suspicion of a possible fulminating hemorrhagic pancreatitis, it becomes imperative to resort to emergency surgery. Decompression of the common bile duct as well as the gallbladder is indicated; surgery allows free drainage to the exterior. Antibiotics are an important adjunct in such cases, but the morbidity and mortality still remain high. Recurrent attacks of pain despite T-tube drainage are possible. It is also conceivable that after the T-tube is removed the patient may still continue to suffer recurrent bouts of pancreatitis. These chronic forms of pancreatitis with acute exacerbations are usually related to alcoholism; it is common for pancreatic lithiasis to exist or to develop subsequently. Charles Puestow[1] had devised an operation for the drainage of these dilated, obstructed pancreatic ducts; it is a pancreaticojejunostomy. The success of this operation is still controversial. At present, some authors recommend subtotal or even total pancreatectomy as providing the best chance for curing chronic recurrent pancreatitis. The results of total pancreatectomy in the latter forms of recurrent obstructive pancreatitis have been more gratifying than Puestow's pancreaticojejunostomy.

In summary, this writer believes that the errors in diagnosing and operating on biliary tract disease continue to result in operative failures with postoperative complications, both immediate and late. The complications that follow surgery of the biliary tract are almost invariably related to failure to employ the correct procedure, or, lacked the expertise required in biliary surgery. In rechecking the failures and the complications that develop after biliary surgery, one frequently finds that the patient should not have been operated on in the first place. Mistaken diagnosis is often the problem. Failure to make a careful anatomical dissection and failure to carry out gentle and detailed technique result in most operative accidents. The quality and experience of the surgeon are paramount when evaluating the ultimate results of biliary surgery. The great majority of postoperative complications are remediable or curable if suspected and expertly corrected soon after their onset.

Subphrenic abscess is another dreaded and serious complication that can occur after an extensive biliary procedure. It has always been associated with high morbidity and mortality. The diagnosis at times is elusive, but in a short time it usually becomes apparent and will be recognized on X-ray studies. Most often, these abscesses (subhepatic and subphrenic) occur in the postoperative period and take about 1 or 2 weeks to develop. With present-day techniques, broad-spectrum antibiotics, and good surgical management, we have reduced the incidence of this complication. With the aid of antibiotics, we have significantly changed the pattern and outcome of subphrenic abscess and its complications. Despite all recent advances in antibiotic therapy, and fluid and electrolyte replacement, morbidity and mortality still remain too high. Ochsner and DeBakey[2] in 1938 reported a collective series of 3,608 cases with a mortality of 32.8%. Though the mortality in recent years has improved, the improvement has not been dramatic. Diagnosis of subphrenic abscess is often missed until late, but is usually recognized after an X-ray study is done for unexplained fever and persistent RUQ pain. The fever may or may not be intermittent or associated with chills. Subdiaphragmatic abscess still goes unrecognized in many instances and may persist for months or even years.

Though a subdiaphragmatic abscess may occur on the right and/or left side, that which follows biliary surgery is almost invariably found on the right side. The abscess may be subhepatic, but more often it will be subphrenic in location. Not infrequently, it may be necessary to differentiate subphrenic abscess from other conditions of the lung and liver. In the latter instance, a computed tomography (CT) scan has proven to be of value; arteriography and ultrasonography have also been useful. The gallium scan is also helpful, and tomography is diagnostic. A fluid level with air in the suspected subphrenic abscess on the right or left side is pathognomonic of subdiaphragmatic abscess. This writer has reported[3] on a "pseudo-subdiaphragmatic abscess" that occurred in the postoperative period after cholecystectomy, where the signs and symptoms appeared approximately 10 days after surgery. Routine chest X-rays revealed a typical right-sided subphrenic abscess. The patient returned to the hospital, and broad-spectrum antibiotics were immediately administered (high-dosage ampicillin and garamicin). These antibiotics did not affect the fever, nor did they alter the typical clinical picture of subdiaphragmatic abscess. The writer felt it necessary to reoperate on this patient. At surgery, nothing but air was discovered under the diaphragm. A systematic search was made for pus by a direct right approach through the abdomen, but again there was no evidence of suppuration anywhere. All cultures made at surgery showed no growth. Even the dome of the liver was needle aspirated to see if a top-side liver abscess existed, but it proved negative. All spaces (subdiaphragmatic, subhepatic, and Morison's) were drained with Penrose-wick drains, transpeitoneally. The patient made an uneventful recovery and left the hospital in excellent condition—symptom free. This writer cautions that air can easily get under the diaphragm and be trapped quickly by fibrinous deposits between the liver and diaphragm; for some reason, a fluid-like level develops. Whether this process results from fibrin and a slight serous accumulation cannot be determined, but the clinical and roentgenological pictures both simulated a typical subdiaphragmatic abscess. This entity was labeled *pseudosubdiaphragmatic abscess* (see "Pseudo-subdiaphragmatic Abscess" at the end of this chapter).

Interventional surgery was performed to prevent serious complications that often develop from subdiaphragmatic abscess—extension of pus through the diaphragm and into the lung and bronchus. The high mortality rate is primarily due to the extension possibilities of this form of infection. There are several techniques for approaching a subdiaphragmatic abscess. One is the retroperitoneal approach; the second is the posterior approach. This writer finds that the direct abdominal approach, entering directly through the peritoneal cavity, is quicker, safer, and more effective. This approach safely exposes all the structures, and readily allows better vision and more information without resulting in complications. Since a subdiaphragmatic abscess is not easily discovered in the immediate postoperative period other than by obvious signs and symptoms, the surgeon must maintain a high degree of suspicion for this complication in order to make the quickest diagnosis and operate at the earliest moment. Multiple drainage is mandatory through the direct abdominal approach. Patients who have been treated surgically with this method have benefited, but the mortality, though reduced, still remains high—approximately 15–20%. If the earliest possible drainage of pus is not instituted, mortality may approach 100%.

It is significant that subphrenic abscess continues to occur despite the use of broad-spectrum antibiotics both pre- and postoperatively. Many surgeons have limited experience with this disease, yet they must maintain a high clinical index of suspicion for it. It is believed that the typical clinical picture of subdiaphragmatic abscess may have been altered by the preoperative use of antibiotics; it is also claimed that antibiotics may have increased the incidence of this complication. *Unquestionably, antibiotics have served to mask the typical clinical picture and course of this disease entity.*

When the surgeon anticipates that there will be a fistulous tract between the gallbladder and the duodenum, he should prepare the bowel preoperatively with an antibiotic so that when the abdomen is entered, the surgeon can separate the two structures, remove the gallbladder, and close the duodenal defect with some degree of certainty. When a large, acutely inflamed fistula exists between the duodenum and gallbladder, it may be wiser to leave it alone with the hope that it will ultimately close spontaneously. After the stone is removed, the fistulous continuity between the gallbladder and duodenum may prove to be beneficial. Here, then, is a case of judgment, in the opinion of the writer: whether to preserve a cholecystoduodenal fistula after the stone has been removed or to risk the recurrence of a duodenal fistula.

If a biopsy specimen is taken from the pancreas, it is advisable to place a Penrose drain near the duodenum to allow for the possibility of pancreatic leakage. If there is a question about a cut into the pancreatic duct made inadvertently during a sphincterotomy, a small polyethylene tube can be inserted into the pancreatic duct to assure egress of the pancreatic juice into the duodenum. If a carcinoma of the ampulla is recognized and found to be early, with no evidence of metastatic lesions elsewhere, i.e., in the lymph glands in the portahepatis, along the lesser and greater curvatures, and behind the duodenum, a pancreaticoduodenectomy (Whipple) may be undertaken with the possibility of a favorable outcome. This, of course, assumes that no other contraindications exist. It

must be understood that this formidable operative procedure carries a high morbidity and mortality, and that medical-legal permission, after explanations, must be obtained before operating. The best possible results for carcinoma of the ampulla of Vater are obtained with Whipple's operation when there is no existing evidence of any metastases, local or distal.

References

1. Puestow CB: *Surgery of the Biliary Tract: Pancreas and Spleen.* Kingsport, TN, Year Book Publishers, 1953, p 85.
2. Ochsner A, DeBakey ME: *Christopher's Minor Surgery.* Philadelphia, WB Saunders, 1959.
3. Glassman JA: Pseudosubdiaphragmatic abscess. *Int Coll Surg* 61:57, 1976.

Cholecystectomy in Patients with Coronary Artery Disease

Chronic gallbladder disease and coronary heart disease frequently coexist in the same patient, and the following questions arise:

1. What is the operative risk of cholecystectomy in a patient with coronary artery disease?
2. Will cholecystectomy influence the subsequent course of the coronary patient?

At the Mayo Clinic, J.R. Keyes and W. Walters[1] selected 100 patients (ages varying from 40 to 79); each patient (male and female) was diagnosed as having coronary disease associated with established cholecystic pathology. Cholecystectomy was well tolerated, and there were no deaths or complications at the time of surgery. In the postoperative period, one patient died of acute pancreatitis, one from hemorrhagic pancreatitis with necrosis, one from cerebrovascular accident, and one from acute myocardial infarction. The survival rate of this select group after a 6-year follow-up was 70.6%, compared with 83.9% in the normal population. This study established the relatively low risk of cholecystectomy in patients with symptomatic coronary artery disease. The complications that can occur postoperatively, however, were considered to be more serious in the coronary patient.

The writer's experience with coexisting coronary and gallbladder disease has been remarkably similar to the Mayo Clinic report. It is doubtful whether the removal of a diseased gallbladder will directly influence the course of coronary artery disease, but unquestionably the life of the postoperative patient will be extended and made more livable. Certainly, the serious complications caused by unabated biliary disease will be obviated.

Before a middle-age or elderly patient with coexisting coronary and gallbladder disease has a cholecystectomy performed, consultations with the internist and anesthetist are essential. The anesthetist should keep in mind the patient's need for a high oxygen requirement. The anesthesiologist should select the ideal gas mixture that affords the coronary patient the highest percentage of oxygen during the procedure. Fluids must be given cautiously to avoid overloading the patient. The operating team should be ready for any exigency. Early ambulation is recommended, and anticoagulants should be given when deemed advisable.

Note: This writer apologizes to the reader because he is aware that every qualified surgeon is quite cognizant of the seriousness of cholecystectomy in the coronary patient. His prime purpose is to remind and refresh. (See Dr. Louis Lemberg on the differential diagnosis of acute cholecystitis and angina pectoris).

Reference

1. Keyes JR, Walters W: 100 coronary patients operated for cholecystectomy with zero mortality. *Mayo Clin Proc*

Rationale for the Treatment of Chronic Cholecystitis and Cholelithiasis

When chronic cholecystitis and cholelithiasis are diagnosed, the usual treatment is cholecystectomy, and the results are usually very good. The technique for the surgery is described in the section on "Operative Techniques." However, for the present, every patient with cholecystitis with cholelithiasis who goes to surgery should have the abdomen carefully explored, because it is considered an elective procedure, and in each elective operation a complete routine abdominal exploration should be carried out (see "The McNealy-Glassman Round-the-Clock Abdominal Exploration"). Of course, this carries with it the absolute need to examine the entire biliary-pancreatic-hepatic system, which will give the surgeon a more complete understanding of the immediate problem. It will also

give the operator a chance to deal with any associated problem not recognized preoperatively. In regard to the treatment for chronic cholecystitis without stones (the acalculous gallbladder), the surgeon must first firmly decide on that diagnosis. He must determine whether mud, gravel, or sand-like material is present. Oral cholecystograms, ultrasonography, CT scan, and IV cholangiograms can definitely assist in establishing the presence of these entities and whether or not they are responsible for the symptoms and signs that are referable to the gallbladder. This writer recommends that where such a symptomatic problem is encountered and no definite stones are found, elective cholecystectomy is warranted; in addition, common duct exploration may be indicated, depending upon the findings.

Aschoff-Rokitansky bodies or diverticula should have surgery, especially if the signs and symptoms are referable to the RUQ area. Adenomyomatosis of the gallbladder, when found even without the presence of stones, should, contrary to some opinions, be surgically removed, particularly when symptoms and signs point to the gallbladder. If a pathological gallbladder cannot be diagnosed, but the signs and symptoms of cholelithiasis persist in a patient in whom gallbladder disease is a high probability, an abdominal exploration is certainly indicated; and if gallbladder disease is found, cholecystectomy should be carried out. In these instances, the chances are high that the symptoms will disappear, and both the surgeon and patient will have the satisfaction of knowing that a real but elusive pathology has been eradicated. Though this does not occur very often, surgeons must have the courage to speak to patients and inform them that they believe gallbladder disease to be the underlying problem and that surgical intervention and exploration is the proper decision. Surgeons must explain that in gallbladder disease the diagnosis is never a black-and-white, positive or negative finding, that there are many shades of gray, and that surgeons must make their decision in favor of surgery in order to obtain the best, safest, and most lasting result. Every now and then, a normally functioning gallbladder with normal radiographic findings after exploratory surgery, will reveal gravel, mud, or even small stones that have failed to visualize. Most importantly, the surgeon has had the chance to explore the entire abdomen by sight, smell, and palpation, and there is no substitute for that form of study.

Dr. Ken Warren, formerly of the Leahy Clinic, is an exponent of dilating the sphincter of Oddi with Bakes dilators in order to make sure that there is no obstructing lesion or stricture at the level of the ampulla of Vater. This writer also believes that dilating the sphincter is an important diagnostic maneuver, as well as an important overlooked form of treatment. A diagnosis of stricture usually indicates that a fibrotic stenosis of the ampulla exists and that a sphincterotomy may be indicated. If during a careful evaluation no stones, mud, or gravel is found, it is wise to proceed with a careful exploration of the common bile duct, looking for stenosis or spasm of the sphincter of Oddi. If stenosis of the ampulla is found, it should be carefully dilated to no more than 4–5 mm with Bakes dilators. If this cannot easily be accomplished, a duodenotomy and possibly a sphincterotomy are indicated; in most instances of stenosis, a sphincterotomy will improve the patient's condition. There may be instances in which postcholecystectomy symptoms will persist, but further testing and evaluation must be continued. Not infrequently, psychosomatic influences enter into the picture, and the surgeon must be cognizant of them. Psychosomatic therapy should not be excluded from the postoperative treatment in patients who have not been successfully relieved with surgery. Patients who have acute biliary colic without stones, but who have a history of repeated biliary attacks and in whom a diagnosis of cholelithiasis cannot be firmly established, must ultimately be brought to the operating room for abdominal exploration and possible cholecystectomy. Continued medical treatment may result in the misuse of narcotic drugs and the conversion of these patients to drug addiction. *The surgeon must not be guilty of making that mistake.*

Recommended Reading

Colcock BP, Killeen RB, Leach NG: The asymptomatic patient with gallstones. *Am J Surg* 133:44, 1967.
Colcock BP, Perey B: The treatment of cholelithiasis. *Surg Gynecol Obstet* 117:529, 1963.
Comfort MW, Gray HK, Wilson JM: Silent gallstones: 10–20 year follow-up of 112 cases. *Ann Surg* 128:931, 1948.
Crump C: Incidence of gallstones and gallbladder disease. *Surg Gynecol Obstet* 53:447, 1931.
Edholm P, Jonsson G: Bile duct stones related to age and duct width. *Acta Chir Scand* 124:75, 1962.
Glenn F, Hays DM: The age factor in the mortality rate of patients undergoing surgery of the biliary tract. *Surg Gynecol Obset* 100:11, 1955.
Gracie WA, Ransohoff DF: The natural history of silent gallstones: The innocent gallstone is not a myth. *N Engl J Med* 307:798, 1982.
Hays DM, Glenn F: A report on the fate of the cholecystectomy in acute cholecystitis. *Arch Surg* 92:689, 1966.
Hinderleider C, Saperstein L: A review of 814 cases of biliary tract surgery from 1957–1977. *Mt Sinai J Med* 46:243, 1979.
Ibach JR, Hume HA, Erb WH: Cholecystectomy in the aged. *Surg Gynecol Obstet* 126:523, 1968.
Lieber MM: Incidence of gallstones and their correlation with other diseases. *Ann Surg* 135:394, 1952.
Lund J: Surgical indications in cholelithiasis. Prophylactic cholelithiasis: Prophylactic cholecystectomy elucidated on the basis of long term follow-up of (526) non-operated cases. *Ann Surg* 151:153, 1960.
Meyer K, Capos ND, Mittlepunkt AI: Personal experience with 1261 cases of acute and chronic cholecystitis and cholelithiasis. *Surgery* 61:661, 1967.
Schoenfield LJ, Lachin JM, Baum RA, et al: The National Cooperative Gallstone Study. *Ann Intern Med* 95:257, 1981.
Sullilvan DM, Hood TR, Griffen WO: Biliary tract surgery in the elderly. *Am J Surg* 143:218, 1982.
Tangedahl TN: Who gets gallstones and why. *Postgrad Med* 66:175, 1979.
Wenckert A, Robertson B: The natural course of gallstone disease. *Gastroenterology* 50:376, 1966.
Wright HK, Holden WD, Clark JH: Age as a factor in the mortality rate of biliary tract operations. *J Am Geriatr Soc* 11:422, 1963.

Cholecystectomy in the Aged

There is no reasonable appreciation of the age differences of the young and the old. Too often when the patient reaches the age 65 to 70, the physician relaxes his attention, subconsciously assuming that the patient will soon die from other causes. Actually, statistics show that the patients in this age group have a much longer life expectancy and that intensive treatment should be made available to them as diligently and maximally as it would be to the younger patient. It is becoming well established that the elderly patient (aged 75–90) will tolerate major surgery almost as well as the younger one. There have been many instances where this writer has canceled surgery for a young patient to operate on an older one, the reason being that the younger patient was nutritionally deficient and therefore unprepared for safe elective surgery. It is not the age of the patient that is important as much as his or her general condition; whether or not the patient has an associated systemic disease is in itself a vital consideration. Having lived to a ripe old age is an excellent indication that the patient will most likely tolerate the surgery; the quality of his physical makeup has been proved. However, when it comes to the more serious operations, such as extensive surgery for carcinoma of the colon and rectum, the mortality in the aged individuals rises to twice and three times that of the younger patient. Here again, the outcome will depend upon the associated problems that exist in each patient.

The writer is not discounting the importance of the hospital and the qualifications of the surgeon in attaining the best possible results. Elderly patients usually tolerate *emergency major surgical operations* rather poorly. The age of the patient alone is usually not the chief factor in the mortality rate; it is the complications that are prone to develop from the preexisting conditions and associated degenerative systemic diseases. The operating surgeon must make every effort to identify and initially treat all these accompanying disease problems in order to prevent immediate and/or late complications. Postoperative care is also most important. The advent of the surgical intensive care facility has helped greatly to improve the postoperative results in aged patients. Cardiac monitoring and other facilities now available, and constant good, specialized nursing care has significantly improved the postoperative results in high-risk patients.

During surgery, the surgeon, being aware that he is operating on an aged individual with associated cardiovascular-pulmonary problems, diabetes, and genitourinary problems, must pay meticulous attention to all details. He must carry out the surgery with dispatch and with a minimum of trauma, utilizing nontraumatic or noncrushing instruments wherever possible. The wound closure in all carcinoma problems must be fortified with deep-tension nylon sutures because a second surgical procedure should be avoided as much as possible; secure closure is mandatory.

Statistics regarding morbidity and mortality generally show that the mortality for major operations in individuals under 60 is approximately 2.5–3.5%, but when the patient's age rises to 65–75, mortality approximately doubles, to 7–8%, for the same problem. The mortality for emergency operations, of course, is much higher than for elective procedures even in the young, but is significantly higher in the aged patient. Glenn and Hays[1] reviewed their 21-year experience (1932–1953) in patients undergoing cholecystectomy for acute and chronic cholecystitis. In patients less than 50 years of age, the mortality in 2,287 patients was 0.6%; in 1,335 patients between the ages of 50 and 64, it was 2.5%; and in 328 patients over 65, it was 6.7%. In the last group, where the problem was acute cholecystitis, the mortality was 10.7%, while for chronic cholecystitis it was 4.4%. More recent statistics have shown marked improvement. Klingensmith et al.[2] in 1981 reported on 785 patients of all ages undergoing cholecystectomy (acute and chronic), with a mortality rate of 0.64%. Colcock et al.[3] reported 134 consecutive cholecystectomies for symptomatic gallstones without a single death.

Meyer et al., of Cook County Hospital,[4] reported on 1,261 patients operated on for acute cholecystitis, with a mortality rate of 5.3%.* Ibach et al. reported cholecystectomy statistics on 151 patients over 60 years of age. Fifty percent were operated on for acute cholecystitis and 50% for chronic disease. Acute cholecystectomy resulted in a mortality of 2.3%, while elective surgery for chronic cholecystectomy resulted in no deaths. Emergency cholecystectomies carried a mortality of 16.7%. The latter cases involved gangrenous and perforated forms of acute cholecystitis with stones in the common bile duct.

The most common postoperative complications that must be watched for and avoided are cardiac and pulmonary. Cardiac failure, pneumonia, and atelectasis are very serious and frequent complications in major surgery of the aged. Every precaution must be taken to prevent pulmonary embolism; there are surgeons who, in operating on patients 65 years of age and over, routinely employ prophylactic preoperative heparin in small doses (i.e., 5,000 units every 12 hours) to prevent the onset of a thrombotic process that can lead to pulmonary embolism in the postoperative period. The bandaging of both extremities with Ace elastic bandages or fitted elastic stockings before, during, and after surgery has helped to increase the circulatory flow in the lower extremities. Early ambulation after surgery has certainly helped to improve the flow of blood throughout the vascular system. This writer believes that pulmonary embolism has been significantly reduced by these prophylactic precautions. He further recommends his own prophylactic plan: Immediately after the operation is completed, the surgeon and his assistants elevate both lower extremities, and passively exercise and massage them; this helps to return the stagnant blood back into the circulation and replaces it with an inflow of fresh blood. The patient leaves the operating room having already "walked," so to speak, on the operating table, and while asleep under anesthesia. However, the mortality in major operations is still too high for both younger and aged patients.

The advent of advanced knowledge in physiology, biochemistry, anesthesia, effective blood and fluid replacement, and better nursing care, together with electronic monitoring in intensive care units, has helped to lower morbidity and mortality. Broad-spectrum antibiotics and better-trained sur-

---

*Cook County Hospital is a charity hospital. The patients are usually very poor. As a rule, they enter late, most often in the advanced stage of the disease.

geons will continue to make mortality figures fall. The aged patient today goes to surgery with less fear than the patient only a few years ago. This is the goal set by all surgical specialties for all patients of all ages.

Braasch,[5] chief of the Department of Surgery at the Leahy Clinic, writing on cholelithiasis in aged patients, stated that decisions regarding elective cholecystectomy in these patients have been rather confusing for two reasons: (1) The gallbladder calculi can remain silent or make their presence known in a variety of ways. The symptoms may suggest functional gastrointestinal disease or may in fact represent severe gallbladder disease such as acute cholecystitis, with or without jaundice. (2) It is well known that at autopsy examinations of patients 70–90 years of age, 20–30% of the gallbladders studied contain stones in uninvolved gallbladders; these patients had lived without signs or symptoms of gallbladder disease. This raises a question: In a patient over 70, when does one decide to advise an elective cholecystectomy when gallstones have been discovered on a routine choelcystographic study and the patient has slight, minor dyspepsia? Braasch cites two series of cases in which less than half (about 40–45%) of the patients actually went on to develop signs and symptoms of cholecystitis and required surgery. Colcock et al.,[6] in studying 1,356 cases of biliary tract disease that were treated surgically, recorded 859 patients who had a cholecystectomy as the only procedure performed; 8 of these patients died postoperatively. In six of these eight patients, additional surgical procedures of significant magnitude had to be performed at the same time, and unquestionably helped to contribute to the patient's death. There were only two deaths in over 700 operations, representing an operative mortality of 0.3%. This is an unusually low figure, and demonstrates that major surgery can be safely and successfully carried out in the elderly.

Colcock et al. stated that the mortality increases two and possibly three times when complications such as jaundice develop at the time of surgery; this implies that obstructing gallstones add to the risk of the surgery, particularly in the geriatric patient. Gerst reported that 89% of his patients with carcinoma of the gallbladder had concomitant calculi in the biliary tract. These patients fell into the age group in which approximately 30% of the unselected cases might be expected to have asymptomatic gallstones with no complaints throughout their lives. These findings are in agreement with those of most other authors in that we do not yet know what causes carcinoma of the gallbladder. It is conceivable that carcinoma of the gallbladder

might predispose to the formation of gallstones; therefore, this presumably implies that carcinoma of the gallbladder is not caused exclusively by gallstones. It is entirely possible that the association of carcinoma of the gallbladder and cholelithiasis is coincidental.

Nugent and associates, in discussing polyps of the gallbladder and the possibility of their being precursors to carcinoma of the gallbladder, reported that in 115 patients operated on with polypoid lesions of the gallbladder who were followed for at least 15 years postoperatively, not one developed carcinoma. They therefore do not consider it mandatory to advise cholecystectomy for polypoid lesions of the gallbladder in patients over 65 years of age. This is, of course, the opinion of Nugent and associates. It should be mentioned at this time that there are others, including this writer, who feel that a polypoid lesion of the gallbadder found on X-ray may well be an early carcinoma or a lesion that is destined to become malignant; its coexistence with stones should make the diagnosis and the decision for cholecystectomy even easier.

Braasch,[7] reporting on surgical repair of biliary strictures in elderly patients, stated that at the Leahy Clinic, 501 patients were reported in 1959 with benign biliary strictures; of this group, 36 patients were 65 years of age and over. In the patients over 65 years who were operated on for biliary stricture, the commonest cause of failure and mortality was hepatorenal failure or massive hemorrhage in patients with depleted cardiac and hepatic reserves. Braasch firmly believes that acute cholecystitis in the elderly is best managed by earlier surgery, either as an emergency or an elective cholecystectomy, depending upon the patient's general condition. Common duct stones must be removed when found, and any stenotic obstructions of the ampulla of Vater associated with such stones should be relieved by either sphincterotomy or sphincteroplasty. There are many European surgeons who prefer choledochoduodenostomy to sphincterotomy and sphincteroplasty in the aged patients (see "Choledochoduodenostomy, Sphincterotomy, and Sphincteroplasty" in Chapter 17).

References

1. Glenn F, Hays DM: The age factor in the mortality rate of patients undergoing surgery of the biliary tract. *Surg Gynecol Obstet* 100:11, 1955.
2. Klingensmith WC, et al: Complementary role of Tc99m-

diethyl-IDA and ultrasound in large and small duct biliary obstruction. *Radiology* 138:177, 1981.

3. Colcock BP, et al: The asymptomatic patient with gallstones. *Am J Surg* 113:44, 1967.
4. Meyer K, Capos N, et al: Personal experience with 1261 cases of acute cholecystitis and chronic cholecystitis and cholelithiasis. *Surgery* 61:661, 1967.
5. Braasch JW, et al: Acute cholecystitis. *Surg Clin North Am* 44:707:16, 1964.
6. Colcock BP, McManus JF, et al: Experience with 1356 cases of acute cholecystitis and cholelithiasis. *Surg Gynecol Obstet* 101:161, 1955.
7. Braasch JW, Warren K, et al: Progress in biliary stricture repair. *Am J Surg* 129:134, 1975.

Cholecystectomy in Childhood

Ternberg and Keating,[1] in *Swenson's Pediatric Surgery*,[2] discuss the etiology of gallbladder disease in children and call our attention to certain problems. They state that one group of surgeons may, based on their own limited experience, attribute biliary disease to infections, congenital anomalies, and hemolytic diseases. Another group, active in hemolytic centers, may be led to believe that hemolytic diseases are the primary causes of gallbladder diseases. Ternberg and Keating believe that making a distinction between calculous and acalculous disease of the gallbladder can clarify the overall etiological picture.

CALCULOUS DISEASE

The signs and symptoms of calculous cholecystitis and other forms of cholecystitis are essentially similar. Abdominal pain is the main complaint. The common complaint is epigastric or RUQ pain that radiates to the back (interscapular) and to the right shoulder. Of equal frequency is RLQ or diffuse umbilical pain. Younger children offer the greater difficulty in localizing the pain. Patients with sickle cell disease who complain of having abdominal pain are apt to be considered as suffering from sickle cell abdominal crisis. Ternberg and Keating state that cholecystectomy in sickle cell patients who had calculous disease results in a lower frequency of recurrent abdominal pain. The most frequent physical finding is tenderness (local or diffuse), along with a moderate fever and a 20% chance of developing jaundice. Stones can be located by flat films of the abdomen, by cholecystogram, and by ultrasonography.

The stones are usually of pigment, cholesterol, or mixed types. Pigment stones are usually associated with repeated attacks of hemolysis. Any patient who has a hemolytic disease is subject to the development of pigment stones. Hemolytic episodes accompanied by sepsis can also predispose to stone formation. Ternberg and Keating state that nonconjugated bilirubin, being insoluble, can contribute to stone formation. Other factors leading to stone formation in the gallbladder are obesity, familial tendencies, cystic fibrosis, and a decrease in ileal function.

The role of stasis may be a factor in stone formation. In such anomalies as choledochal cysts, cystic duct obstruction, and hormone-induced influence on motility, stasis is the feature that leads to stone formation. This may be the reason why, in females at puberty, the incidence of gallstone formation is increased.

ACALCULOUS DISEASE

Infection is most often cited as the cause of noncalculous (acalculous) disease in children. Hydrops of the gallbladder may follow severe trauma, operation, illness, and congenital anomalies. Secondary infection may superimpose on a primary infection. In Ternberg's and Keating's patients, 60% had an illness that preceded cholecystitis. In about 50%, a culture was obtained. In one patient with burn sepsis, *Pseudomonas* was cultured. Abdominal pain may start acutely or may cause sudden worsening of pain. Fever and jaundice are more frequent in acalculous than in calculous disease of the gallbladder. An abdominal mass is frequently palpated, but as in adults, muscle guarding can mask it. However, X-ray films may show the mass. CT scans and ultrasonography are also useful in such problems.

DIAGNOSIS

The most important factor in diagnosing gallbladder disease in children is the awareness of the pediatrician and surgeon that cholecystitis and cholelithiasis do occur in children, as in adults. The differential diagnosis includes appendicitis, intussusception, and volvulus. Ternberg and Keating state that sickle cell abdominal crisis, hepatitis, and abdominal epilepsy are frequent causes of delay.

TREATMENT

The treatment of cholecystitis and cholelithiasis is cholecystectomy. Cholecystectomy, as in the adult, is reserved for special situations, such as the patient who will not tolerate a longer procedure. Cases have been reported where, after a cholecystectomy, relief was attained without further surgery. It should be kept in mind that in a patient with chronic hemolytic disease, failure to remove the gallbladder will result in repeated episodes of stone formation. Ternberg and Keating state that if hemolytic disease can be treated with the expectation of reducing recurrent episodes, cholecystostomy and removal of stones may be all that is required. They recommend cholecystectomy in cases where cholesterol stones are found. The reason is that the primary cause in cholesterol stone formation is the presence of cholesterol-saturated bile, and that recurrences will occur if the gallbladder is allowed to remain.

In acalculous cholecystitis, the treatment will depend on the patient's condition. If the patient presents no complications, cholecystectomy is considered a reasonable treatment. If the patient is not in ideal condition, cholecystostomy may be preferred. If the surgeon recognizes that the gallbladder is not chronically inflamed, and that the underlying cause of stone formation may be remedied, then cholecystostomy with drainage may be all that is required. If, after follow-up studies on a cholecystostomy the patient indicates that the gallbladder is functioning normally, Ternberg and Keating see no reason to follow up with a cholecystectomy. The common duct should not be explored without good reason. An initial cystic duct cholangiogram should be carried out, and if a common duct problem exists or if stones are discovered, a common duct exploration is indicated. The common duct in infants and children is very small, and as in adults, its exploration can induce stenosis. As in adult cholecystitis, early cholecystectomy may prevent complications.

Recommended Reading

Ariyan S, Shessel FS, Pickett LK: Cholecystitis and cholelithiasis masking as abdominal crises in sickle cell disease. *Pediatrics* 58:252, 1976.

Brenner RW, Stewart CF: Cholecystitis in children. *Rev Surg* 21:327, 1964.

Brunet C, Jacques G, Tremblay R: La cholecystite et la cholelithiase chez l'enfant. *Can Med Assoc J* 91:1354, 1964.

Burrington JD, Smith MD: Elective and emergency surgery in children with sickle cell disease. *Surg Clin North Am* 56:55, 1976.

Forshall I, Rickham PP: Cholecystitis and cholelithiasis in childhood. *Br J Surg* 42:161, 1954.

Grace N, Rodgers B: Cholecystitis in childhood. *Clin Pediatr* 16:179, 1977.

Hanson BA, Mahour GH, Woolley MM: Diseases of the gallbladder in infancy and childhood. *J Pediatr Surg* 6:277, 1971.

Holcomb GW, O'Neill JA, Holcomb GW III: Cholecystitis, cholelithiasis and common duct stenosis in children and adolescents. *Ann Surg* 191:626, 1980.

Karayalcin G, Hassani N, Abrams M, et al: Cholelithiasis in children with sickle cell disease. *Am J Dis Child* 133:306, 1979.

Lachman BS, Lazerson J, Starshak RJ, et al: The prevalence of cholelithiasis in sickle cell disease as diagnosed by ultrasound and cholecystography. *Pediatrics* 64:601, 1979.

Leo WA: Acute calculous cholecystitis in childhood. *Mo Med* 58:564, 1961.

Lorvenburg H, Mitchell A: Cholecystitis in childhood. *J Pediatr* 12:203, 1938.

References

1. Ternberg JL, Keating JP: Acute acalculous cholecystitis. *Arch Surg* 110:543, 1975.
2. Swenson O: *Swenson's Pediatric Surgery*, ed 4. New York, Appleton-Century-Crofts, 1980.

Cholecystectomy in Adolescents and the Aged

It was Potter[1] who first created an interest in the number of reports of cholecystitis and cholelithiasis in children and adolescents. Since 1928 many reports have been recorded. In 1924 Blalock[2] reviewed 883 cases of biliary tract disease at the Johns Hopkins Hospital and recorded 11 cases in patients younger than 20 years of age—an incidence of 1.2%. In 1954 Glenn and Hill,[3] after reviewing a 20-year experience with 3,222 cases of biliary tract disease, recorded 7 cases of cholecystitis and cholelithiasis in children 15 years of age or younger—an incidence of 0.22%. A report by Andrassy et al.[4] reported 1,803 primary cholecystectomies performed for gallbladder disease at the Santa Rosa Medical Center. Seventy-nine patients were 20 years old or younger—an incidence of 4.3%. Thirteen of these patients were 15 years of age or younger—an incidence of 0.72%. Wingert et al.,[5] from the Department of Pediatrics and Radiology of the University of Southern California School of Medicine, reported six cases of cholecystitis and cholelithiasis, all confirmed by X-ray studies and surgery. These patients were observed over a 10-year period. In the 79 patients recorded by Andrassy et al., cholecystitis was the diagnosis for which a cholecystectomy was performed. Invariably there was a marked delay in diagnosis in many cases. The etiological factors were considered different in the different races and age groups; however, they appeared to be quite similar in the adolescents and young adults. Hemolytic disease was present in all 5 black patients, but in none of the remaining 74. The patients who were younger than 10 years of age were more likely to have congenital anomalies or an infectious etiology for their gallbladder disease. Cholecystectomy was performed, with a minimum of morbidity and no mortality.

Cholecystitis must be considered in the childhood and adolescent period whenever an unexplained abdominal pain exists, and especially after a cholecystogram or sonogram proves the existence of cholecystitis. Cholecystograms and sonograms are safe and reliable methods for establishing a diagnosis. Wingert et al.[5] concluded that gallbladder disease is uncommon in childhood, and the etiology of cholelithiasis, with the exception of hemolytic disease, still remains indefinite and rather obscure. Classical signs and symptoms of gallbladder disease were usually lacking in the children in this group study, but with a high index of diagnostic suspicion and with X-ray examinations, the diagnosis ultimately became apparent. Since the diagnosis is not obvious, and is not easily suspected in children and adolescents, gallbladder disease must always be included in the differential diagnosis wherever vague abdominal pain and jaundice coexist. An intermittent colicky abdominal pain occurred in about 95% of the cases; nausea, vomiting, and pain occurred in about 75%. Though jaundice occurred in about 66% of the cases, common duct stones were present in only 6%. Tenderness in the RUQ is often found. Slight enlargement of the gallbladder may be palpated, and at times a true acute surgical abdomen may exist; however, a positive diagnosis will still depend upon demonstrating stones on the cholecystogram or sonogram.

These authors further found that in their adolescent patients, females were more predominant than males; this pattern also held in obese patients. In a sense, there was a great resemblance to the cholecystitis in the adult population. Since a diagnosis of acute cholecystitis and cholelithiasis is uncommon to rare in young individuals, there is a greater likelihood for a delay in diagnosis, as well as a great hesitancy to consider cholecystitis and cholelithiasis as the diagnosis. Appendicitis was considered most often as the preoperative diagnosis despite the RUQ pain. About 15% of the patients underwent surgery with a preoperative diagnosis of acute appendicitis. These authors also recognized that in many of their patients less than 10

years of age, cholecystitis without cholelithiasis existed. In these latter cases, they recommended that appropriate bacterial cultures be made and that a more careful search be carried out for congenital anomalies. They concluded that cholecystectomy is a safe procedure for these young patients, and no mortality was recorded. This writer had had two young adult patients, 17 and 20 years of age, who presented with acute cholecystitis and acute appendicitis.

Morbidity and mortality following surgery in aged patients, especially those over 70 years of age, has been falling progressively because of better preoperative and postoperative care, better anesthesia, and the availability and use of blood when needed. Another great advance in surgery for the aged has been the introduction of various broad-spectrum antibiotics administered pre- and postoperatively. The U.S. population is constantly growing; it is now over 235 million. It is believed that close to 20 million Americans are over 65 years of age. Approximately 15% of the total adult population have gallstones, and that the incidence continues to increase with age, especially over 65. Cholecystitis and cholelithiasis usually have a long history, but their complications generally develop as the person grows older. The associated systemic diseases that ultimately develop with the aging process render patients over 65 somewhat more vulnerable to the consequences of complications and to the trauma of the surgical procedure itself. With the better understanding of the physiology of the body and its aging process, there is also a greater awareness of coexisting systemic problems such as generalized arteriosclerosis, cardiovascular-pulmonary problems, diabetes mellitus, and hypertension. Measures are now routinely taken preoperatively to control possible complicating problems, especially in elective cases, and, to a smaller degree, even in emergency cases. The surgeon is now fully aware of the coexistence of cancer with cholelithiasis and knows that approximately 1 in every 100 patients with cholelithiasis will develop carcinoma in the bilary tract. We are now advising older patients with known gallbladder disease (cholelithiasis) that elective surgical procedures performed prophylactically will prevent advanced complications such as fistulous tracts, gallstone ileus, jaundice, liver changes, and finally, carcinoma. Because the potential complications are more likely to occur in advanced age, the surgeon should recommend prophylactic elective cholecystectomy.

In the future, it is conceivable that there will be preventive measures other than surgery to interrupt the progress of biliary tract disease. This problem is now being researched, and it is possible that with a better understanding of the pathophysiology of gallstone formation, greater preventive measures may be developed (see "Pathogenesis of Cholesterol Gallstones" in Chapter 3). In the meantime, the present status of gallbladder disease in the aged should be dealt with if possible by elective cholecystectomy. There are surgeons who perform emergency cholecystectomies and routine common duct explorations at the same time. This writer advocates that in emergency situations in the aged patient, one should keep in mind that temporary procedures such as cholecystostomy may be wiser; and that more will be learned about a particular patient following a secondary elective operation, which is preferable because elective surgery and preoperative preparation make it safer.

When the patient is fully evaluated preoperatively and all preparations are made for an elective operation, it is likely that a longer operation will be better tolerated. In reviewing the geriatric field, particularly biliary tract surgery in the older age group, we find that the number of older patients coming to surgery with gallbladder disease is increasing; even patients from 70 to 90 and over are now being routinely operated on. The fact that the patient has lived to this age demonstrates his or her ability to survive, and shows that the tissues are of good quality and most likely will heal well. The elderly patient has already demonstrated the ability to withstand extensive surgical procedures when necessary. Therefore, when surgery is indicated, we have shown that prophylactic or emergency surgery can be tolerated. It is, of course, preferable to perform an elective procedure in the patient who is well prepared physiologically; all associated systemic problems must be evaluated and corrected. Anesthesia today is considered relatively safe, especially when a qualified anesthetist and surgeon are working together with proper medical facilities and assistants.

Today, just like neonates, adolescents and middle-aged patients can withstand extensive surgery—so can the elderly, when surgery is indicated. It is important to reemphasize that there should be no controversy among general surgeons regarding emergency, elective, delayed, or secondary biliary tract surgical procedures. Each case must be individualized and carefully evaluated, and the surgeon's judgment must be final. It is imperative that proper timing be observed and that consultation be sought whenever indicated. Above all, conservative surgical judgment should be practiced. *It must be remembered that there is only one cure for carcinoma of the gallbladder, and that is prophylactic elective cholecystectomy.* The final word is that if the geriatric patient who requires biliary tract surgery is given a proper preoperative evaluation and a correct surgical procedure at the right time, he or she will have a good chance for complete recovery without complications.

There will be instances where the mortality will be elevated, but this will most likely occur in the dire emergencies, where the disease process and the surgery cannot wait. Cholecystostomy, though a less extensive procedure than cholecystectomy, is usually selected for those individuals at high risk; that is, the patient with an emergency problem or advanced pathological state will not safely tolerate an extensive form of anesthesia and surgery. Even though cholecystostomy (only drainage of the gallbladder) is employed, the advanced state of the disease, the advanced age of the patient, and associated systemic diseases will be the main causes of higher mortality. Here again the writer makes a plea for careful elective evaluation and the use of minimal surgery in each case. A patient with severe gallbladder disease who has an implanted pacemaker and is controlled with cardiac and renal medications presents no contraindication to either emergency cholecystostomy or even elective cholecystectomy.

Recommended Reading

Grace N, Rodgers B: Cholecystitis in childhood. *Clin Pediatr* 16:179, 1977.

Hanson BA, Mahour GH, Woolley MM: Diseases of the gallbladder in infancy and childhood. *J Pediatr Surg* 6:277, 1971.

Holcomb GW, O'Neill JA, Holcomb GW III: Cholecystitis, cholelithiasis and common duct stenosis in children and adolescents. *Ann Surg* 191:626, 1980.

Karayalcin G, Hassani N, Abrams M, et al: Cholelithiasis in children with sickle cell disease. *Am J Dis Child* 133:306, 1979.

Leo WA: Acute calculous cholecystitis in childhood. *Mo Med* 58:564, 1961.

Lorvenburg H, Mitchell A: Cholecystitis in childhood. *J Pediatr* 12:203, 1938.

Lachman BS, Lazerson J, Starshak RJ, et al: The prevalence of cholelithiasis in sickle cell disease as diagnosed by ultrasound and cholecystography. *Pediatrics* 64:601, 1979.

MacMillan RW, Schullinger, JN, Santulli TV: Cholelithiasis in childhood. *Am J Surg* 127:689, 1974.

Morales L, Taboada E, Toledo L, et al: Cholecystitis and cholelithiasis in children. *J Pediatr Surg* 2:565, 1967.

Pellerin D, Bertin P, Nhoul-Fekete C, et al: Cholelithiasis and ileal pathology in childhood. *J Pediatr Surg* 10:35, 1973.

Roslyn JJ, Berquist WE, Pitt HA: Increased risk of gallstones in children receiving total parenteral nutrition. *Pediatrics* 71:784, 1983.

Sarnaik S, Slovis TL, Corbett DP, et al: Incidence of cholelithiasis in sickle cell anemia using the ultrasonic grayscale technique. *J Pediatr* 96:1005, 1980.

Sastic JW, Glassman CI: Gallbladder disease in young women. *Surg Gynecol Obstet* 155:209, 1982.

Sneider SE, Winslow OP Jr: Cholecystitis and cholelithiasis associated with pancreatitis in a child. *JAMA* 182:302, 1962.

References

1. Potter AH: Biliary disease in young subjects. *Surg Gynecol Obstet* 66:604, 1938.
2. Blalock A: A review of 883 cases of biliary tract disease in younger patients. Johns Hopkins Hosp, Baltimore, MD, 1924.
3. Glenn F, Hill HR Jr: Primary gallbladder disease in children. *Ann Surg* 139:302, 1954.
4. Andrassy RJ, Treadwell TA, Ratner IA, et al: Gallbladder disease in children and adolescents. *Am J Surg* 132(1), 1976.
5. Wingert, Willis, Mikity: Dept. of Pediatrics and Radiology, University of Southern Calif.

Cholecystectomy in Pregnancy

Cholecystitis occurs infrequently in pregnancy—about 0.8 cases per 1,000 pregnancies. The mean age of these patients is 26, varying between 15 and 40 years. The signs and symptoms of acute cholecystitis are the same as those of nongravid patients. Ultrasound has become an important diagnostic tool for differentiating other conditions that present with RUQ pain and tenderness during pregnancy. Ultrasound, being noninvasive, may be employed in all three trimesters, without harm to the fetus. It has proven to be very accurate. Gallstones were identified in 25 of 26 patients with 96% accuracy, as substantiated at surgery.

Conservative medical management must be tried first, primarily because of the high percentage of successes (84%). In addition, surgery is not without risk, depending upon the trimester of pregnancy. Surgery may lead to spontaneous abortion or preterm delivery. The surgeon must also keep in mind that anesthetic agents pose a special risk to the fetus, especially in the first trimester. In the third trimester, every effort should be made to prolong the pregnancy.

Landers and Carmona[1] reviewed 30 cases of acute cholecystitis during a 12-year period. Twenty-one patients were successfully managed with medical therapy, nine underwent cholecystectomy, four failed to respond to conservative management, and five went directly to surgery. One patient underwent cholecystectomy during the first trimester and aborted thereafter. Two patients had to undergo cholecystectomy in the early third trimester; both were complicated by preterm labor and delivery. Those patients who underwent surgery in the second trimester did not experience any complications. *These writers concluded that conservative surgical management for diagnosed cholecystitis in pregnancy is the proper approach, and that surgical intervention should be reserved for patients who fail to respond to medical therapy.*

Glenn and McSherry[2] reported on 300 women who had cholecystectomy for symptomatic cholelithiasis. Of these patients, 219 were definitely pregnant prior to their surgery; 218 of the 219 had biliary calculi at surgery; 5 had symptoms prior to their pregnancy; 89 had symptoms during pregnancy, usually in the second trimester. In 67 patients, signs and symptoms occurred within 6 months after their pregnancy; in 23 patients they occurred 6–12 months after pregnancy. In three patients, cholelithiasis was associated with jaundice.

Printen[3] sums up a 10-year experience with cholecystitis during pregnancy. If repeated attacks occur or severe complications such as pancreatitis develop, surgical intervention is indicated. Fetal morbidity is less than 5% following cholecystectomy, especially in the second and third trimesters; it is 60% when pancreatitis is left untreated.

References

1. Landers D, Carmona R: Acute cholecystitis in pregnancy. 69:131, 1987.
2. Glenn F, McSherry C: Gallstones and pregnancy among 300 young women treated with cholecystectomy. *Surg Gynecol Obstet* 127:1067, 1968.
3. Printen KJ: Cholecystectomy during pregnancy. *Am Surg* 44:432, 1978.

Cholecystectomy in the Diabetic

INTRODUCTION

Elliott P. Joslin, in his lifetime a world authority on diabetes mellitus, in his book, *Treatment of Diabetes Mellitus*, emphasized certain conclusions based upon a lifetime of observations. These conclusions were as follows:

1. "The subsidence of symptoms of gallbladder infection (after cholecystectomy) reacts quickly upon the diabetic."
2. "If you could choose the type of diabetes you are likely to acquire, I would recommend the *gallstone variety*. It is the best of all types of diabetes."
3. "I recommend removal of gallstones both in the diabetic and nondiabetic when the danger is slight (elective surgery), first for the prevention of diabetes, and second because if diabetes is present an operation may alleviate it."
4. "Surgeons who operate on a non-diabetic, hereditarily predisposed to diabetes, may well prevent the disease."

Cholecystectomy in the Diabetic

How should the surgeon treat acute cholecystitis in a diabetic patient under 65 years of age? Over 65 years?

How should the surgeon deal with *asymptomatic chronic cholelithiasis* in a diabetic under 65 years of age? Over 65 years?

How should the surgeon deal with *symptomatic chronic cholelithiasis* in a diabetic patient? With jaundice?

How should fulminating acute cholecystitis be treated in a diabetic?

It is well established that peri- and postoperative complications in the diabetic patient are more frequent and certainly more serious than in the nondiabetic. The writer's experience with acute cholecystitis in a diabetic patient has taught him the following:

1. Morbidity and mortality rates are higher.
2. Before surgery is decided upon, an internist should be consulted.
3. The sugar-insulin balance must be managed stat.
4. Acidosis must be corrected stat.
5. Electrolytes and IV fluids must be corrected stat.
6. Broad-spectrum antibiotics must be ordered stat and administered (IM and IV), and then continued peri- and postoperatively.

The surgeon should order the antibiotics, because he knows best which ones are most effective against organisms common to the biliary tract and bile.

All diabetics, regardless of age, and whether or not their insulin is controlled, receive prophylactic preoperative broad-spectrum antibiotics (see Chapter 15). *Preoperative complications* most often encountered at surgery are:

1. Localized or extensive gangrene of the gallbladder wall.
2. Empyema.
3. Perforation.
4. Localized abscess.
5. Generalized peritonitis.
6. Fistulous tracts.

Postoperative complications most frequently encountered are:

1. Wound infections.
2. Wound dehiscence.
3. Uncontrolled sugar-insulin imbalance, hyperglycemia, stupor, coma, and death.

A *nondiabetic*, 65 years of age, with associated degenerative disease (i.e., arteriosclerosis, chronic renal disease, and hypertension), is less likely to develop complications in the postoperative period than a 65-year-old diabetic with the same degenerative pathology. One of the reasons may be that a 65-year-old diabetic develops degenerative changes that are further advanced physiologically than the patient's chronological age, possibly by 5 or 10 years. For this reason, the sugar-insulin balance must be carefully monitored pre-, peri-, and postoperatively. Failure to do so can result in hyperglycemia, stupor, coma, and death.

In the writer's experience with diabetic patients *under 65 years of age*, who are in fairly good condition but who also have associated degenerative changes, a *nonsymptomatic chronic cholelithiasis* would most likely benefit from a prophylactic elective cholecystectomy. It is well known that asymptomatic cholelithiasis will ultimately become symptomatic when a gallstone suddenly obstructs the neck of the gallbladder or the cystic duct, and produces inflammatory changes that will require emergency cholecystectomy.

Acute cholecystitis in a diabetic requiring emergency cholecystectomy predisposes that patient to increased morbidity and mortality. Comparative statistics on morbidity and mortality in diabetic and nondiabetic patients were presented by Sandler et al.[1] Complications developing in diabetic compared to nondiabetic patients following elective surgery were 18.7% vs. 10.2%, and in emergency surgery, 57.9% vs. 39.1%. The mortality was higher in diabetics compared to nondiabetics, 7.9% vs. 3%. The highest incidence of complications occurred in older diabetics—those with associated degenerative diseases. The inability of the diabetic to limit the spread of infection was shown in the statistics published by Turner et al.[2] from Charity Hospital, New Orleans; perforations of the gallbladder occurred in 17% of diabetics compared to 8.3% of nondiabetics.

Diabetic patients under 65 years with *nonsymptomatic* chronic cholelithiasis and associated disease usually tolerate elective surgery as well as equivalent nondiabetics. This same diabetic patient who suddenly develops an acute *symptomatic* cholelithiasis should, in this writer's opinion, be advised not to procrastinate but to decide on elective cholecystectomy. Statistically, this patient's chances of avoiding postoperative complications will be significantly reduced. In choosing to delay surgery by adopting the "if it doesn't bother you, don't bother it" philosophy, the diabetic patient is inviting a sudden acute cholecystitis that will require emergency surgery, with its attendant potential for increased morbidity and mortality.

In the majority of cases, the diabetic patient with chronic cholelithiasis, when carefully prepared for prophylactic elective cholecystomy, is expected to do as well, and obtain the same good results, as the equivalent nondiabetic. Dr. E.P. Joslin,[3] in his book *Treatment of Diabetes Mellitus*, states, "*To diabetics my advice is to have the gallstones removed when the conditions of the time, place, surgeon, and physician are propitious.*" Today there are two schools of thought regarding the question of whether or not to recommend cholecystectomy in a diabetic with asymptomatic cholelithiasis. Should the surgeon do as Joslin recommends? Unfortunately, opinon remains divided. *This writer wholeheartedly sides with Joslin.*

The age of the patient has become an important factor in asymptomatic diabetics. In a patient *under 65 years* of age, with a normal blood sugar level and no associated degenerative changes, this writer would elect to be conservative and treat the condition medically. Strict attention to the sugar-insulin balance and to diet (no fatty or fried foods, etc.). A similar diabetic patient *over 65 years of age,* with degenerative disease but *asymptomatic,* would be advised to have elective surgery. The patient would be cautioned tactfully, yet realistically, about the higher risk of morbidity and mortality. The patient should decide in favor of cholecystectomy. Should this same patient change from *asymptomatic* to *symptomatic* cholelithiasis, this writer would unequivocally recommend prophylactic elective cholecystectomy. If jaundice were to become evident, surgical intervention would be mandatory.

A fulminating toxic acute cholecystitis in a diabetic patient, regardless of age, calls for a very short period of intensive preoperative management followed by emergency surgical intervention. The internist must do his best to control any sugar-insulin imbalance that exists, while at the same time supplying IV electrolytes to avoid acidosis and correct any electrolyte imbalance. The surgeon should order broad-spectrum antibiotics known to be most effective against biliary and colonic organisms. After the best possible medical improvement attainable, the patient should be taken to surgery.

The surgeon, anesthesiologist, and internist must decide whether general or local anesthesia is best for the patient. This writer prefers general anesthesia (mixed gases), with the highest possible oxygen levels. General anesthesia allows faster surgery, better exposure, and minimal shock to the patient. The surgery should be minimal and restricted to a lifesaving procedure, namely cholecystostomy with evacuation of gallstones, pus, and debris. A mushroom catheter is sewn into the fundus of the gallbladder (see Chapters 10 and 15) and brought out through a stab wound. Postoperatively, the treatment must focus on maintaining the sugar-insulin balance, correcting acidosis, maintaining the electrolytic balance, and continuing the administration of broad-spectrum antibiotics. Mask or intranasal oxygen is advised.

References

1. Sandler et al: Factors associated with postoperative complications in diabetes after biliary tract surgery. *Gastroenterology* 91:157, 1986.
2. Turner et al: Charity Hospital, New Orleans, LA.
3. Joslin EP: *Treatment of Diabetes Mellitus.* Philadelphia, Lea and Febiger, 1937.

Cholecystectomy in Patients with Cirrhosis of the Liver

Garrison et al.,[1] in reporting on their study of 39 patients with cirrhosis of the liver who had undergone biliary surgery, reached the following conclusions:

Operations on the biliary tract in these patients resulted in a higher morbidity and mortality than in normal-risk patients. Eight patients (21%) died, and major postoperative complications developed in 35% of the survivors. Local and systemic infections and massive bleeds were the major causes of all deaths. Choledochotomy was performed on 10 patients; 3 (30%) died, and nine major complications developed in 5 surviving patients. Preoperative risk factors found to be predictive of high morbidity and mortality were (1) ascites, 50% mortality and 50% morbidity; (2) prolonged prothrombin time, 29% mortality and 28% morbidity; and (3) a serum albumin level of less than 3.5 μg/%, 33% mortality and 40% morbidity.

The coexistence of major systemic disease made no significant difference between those who survived and those who did not. In 12 patients with no ascites and normal blood chemistries, no deaths occurred; 1 patient developed complications. The authors concluded that biliary surgery in cirrhotic patients carries a high mortality and morbidity, and that the risk of such patients can be assessed preoperatively. There is a subgroup of patients with liver cirrhosis and cholelithiasis that can have a favorable outcome. Operative intervention in these patients should preferably be reserved for the complications of biliary tract disease.

Block et al.[2] reported on 49 patients with cirrhosis of the liver in whom they performed cholecystectomy or cholecystostomy. The mortality was 10.2%. The complications included massive interoperative blood loss in 16.3%, wound problems such as dehiscence, and infection in 12.2%. The authors evaluated their operative results using Child's classification; that is, they divided their patients into three classes of liver involvement: A, B, and C. In class A, the patient was able to respond very satisfactorily to preoperative management; that is, prothrombin time was reduced; albumin was increased; bilirubin fell; and alkaline phosphatase and ascites improved. Class A patients tolerated the surgery of cholecystectomy and recovered. No deaths were reported in this class. In class B, the patient responded, but not as satisfactorily as the patient in class A. Of 11 patients operated on, 1 (9%) died. Of 17 patients in class C, 4 (23.5%) died. The overall mortality was 10.2%, but in class C it rose to 23.5%. The complications in class A consisted of wound infections; one patient suffered hemorrhage. In class C, all deaths were due to liver failure and/or sepsis.

Massive blood loss occurred in 1 patient in class B, but in class C, 7 of 17 suffered massive blood loss. At operation, the average blood loss was 1 liter. Stone's[3] contention is that Child's criteria can be applied to all cirrhotic patients considered for major surgery, and not just for portal decompression procedures in cirrhotic patients. Garrison et al. confirmed Stone's recommendations; he re-

ported his mortality rates for abdominal procedures in cirrhotic patients as 10, 31, and 76%, respectively, for Child's classes A, B, and C.

Block et al. concluded that operative intervention for symptomatic cholelithiasis is acceptable for Child's class A and B patients; this procedure should be carried out at the earliest appropriate time; one should not wait too long, because the patient's liver function may deteriorate to Child's class C. This would be most unfortunate if the need for emergency intervention arose. The Child's class C patient, because of associated considerable blood loss both inter- and postoperatively, should be operated on only as an urgent or emergent case. If this patient is symptomatic and requires cholecystectomy, it is possible to prepare the patient electively by improving the nutrition, controlling ascites, and requiring the patient to abstain from alcohol.

In other words, it is possible to electively convert a Child's class C patient to a class B in order to improve the patient's chances for survival. In emergency circumstances, if at all possible, local anesthesia is preferred to general anesthesia, because the serious complications of massive hemorrhage and anesthetic toxicity may be avoided. Aranha et al.[4] recommend preoperative endoscopic retrograde pancreatography to evaluate an existing jaundice; it is possible that the jaundice is not related to extra-hepatic stones but is actually due to parenchymatous liver disease. Aranha et al. also suggest that, if possible, cholecystostomy should be considered even when the first choice is to perform a cholecystectomy. To prevent a major bleed from the liver bed, Aranha et al. also recommend that in certain instances a partial or incomplete cholecystectomy be performed, with electrocoagulation of the leftover posterior wall of the gallbladder. This operation was originally performed by Pribram[5] in Germany and by Thorek in the United States. Thorek[6] named the procedure *cholecystoelectrocoagulectomy.*

Recommended Reading

Castaing D, Houssin D, Lemoine J, et al: Surgical management of gallstones in cirrhotic patients. *Am J Surg* 146:310, 1983.

Cayer D, Sohmer MF: Surgery in patients with cirrhosis. *Arch Surg* 71:828, 1955.

Doberneck RC, Sterling WA Jr, Allison DC: Morbidity and mortality after operation in nonbleeding cirrhotic patients. *Am J Surg* 146:306, 1983.

Glenn F: Biliary tract disease. *Surg Gynecol Obstet* 153:401, 1981.

Henrikson EC: Cirrhosis of the liver: With special reference to the surgical aspects. *Arch Surg* 32:413, 1936.

Hughson W: Portal cirrhosis with ascites and its surgical treatment. *Arch Surg* 15:418, 1927.

Lindenmuth WW, Eisenberg MM: The surgical risk in cirrhosis of the liver. *Arch Surg* 86:235, 1963.

McSherry CK, Glenn F: The incidence and causes of death following surgery for nonmalignant biliary tract disease. *Ann Surg* 191:271, 1980.

Schwartz SI: Biliary tract surgery and cirrhosis: A critical combination. *Surgery* 90:577, 1981.

References

1. Garrison RN, Cryer HM, Howard DA, et al: Clarification of risk factors for abdominal operations in patients with hepatic cirrhosis. *Ann Surg* 199:648, 1984.
2. Block, Alleban, Walt: Reported 49 cases of cirrhosis.
3. Stone HH: Reliability of criteria for predicting persistent or recurrent sepsis. *Arch Surg* 120:17, 1985.
4. Aranha GV, Sontag SJ, Greenlee HB: Cholecystectomy in cirrhotic patients: A formidable operation. *Am J Surg* 143:55, 1982.
5. Pribram BOC: The method for dissolution of the common duct stones remaining after operation. *Surgery* 22:806, 1947.
6. Thorek M: Cholecystoelectrocoagulectomy, 4-vol. set, in *Modern Surgical Technique*. Philadelphia, JB Lippincott Co, Vol. 3, 1949, pp 2304–2328.

Factors Influencing Long-Term Results of Cholecystectomy

Stefanini et al.[1] reviewed 800 postcholecystectomized patients in order to establish the frequency and severity of postoperative symptoms and the factors that influence them. From a total of 551 patients reported as symptomatic cure, 217 continued to complain of mild symptoms, and 32 suffered from severe symptoms. These figures will be compared later on with a computer analysis of postcholecystectomized patients by Bodvall and Overgaard[2,3] of Goteborg, Sweden. Stefanini et al. found that residual stones in the common bile duct and stenosis of the sphincter of Oddi were the main underlying causes of severe postcholecystectomy distresses. They felt that sphincteroplasty is the procedure of choice in both retained stone and common duct stenosis. These writers found that mild postcholecystectomy symptoms were more related to preexisting hepatic damage caused by concomitant gallstone disease. Patients with a long interval between the onset of severe cholecystitis and cholecystectomy had the higher incidence of mild distress. Stefanini et al. concluded that early cholecystectomy is best.

COMPUTER ANALYSIS

Common causes of postcholecystectomy symptoms are retained common duct stone, cystic duct remnant, so-called dyskinesia, and stenosis of the sphincter of Oddi.

In a study with computer analysis of 1,930 patients with postcholecystectomy symptoms, Bodvall and Overgaard divided their patients into two groups. Group 1 consisted of 938 patients with 5- to 9-year follow-up; group II consisted of 992 patients with a 2-year follow-up. Patients with postcholecystectomy biliary distress (39.6%) were divided according to the severity of their symptoms into four categories: dyspepsia, 10.7%; attacks of mild pain, 23.5%; occasional attacks of severe pain, 3%; and postcholecystectomy biliary distress, 2.4%.

Group I patients, with a long interval between cholecystectomy and follow-up, had a significantly higher frequency of distress than group II, with a short interval.

1. Women had a significantly higher frequency of postcholecystectomy distress than men.
2. A decreasing frequency of distress was noted with advancing age. This pattern was found in both sexes except in women aged 40–49, in whom the highest frequency of symptoms were 53.5%.
3. Patients with choledocholithiasis had a significantly higher frequency of postcholedochostomy symptoms than those who had mild to severe cholecystitis.
4. The longer the preoperative history, the higher the frequency of postcholecystectomy distress.
5. The factors of sex, age, and type of gallbladder disease were independent of each other, and each influenced the frequency of postcholecystectomy distress.
6. The later in the course of acute cholecystitis that cholecystectomy was performed, the lower the frequency of postcholecystectomy distress.
7. Patients who had had common duct exploration for stones had a significantly lower frequency of postcholecystectomy distress than those who had not undergone choledocholithotomy.
8. Patients who had a functioning gallbladder preoperatively had a greater frequency of postcholecystectomy distress than those who had a nonfunctioning gallbladder.
9. The size or number of calculi in the gallbladder did not influence the frequency of postcholecystectomy distress.
10. Patients with an acalculous, functioning gallbladder had a significantly higher frequency of

postcholecystectomy distress than those with stones in a functioning gallbladder.

11. The gallbladder disease per se, not the presence of a stone, influences the frequency of postcholecystectomy distress.

12. Patients with dyspepsia and mild attacks of pain considered themselves improved by the cholecystectomy; this group constituted 34.2% of the entire series.

13. Patients with occasional attacks of severe pain made up 3% of the series.

14. Finally, 2.4% of the patients had disabling symptoms of severe postcholecystectomy distress.

References

1. Stefanini P, Carboni M, Petrassi N, et al: Factors influencing the long term results of cholecystectomies. *Surg Gynecol Obstet* 139:734, 1974.
2. Bodvall B, Overgaard B: Computer analysis of postcholecystectomy biliary tract symptoms. *Surg Gynecol Obstet* 124:723, 1966.
3. Bodvall B, Overgaard B: The postcholecystectomy syndrome. *Clin Gastroenterol* 2:103, 1973.

Complications of Cholecystectomy

Larry C. Carey, M.D., F.A.C.S., I.B.A.

Complications occur in about 10%, and the great majority of those are minor complications such as atelectasis, minor wound infections, and transient fever, often unexplained. The major complications of cholecystectomy can be divided into those occurring early, either during or soon after operation, and those occurring late, weeks to years after the surgical procedure.

INTRAOPERATIVE COMPLICATIONS

The variations of anatomy in the area of the cystic duct and artery are numerous. Care must be taken to identify the cystic artery at its origin and to dissect it well on to the gallbladder surface. In elderly patients with arteriosclerotic vessels, one must be particularly careful to avoid a tortuous right hepatic

From Henry ML, Carey LC: Complications of cholecystectomy. *Surg Clin North Am* 6:, 1983. With permission of Dr. Larry Carey.

artery, which at times comes very close to the wall of the gallbladder. Until the last few years, hepatic artery injury was thought to be a highly lethal injury. *The use of hepatic artery ligation to control bleeding from hepatic trauma has made it clear that hepatic necrosis is not common with hepatic artery ligation.* Nonetheless, the arteries deserve the respect of the surgeon, and injury should be avoided. Should bleeding develop during gallbladder dissection, careful control is indicated. Blind clamping in the depths of the surgical field increases the risk of injury to the structures in the porta hepatis. Bleeding can be controlled first with finger compression, but this maneuver may obscure the field; a vascular clamp allows better exposure. The clamp can be released slowly, the site of bleeding identified, and the bleeding controlled safely. If the right hepatic artery has been injured, repair is very difficult, and ligation is preferred. Broad-spectrum antibiotics are indicated, and hepatic enzymes (SGOT, SGPT) should be monitored postoperatively to assess hepatic necrosis.

Several recent reports have stressed the extremely high risk of cholecystectomy in the patient with portal hypertension. The loss of blood in these patients is enormous, and if at all possible, cholecystectomy should be avoided. Without question, the most devastating operative complication of cholecystectomy is injury to the ductal system. Hermann's[1] review cites the incidence of bile duct injury to be 0.5%. One often gets a clue to exercise more caution in the cystic duct dissection when there is a very short cystic artery. It is alarming that in many instances of common duct injury the surgeon describes a very easy and uncomplicated operation, and the first clue that ductal injury has occurred comes when jaundice becomes evident in the early postoperative period.

The best time to deal with common duct injury is at the time of its occurrence. The injuries are complete transections, partial transections, or avulsion in type. If one finds that a ligature, a clip, or a surgical clamp has been placed partially or completely across the duct, removing the offending cause is all that is required. Careful postoperative observation is necessary for 12 to 24 months, with serial alkaline phosphatase determinations at 2- to 3-month intervals. In the case of avulsion injuries, they most often occur as a result of pulling too hard on the cystic duct. These tears can be repaired by carefully suturing the flap of avulsed duct back in place. Traditionally, 000000 silk suture has been used, but the recent availability of synthetic monofilament absorbable sutures may change the suture material of choice. In either event, the sutures are placed with the knots on the outside, and a small T-tube is used to stent the repair for 10 to 15 days. A soft drain is left in the area of repair until all evidence of bile leak has stopped. When the avulsed flap of duct is not available, autogenous vein will substitute as an acceptable patch.

When the duct has been completely divided, an end-to-end repair is preferred. If there is traumatized tissue at the site of transection, the ends of the duct are debrided and carefully approximated with delicate technique and fine suture. Modest magnification ($2\times$) is very helpful when anastomosing bile duct of normal caliber. A small tube is placed prior to beginning the repair, with exit site proximal or distal to but never through the repair. The stent is left for 10 to 15 days if there is no bile leak, and the cholangiogram shows no extravasation. Terblanche[2] has recently stressed the importance of preserving the blood supply to the common duct, but the work awaits confirmation. Attempts at other than end-to-end anastomosis are not advisable unless implantation of the proximal duct into bowel is considered. This probably should be reserved for instances in which a segment of duct has been resected, making reconstruction without tension impossible. In such cases, either choledochoduodenostomy or choledochojejunostomy Roux-en-Y may be considered. The Roux-en-Y technique is probably better for avoiding reflux of chyme into the ductal system and lessens the chance of infection. One of the most important factors in managing bile duct reconstruction is the continued observation of the patient. Bile duct strictures may occur years after reconstruction. There will be a rise in alkaline phosphatase levels prior to symptoms or jaundice in most cases. As the alkaline phosphatase level rises, stricture should be suspected and proper imaging studies of the bile duct performed. Endoscopic retrograde cholangiography (ERC) is the diagnostic study of choice. It is fast, safe, and accurate, and it provides the detail needed to make decisions about therapy. Although common duct injury should be considered an unfortunate complication, unrecognized common duct injury is a disaster. If drains have been left in, bile drainage may be copious. If there is no drainage, the onset of jaundice is rapid and progressive. Evidence of sepsis is common, with fever accompanying the jaundice. These findings should quickly lead to the appropriate diagnostic studies, and again ERC is very helpful. Occasionally, radiopaque material injected into the biliary fistula will show the lesion, but it is wise to delay sonogram for 8 to 14 days. Recent advances in radionuclide imaging may be helpful in defining the anatomic abnormality.

Laboratory tests will show elevated levels of bilirubin and alkaline phosphatase. The level of transaminase enzymes may be slightly elevated but usually do not suggest hepatitis. Once the problem is recognized, repair should proceed. To delay correction awaiting dilatation of the proximal ducts is not prudent. Primary choledochocholedochostomy is almost never preferred if not done at the time of the injury. Delayed reconstructions are best done with choledochojejunostomy Roux-en-Y. The injury is nearly always closer to bifurcation of the common hepatic duct than one would expect based on radiographic findings. A careful single-layer anastomosis is done without stent. Great attention is paid to making a watertight anastomosis. Bile leak may be more important in bile duct stricture after repair than is appreciated. The reconstruction without a stent works quite well if carefully and precisely performed. Perforation of the common duct in the course of a cholangiogram is an infrequent but worrisome complication that usually becomes apparent when the cholangiogram is seen. It is best managed by T-tube drainage. Attempts at exposing and repairing the injury may produce more harm, and simple drainage is all that is required. The same is true when a false passage is created during common duct exploration. Unless the injury is easily seen or is very extensive, it can be managed quite well with simple T-tube drainage. When the postoperative cholangiogram shows no extravasation, usually about 10 to 12 days the T-tube may be removed. In either event, subsequent stricture is unlikely unless the injury has been extensive.

EARLY POSTOPERATIVE COMPLICATIONS

Wound Complications

Wound infections occurring after cholecystectomy are not common: it is 2% with cholecystectomy and almost 8% with associated common duct exploration. Certain factors such as obstruction, advanced age, and acute inflammation have been shown to be associated with an increase in the incidence of infection. Furthermore, positive cultures of bile and gallbladder wall are associated with an increased incidence of wound infection. Of interest is that when bacteria are found in the bile and a wound infection develops, it is likely to be from one of the same organisms present in the bile. This observation is the argument used to support routine intraoperative cultures of bile. The most common organisms are *E. coli*, staphylococci, *Klebsiella*, and *Aerobacter*. Any one of several of the cephalosporin drugs is effective. In patients at increased risk, such as the elderly (over 70), those with obstruction, and those with acute cholecystitis, the use of prophylactic antibiotics is rational. The drug is given a short time preoperatively, and its administration is continued for one or two doses postoperatively. If prophylaxis is unsuccessful, surgical drainage may be necessary. The proper timing of the drainage procedure is important. To attempt drainage too early fails to solve the problem; to wait too long exposes the patient to excess risk of systemic infection. The timing of drainage is based on clinical observation, which includes the temperature, local physical findings, and general state of the patient. Additional help may be gained from an abdominal ultrasonogram, which can help to locate the abscess. Depending on the ability of the radiologist, percutaneous drainage may be performed with ultrasonograpic control. Occasionally, bile may accumulate in the subhepatic space. Bile in the abdomen may or may not produce dramatic symptoms. In some patients, it is quite well tolerated and produces few symptoms. Again, an ultrasonogram will localize the lesion to allow surgical or percutaneous sonographically controlled aspiration. If no source of continuing bile leak is present, a single episode of aspiration may be all that is required. If there is evidence of continued leak, surgical drainage should be performed.

Premature T-Tube Removal

When it is necessary to place a T-Tube in the common bile duct, care should be taken to secure the tube to avoid accidental dislodgement. A drain should be left near the site of choledochotomy. The previous recommendation for leaving a redundant segment of the T-tube in the abdomen is no longer appropriate since the T-tube tract may be needed for percutaneous stone extraction. This practice further strengthens the need for careful security of the internal portion of the tube. If the T-tube does become dislodged, the associated drain may be adequate to allow escape of the bile. If drainage is not adequate, or if clinical signs of peritonitis or infection develop, surgical drainage is indicated. The delay should be minimal if systemic sepsis is to be avoided.

Retained Common Duct Stone

Glenn[3] has noted that 1.1% of patients undergoing cholecystectomy have retained common duct stones; those having a common bile duct exploration have a 4.3% incidence. As operative cho-

langiography and choledochoscopy have become more commonly used, the incidence of retained common duct stones has diminished. Routine operative cholangiography helps to identify those patients requiring common duct exploration. Common bile duct exploration with a choledochoscope lessens the incidence of retained stones, compared with those explorations without intraoperative endoscopy. Using both techniques helps eliminate the risks.

When a stone is found prior to removal of the T-tube, two options are considered. One is to attempt to dissolve the stone. Different compounds have been used. A heparinized saline solution was used early, but the one in vogue is a medium-chain triglyceride called monooctonoin (Kapmul). The material is infused into the T-tube over a period of 4 to 6 days, and repeat cholangiograms are performed to look for the stone. Although several authors have reported good results, especially in stones high in cholesterol content, our results have been poor, with only 1 stone in 10 being satisfactorily treated. Diarrhea and abdominal cramps have been serious enough to terminate treatment in 50% of our patients.

Percutaneous stone extraction using the T-tube site has been safe and successful. The T-tube must remain in place 5 to 6 weeks to allow sufficient time for the tract to mature. The tube should be placed to provide the most direct path from the skin to the choledochotomy and should be of sufficient size to allow future instrumentation (at least 16 to 18 Fr). The T-tube is removed, and one of two methods can be used. Early reports of a fluoroscopically controlled passage of wire baskets through the tract have led to general acceptance of this procedure as both safe and efficient. More recently, the use of a pediatric bronchoscope or choledochoscope through the tract has allowed direct visualization of the retained stone. Once this has been accomplished, a similar basket can be passed through a channel in the scope for retrieval of the stone. This method is becoming more accepted and has nonoperative success rates of greater than 90%.

LATE COMPLICATIONS

Bile Duct Stricture

Benign stricture of the extrahepatic biliary ducts is most often related to an intraoperative accident. Most ductal injuries with subsequent stricture and obstruction occur at or proximal to the cystic duct–choledochal junction. The stricture may develop within a few months or as long as many years after the initial cholecystectomy.

222

CASE REPORT. A 45-year-old morbidly obese woman underwent cholecystectomy in February 1982. The operation was uncomplicated, and a pre-existing ventral hernia repair was performed. Postoperatively, a segment of transverse colon at the margin of the hernia repair became herniated and necrosed. This complication resulted in intestinal fistula and wound infection with wound disruption requiring a 2-month hospitalization. Before discharge, the patient was noted to have an unexplained elevation in her alkaline phosphatase level but had no biliary tract symptoms, and no diagnostic studies were performed. The patient was readmitted in July 1982 because of bleeding at the site of a prolapsed colostomy, and again the alkaline phosphatase level was elevated, but in the absence of symptoms, no further diagnostic studies were done. Not until jaundice developed in October 1982 was an investigation of the biliary tree conducted. The jaundice was painless and associated with no symptoms. A retrograde cholangiogram showed two surgical clips to have been placed across her common hepatic duct, producing near total obstruction. A hepaticojejunostomy was performed (Roux-en-Y), and she got well, with normal liver enzyme studies. Remarkably, she had near total obstruction of her hepatic duct for 8 months, with no symptoms and no jaundice. As is so often true, the elevation of the alkaline phosphatase level was the first clue to common duct occlusion.

While bile duct strictures develop, the only clue may be painless jaundice. Occasionally, and more often with partial than complete obstruction, cholangitis may develop. The infection may be severe and require an emergency decompression of the obstructed duct. Antibiotics should always be given, but decompression may be the only effective treatment if sepsis continues despite maximal medical therapy. If one looks closely enough, over one half of these patients will have had a previous episode of cholangitis. If that is the case, when one suspects ductal stricture, percutaneous transhepatic decompression may be helpful. This technique may allow management of the sepsis without a surgical procedure, permitting correction of the stricture under more ideal circumstances. This procedure was first described by Molnar.[4] It not only allows for immediate decompression of the biliary tract but also may allow for further anatomic definition radiographically and even postoperative decompression after definitive repair. Certain bile duct strictures can be treated with balloon dilatation via the percutaneous route. Although most success has been with dilating strictures of bilioenteric an-

astomoses, in some instances long-term patency has been possible with strictured ducts, with or without previous repair. If percutaneous drainage is not successful, the definitive treatment with choledochojejunostomy Roux-en-Y is preferable to an operative temporizing procedure that may make definitive treatment more difficult. *In patients with severe jaundice, preoperative decompression of the bile ducts may reduce postoperative complications.* In our experience, reducing the bilirubin below 6 mg/100 ml lessens postoperative morbidity, especially those of infection. This not only allows for decompression but also gives the surgical team ample time to assess and correct other abnormalities, especially those of nutrition and fluid status. Others have found significant differences with preoperative decompression techniques. If the percutaneous technique is to be used, it must be accomplished with minimum complications. Some have suggested that preoperative decompression may reduce the size of dilated ducts, making ultimate reconstruction more difficult. Though this is a theoretical consideration, in practice it has not been a factor of importance.

Roux-en-Y hepatico- or choledochojejunostomy is preferred for managing bile duct stricture rather than loop choledochojejunostomy or duodenostomy. The Roux-en-Y technique avoids tension and prohibits reflux of gastrointestinal contents into the ductal system through its defunctionalized nature. The technique described by Wexler and Smith[5] using a nonsuture technique of mucosal patch has proved to be of little merit. The incidence of recurrence is high, and in fact nearly all strictures can be dealt with by careful dissection even into the substance of the liver. The technique described by Hepp[6] and popularized by Bismuth[7] involves extending an incision into the left hepatic duct, which is quite superficial. This maneuver allows one to enlarge the left hepatic duct orifice, and facilitates a hepaticojejunostomy. Because of the proximal nature of the majority of these strictures, they present the greatest challenge for the surgeon regarding exposure and operative repair, as well as long-term results. Warren [8-11] notes a 78% successful repair rate over a 27-year period, with a 13% mortality. He also states that there has been a progressive decrease in mortality when the data for this time period are inspected over divided time intervals, progressing toward the present. Improved techniques in anesthesia, increasing familiarity with surgical procedures, newer antibiotics, and better postoperative care are at the root of the improvement. Warren recently reviewed 34 collected series with over 5,500 patients and observed a 72% rate of satisfactory results, with an 8% mortality. This problem continues to challenge the best surgeons.

Retained Common Duct Stone

With the advent and common usage of ERC, the diagnosis of retained common duct stones has become much easier. When a common bile duct stone is found remotely after cholecystectomy, two possibilities exist. The stone may have formed in the duct, or it may have been left in the common duct. It is important, if possible, to distinguish these possibilities, since there is a considerable difference in approach to the two problems. It is not always possible to discern retained stones from primary common duct stones. In general, primary stones are softer, less well formed, and darker than retained stones. When there is strong evidence that the stone is retained, then the only treatment required is the removal of the stone. While there is considerable feeling that surgical removal is preferred in the United States, in many parts of the world the problem is managed by endoscopic papillotomy with extraction of the stone or simply allowing it to pass. This procedure is safe and effective but is less widely available in this country than in Europe. Success rates of 80 to 95% have been reported in the recent literature, and this procedure may be an effective alternative to surgery as familiarity with the procedure increases. When it seems likely that stones have formed in the duct, then an element of stasis may be presumed. In those cases, failure to relieve the stasis will result in further stone formation. Either sphincteroplasty or choledochoduodenostomy will effectively relieve the stasis. Good results can be obtained in nearly 100% of cases for retained stones with minimal morbidity. Since both procedures are effective, the surgeon should choose the one with which he or she is most comfortable. In neither instance is a T-tube or stent necessary. In both procedures, an opening of 2.5 cm in the common duct is preferred since that seems to minimize the risk of cholangitis.

Retained Cystic Duct Stump

Whether a retained cystic duct may be a source of recurrent symptoms after cholecystectomy is controversial. Occasionally, a subtotal cholecystectomy may have been performed and a very confusing situation results. In such cases, the original operation was usually performed three to four decades previously when many surgeons were fearful of dissection about the common duct. As a result, only the portion of the gallbladder that was easily accessible was removed. Later, the patient developed symptoms typical of cholecystitis or biliary colic but had a history of previous cholecystectomy. Occasionally, an oral cholecystogram will show what appears to be a gallbladder, and at operation it is obvious that only a portion of the gallbladder had been removed. If an oral cholecystogram fails to demonstrate the gallbladder remnant, an ultrasonogram or retrograde cholangiogram may establish the diagnosis. In such patients, the treatment is completion of cholecystectomy. More often, one encounters patients who have recurrent symptoms suggestive of biliary tract disease and who are found to have a remnant of cystic duct. This problem can be eliminated if at the first operation care is taken to carefully identify the junction of the cystic duct and common duct and to divide the cystic duct no more than 3 mm from the junction. When this careful dissection is not done, the result is a remnant of cystic duct that may be a few millimeters or several centimeters in length. With the long ducts, stasis occurs, and stones tend to reform and produce symptoms. The problem is in trying to decide, in the absence of stones, whether a cystic remnant is of sufficient length to be symptomatic. In general, if the remnant is less than 1 cm, symptoms are almost never a consequence of the stump. For those cases in which the remnant is larger than 1 cm, recurrent stones are likely to be the source of the symptoms. Cystic duct neuromas can nearly always be found at the end of the cystic duct and have never been convincingly shown to produce symptoms.

Papillitis

Zollinger[12] showed many years ago that forcible dilatation of the sphincter of Oddi produced hemorrhage with subsequent fibrosis. This led to the saying, "The surgeon should explore the common bile duct with the same temerity he would explore his own urethra." Vigorous stretching of the distal common duct and sphincter is to be deplored. There is little to defend the notion that useful information is garnered by "calibrating" the sphincter with dilators. We have condemned the use of Bakes dilators in common duct exploration and prefer the use of softer, tapered silk woven catheters, which allow irrigation as well as exploration. The passage of a 6 or 8 Fr catheter is harmless and provides the necessary information about common duct patency. Passage of stones through the sphincter may produce damage similar to forcible dilatation. Acosta[13] recovered large stones from the stool of patients recovering from pancreatitis, demonstrating passage through the intact sphincter. When sphincteric trauma is followed by fibrosis, partial obstruction of the common duct results. Stones may form proximal to the obstruction, and in some instances pancreatitis may occur. The diagnosis may be suggested by radionuclide scan and confirmed by ERC or transhepatic cholangiogram. The treatment is sphincteroplasty with relief of the obstruction.

Pancreatitis

The occurrence of hyperamylasemia after cholecystectomy is not an unusual event. After operative cholangiography, it can be demonstrated that to 4 to 8% of patients are hyperamylasemic; however, similar elevations have been noted after cholecystectomy without cholangiogram. This suggests that the elevation of the amylase level is secondary to other events, not related to increased ductile pressures during injection of contrast medium, as noted previously. Pancreatitis, however, is an uncommon occurrence. Between 0.7 and 2.4% of patients undergoing biliary tract surgery develop this complication. Mortality is notably high (29% and 50%) in retrospective studies of those patients undergoing cholecystectomy. In both series, there was aggressive manipulation of the sphincter of Oddi at surgery. If pancreatitis develops postoperatively, early diagnosis and aggressive fluid and electrolyte replacement are mandatory.

Postcholecystectomy Syndrome

One of the most disturbing situations we face as surgeons is performing a cholecystectomy for presumed symptomatic gallstones and then having the patient return in 3 months to many years later with symptoms identical to those for which the operation had been done. This syndrome has been noted to occur in up to 5% of patients operated on for stone disease of the biliary tract. Several possibilities exist. (1) The symptoms for which the operation was performed were unrelated to the gallstones. (2) An operative error may have produced a situation that leads to recurrent biliary tract disease. (3) The patient may have developed new disease of the biliary tract. Persistence of symptoms unrelated to biliary tract disease can usually be avoided by a careful history. Certain conditions such as peptic ulcer, reflux esophagitis, transverse colon cancer, retrocecal appendicitis, and others may mimic biliary colic or acute cholecystitis. The

surgeon must remember that the disease process may be outside the biliary tree, as shown in up to one-third of patients in some series studying postcholecystectomy syndrome. The surgeon must recognize these possibilities, exclude them by a careful history, and, when indicated, perform appropriate diagnostic tests. This is not to say that every patient requiring cholecystectomy should have an upper gastrointestinal series, barium enema, and intravenous pyelogram. The experienced clinician should, by a careful history, be suspicious enough so that he or she can interpret the patient's symptoms and pursue alternative diagnoses when warranted.

ERC has become valuable in the diagnosis of anatomic abnormalities associated with this syndrome. Cooperman[14] noted that over 50% of patients had demonstrable abnormalities, including choledocholithiasis, papillary stenosis, pancreas divisum, and pancreatic carcinoma. The majority of those studied by Gregg[15] had definable abnormalities as well, including 70% of their patients who were believed to have ampullary stenosis. These series should alert the clinician that symptoms occurring after biliary tract surgery may have a definite cause and that pertinent studies should be pursued. It is equally important not to raise unrealistic expectations about what cholecystectomy will accomplish. The patient should be told that if the intermittent right upper quadrant pain is caused by gallstones, removing the gallbladder will relieve the symptoms. Food intolerances, dyspepsia, flatulence, and vague nonspecific abdominal complaints will probably not be affected.

Recommended Reading

Aranha GV, Sonta SJ, Greenlee HG: Cholecystectomy in cirrhotic patients: A formidable operation. *Am J Surg* 143:55, 1982.

Bean WJ, Mahorner HR: Removal of residual biliary stones through T-tube tract. *South Med J* 65:377, 1972.

Bodvall B: The postcholecystectomy syndrome. *Clin Gastroenterol* 2:103, 1973.

Boey JH, Way LH: Acute cholangitis. *Ann Surg* 191:264, 1980.

Caride VJ, Gibson DW: Noninvasive evaluation of bile leakage. *Surg Gynecol Obstet* 154:517, 1982.

Chetlin SH, Elliot DW: Preoperative antibiotics in biliary surgery. *Arch Surg* 107:319, 1973.

Conn JH, Chavez CM, Fair WR: Bile peritonitis. *Am Surg* 36:219, 1970.

Cruse PJE: Incidence of wound infections on general surgery services. *Surg Clin North Am* 55:1269, 1975.

Denning DA, Ellison EC, Carey LC: Preoperative percutaneous transhepatic decompression lowers operative morbidity in patients with obstructive jaundice. *Am J Surg* 141:161, 1981.

Fartha GJ, Ammar AD, Change FC: The incidence and significance of elevations of serum and urinary amylase levels following transcystic duct cholangiography. *Surg Gynecol Obstet* 151:769, 1980.

Flint LM, Mays GT, Aaron WS, et al: Selectivity and management of hepatic artery ligation. *Ann Surg* 185:613, 1977.

Gardner B: Intracholedochal heparinized saline from treatment of retained common duct stones. *Ann Surg* 170:24, 1973.

Garlock JH, Hurwitt ES: The cystic duct syndrome. *Surgery* 29:833, 1951.

Glenn F, Johnson G: Cystic duct remnant. *Surg Gynecol Obstet* 101:331, 1955.

Glenn F: Retained calculi within the biliary ductal system. *Ann Surg* 179:528, 1974.

Glenn F: Iatrogenic injuries to the biliary duct system. *Surg Gynecol Obstet* 146:430, 1978.

Hess W: *Surgery of the Biliary Passages and the Pancreas.* New York, D Van Nostrand Co, 1965.

Imrie CW, McKay AJ, BAenjamin IS, et al: Secondary acute pancreatitis: Etiology, prevention, diagnoses and management. *Br J Surg* 65:399, 1978.

Jakimowicz JJ: Postoperative choledochoscopy. *Arch Surg* 118:810, 1983.

Jones SA, Steedman A, Keller TB, et al: Transduodenal sphincteroplasty (not sphincterotomy) for biliary and pancreatic disease. *Am J Surg* 118:292, 1962.

Kappes SK, Adamas MB, Wilson SD: Intraoperative biliary endoscopy. *Arch Surg* 117:603, 1982.

Lygidakis NJ: Operative risk factors of cholecystectomy-choledochotomy in the elderly. *Surg Gynecol Obstet* 157:15, 1983.

Mack E, Patzer EM, et al: Retained biliary tract stones: Nonsurgical treatment with Capmul 8210. *Arch Surg* 116:341, 1981.

Madden JL: Primary common bile duct stones. *World J Surg* 2:463, 1978.

Mazzariello R: Review of 220 cases of residual biliary calculi treated without reoperation. *Surgery* 73:299, 1973.

Mazzeo FJ, Jordan FT: Endoscopic papillotomy for recurrent common duct stones and papillary stenosis. *Arch Surg* 118:693, 1983.

McSherry CK, Glenn F: The incidence and causes of death following surgery for nonmalignant biliary tract disease. *Ann Surg* 191:271, 1980.

Moody FG, Becker JM, Potts JR: Transduodenal sphincteroplasty and transampullary septectomy for postcholecystectomy pain. *Ann Surg* 197:627, 1983.

Moss JP, Whelan TG, Dedman TC, et al: Postoperative choledochoscopy through the T-tube tract. *Surg Gynecol Obstet* 151:807, 1980.

Nardi GL, Acosta JM: Papillitis as a cause of pancreatitis and abdominal pain. *Ann Surg* 164:611, 1966.

Passi RB: Endoscopic papillotomy. *Surgery* 92:581, 1982.

Robson MC, Bogart JM, Heggers JP: An endogenous source of wound infections based on quantitative bacteriology of the biliary tract. *Surgery* 86:471, 1970.

Schwartz SE: Biliary tract surgery and cirrhosis. *Surgery* 90:577, 1981.

Sharp KW, Gadacz TR: Detection of patients for dissolution of retained common duct stones with mono-octonin. *Ann Surg* 196:137, 1982.

Stout DJ, Sirak MV, Sullivan BH: Endoscopic sphincterotomy and removal of gallstones. *Surg Gynecol Obstet* 150:673, 1980.

Strom PR, Stone HH: Technique for transduodenal sphincteroplasty. *Surgery* 92:546, 1982.

Stuart M, Hoer S: Late results of choledochoduodenostomy and sphincterotomy for benign disorders. *Am J Surg* 123:67, 1972.

Sullivan DM: Biliary tract surgery in the elderly. *Am J Surg* 143:218, 1972.

Thompson JE, Tompkins RK, Longmire WP: Factors in management of acute cholangitis. *Ann Surg* 195:137, 1982.

Vogt DF, Hermann RE: Choledochoduodenostomy, choledochojejunostomy or sphincteroplasty for biliary and pancreatic disease. *Ann Surg* 193:161, 1981.

White TT, Morgan A, Hopton D: Postoperative pancreatitis. *Am J Surg* 120:132, 1970.

References

1. Hermann RE: A plea for a safer technique of cholecystectomy. *Surgery* 79:609, 1976.
2. Terblanche J: An ischemic basis for biliary structures. *Surgery* 94:52, 1983.
3. Glenn F, McSherry CK: Secondary abdominal operations following biliary tract surgery. *Surg Gynecol Obstet* 121:979, 1965.
4. Molnar W, Stockum AE: Relief of obstructive jaundice through percutaneous transhepatic catheter: A new method. *AJR* 122:356, 1974.
5. Wexler M. Smith R: Jejunal mucosal graft. *Am J Surg* 129:204, 1975.
6. Hepp J, Couinaud C: L'abord et l'utilisation du canal hepatique gauche dans le reparation de la voie biliare principale. *Presse Med* 64:947, 1956.
7. Bismuth H, Lazorthes F: *Les traumatismes operative de la voie behaire prinicpale.* Paris, Masson, 1981.
8. Warren KW, Cristophi C, Armendariz R: The evolution and current prospectives of the treatment of benign duct strictures: A review. *Surg Gastroenterol* 1:141, 1983.
9. Warren KW, Jefferson M: Prevention and repair of strictures of the extrahepatic bile ducts. *Surg Clin North Am* 53:1169, 1973.
10. Warren KW, McDonald WM: Facts and fiction regarding strictures of the extrahepatic ducts. *Ann Surg* 159:996, 1964.
11. Warren KW, Mountain JC, Midell AI: Management of strictures of the biliary tract. *Surg Clin North Am* 51:711, 1971.
12. Zollinger RM, Branch CD, Bailey OT: Instrumental dilatation of the papilla of Vater: Experimental and clinical observations. *Surg Gynecol Obstet* 66:100, 1938.
13. Acosta JM, Ledesma DL: Gallstone migration as a cause of acute pancreatitis. *N Engl J Med* 290:484, 1974.
14. Cooperman M, Ferrara JJ, Carey LC, et al.: ERCP, its use in the evaluation of nonjaundiced patients with the postcholecystectomy syndrome. *Arch Surg* 116:606, 1981.
15. Gregg JA: Postcholecystectomy syndrome and its association with ampullary stenosis. *Am J Surg* 139:374, 1980.

Serious Complications Following Biliary Tract Surgery

BILIARY FISTULAE

Whether a cholecystectomy has been performed, or the common duct opened for exploration, or a cholecystostomy done, a biliary fistula may sometimes develop. A biliary fistula usually comes from the site of an inadvertent tear or perforation created during the time of surgery; alternatively, it may be due to a leakage occurring from the liver bed caused by a tiny canaliculus draining bile. We usually hope that serosalization will produce hemostasis and prevent canalicular oozing of bile. A Penrose drain (with wick) placed in Morison's fossa assists lateral drainage of bile to the exterior. However, when the drainage become excessive, it must be considered abnormal, and distal obstruction must be suspected and immediately sought. Biliary fistulae that develop during surgery should preferably be dealt with at surgery for the best results. If there is a perforation, as stated previously, it should be repaired immediately and drained with a Penrose (wick) drain. If deemed necessary, a bypass operation should be carried out to decompress and redirect the flow of bile into the jejunum or duodenum. A persistent biliary fistula is a serious complication which requires reevaluation with cholangiographic studies; the latter may help establish a diagnosis for persistence of a biliary fistula. Depending upon the cholangiogram, a secondary operative procedure may be required to deal with the distal obstruction, which, not infrequently, may be a stenotic sphincter of Oddi or a missed, retained, or impacted stone. It is possible that an overlooked tumor of the biliary tree, i.e., ampullary carcinoma or carcinoma of the head of the pancreas, may have been the cause of distal obstruction.

The drainage that follows removal of a Penrose drain may be slight, intermittent, diffuse, or persistent. It, too, must be considered to be the result of a fistula and must be doubly checked with cholangiographic studies. It is conceivable that an incomplete cholecystectomy may give rise to a fistula. At times during surgery, what was thought to be a large cystic duct turns out to be a good portion of Hartmann's pouch. These situations call for reoperation, when possible, when the cholecystectomy must be completed. The preferable site of ligation of the cystic duct is about 3 to 5 mm from the common duct wall, depending upon traction, the size of the cystic duct, and the size of the common duct. A cholecystectomy inadvertently performed in the presence of a carcinoma of the head of the pancreas with jaundice, and not discovered at surgery, will result in a disastrous situation. A back pressure created at the common duct outlet will inevitably blow out the cystic duct, producing a biliary peritonitis or, if one is fortunate, a biliary fistula to the exterior.

Wherever a fistula develops, we must think in terms of a distal obstructive lesion or the possible loss of some degree of continuity of the wall of the common duct. It should be kept in mind that a patient may secrete 1,000 to 20,000 cc of bile in 24 hours, and that a continuous or complete diversion of the bile from the common duct to the exterior can result in a serious electrolyte and fluid imbalance. Bile, of course, whenever left in the abdomen, establishes a biliary peritonitis that cannot be dealt with in any way other than by opening the abdomen and draining it. One must not depend on absorption of the bile because a chemical peritonitis is the forerunner of a bacterial peritonitis and subsequent death.

Continuous loss of bile, which contains fluids, electrolytes, and bile salts, can readily deplete the body of these nutrients. While the surgeon must always be cognizant of the fact that fluids and electrolytes must be replaced, he must not forget that the ideal replacement for bile loss is bile itself. This is very difficult to do because of its bilious or bitter taste; even trying to reinstill it directly into the stomach via a Levin tube results in gastric irritation, nausea, and vomiting. To have the patient drink bile is also a nauseating experience which is invariably rejected.

An ileostomy bag with a Karaya gum ring can be placed around the fistula; it serves as an ideal collector of draining bile and prevents irritation to the skin. The ileostomy bag helps to control infection around the stoma; it also collects and measures the bile, thus helping to establish the amount of fluid and electrolytes that must be replaced before the patient can be considered ready for surgical correction of the cause of the fistula.

The ideal procedure after electrolyte and fluid replacement is to inject radiopaque dye into the fistula and visualize the entire biliary tree; this helps to locate the site of injury and/or the site of obstruction. If direct dye injection cannot be performed, it may be more convenient to do an IV cholangiogram, which may also be helpful. There is no more effective procedure than a direct retrograde instillation of dye. An upper gastrointestinal study will at times help in diagnosing a pathological duodenal shadow which may indicate that the ampulla of Vater or the head of the pancreas is involved, causing an obstruction overlooked during the cholecystectomy. This type of obstruction is usually complete, and the surgeon may have to turn finally to laparotomy or percutaneous transhepatic cholangiography. One must also keep in mind that ERCP is capable of obtaining a retrograde endoscopy cholangiogram. This is not always available, but it should be utilized if the facilities and talent are available.

Another cause of biliary fistula is a defect in the continuity of the duodenal wall. Wherever a duodenostomy is performed for inspection and evaluation of the sphincter, ampulla, or duodenum itself, a faulty closure can result in a duodenal fistula that results in a serious loss of duodenal content and bile. This is a serious combined biliary and duodenal fistula because the fluid and electrolyte loss is greater than the bile loss alone. For this reason, this writer recommends using two rows—not one—for closure of a duodenotomy. *In duodenal closure, it is important not to rely on just one row of interrupted sutures. A second row of interrupted (000) silk is more suitable for an effective closure.* A transverse closure is best if the incision was made vertically. In a duodenal fistula, the surgeon must recognize that not only are duodenal and intestinal fluids lost, but also pancreatic enzymes, electrolytes, and bile; the nutritional loss is greater than that occurring with a pure biliary fistula.

A central venous pressure (CVP) line may be necessary for hyperalimentation feeding in order to bring the patient up to the proper nutritional level before any surgery is contemplated. With a strict NPO regimen and a CVP line with intravenous hyperalimentation, it is now possible to have the duodenal fistula close spontaneously. During this management, one must be sure that the patient receives the full daily nutritional requirement without allowing complications to interfere with the progress. This writer does not employ an irrigation sump drain, but merely places a tube at the biliary drainage site and collects the bile with a low-pressure suction apparatus; an alternative procedure is merely to add an ileostomy-type bag to collect the bile and protect the stoma. Irrigation, in the writer's experience, is a stimulus that interferes with healing. To dissect out a fistulous tract and anastomose it into the intestine is passe; it does not work. This fistulous tract in most instances will close spontaneously.

HEMORRHAGE

We must consider the importance of preoperative preparation of the patient. Usually a jaundiced patient will have liver damage, a faulty production of prothrombin, and a deficiency of vitamin K; hence, a prolonged bleeding time. If a patient goes to surgery for gallbladder disease, it is imperative that the preoperative prothrombin time be brought up to a normal level. The coagulation time and partial thromboplastin time (PTT) should also be brought up to approximately normal levels. In longstanding liver disease caused by chronic biliary disease, the bleeding tendency may not only become a difficult problem during surgery but may also become a very serious drawback in the postoperative period. Mephyton or vitamin K_1 (aqueous) is employed intravenously as well as intramuscularly to improve coagulation and bleeding times as well as liver function. A high-protein, high-carbohydrate, low-fat diet is given preoperatively if the patient will tolerate it; if not, a CVP line is utilized for hyperalimentation. The latter will usually bring the patient up to the ideal preoperative level for surgery.

In a poorly prepared patient in whom the prothrombin time has been seriously impaired, the surgeon should not proceed with elective surgery. He may find that though active bleeding is not obvious, continuous oozing that does occur, especially from the liver bed, can become serious. On occasion, this situation requires transfusions during the surgery to make up for the blood loss. A serious laceration of the liver at this time could be disastrous, since the liver already lacks its usual capability to manufacture prothrombin. The greatest preventive care must be given to the patient to prevent undue bleeding. Of course, there will be instances where portal hypertension may be a coexistent factor; here the surgeon has no way to control the situation except to take every precaution possible. One may have to delay surgery as long as possible, reduce the surgery to a minimum, and, in a high-risk patient, do a cholecystostomy as the safest operation.

Whenever an inadvertent cut or tear of the biliary or vascular tree takes place, an immediate repair or ligation must be done as soon as it is discovered. Finger manipulation and careful application of fine noncrushing forceps is the preferred technique. With a specific arterial ligation or a metal clip, the surgeon can save a patient's life. With proper light, trained assistants, and good exposure, the well-trained surgeon, using good judgment, will at this time attain the best possible result, as well as a living patient. The common signs and symptoms after surgery that suggest bleeding are pallor, falling hemoglobin, coldness, sweating, wet skin, restlessness with a rapid pulse, and low blood pressure that continues to fall. Any combination of these early signs and symptoms provides a strong indication that a postoperative patient is bleeding. The dressing should immediately be checked to see if bile alone is draining or whether blood too is present. We look for a "wet" dressing. These factors will help to establish the fact that active bleeding is going on.

The commonest source of bleeding at this early period is from the cystic artery or gallbladder bed. Another source may be from the cystic artery's junction with the hepatic artery or from the right hepatic artery itself. Not infrequently, the portal vein may be torn, perforated, or lacerated sufficiently to produce serious hemorrhage. The patient's hematocrit and hemoglobin begin to fall rapidly, often to a dramatic degree that is usually seen in the postoperative period of cholecystectomy. It is also possible that a hematoma may be forming in the RUQ which can be palpated as a rigid mass in that area. Since the blood is being actively evacuated through the drain, one must not hesitate to reoperate soon. The blood must be replaced and the patient gotten out of shock; only then can the patient be rapidly prepared for reoperation and explored.

The hematoma must be evacuated because, if left, it may become infected and lead to subhepatic and/or subdiaphragmatic abscess. *The writer insists that hemostasis be complete before the abdomen is closed; everything must be rechecked, with all assistants looking to see if the surgeon is correct in proclaiming the field dry.* There are many little tricks that can be utilized to achieve an absolutely dry field before closing the abdomen. One is compression with a warm pack, using a Deaver retractor for added pressure; another is the use of Surgicel, Gelfoam, or sheets of Avitene over the liver surface. Serosalization, when possible, is the best procedure, using a continuous lockstitch. All oozing and arterial and venous bleeding should be stopped with coagulation or clips. When hemostasis is finally secured, a Penrose (wick) drain or Jackson-Pratt suction drain is placed in Morison's fossa and brought out through a lateral subcostal stab wound.

SUBDIAPHRAGMATIC ABSCESS

Still another serious complication is subhepatic and/or subdiaphragmatic abscess. Generally in gallbladder operations, as soon as the abdomen is opened, it is possible for air to travel or dissect above the liver and under the diaphragm, creating a closed air space between the diaphragm and the dome of the liver. This is common, and in time this pneumoperitoneum will absorb. Every now and then, however, a pseudosubdiaphragmatic abscess may form (reported by this writer) in which a definite subdiaphragmatic air bubble with a fluid level will be found on X-ray, associated with elevated temperature and a slight chill. All antibiotics will fail to change the picture. The fluid level may remain despite therapy and surgical intervention, as in the writer's case. In the latter case, this turned out to be nothing but air and serum trapped and sealed between the liver and the diaphragm. The fluid level was created by serosanguinous fluid trapped by trabeculation that occurred soon after opening and exploring the abdomen. When no abscess was discovered, the liver was punctured at its apical portion to see if the abscess was enclosed within the liver itself, but here again, no pus was found.

One must be most hesitant before attempting surgery to look for a late postoperative subdiaphragmatic abscess. Nevertheless, one cannot procrastinate because subdiaphragmatic abscess is a serious condition and can lead to many complications. For example, there may be perforation through the diaphragm into the chest, where a pleuritic abscess or empyema may develop, or the pus may spread, producing severe toxicity. In either case, the patient may die if the pus is not drained by an intervening surgical procedure. However, the greatest precaution that this writer can advise in the prevention of subdiaphragmatic abscess is to avoid passing the hand routinely between the liver and diaphragm, looking for metastatic lesions, when there is no evidence of carcinoma. Routinely passing the hand over the liver and under the diaphragm can create a pneumoperitoneum underneath the diaphragm, and if small amounts of blood or serum move up by gravity, they can be quickly trapped by the rapidly forming fibrinous exudate; in the subsequent postoperative period, a perfect picture of subdiaphragmatic abscess with a fluid level is found. The technique of bringing the liver down routinely with the hand, pushing it down into the abdominal field, also invites infection, especially where there is leakage of infected bile. This writer brings the liver down into the field by applying a clamp to the round ligament and bringing the liver and gallbladder gently into the operative field. The surgeon's hand need not enter the subdiaphragmatic space because one can easily find evidence of metastasis by superficially looking and touching.

Drains should not be placed into the subdiaphragmatic area routinely; only where extensive manipulation was carried out and a suspicion that infectious material exists should subdiaphragmatic drainage be instituted. The subhepatic space should be drained routinely; that is, Morison's fossa should be drained with one or two Penrose (wick) drains brought out through a lateral subcostal stab wound. All drains should be gently removed, starting on the third or fourth day and ending on about the seventh day, depending upon whether bile is still draining. The drain (whether Penrose or Jackson-Pratt) should be removed gently so that it doesn't drag bowel or omentum into the subcostal wound.

Subdiaphragmatic abscess is not a common complication after cholecystectomy, but it must be looked for in every case as a potential complication; and though it is seen in about 5–10% of patients in various clinics and in varying geographic locations, one should presume that it is a potential complication everywhere and at all times. There are certain signs and symptoms that accompany subdiaphragmatic collections of bile and blood: tenderness, palpable mass, leukocytosis with a shift to the left, and an elevated temperature that may or may not be hectic. If the symptoms and signs become more severe with time, jaundice may become an added factor. When infection sets in, the bile and blood convert to abscess formation, and toxic effects become enhanced. The infection may lead to pericholangitis, which becomes a superimposed complication. Whenever there is leakage of bile and blood from the liver bed or from the biliary tree itself, it may be expected to drain by gravity and/or by diaphragmatic action in any direction. Usually blood and bile drain along the liver surfaces and under the diaphragm, so that a subhepatic abscess forms over the liver and under the diaphragm, resulting in a subdiaphragmatic abscess.

Immediate surgical intervention to drain the abscess must be undertaken as soon as the diagnosis is established, or the patient will become more toxic as the morbidity increases. The techniques for subhepatic and subdiaphragmatic drainage are described in the section under "Pseudosubdiaphragmatic Abscess" at the end of this chapter.

BILIARY PERITONITIS

Another serious complication of postoperative biliary tract surgery is biliary peritonitis. Whenever there is leakage of bile into the peritoneal cavity that cannot escape, the bile will extravasate and accumulate to produce local or general biliary peritonitis, which is a chemical form of peritonitis that is unresponsive to medical treatment. In 12 to 24 hours the biliary peritonitis will develop into a suppurative peritonitis, which results in increased mortality. Whenever bile is freed and pours into the free abdominal cavity, it can be dealt with only by surgical intervention. Immediate and appropriate surgery must be carried out to drain off the

accumulating bile; biliary peritonitis does not respond to antibiotics. Any tear or disruption of the biliary tree, including continued leakage from the postoperative gallbladder bed of the liver, may result in a biliary peritonitis. Biliary peritonitis may develop by slow oozing from the liver bed. Peritonitis will also occur when a suture slips off the cystic duct; here the bile pours into the peritoneal cavity, and the situation is worsened because of an unsuspected distal obstruction lower down in the biliary tree exists, i.e., carcinoma of the ampulla or of the head of the pancreas. *Unfortunately those surgeons who sponsor no T-tube or Penrose drainage are not fully convinced of these facts.* If the bile leaks out slowly and accumulates locally, a lesser reaction may still produce pain and rebound tenderness. The overall response will depend on the rate of bile leakage, the location and extent of the peritoneal surface involved, and the condition of the patient. For example, bile escaping around a loosely sewn-in T-tube may invoke an immediate response of pain and tenderness, but if the T-tube and the accessory drains (i.e., Penrose, and Jackson-Pratt) are draining well, the bile leak will be contained and probably correct itself. If a spastic sphincter develops, or if a carcinoma of the head of the pancreas is overlooked, the leak in the common duct will become aggravated, demanding immediate surgical intervention.

Should a surgeon be so unfortunate as to do a cholecystectomy and fail to identify a concomitant carcinoma of the head of the pancreas, the ligated cystic duct will experience undue back pressure and blow out. The backed-up bile will then spill out into the peritoneal cavity. Just such a calamitous case was referred to me many years ago, by another hospital. The patient arrived by ambulance, in shock, intensively jaundiced, and stuporous, with a markedly distended abdomen. No history was obtainable other than that her gallbladder had been removed at the referring hospital. There was no time to remove the patient from her cart and certainly no time for discussion.

The abdomen was quickly prepared for immediate exploration. Anesthesia was contraindicated because of the shock. The recent incision was opened, and out poured a gallon of bile. The abdominal cavity was stained deep green. All the free bile was aspirated, and the remainder was walled off by pockets sealed by multiple synechiae. Visual exposure was impossible until all the synechiae were broken down by finger manipulation and the trapped bile released. Finally, under a reasonably dry field, an obvious hard mass was palpated in the head of the pancreas. Metastatic glands were palpated in the porta hepatis and along the splenic artery. The cystic duct was wide open and still los-ing bile. This duct was religated, and a T-tube was placed in the common duct. The long arm of the T-tube was brought out through a subcostal stab wound. Two Penrose drains (wick) were employed, one below the diaphragm and one in Morison's fossa.

The patient improved rapidly, the jaundice began to disappear, and full consciousness returned. After several days, she was up and around, showing only faint jaundice, feeling no pain, and eating well.

The T-tube drained profusely, and the bile was collected in a receptable at the patient's side. Cobalt therapy was all we had to offer at the time. The patient ultimately died (in less than 1 year).

The moral of this story is: Always do a routine, complete around-the-clock abdominal exploration before proceeding with a so-called routine cholecystectomy.

Recommended Treatment

Biliary peritonitis, when caused by a continuous flow of bile into the peritoneal cavity, is a true surgical emergency. In other words, there is no way of removing bile from the free abdominal cavity unless it is removed physically. Antibiotics cannot help to relieve biliary peritonitis; they can only serve as an adjunct to prevent possible secondary infection. Only surgical intervention can remove the bile, locate its source, and correct the immediate problem. Multiple drains should be placed at the sites where the bile is most likely to collect.

Adjunctive treatment consists of replacement of fluid loss, correction of electrolyte imbalance, and replacement of lost protein. The fluid volume must be restored, and if necessary, a CVP line should be inserted for continuous hyperalimentation. The urinary output and the patient's general condition should be monitored. Hemoglobin and hematocrit studies should be done every 3 hours. The patient will ultimately improve if properly managed in the manner described. However, if the underlying cause is neither an impacted stone nor a spastic sphincter, but rather a persistent obstructing carcinoma of the head of the pancreas, the patient's outlook remains grim. Cholecystojejunostomy, or choleystodirodenostomy may temporarily alleviate the obstructive jaundice.

SPONTANEOUS PERFORATION

Spontaneous perforation of the extrahepatic biliary system is extremely rare. It was reported in isolated individuals as early as 1912. McWilliams[1] reported 90 cases of biliary peritonitis, approximately 10%

of which were nontraumatic perforations of the biliary system. The recommended treatment of course is (1) closure of the perforation when the leak is recognized, (2) cholecystectomy when necessary, (3) operative cholangiography when essential for exploration of the biliary tree to look for additional pathology, and (4) T-tube choledochostomy. Depending upon the findings, these are the possible treatments of spontaneous perforation. Besides taking care of whatever specific causes may exist, this writer places a Penrose (wick) drain into Morison's fossa and brings it out through a lateral subcostal stab wound. A Jackson-Pratt drain may be superior because of its constant suction.

COMMON CAUSES OF BILE LEAKAGE

1. *T-tube* when not hermetically sewn into the common duct.
2. *Anastomotic sites* between the common duct and common duct (end-to-end); common duct and duodenum; common duct and jejunum (Roux-en-Y); hepatic duct and jejunum (end-to side); and intrahepatic duct and jejunum (Longmire operation).
3. *Repair sites* of the common duct (primary closure of a choledochal stoma).
4. *Cystic duct* blowout or faulty ligation; cholecystectomy in the presence of overlooked carcinoma of the head of the pancreas, sphincter of Vater, and lymphomas.
5. *Traumatic* accidents (penetrating or nonpenetrating) or lacerations anywhere in the biliary tract or liver.
6. *Iatrogenic*, i.e., tears or cuts that take place inadvertently at surgery.
7. *Liver biopsy* resulting in bile leakage via the needle tract; bile leakage from overloaded, severed, or anomalous bile ducts during cholecystectomy; cirrhosis of the liver with portal hypertension.
8. *Percutaneous transhepatic cholangiograms;* skinny needles.
9. Failure to recognize active oozing from the gallbladder liver bed; also failure to identify congenital unligated small bile ducts.

Recommended Reading

Jules GI, Conroy PM, Fuelleman RW: Bile leakage following percutaneous transhepatic cholangiography with Chiba needle. *Arch Surg* 112:954, 1977.
McKinzie G: Extravasation of bile after operations on the biliary tract. *Aust NZJ Surg* 24:181,1954.

Reference

1. McWilliams CA: Acute spontaneous perforation of the biliary system into the free peritoneal cavity. *Ann Surg* 55:235, 1912.

PSEUDOSUBDIAPHRAGMATIC ABSCESS

The following is a case report published by this writer that best exemplifies this unusual pathological entity. The etiology, pathogenesis, and treatment are described, as well as recommended precautions to prevent this condition.

A white man, aged 58, was hospitalized on October 15, 1972,[1] with pain in the epigastrium and RUQ, nausea, and vomiting. The only notable past history was cauterization of an anal fissure. His physical examination was unremarkable except for slight tenderness in the RUQ; there was no jaundice at any time. The diagnosis on admission was chronic cholecystitis and cholelithiasis.

On October 18, a laparotomy and cholecystectomy were performed. The lower liver edge was concealed high under the costal margin, and the liver had to be displaced downward before the gallbladder could be removed. A Penrose drain was placed into Morison's fossa and brought out through a subcostal stab wound.

The histopathological report confirmed chronic cholecystitis with cholelithiasis and partial fibrous obliteration of the appendix. The patient was given cephalothin for a low-grade fever after the first postoperative day. The highest rectal temperature was 101.8°F. A chest X-ray on October 21 showed clear lung fields. He was discharged on the 10th postoperative day. Five days later, he was readmitted because of chills, fever, cough, and a sharp pain in the right anterior thoracoabdominal region.

The patient appeared to be slightly ill, but not toxic or jaundiced. His temperature was 100.8°F orally, and his pulse rate was 80 per minute. The right side of the diaphragm did not move on inspiration. Tenderness was elicited approximately at the level of the eighth interspace just anterior to the midaxillary line. Percussion over the right costal area also revealed some tenderness, and there was definite tenderness on deep pressure in the upper quadrant just under the right costal margin. The liver and spleen were not palpated. A chest X-ray showed the lungs to be essentially clear (see Fig. 91). The right hemidiaphragm was higher than the left, with a large air bubble and an obvious fluid level beneath it. X-ray of the abdomen showed the same large air-fluid level on the right side, just beneath the hemidiaphragm. Numerous small air

bubbles were seen around the liver. A barium swallow contrast X-ray showed that the air-fluid level was not related to the nearby bowel. The white blood cell count was 10,000/mm,[3] with a slight shift to the left. The patient was given 80 mg of aminoglycoside (gentamicin) intramuscularly every 8 hours in an attempt to shrink the abscess. After 4 days, his temperature dropped only slightly and the X-ray pictures of the mass remained unchanged.

Surgical intervention using an anterior retroperitoneal approach did not reveal any pus. Intraperitoneal exploration revealed blood clots within a wall of fibrous tissue, with absolutely no evidence of pus. We then thought that an existing mass within the top of the liver which had been interpreted as subphrenic, perhaps a liver abscess, was the cause. But investigation by instrument and finger perforation into the dome of the liver at its softest apical spot still showed no evidence of pus. We then realized that a hemopneumoloculation had rapidly developed under the right diaghragm, simulating a subdiaphragmatic abscess. The area was drained with four separately placed Penrose drains extending from the apex of the liver and brought out through a subcostal stab wound. Culture specimens were taken from many subdiaphragmatic sites.

Postoperatively, the patient's temperature dropped to normal. He felt much better and progressed to complete recovery. X-ray follow-up studies subsequently showed that the gas and fluid levels had completely disappeared. The patient was discharged in excellent general condition.

All culture and sensitivity studies performed at surgery were negative for pathogenic organisms.

Discussion

Subdiaphragmatic or subphrenic abscess is not an uncommon postoperative complication following abdominal surgery for a suppurative pathological process. Occasionally a subphrenic abscess occurs after surgery for a relatively nonsuppurative or noninfected process, e.g., cholecystectomy or gastrectomy. In this case, we found no specific reports of a pneumohemoencapsulation in the subdiaphragmatic space after laparotomy associated with clinical symptoms and signs similar to those of a subphrenic abscess.

Bryan et al.,[2] in reviewing a series of 194 patients who had had extensive major operations, found 4 patients with relatively large volumes of trapped air associated with fluid levels that had to be evacuated. These cases mimicked diaphragmatic abscess but showed no evidence of infection, and the air spontaneously disappeared without sequelae.

Postoperative pneumoperitoneum may be bilateral, but usually localizes in the right subphrenic space. In most instances, the hand separates the liver from the undersurface of the right dome of the diaphragm, and since it is the heaviest upper abdominal viscus, it falls away from the diaphragm, leaving a large air space which persists even when the abdomen is tightly sutured.

Certain operative procedures also affect the distribution of the air; for example, dividing the falciform ligament evenly distributes air under both domes of the diaphragm. According to Bryan et al., the falciform ligament is mainly responsible for maintaining a unilateral pneumoperitoneum. Unilateral distribution of air, with a preference for the right subphrenic space, is subsequently correlated with right-sided pulmonary complications. These include right basal pulmonary collapse (basal atelectasis), dehiscence of the abdominal wound, and delayed restoration of gastrointestinal function. Drains inserted through the abdominal wall have little effect on the incidence of postoperative pneumoperitoneum, but free air can enter the peritoneal cavity along the path of the Penrose drain.

In this case, the unusually high liver had to be displaced downward to facilitate the cholecystectomy. Air must have quickly entered the abdominal cavity and localized in the right subdiaphragmatic space with blood or serum that rolled upward during the operation and accumulated in one area. The latter immediately formed adhesions or fibrosis, or serum producing an encapsulation of air and blood in the subphrenic space and clinically simulated a subdiaphragmatic abscess.

Recommended Reading

Brown DW: Combined lung-liver radioisotope scan in the diagnosis of subdiaphragmatic abscess. *Surg Gynecol Obstet* 1:145, 1963.

Ryan GB, et al: Postoperative peritoneal adhesions: A study of the mechanisms. *Am J Pathol* 65:117, 1971.

References

1. Glassman JA, Kurzer O, Pieck C: Pseudosubdiaphragmatic abscess. *Int Coll Surg* 61:57, 1976.
2. Bryan LA, et al: A study of the factors affecting the incidence and duration of postoperative pneumoperitoneum. *Surg Gynecol Obstet* 117:145, 1963.

11

LAST-RESORT TECHNIQUES FOR THE REMOVAL OF IMPACTED GALLSTONES FROM THE COMMON BILE DUCT

Many articles have been written about the leftover or residual stone in the common bile duct. Even more attention has been devoted to the many techniques devised to remove the residual stone after the failure to remove it at the first surgery. Burhenne's technique involves operating via the fistulous tract created by the T-tube. He employs a long Dormia basket, which he threads along the fistulous tract into the common bile duct. Once he is able to bypass the retained stone, he opens the basket and manipulates it until he traps the stone and lifts it up and out of the common duct. The Burhenne technique is carried out in the X-ray department or the operating room, where, under sedation and light intravenous anesthesia, the procedure is monitored on a TV screen. The helix basket either traps the stone, fragments it, or misses it entirely. Failure to remove the stone calls either for a repeat search operation or a secondary abdominal operation. Though a good percentage of stones are successfully retrieved, one has to contend with the loss of time, psychic trauma, extra hospitalization, and additional expense. A second operation may involve morbidity and even possible mortality. A secondary nonoperative procedure commonly attempted is systemic or local dissolution of the stone. Chenodeoxycholic acid and its related compounds have been employed to dissolve gallstones, but without significant success. Finally, after every possible secondary nonoperative procedure has been tried without success, a second operation must be undertaken with the hope of finally locating and removing the leftover stone. This operation involves greater hospital expense, higher morbidity, and, not infrequently, mortality. Any of these secondary "too late" procedures could conceivably have been avoided. The surgeon, by making certain that all gallstones recognized at the first surgery are completely removed, will do much to prevent the so-called "recurrent" stones in the common duct.

This writer wishes to stress the need to recognize the elusive or impacted gallstone at the first surgery and to resort to every possible trick, tactic, and technique to remove it. Systematic hepatic duct exploration must be carried out routinely to prevent unrecognized leftover hepatic duct calculi from rolling down into the common duct at a later date. Often the surgeon prematurely gives up the attempt to remove an impacted stone, and far too often he resorts to an alternative procedure such as a choledochoduodenostomy (or -jejunostomy). To employ the latter procedure is considered good judgment, but only after every other possible means has been tried to extricate the gallstone without success.

The techniques and instruments employed for removing impacted stones from the common bile duct are varied and at times sophisticated, but never predictably effective. For this and other reasons, biliary instruments have never been standardized or universally accepted. The most frequent causes of postcholecystectomy signs and symptoms such as persistent or recurrent pains and jaundice are (1) retained stone in the common duct; (2) stricture; (3) neoplasm of the papilla of Vater; and (4) infection, usually cholangitis. A recommended procedure for common duct exploration is one that does not allow omissions or margins of error when attempting to remove gallstones from the common and hepatic bile ducts at the initial surgery. If Confucious were alive today, he would say:

First look is best look,
Second look is "too-late" look!

This writer demonstrates (diagrammatically) how a routine common duct exploration is conducted on the uncomplicated choledocholithiasis. Figs. 109 1-2-3-4-5-6-7-8-9. This writer believes that failure to remove all stones from the biliary tract at the first surgery is usually due to the following reasons: (1) The surgeon does not have the patience to locate the stone and remove it. (2) The surgeon may have to end the surgery because a high-risk patient is suddenly not doing well. (3) The hospital may be remiss in not providing the surgeon with the latest well-known and available surgical instruments especially devised to assist him in removing obstinate or impacted stones from the common duct. (4) It is possible that the surgeon may be inexperienced in dealing with unusual and difficult gallstone impactions. Today every hospital should have the various specialized gallstone extractor instruments that are easily available to help the surgeon overcome the formidable gallstone impaction problems and thus simplify whatever procedure is selected to extricate the obstinate calculus. Examples of such specialized instruments are (1) the Glassman-Dormia[1-6] unipolar set; (2) the Glassman bipolar helix basket set; (3) the Storz rigid choledochoscope; (4) the Machida flexible choledochoscope; (5) the Fogarty balloon biliary catheter; (6) the Glassman double-barreled biliary balloon catheter with multiple flexible filiform probes; and (7) Mazzariello-Cipriana forceps. All Glassman gallstone extractor instruments have screw-on attachments that allow them to function singly or in combination with one another. All instruments screw on to the fine, flexible filiform lead probe (see Technique for Removal of Impacted Gallstones). The Storz and Machida choledochoscopes allow the surgeon to look inside the biliary tree; Fogarty was first to employ the bil-

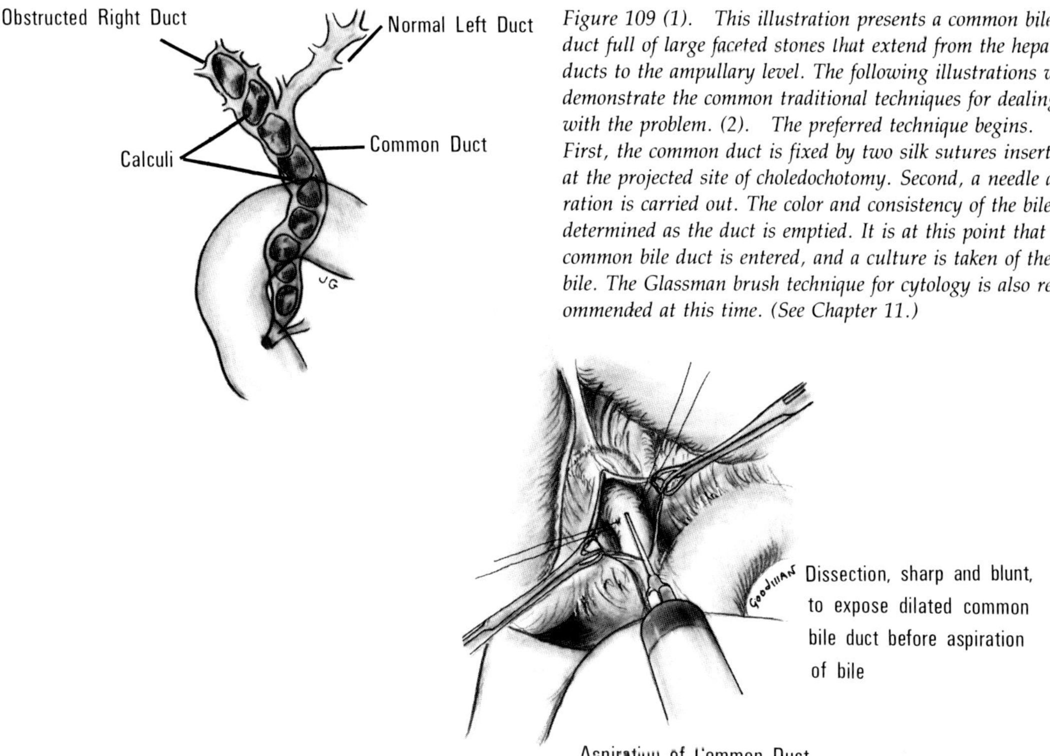

Figure 109 (1).   This illustration presents a common bile duct full of large faceted stones that extend from the hepatic ducts to the ampullary level. The following illustrations will demonstrate the common traditional techniques for dealing with the problem. (2).   The preferred technique begins. First, the common duct is fixed by two silk sutures inserted at the projected site of choledochotomy. Second, a needle aspiration is carried out. The color and consistency of the bile is determined as the duct is emptied. It is at this point that the common bile duct is entered, and a culture is taken of the bile. The Glassman brush technique for cytology is also recommended at this time. (See Chapter 11.)

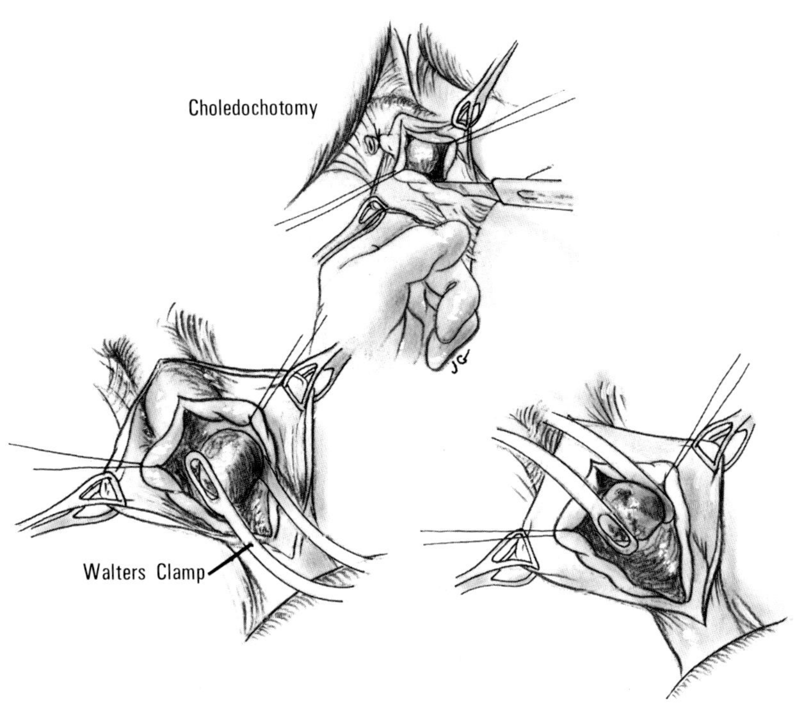

Figure 109 (3).   The common bile duct has been entered and the edges retracted using noncrushing forceps. Since the gallstones are found to be large they are easily grasped by a suit- *able forceps and removed one at a time. The common duct can be "milked" upwardly to more easily deliver the stones lower down in the duct.*

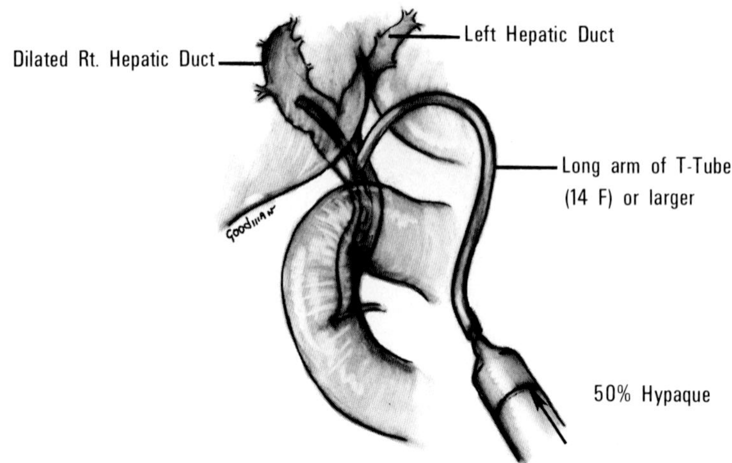

Figure 109 (4). After the common duct is cleared of all the stones, the duct is irrigated with warm saline to wash out the existing debris and small stones. It is here that the author recommends that the common duct be brushed out gently from the right and left hepatic ducts all the way down to the ampulla of Vater. The brush is then sent sterilely to the bacteriology department for culture and sensitivity studies; and from there to the pathology department where, by centrifuging, a cell-block is made for the cytology department. It is now possible to make the earliest diagnosis of carcinoma of the liver, common duct, ampulla, duodenum, and pancreas.

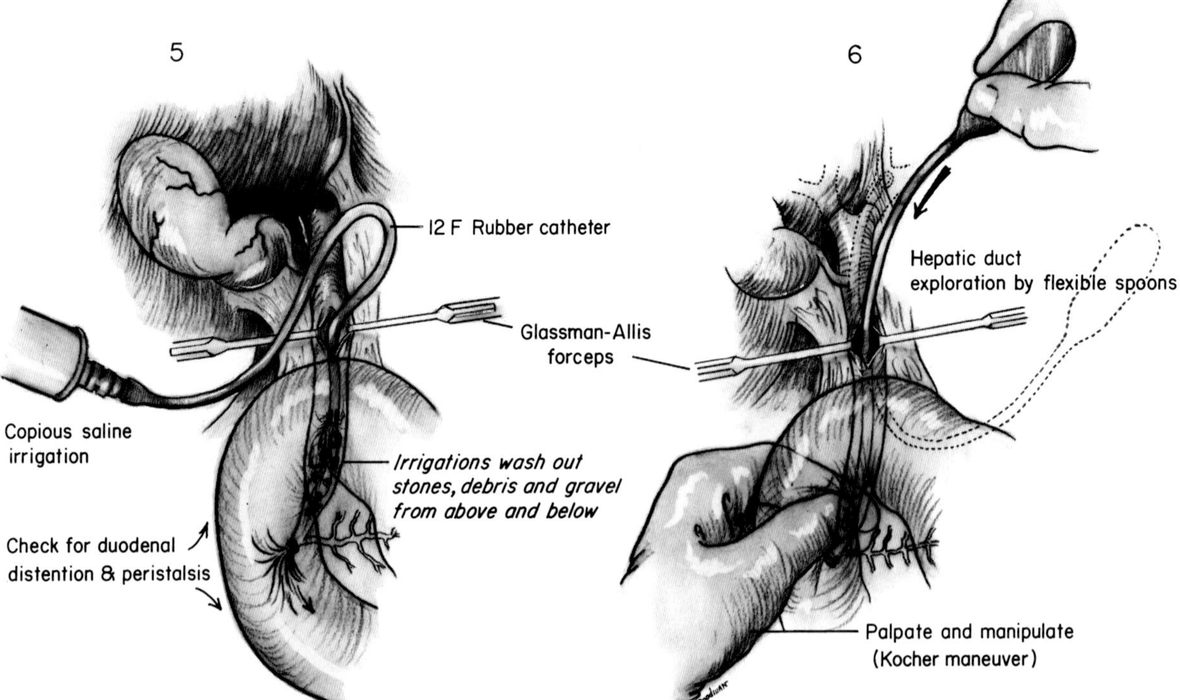

Figure 109 (5) and (6). illustrate the method of common duct irrigations. It is most important to repeat the irrigations and they should consist of copious amounts of warm saline. Probing and spooning the right and left hepatic ducts are most important, yet are frequently overlooked. When the usual and traditional techniques for removing stones from the common duct fail, the surgeon should waste no more time; he should switch immediately to other alternate techniques for removing intractible and impacted gallstones. (See Chapter 11.)

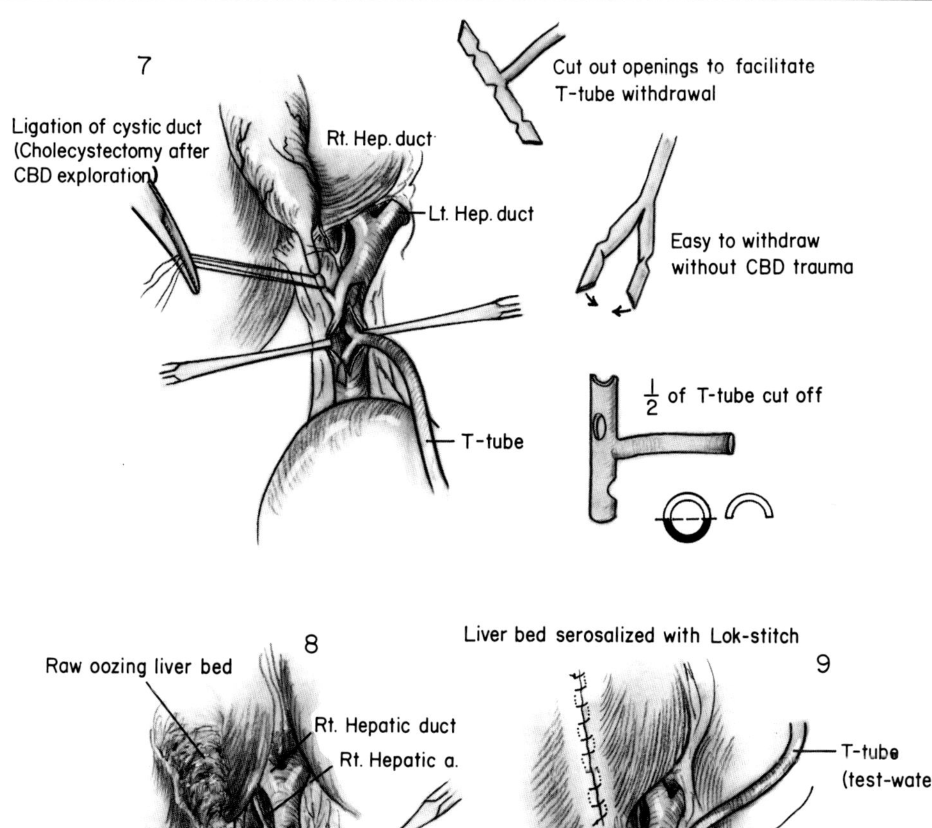

Figure 109 (7), (8), (9).   Ligation of the cystic duct (chole-cystectomy after CBD exploration) and the T-tube brought out through a subcostal stab-wound and anchored with black silk sutures. See Chapter 12 on choledochotomy and common bile duct exploration for more indications for T-tube drainage.

iary balloon catheter; the Mazzariello clamp permits wider separation of its jaws within the common bile duct.

By employing any one or any combination of these modalities, the surgeon can significantly simplify and overcome almost any impacted gallstone problem. Unquestionably, the surgeon will lower the present unacceptably high percentage of leftover stones in the common duct. During the past several years, the probe, basket, and brush technique has been improved and a new and improved set of interrelated instruments has been developed, as well as new techniques that will further assist the surgeon in removing the more elusive and impacted ductal stones at the first operation. Thus, the number of secondary operations will, hopefully, be reduced. The wire basket is shaped like a helix and can be opened, closed, or contracted at either end of the instrument. This means that the basket is bipolar and can be manipulated simultaneously from the choledochotomy stomal site above and at the duodenotomy below. With this new technique, a unique set of interrelated instruments are used that were first introduced by the author in 1964. Since then, the Dormia basket has been modified by the writer so that it now serves a double role in trapping the elusive gallstone in the common bile duct from either above or below. The new instruments are designed to work between these two openings; the maneuvers used are up-and-down movements and twisting back-and-forth manipulations. The impacted stone is first dislodged, then trapped, and finally removed while still in the grasp of the contracting basket. The instruments are used either singly or in combination. A most significant feature of these instruments is that they employ mechanical forces that are opposite of those used by the older flexible spoons, probes and forceps: namely, an upward *uncorking* maneuver.

Since 1964, when this writer first introduced the interrelated set of probe, basket, brush instruments, and combined choledochoduodenotomy technique, both instruments and technique have undergone significant modifications—so much so that they now offer even greater opportunities for effective removal of subborn impacted gallstones at the first surgical attempt. The uni- and bipolar baskets remain essentially the same, except that they now screw onto multiple 4-, 8-, or 10-inch long fine, flexible filiform probes that precede them in order to bypass the impacted stone more effectively. Where the Glassman flexible probe and Fogarty biliary balloon catheter have previously failed to bypass the occasional impacted stone, the new fine, flexible filiform probes will successfully do so. Failure to bypass the impacted stone means that the gallstone must inevitably be *approached from below via duodenotomy* rather than from above via choledochotomy. This, of course, means additional surgery (Fig. 110).

If the surgeon decides to remove the impacted gallstone from below via duodenotomy, he has a choice of two techniques.

Technique 1

The surgeon employs a metallic malleable probe with a screw-on blunt tip that can be unscrewed once it emerges from the ampullary (duodenotomy) stoma. A Glassman-Dormia basket is now screwed

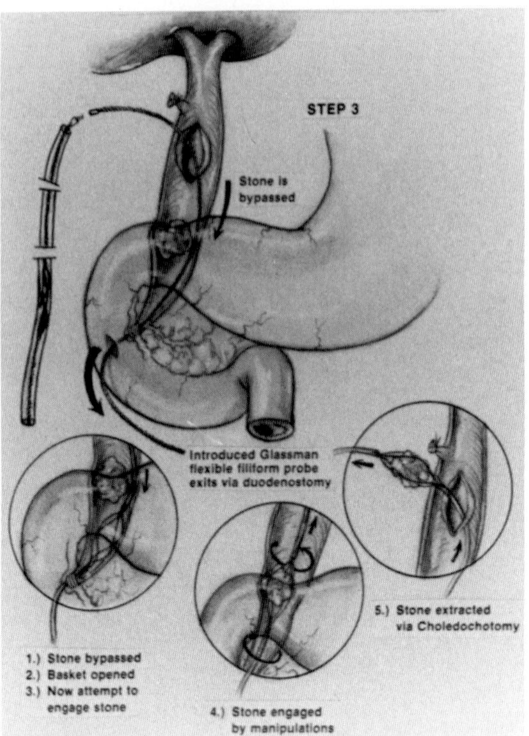

Figure 110. Demonstration of the filiform probe passing out of the ampullary stoma and the basket opened below the gallstone. By up and down, side-to-side movements as shown with arrows the helix basket entraps the stone and removes it via the choledochotomy stoma. See inserts.

on to the bare tip, and the collapsed basket is gently drawn up into the lumen of the common bile duct. The basket is opened and maneuvered until the stone is trapped in the basket and removed via the choledochotomy stoma (Figs. 110, 111).

Technique 2

The surgeon employs a metallic malleable probe that has a fine, blunt tip at its lead end and a female screw-on attachment at its rear end (Fig. 112). The fine, blunt-tipped end is inserted into the ampullary stoma and directed upward to reach the impacted stone. By gentle upward thrusts, the stone is disimpacted. Once the stone is freed, the probe continues upward and bypasses the stone to emerge from the choledochostomy stoma. A Glassman uni- or bipolar basket instrument is screwed onto the end of the probe and drawn upward into the lumen of the common duct. The basket is opened and manipulated until the stone is engaged within the basket and lifted out through the choledochotomy

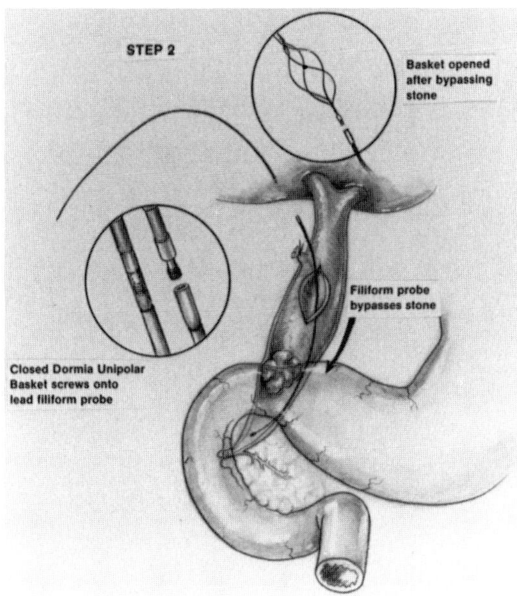

Figure 111. Illustration showing both a unipolar basket (a single basket at the end), and a bipolar basket (the basket is situated in the middle). The filiform No. 4 is gently advanced so that it exits the ampullary stoma; by palpating the common duct and duodenum, one determines that the collapsed basket is ready to be opened and manipulated to entrap the stone.

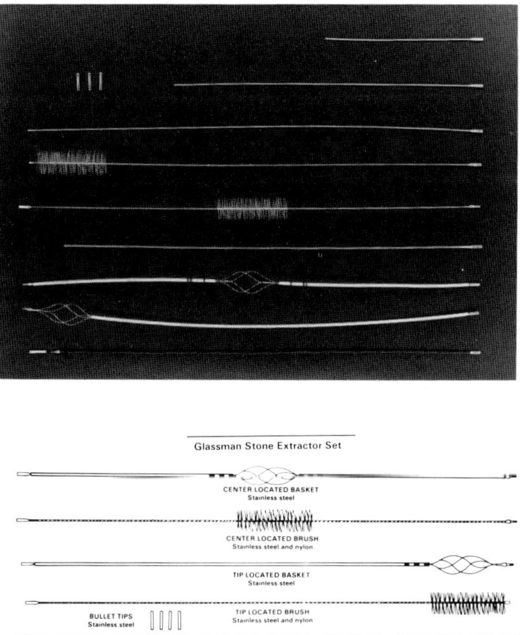

Figure 112. The Glassman Stone Extractor Set.

stoma. If the stone is best removed from below via the ampullary stoma, a preliminary sphincterotomy should be performed.

Gallstone Extractor Instruments

The flexible, semirigid guide probe has two screw-on attachments, male and female, one at either end. A special helix-designed spring basket has been devised to be manipulated, i.e., completely opened, partially opened, or closed by a newly created bipolar sleeve mechanism in which the centrally placed helix-type basket may be manipulated and controlled from either end. This basket is made of fine stainless steel spring wire and has male and female screw-on attachments at either end (see Figure 112). The basket trap was given a helix shape on purpose so that, by being twisted back and forth, it ensnares and traps the gallstones. When the plastic sleeves are manipulated, either from above or below (choledochotomy stoma or

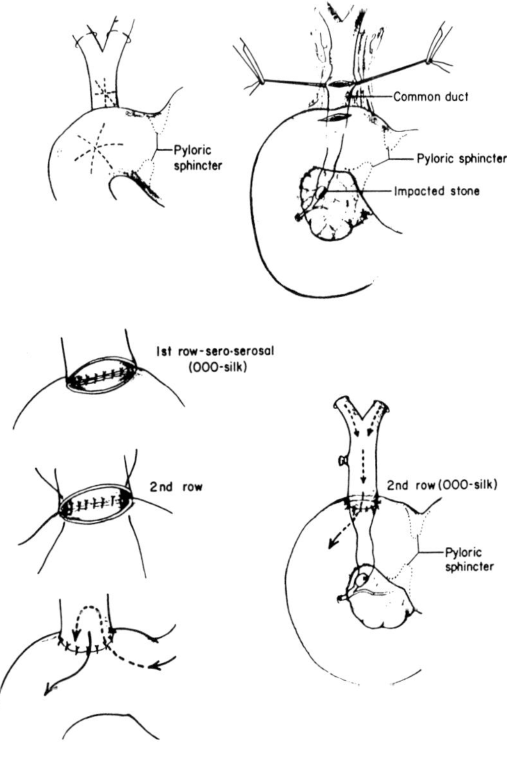

Figure 113. The technique for a recommended choledocho-duodenostomy. When all measures fail to remove the impacted gallstone from the common duct, this procedure is considered acceptable. It is not without certain drawbacks.

240

ampullary stoma), whichever is considered best. The basket is opened to any desired size. Manipulation of the basket should preferably begin at the lower end of the common bile duct. Since the lowest portion of the common bile duct narrows to an extremely small semifixed diameter, the basket is minimally expanded. As the diameter widens, the basket opens as it is drawn up higher into the wider portions of the common bile duct. By manipulating both ends of the nylon brush, the surgeon can (for the first time in biliary history) gently and safely "sweep" the lumen of the common bile duct of all its debris, small stones, and gravel. The male and female end portions of the nylon brush permit it to be attached to any of the other interrelated instruments that enter or exit the common bile duct, either through the choledochotomy stoma site or via the ampullary stoma.

It should also be mentioned here that there is a prophylactic value in routinely but carefully dilating the ampulla of Vater during exploration of the common duct. To omit this procedure may mean a failure to ascertain whether or not an organic obstruction, such as a stricture, carcinoma, or impacted stone, is present. Unfortunately, the small stones and gravel particles that are left over in the biliary tree may not easily pass through the ampulla of Vater in the postoperative period. Gentle dilation of a mild stenosis of the sphincter of Oddi is considered a good prophylactic measure against postcholecystectomy syndrome and pancreatitis. Failure to dilate an ampullary stricture successfully may necessitate a secondary procedure requiring either a transduodenal or an endoscopic approach for sphincterotomy. The latter procedure has strict indications and should not be carried out routinely.

The writer concedes that for one reason or another it may become necessary for the surgeon and/ or the anesthetist to terminate the procedure, in which case the surgeon may decide to quickly sew in a T-tube and close the abdomen. Alternatively, the surgeon may decide to do a palliative choledochoduodenostomy (or - jejunostomy) (Fig. 113); in either instance, a follow-up plan may be contemplated, in which case an attempt to dissolve the stone will be made. If there is an impacted gallstone that is resistant to removal by any of the traditional techniques (i.e., spooning, forceps, irrigations, and probes), the surgeon should proceed at once with the writer's recommended standard operating procedure:

1. The Glassman-Dormia unipolar multi-filiform basket, probe, and brush technique; if this technique fails, the surgeon should try:

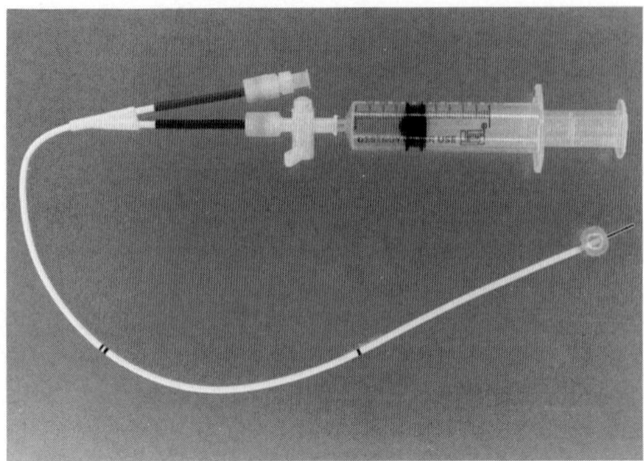

Figure 114.   The Glassman-Fogarty biliary balloon is attached to the hypodermic syringe containing water; note stopcock that allows balloon to remain distended without the hand on the plunger. Note the two channels within the single catheter. The balloon is shown distended to more clearly show its position relative to the proximal two openings and the distal screw-on tip.

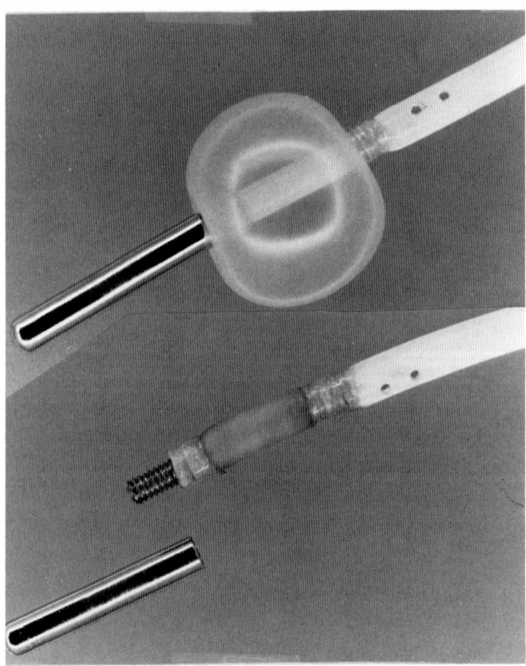

Figure 115.   Enlargement of the Glassman-Fogarty biliary balloon catheter tip. The blunt metal tip is screwed onto the male screw-on end of the portion of the catheter. The balloon is collapsed and the two stomata are clearly shown proximal to the balloon.

2. The Glassman double-barreled biliary balloon with filiform catheter technique; if this technique fails, the surgeon may try (Figs. 114, 115):
3. The Storz rigid choledochoscope, if the hospital has one and if the surgeon knows how to use

it. If this instrument does not work, the surgeon may try the flexible Machida choledochoscope. If it is not available, or if it cannot free and remove the impacted stone, then the writer recommends (Figs. 116, 117, 118):

4. The Glassman combined choledochoduodeno-tomy procedure, in which the surgeon employs the Glassman uni- or bipolar helix basket and brush technique. The procedure involved here is known as the *uncorking principle* or the *retrograde technique*, in which the gallstone is disimpacted from below upward and removed either from above or below (see Fig. 119).

The new gallstone extractor instruments were not intended for routine explorations of the common duct; their

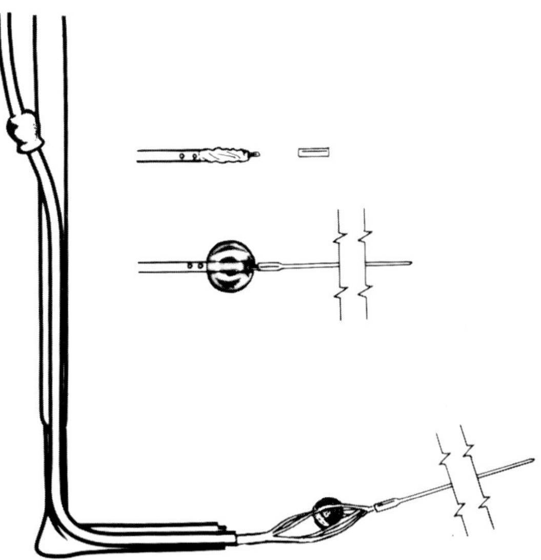

Figure 117. Shown here is the collapsed balloon with screw-on end. Insert illustrates the tip itself.

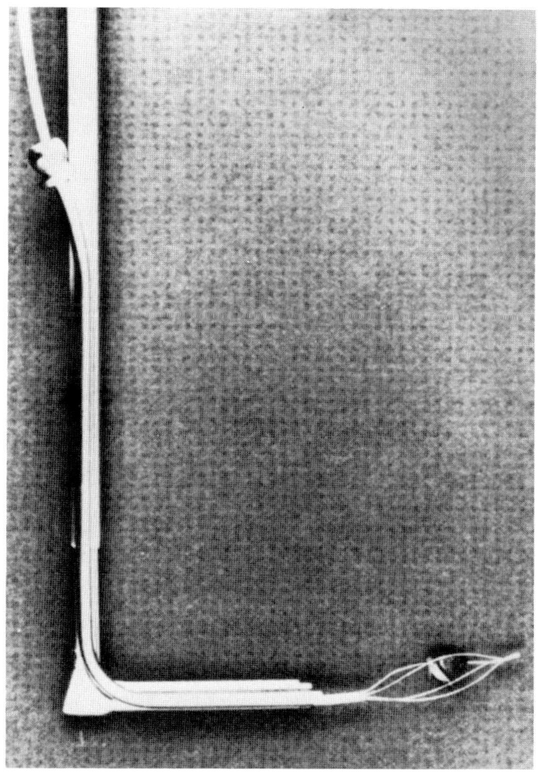

Figure 116. This photograph illustrates how as a last-resort technique, the flexible filiform probe may be passed through the large channel in the choledochoscope under direct visualization in order to successfully bypass the impacted gallstone. The Glassman-Dormia basket is screwed onto the female portion of the filiform probe, and in its collapsed form is advanced beyond the stone. At this time the basket is manipulated from above until the stone is entrapped. When it is time for the withdrawal of the trapped stone, all the instruments—namely, choledochoscope, basket instrument, and filiform probe—are removed in one maneuver.

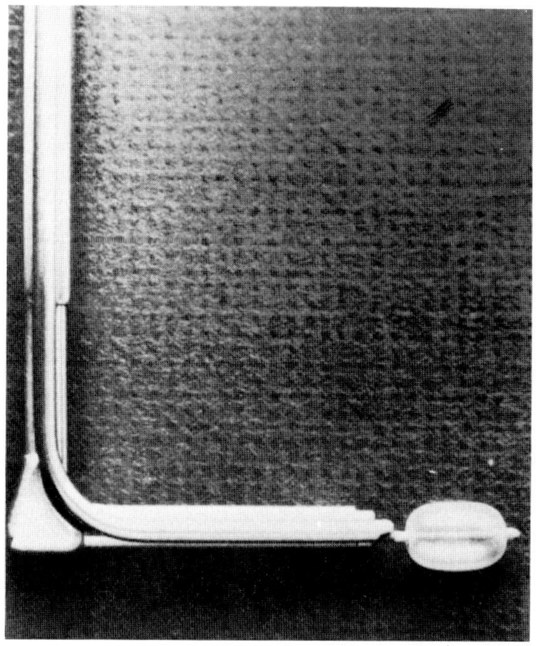

Figure 118. The flexible filiform probe is passed through a channel on the side of the choledochoscope and under direct vision, attempts are made to bypass the impacted gallstone. The balloon catheter is screwed onto the female portion of the filiform lead probe, and advanced beyond the stone. The balloon is inflated to about 3 ml of water or air. The Glassman biliary catheter provides a stop-cock to close-off the balloon channel to free both hands. When the stone has been bypassed, the balloon is lifted up with the stone, and choledochoscope. If there is a question regarding positions of the stone and balloon, a 50% Hypaque solution is instilled into the second channel of the catheter and an x-ray will reveal their exact relationship.

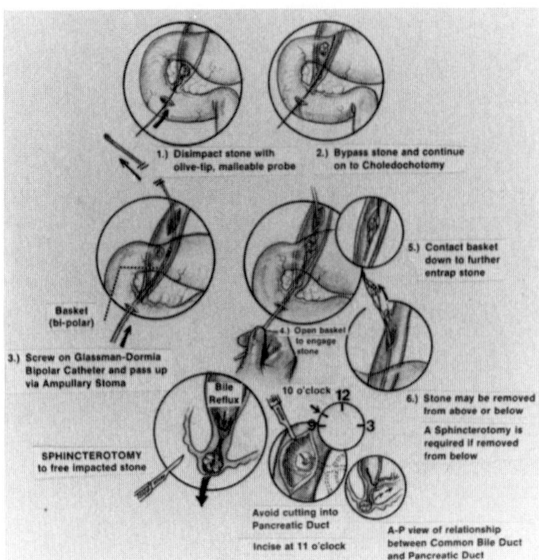

Figure 119. Illustrated here is the author's retrograde technique for removing a low-lying impacted gallstone in the common duct. A duodenotomy is performed. A fine, flexible blunt-tipped probe with a female screw-on attachment at the other end is employed to gently pass through the ampullary stoma and disimpact the stone upwardly into a wider diameter of the common duct. Having displaced the stone upwardly the probe continues to advance in an upward direction bypassing the stone as it makes its way out of the choledochotomy stoma. At this point the male screw-on portion of the bipolar basket catheter is screwed onto the female screw-on portion of the blunt-tipped probe. The flexible probe is now ready to draw up the bipolar basket catheter into the common bile duct. As the basket portion passes into the duct at its lowest level, the baskets are allowed to open gradually either from above or below. The open basket is now manipulated back and forth and up and down in order to ensnare the stone. After the stone is entrapped it may be removed either from above (choledochotomy stoma) or from below via the ampullary stoma. If it appears to be more preferable to remove the stone from below then a preliminary sphincterotomy should be done.

use is recommended only in specific last-resort instances such as the following:

1. Whenever an elusive stone or stones are discovered on the operative cholangiogram, and all the usual extraction methods and instruments have failed.
2. Whenever an operative cholangiogram reveals the existence of a resistant second- or third-degree impacted gallstone.
3. Whenever a duodenotomy is performed in order to extract a gallstone via the ampullary stoma.
4. Whenever multiple smaller stones are found in the common duct and the usual extraction methods have failed to remove all of them.
5. Whenever great amounts of debris, gravel, and smaller stones cannot be completely removed by irrigations alone. "Sweeping" the common duct with the nylon brush will help to accomplish it.
6. Whenever a stone is suspected or palpated but the cholangiogram fails to reveal it, and routine extraction measures have failed.
7. Whenever an operation is performed for extrahepatic obstructive jaundice and no pathology is found, yet an elusive or missed stone is suspected.
8. Whenever a second or third operation is performed for postoperative, recurrent, or persistent jaundice with colic or chills and an impacted or ball-valve stone is suspected.

Before exploring the common bile duct, the surgeon should consider the prerequisites. He should know that the common bile duct may be angulated, curved, or kinked. The duodenum should be reflected medially, and the descending fixed portion of the duodenum should be freed and depressed downward. This maneuver, known as the *Kocher maneuver*, will help to straighten out most existing angulations and allow easier and more accurate manipulation within the common bile duct. The surgeon must first determine whether the gallstone is truly fixed or impacted and whether it is or is not movable. The most likely site of obstruction must be ascertained; this is vital in deciding whether the impaction should be considered first-, second-, or third-degree impaction.

The classification of impaction is as follows:

First-degree impaction of the gallstone refers to an incompletely obstructed stone. With judicious and expert manipulations utilizing traditional biliary instruments, the surgeon can remove it with the further aid of irrigations. Fogarty's biliary balloon catheter has been used effectively in non-impacted gallstones of the common duct. (Fig. 120).

Second-degree impaction of the gallstone indicates that the calculus is fixed in the narrow portion of the common duct. The stone may or may not be capable of disimpaction but every effort should be made. By utilizing the more sophisticated biliary instruments that are now available, the stone can more readily be extracted. This, of course, requires the use of special biliary balloon catheters, the helix basket, and brush instruments.

If every effort has been made to disimpact the stone without success, then the impaction must be labeled a *third-degree impaction*. Once a reasonable effort has been made to disimpact and remove the stone using the procedures described above, but without success, the procedure recommended below should be employed (Figs. 121, 122, 123). These procedures are known as *multi-filiform-helix basket*

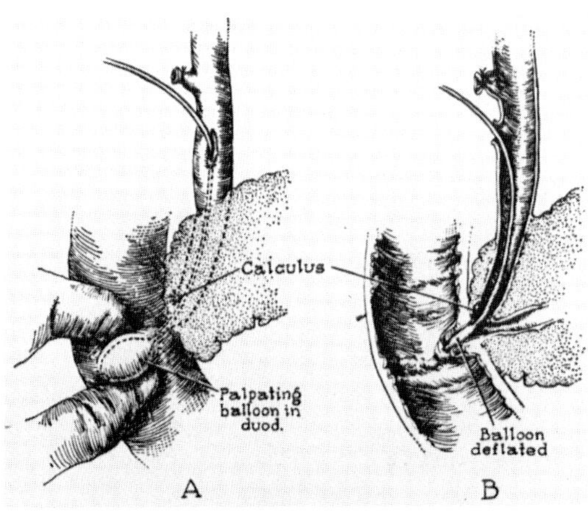

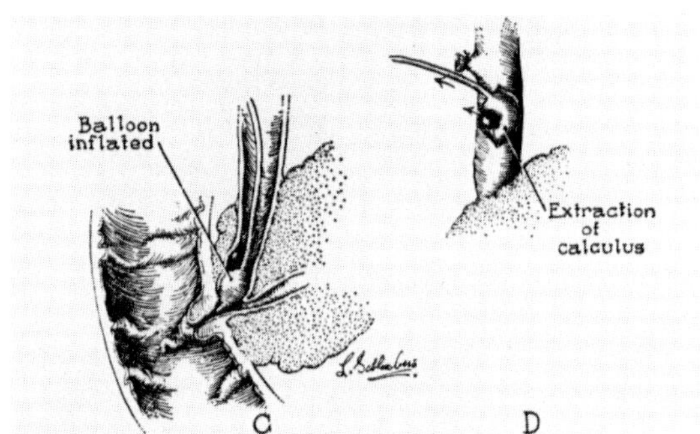

Figure 120.   Confirmation of patency of the ampulla of Vater and removal of a free-floating calculus (Fogarty technique).

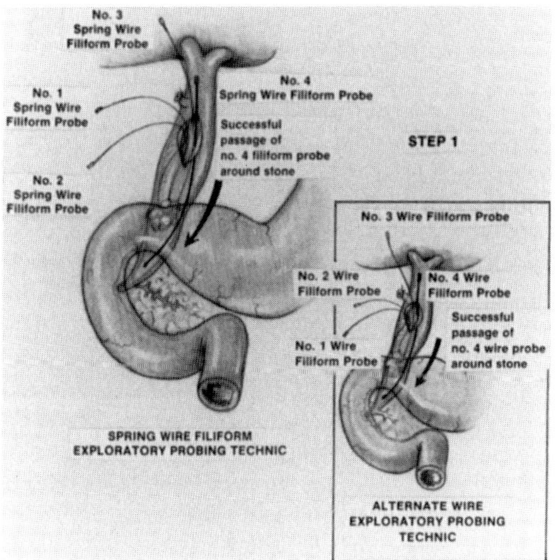

Figure 121.   Step 1—illustrated here is the new technique of employing multiple fine filiform probes via the choledochostomy stoma in order to bypass the impacted gallstone. Shown also is the filiform probe passing the stone. It is at this point that the basket is slowly opened and manipulated.

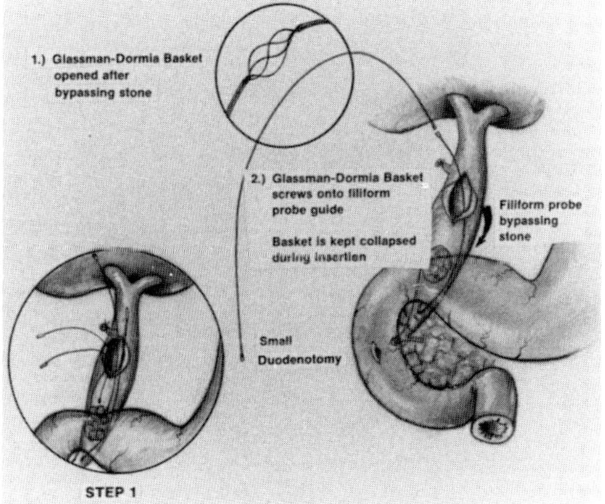

Figure 122.   Illustration shows the variable ways that the fine flexible filiform probes may bypass the stones or pass between them. Should the filiform probe extend in between the stones, it is considered acceptable to proceed with removing them. All that is required is that the basket be able to bypass the stones to entrap them.

Figure 123.   Illustrated here is a Glassman unipolar type helix basket that screws onto the female-end portion of the remaining filiform probe. A unipolar basket has only one basket located at the end of the instrument and is manipulated from the opposite end. The bipolar basket is in the middle and may be operated from either end. See inserts.

and *multi-filiform biliary-balloon catheter* techniques. They will be fully described in detail under their headings below.

Technique 3

For second- and third-degree gallstone impaction, the first procedure should be the combined Glassman-Dormia-basket (uni- or bipolar) and multi-filiform probe technique (Figs. 121, 122, 123).

An 8- or 10-inch fine, flexible filiform probe is inserted into the choledochotomy stoma and gently manipulated downward until the stone is encountered. Manipulations are continued in order to bypass the stone. If the fine, flexible probe fails to bypass the stone, then the probe is left in place, and a second probe is inserted and manipulated to bypass the stone. If this probe cannot bypass the stone, a third probe is inserted and manipulated. The fourth and fifth probe are then employed while the other probes remain in place. This form of probing must be continued until one flexible filiform probe bypasses the stone. All filiform probes except the one that has bypassed the stone are then removed. To the end portion of the filiform probe, a unipolar Glassman-Dormia helix basket is screwed on, and the combined two instruments are gently advanced downward until the collapsed basket is felt to be beyond the level of the stone and the tip end of the filiform probe has advanced into the duodenum (Figs. 121, 122, 123).

The basket is now opened and manipulated up and down, and twisted around and around, until the surgeon feels that the stone has been unsnared. At this point, the basket is tightened in order to better grasp the stone and more easily lift it out. The basket containing the stone is carefully and gently lifted out of the common duct. Do not remove the filiform lead probe completely; it should remain in its advantageous position, i.e., below the stone level, in case repeated attempts are required to engage and extract the stone. If the stone is not ensnared, this procedure should be repeated until it is finally trapped and removed. If it is decided that a kinked or angulated common duct is interfering with the delivery of the stone, a Kocher procedure should be carried out with the expectation that instrumentation will be more accurate and effective. After the descending duodenum is undermined, it is reflected medially and straightened out by being pressed downward. If the stone cannot be ensnared by the basket, the balloon technique or the Glassman double-barreled biliary balloon

catheter with multiple flexible filiform probes should be tried.

Technique 4

The second technique used for second- and third-degree gallstone impactions should be with a combined *Glassman double-barreled balloon catheter with multiple flexible filiform probes* (Figs. 124, 125, 126, 127, 128, 129). An 8- to 10-inch fine, flexible filiform probe is inserted into the choledochotomy stoma and gently manipulated downward until the stone is encountered. Manipulations and probings are carried out with the hope of bypassing the impacted stone. If the flexible filiform probe cannot bypass the stone, it is left in and a second filiform probe is inserted with the same purpose. The same procedure is repeated with a third and a fourth probe, if necessary. If the surgeon feels that it is still possible to bypass the stone, he should continue to probe for a successful bypass by removing filiform 1 and reinserting it. Failing to bypass again, the surgeon should remove filiform 2 and reinsert it. If one probe succeeds in bypassing the gallstone, all the others are removed. The Glassman double-barreled balloon catheter should be screwed onto the female end portion of the filiform probe and the united two instruments advanced downward gently but firmly until the flexible probe passes out of the ampulla into the duodenum and the collapsed balloon bypasses the stone (Figs. 124, 125, 126, 127, 128). If the exact position of the balloon is uncertain, the catheter is provided with another inlet (blue color), which will allow the surgeon to instill 2 or 3 cc of Hypaque dye in order to double-check the location of the stone (or stones) in relationship to the balloon (Figs. 125, 126). If no adjustment is necessary, the balloon is inflated with 3, 4 and 5 cc of air or saline. A stopcock is provided to lock the inflated balloon in order to permit the surgeon to use both hands (Figs. 114, 115). The catheter is now gently and firmly raised out of the common duct, and with it the impacted stone (or stones). At this point, the common bile duct is irrigated and followed by a sweeping out of any existing tiny stones, mud, or gravel from the common bile duct (Fig. 128). The Glassman nylon brush is ideal because its centrally placed nylon bristles are most suitable for this problem. The new common bile duct brush is made of soft nylon and comes in several diameters to accommodate various common duct sizes (Fig. 112 b. and d.). This brush is disposable, and serves new and important func-

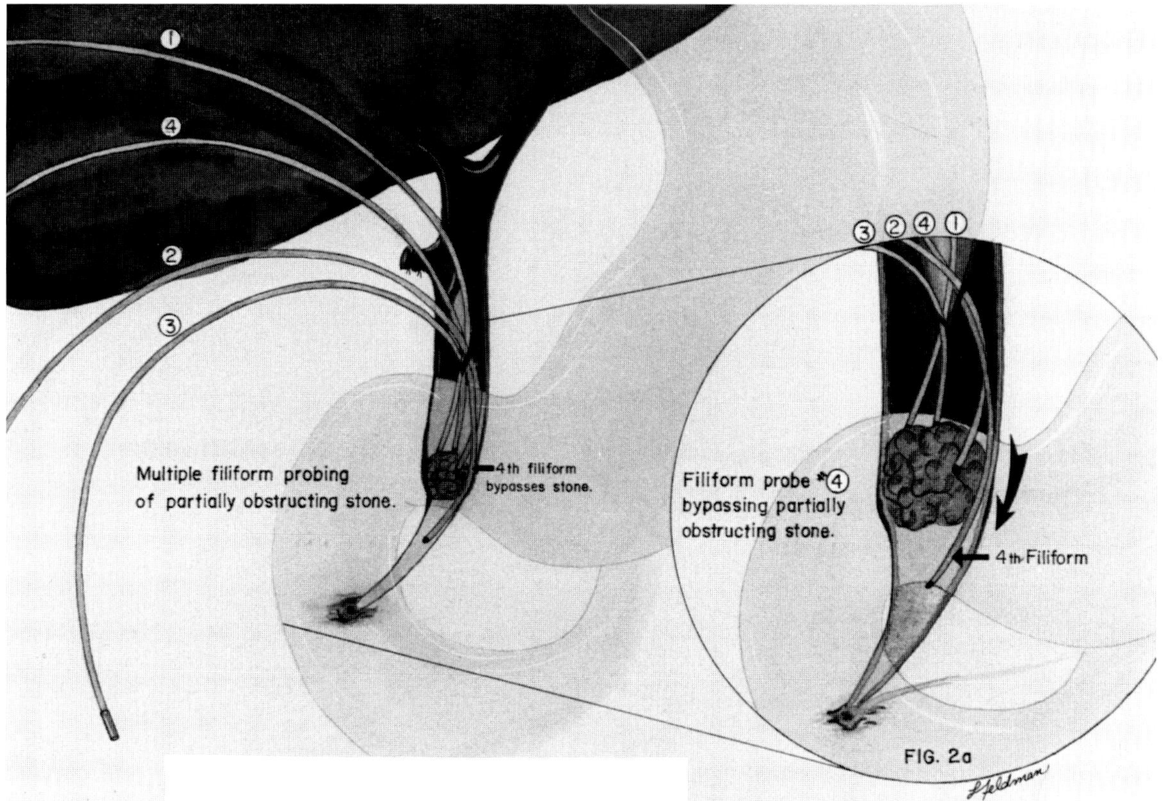

Figure 124.   Multiple flexible filiform probes (1, 2, 3, and 4) are probing the common duct stone in order to bypass it. If one filiform probe successfully bypasses the stone, the rest of the filiform probes are removed. Note that #4 filiform probe has bypassed the stone, and is ready to be connected with the screw-on end of the biliary balloon catheter.

tions. Besides sweeping out the debris from the lumen of the common bile duct quickly and efficiently, it is also used for culture and sensitivity studies, as well as for cell block biopsy. The brush, being disposable, is sent to the department of bacteriology under sterile conditions for culture and sensitivity. From the laboratory, the brush is sent on to the pathology department, where the bristles are immersed in sterile saline and shaken to loosen the attached cells. The fluid is then centrifuged to produce a cell block for a possible unrecognized pathological diagnosis related to the common bile duct, liver, papilla of Vater, duodenum, or pancreas (Fig. 129). *The brushing procedure must become routine whenever the common bile duct is opened and explored.* No one can dispute the contention that a routine precaution against infection and neoplastic changes of the common duct, ampulla, duodenum, and pancreas is useful. It is this writer's routine after the common duct has been cleared of all stones, gravel, and mud. Proceed now in indicated cases to gently dilate the sphincter of Oddi. To omit this procedure could mean the failure to ascertain

whether or not an organic obstruction, i.e., stricture, carcinoma, or impacted stone, is present. There are several advantages to minimal but careful dilation of the ampulla: (1) Small stones and gravel particles inadvertently left over in the tree will pass more easily through a dilated ampulla of Vater, especially when assisted with adequate irrigations. (2) Dilatation of a stenosis of the sphincter of Oddi is considered a good prophylactic measure and treatment against postcholecystectomy syndrome and pancreatitis. Gentleness and a maximum dilatation of 3–5 mm are recommended. (3) Failure to dilate an ampullary stricture successfully may necessitate a secondary procedure requiring a transduodenal or endoscopic sphincterotomy. The latter procedure has strict indications and should not be carried out routinely.

If the T-tube choledochogram reveals a missed stone, the same exploratory procedures must be repeated. The T-tube should be removed and the stone diligently searched for and removed. If there are extenuating circumstances that contraindicate continuation of the surgery, the operation should

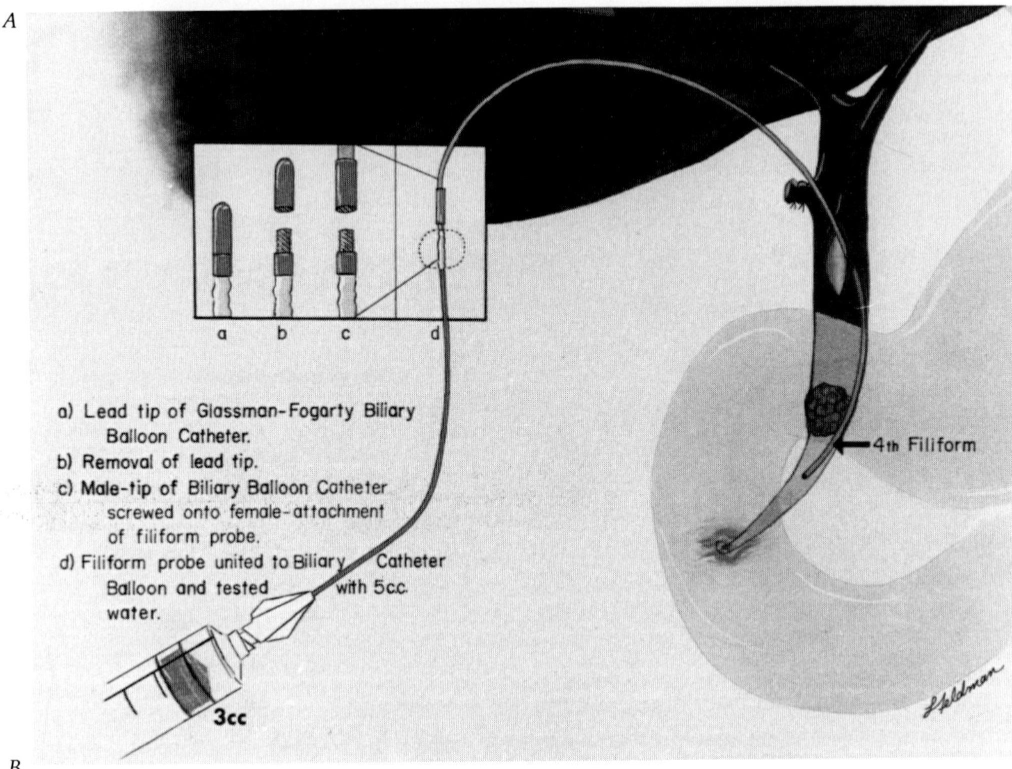

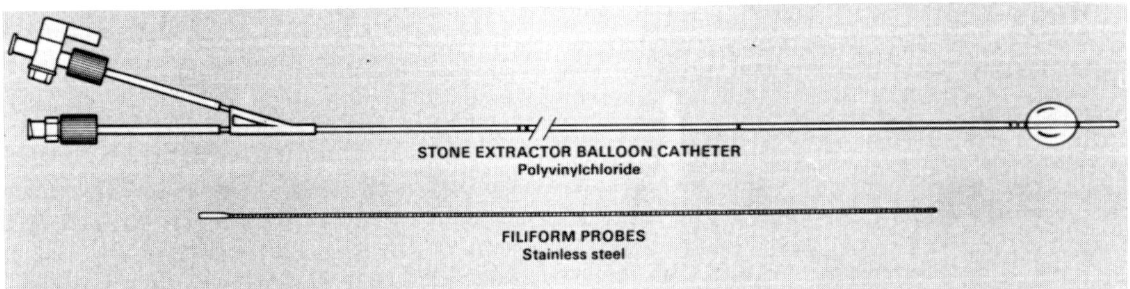

Figure 125.   A. Illustrates the filiform catheter leading the Glassman biliary balloon catheter beyond the stones, where the balloon is inflated. B. Illustrated also is the withdrawal of the inflated ballon and with it the gallstone.

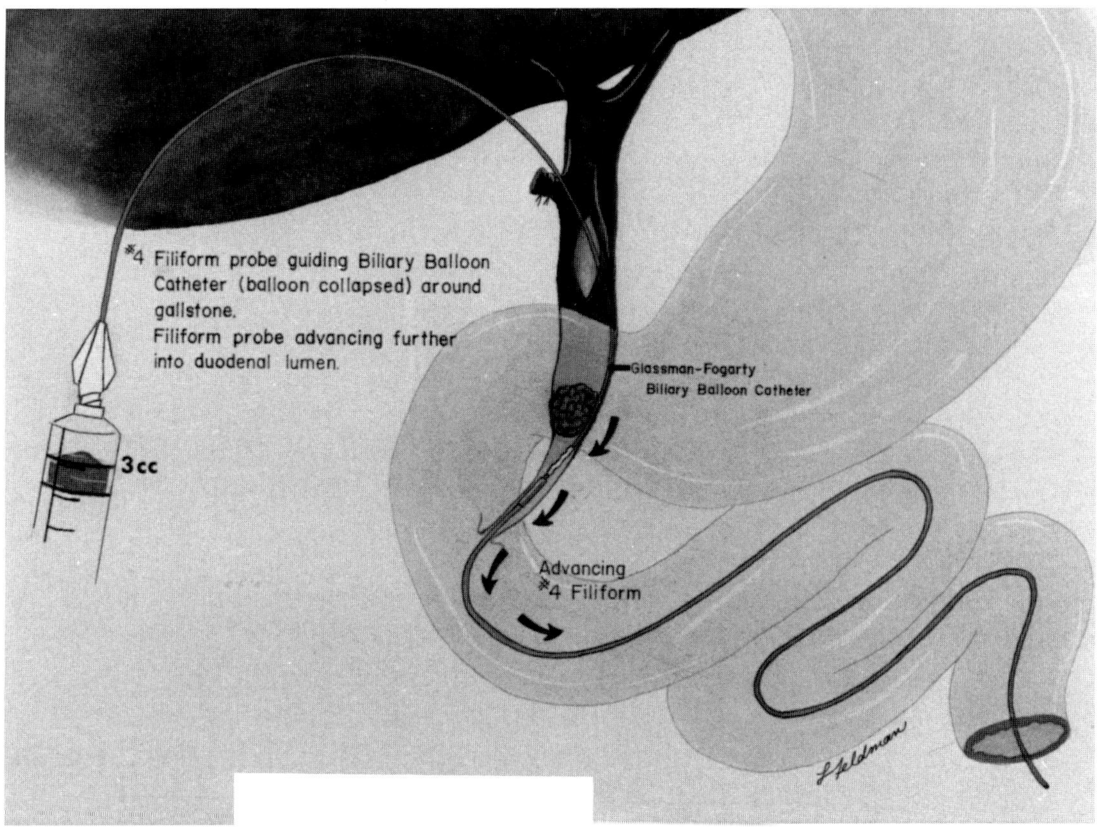

Figure 126. The biliary balloon catheter now attached to the No. 4 filiform probe is advanced downwardly so that it *passes through the ampullary stoma and threads itself along the duodenal lumen.*

be stopped. At this point, based upon the best judgment of the surgeon, the operation is either terminated with the placement of the T-tube into common duct, or a palliative choledochoduodenostomy or (-jejunostomy) is performed, provided the procedure can be tolerated (see Figure 113).

Sewing a 16 Fr T-tube into the common duct is the last step before closing the abdomen. Before bringing out the long arm of the T-tube, a cholangiogram is taken as a last check. If the entire biliary tract is negative for retained stones, the abdomen may be closed and the tube anchored to the subcostal stab wound. Before the patient leaves the operating room, the long arm of the T-tube is connected to a receptacle or rubber glove so that drainage is unimpeded until it is finally connected to a side container in the recovery room. *This writer strongly cautions against primary closure of the common bile duct in order to avoid inserting a T-tube.* Without a T-tube in place, a subsequent cholangiogram cannot be taken. Without a T-tube, local dissolution therapy is impossible. Also, secondary surgery for any reason becomes extremely difficult and haz-

ardous without a T-tube to guide the operator. Most of all, one must not lose track of the fact that the fistulous tract created by the long arm of the T-tube offers the surgeon another opportunity to fish out a retained stone with a long-arm Dormia basket via the T-tube fistulous tract. One should also mention the fact that primary closure of the common duct can result in unexpected and unrecognized serious leakage of bile or blood (hemobilia), without having recourse to an established tract for exit. Always leave a line of retreat with options. *There is no antibiotic for bile peritonitis other than to prevent secondary infection or bacterial peritonitis.*

The recommended *last-resort technique* is the choledochoduodenostomy procedure.

As stated previously, this procedure is based on the principle of "uncorking" the gallstone or removing it by the retrograde technique. A duodenotomy is performed at the projected level of the ampulla of Vater. The papilla is located through a small incision (about 2.5 cm). After duodenotomy is performed, the papilla of Vater is located by pal-

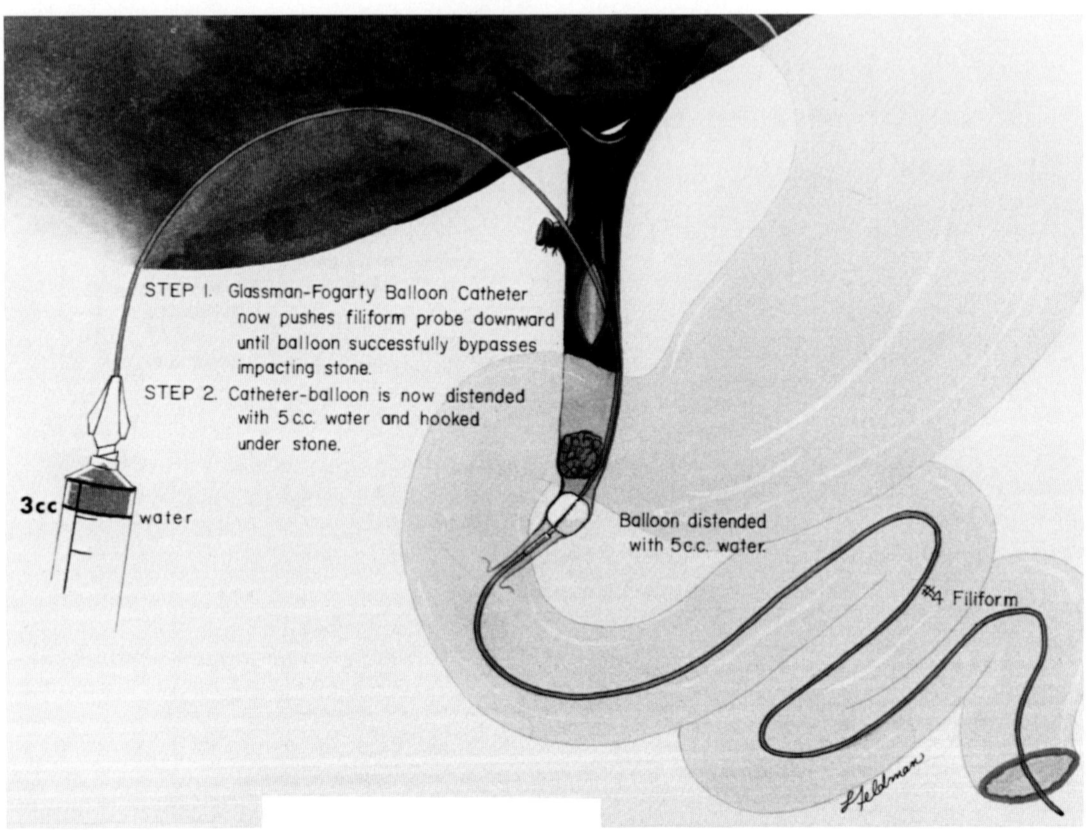

Figure 127.   When the filiform probe can be palpated in the lower portion of the duodenum, the balloon may then be inflated with 3–5 ml of water depending upon the diameter of the common duct. Pull the balloon upwardly and with it should come the incarcerated stone. If the surgeon is unsure of the balloon-stone relationship, he may instill 3–5 ml of Hypaque dye via the blue inlet of the catheter and X-ray the balloon-stone relationship. The X-ray may reveal an unusual relationship, multiple stones, or perhaps some abnormality. Irrigations are possible via this blue channel, and instillations of glycerin or mineral oil may improve the stone extraction by decreasing surface tension within the common duct.

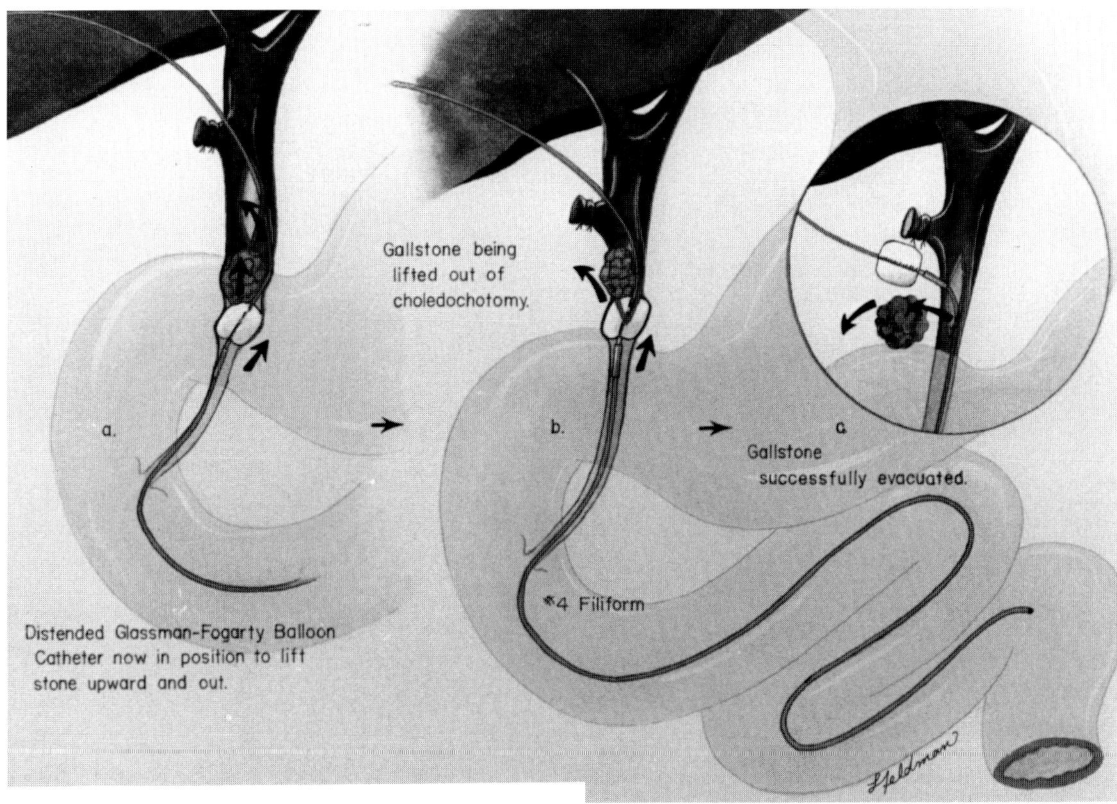

Figure 128.   The distended Glassman-Fogarty balloon catheter is now in position to lift the stone upward and out.

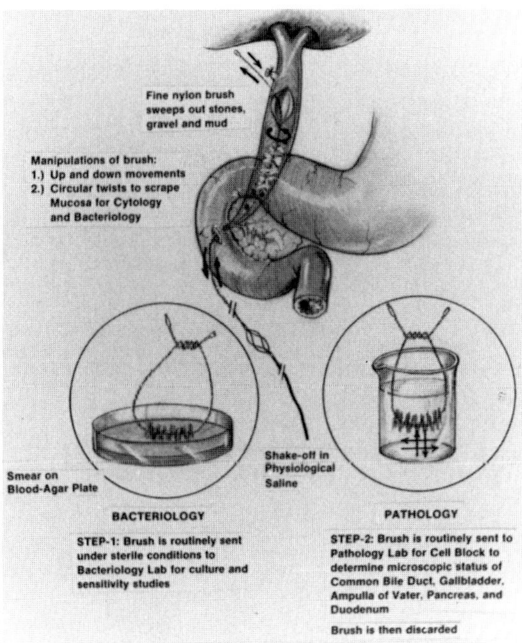

Figure 129.   Illustration shows how after the stones are removed the introduction of a fine nylon brush will, when used
as directed, sweep out the debris and mud that remains after
stone removal. The irrigations with saline should be employed last. The nylon brush is disposable and, therefore, it
should be sent sterilely to the bacteriology department for
culture and sensitivity; from there it is sent on to the pathology department for centrifuge and cell-block studies. The author recommends that sweeping the common bile duct and re-
questing bacteriological and pathological studies should be a
routine procedure in every instance where the common duct
is opened for exploration.

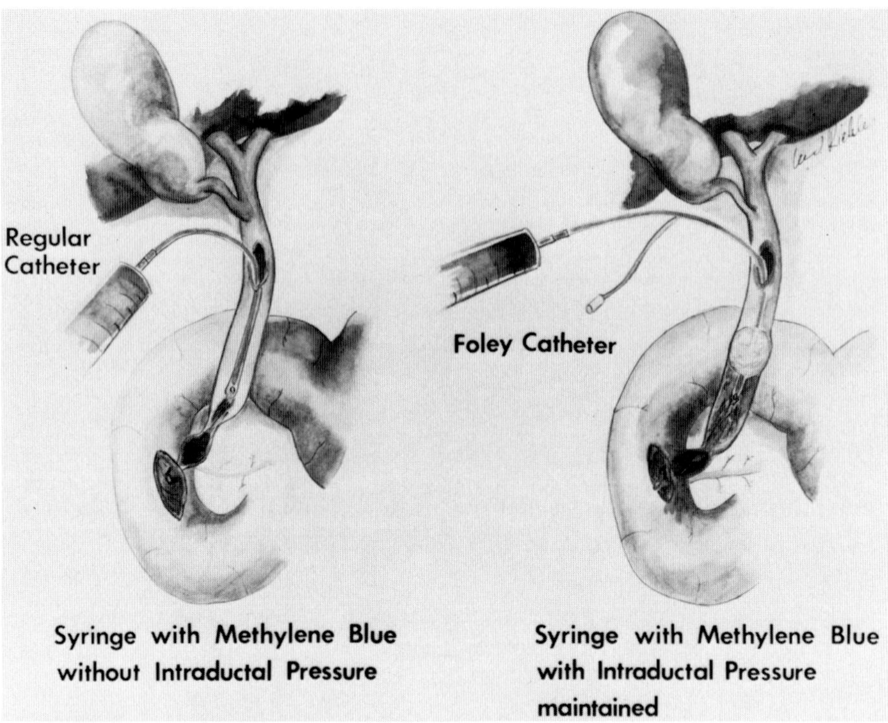

Figure 130.   The author's injection method of methylene blue dye. This method will identify the stoma of the ampulla of Vater during a duodenotomy and planned common duct explorations.

pation or visualization. If the papillary stoma cannot be found (even with the aid of magnification), a trick utilizing the author's injection method of methylene blue may be tried. The dye solution is made up of nine parts hydrogen peroxide to one part methylene blue and is gently instilled into the common duct via a 12 Fr rubber catheter, using a 5-cc syringe (Fig. 130).

The dye seeping out of the ampullary stoma localizes the exact site for entrance. If the dye fails to pass through the stoma, the surgeon may employ a small Foley catheter with a 5-cc bag to obstruct the lumen of the duct before injecting the dye under slight pressure. This procedure often helps to localize the site of the ampullary opening (Figs. 128, 130, 131, 132, 133). Betadine solution may be tried instead of methylene blue solution. Once the stoma of the ampulla is located through a duodenotomy incision, a fine Glassman blunt-tip flexible probe is gently inserted into the ampullary opening. The purpose here is to dislodge the second- or third-degree impacted gallstone upwardly and to the side. The stone is disregarded and bypassed, and the fine blunt tip is brought out through the choledochotomy stoma. Either the bipolar or unipolar helix basket instrument may now be screwed onto the female end portion of the fine probe, manipulated upward into the lumen of the common duct, and then directed toward the choledochotomy stoma (see Figures 110 and 111). The probe now draws the basket upward until the top end of the basket is outside the choledochostomy stoma. At this point, the stone may be lifted out of the common duct from either above or below. If for any technical reason it is more feasible to remove the calculus from below (via the ampulla), a prophylactic sphincterotomy should be performed before the stone is extracted. This search-and-ensnare procedure may be repeated until the impacted gallstone is successfully trapped and removed. The common duct is now swept out with the Glassman bipolar nylon brush, holding one end outside the choledochotomy stoma and the other end outside of the duodenotomy stoma (Fig. 129). Up-and-down gentle brushing, combined with saline irrigations, is advisable. The disposable brush is routinely sent sterilely to the bacteriological laboratory for culture and sensitivity studies; from there it is sent to the pathology laboratory for a "shake-off" in saline and then centrifuged for cell block biopsy (Fig. 129).

The writer again wishes to emphasize that whenever the common duct is opened, a routine brushing for cytological and bacteriological studies should be made. One

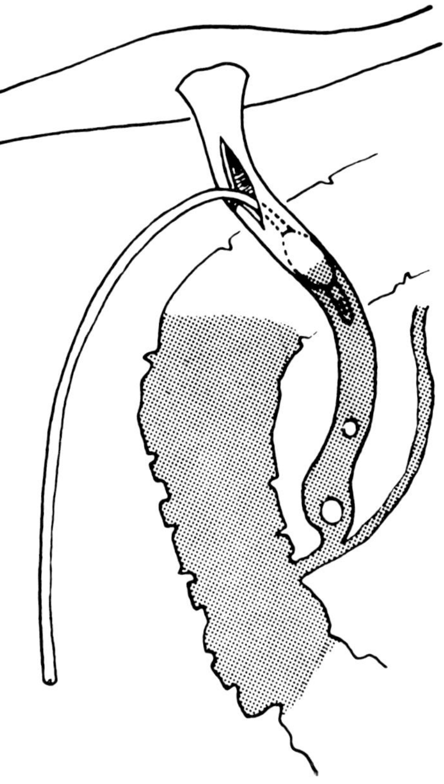

Figure 131.   The author uses this pressure method for opening and/or locating the site of the ampulla of Vater during a duodenotomy exploration. This illustration shows two stones floating in the distal common duct, a normal functioning ampullary stoma, and the duct of Wirsung.

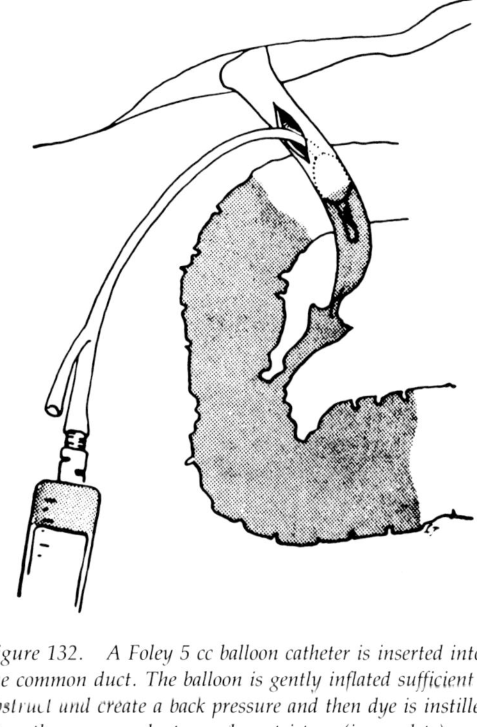

Figure 132.   A Foley 5 cc balloon catheter is inserted into the common duct. The balloon is gently inflated sufficient to obstruct and create a back pressure and then dye is instilled. Here the common duct reveals a stricture (incomplete), no stones, and a patent ampullary stoma as evidenced by a good filling out of the duodenum. This writer employs the same technique during a common duct exploration and duodenotomy to localize the exact site if the ampullary outlet when it fails to show.

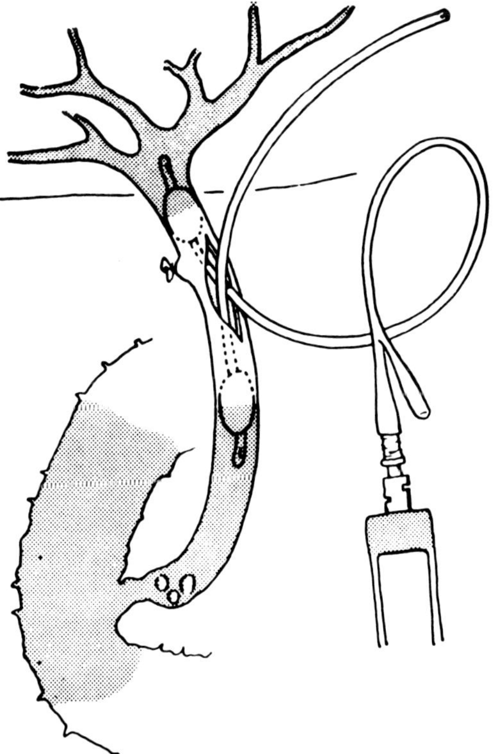

Figure 133.   Though this pressure method with a 5-cc Foley catheter was originally used to visualize the common and hepatic ducts, this writer has employed the same technique for locating the site of an obstructed ampulla of Vater during duodenotomy exploration.

never can tell when an unexpected additional finding can improve the diagnosis and treatment. The dilatation of the sphincter of Oddi should be done gently whenever the indication exists. At this point the T-tube (perferably 16 Fr) is sewn into the common duct and a final cholangiogram performed. If the biliary tree is clear of all stones, the long arm of the T-tube is brought out through a stab wound and sutured to the skin. The gallbladder bed (Morison's fossa) should be routinely drained with a Penrose (wick) drain or Jackson-Pratt constant suction drain (see "Cholecystectomy—Drain or No Drain?" in Chapter 10).

If this last-resort procedure fails to recover the impacted gallstone, the indication for a last-resort choledochoduodenostomy clearly exists. The surgeon may elect to do a choledochoduodenostomy or -jejunostomy, whichever appears to be more suitable to the anatomical situation. The surgeon must also keep in mind that certain serious complications may develop with the above palliative procedures: (1) stenosis and obstruction, (2) reformation of gallstones with obstruction, (3) fistulous formation, and (4) infection (cholangitis). A recommended procedure is shown in Figure 113.

References

1. Glassman JA: A systematic plan for common duct exploration. *Surgery* 59:685, 1966.
2. Glassman JA: A systematic plan for common duct exploration. *Am J Surg* 112:126, 1966.
3. Glassman JA: Tricks, tactics and techniques for the removal of impacted stones from the common bile duct. *Surg Gynecol Obstet* 151:99, 1980.
4. Glassman JA: Intrahepatic biliary exploration for removal of gallstones. *Int Surg* 68:51, 1983.
5. Glassman JA: Last resort technique for the removal of impacted gallstones from the common bile duct. Presented at the American College of Surgeons Annual Meeting, San Francisco, October 23–28, 1984.
6. Glassman JA: A new technique for the removal of gallstones from the hepatic duct. *Surg Gynecol Obstet* 164:166, 1987.

The Kocher Maneuver

Theodore Kocher described his maneuver in 1903;[1] since then, it has gained acceptance by most surgeons worldwide. Originally Kocher devised this procedure to facilitate a gastroduodenostomy; over time, surgeons extended its use to other gastrointestinal procedures. This maneuver is a perfect example of a bloodless line of cleavage, and for that reason it offers great exposure advantages with a minimum of risk. The Kocher maneuver initially exposes the entire anterior surface of the duodenum while displacing the omentum, colon, and mesocolon downward and to the left. A careful peritoneal curved incision is made parallel to the curvature of the duodenum (Fig. 134). The hand is then placed into the retroperitoneal duodenal space, and with gentle finger manipulations the second and third posterior portions of the duodenum are elevated along a natural line of cleavage. Finger dissection almost bloodlessly lifts the duodenum from its bed and allows it to be reflected to the left. Further careful finger dissection exposes the head of the pancreas and the distal common bile duct. Continued finger dissection exposes the inferior vena cava and possibly the pelvis of the right kidney.

This degree of exposure allows the surgeon greater latitude, better evaluation, and a safer surgical technique. The common duct can be evaluated for its color, size, thickness, and whether or not an impacted gallstone or stones are present. If a stone can be palpated, it can easily be milked upward toward the choledochostomy stoma and removed. If an obstruction is present farther down, a choledochoduodenostomy can be done. The opening made in the distal common duct allows probing up toward the choledochotomy stoma and down toward the sphincter of Oddi.

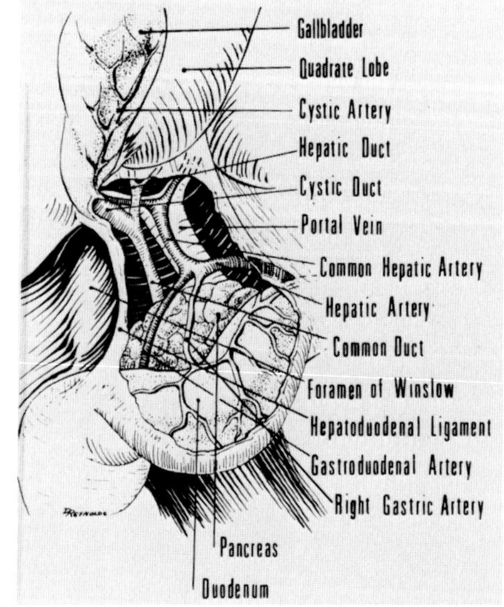

Figure 134. The Kocher maneuver and exposed retroduodenal anatomy. (From Dowdy, G. S., Jr. The Biliary Tract, Philadelphia, Lea & Febiger.)

Whenever the retroperitoneal distal portion of the common duct is opened, it must be drained either with a Penrose (wick) or Jackson-Pratt drain.

Kocher's maneuver has been used to loosen up the first, second, and third portions of the duodenum in order to enable its end to be anastomosed to the esophagus or its side to be joined to the common duct (side-to-side or end-to-side)—choledochoduodenostomy (see Figure 90). Mesenteric-portal vein anastomosis is greatly facilitated by the Kocher exposure; in the Whipple procedure, the Kocher dissection is an integral part of the technique.

Reference

1. Kocher T: Mobilisierung des Duodenum und Gastroduodenostomie. *Zbl Chir* 30:33, 1903.

Choledochoscopy

TECHNIQUE

A standard choledochotomy incision is suitable for the introduction of the scope. The incision should not exceed 10 mm to avoid excessive leakage of irrigating fluid. Endoscopy is best performed from the patient's left side. A suction tube is placed beside the common bile duct to remove the overflow of irrigation fluid. The choledochoscope is assembled by connecting the irrigation tubing as well as the fiberoptic light cable. Introduction of the scope is aided by traction on the stay sutures which open the lumen. The tip of the scope is then advanced gently toward the ampulla. Crossing the stay sutures will approximate the common bile duct walls around the scope, decreasing fluid escape and maintaining intraluminal pressure. The image displayed can be clearly seen from a safe distance without contaminating the eyepiece. The additional eye protector shield is attached to keep the manipulating hand from touching the face mask. Observation is easier if the overhead operating lights are switched off, but the room lights may be left on.

The appearance of a yellow or red circle means that the scope is in contact with the wall; this can be corrected by simply withdrawing or tilting the tip slightly until the lumen is observed. The instrument is then advanced under visual control until the sphincter orifice is seen. This is best achieved by holding the scope with the right hand while applying traction on the distal duct with the left hand on the duodenum. With this maneuver, the common bile duct will assume a straight line, which is the key to successful distal endoscopy. Attempts to pass the tip into the duodenum are not recommended. The best views are generally obtained during the slow withdrawal of the scope, scanning the area in front of the objective. In most instances, distal endoscopy can be completed without resorting to duodenal mobilization by the Kocher maneuver. This may occasionally be necessary if the duct is elongated or angulated.

After satisfactory endoscopy of the distal duct, the scope is withdrawn, rotated 180°, and reintroduced toward the hepatic ducts. After the bifurcation has been identified, the scope is rotated to the left to bring the right main orifice into view. There is a large variation in normal anatomy, but after a few cases one accumulates enough experience to examine each orifice systematically. After slow withdrawal of the scope, the bifurcation returns to view. Slight rotation to the right reveals the orifice of the left main duct, which is then followed peripherally. Upon completion of hepatic endoscopy, the instrument is withdrawn and placed on the small separate sterile table in case reexamination is required.

BILIARY STONE BASKET

Use Medi-Tech models BSB/15/55 and BSB/9/55 with a handle. Other types are too big or will not negotiate the curve. The opening or closure of the basket is carried out by the assistant while the surgeon positions the basket (advances or withdraws it) under visual control. If possible, the surgeon should advance the closed basket beyond the stone, have the assistant open it gently, and withdraw it in an open position. In certain cases, it is easier to catch the stone with this maneuver. If the stone is seen in the open basket, ask the assistant to close it gently, and withdraw the choledochoscope with the stone trapped in the basket.

FOGARTY BILIARY BALLOON CATHETER

When used with the choledochoscope this catheter should preferably be Fr 4 in size. Size Fr. 5 is too large. The surgeon advances the catheter under visual control beyond the stone. The assistant inflates the balloon, and the stone is slowly pulled out together with the instrument and the inflated balloon.

If the Foley balloon catheter fails to bypass the stone and remove it, the Glassman flexible filiform lead probe and basket should be tried in conjunction with the choledochoscope. This calls for the use of the largest tubular passage that is attached to the choledochoscope (see the previous discussion of Glassman's techniques for removal of impacted gallstones).

Technique for the Combined Use of the Choledochoscope with the Glassman Basket Balloon Filiform Lead Probe

The flexible filiform lead probe is passed through the largest curved tube attached to the site of the choledochoscope. Under direct vision, the fine flexible probe is manipulated to bypass the stone. When the probe has passed beyond the stone, the surgeon screws the male screw-on tip of the basket to the female screw-on end portion of the probe. The joined basket and probe are now advanced downward until the collapsed basket bypasses the stone. At this point, the probe threads along the lumen of the duodenum. The basket is now opened and manipulated by being twisted and turned back and forth until the stone is trapped. Once the stone is trapped within the basket, its grip is tightened about the stone and then withdrawn upward; the choledochoscope, the basket with the stone, and the lead filiform are withdrawn together as one maneuver (see the discussion of Glassman's four techniques) (see Figs. 116, 117, 118).

The Mazzariello-Cipriani stone-grasping forceps is a long curved instrument whose distal jaws open widely within the common duct to grasp the stone resistant to ordinary mechanical removal. When this clamp fails to bypass or grasp the impacted stone, it is unable to remove it. Failing to grasp the gallstone, the forceps may be used to crush it. The main feature of this clamp is that its jaws open effectively within a narrow lumen, whereas other clamps fail to do so.

Recommended Reading

Berci G, Shore JM: Advances in cholangioscopy. *Endoscopy* 4:29, 1972.
Berci G, Shore JM, Morgenstern L, et al: Choledochoscopy and operative fluorocholangiography in the prevention of retained bile duct stones. *World J Surg* 2:411, 1978.
Fogarty TJ, Krippaehne WW, Dennis DL, et al: Evaluation of an improved operative technic in common duct surgery. *Am J Surg* 116:177, 1968.
Mazzariello R: Removal of residual biliary tract calculi without reoperation. *Surgery* 67:566, 1970.
Nora P, Berci G, Shore JM, et al: Operative choledochoscopy. *Am J Surg* 133:105, 1977.
Shore JM, Berci G, Morgenstern L: The value of biliary endoscopy. *Surg Gynecol Obstet* 140:601, 1975.

A New Technique for the Removal of Resistant Gallstones from the Hepatic Duct

When carrying out routine biliary tract explorations, it is not uncommon to discover an impacted gallstone in one or both of the hepatic duct radicles. The traditional methods are usually employed to remove them. Techniques for the removal of gallstones trapped in the hepatic duct radicles include blind instrumentation with probes, spoons, forceps, balloons, and copious irrigations with saline. There are many instances in the course of biliary exploration where the surgeon will carefully explore the common bile duct, yet completely fail to search for stones in the hepatic radicles.

A retained gallstone in the hepatic duct radicle may drop or migrate down into the larger common bile duct, and, once there, cause postoperative ductal obstruction, with its usual clinical signs and symptoms. It is also conceivable that a high-lying gallstone in a major hepatic duct radicle may drop down into the common duct and fail to obstruct it completely. In such instances, an incomplete "silent" obstruction ensues, and at a later date, a complete obstruction with symptoms eventually occurs. In the case of parasitic liver disease, i.e., with *Clonorchis sinesis*, true intrahepatic lithiasis develops at multiple obstructive sites accompanied by multiple liver abscesses. Extensive areas of parenchymatous necrosis ultimately form. Stones in the common and hepatic ducts are almost invariably of cholecystic origin. They may be of various types, but almost invariably they are caused by stasis within the gallbladder. The intrahepatic ductal stones are usually formed by local stasis, debris, and infection. It is possible for intrahepatic duct stones to be present even though no calculi are found in the gallbladder or common duct. This is rare. In the latter instance, it is difficult to deny the quality of stone formation originating in the biliary radicles. The present concept of the etiology of intrahepatic stones incriminates stasis, debris, infections, racial factors, and congenital malformations. Not infrequently, parasitic infestations and hemolytic anemias have produced hepatic duct calculi, with obstruction and jaundice.

Recurrent stone formation within the biliary tract of the liver may develop, but it is more probable that a chronic ductal obstruction, i.e., ampullary stricture, has developed into intrahepatic ductal stasis, with subsequent formation of lithiasis. Not infrequently, a chronic ampullary stricture will result in chronic ductal stasis, stone formation, focal liver degeneration, and, ultimately, multiple liver abscesses.

We speak of high-lying stones in a hepatic duct radicle dropping or rolling down into the common bile duct with a larger diameter, but we must not fail to recognize that a gallstone in the common duct may very well roll upward into the hepatic duct radicles, which are of smaller diameter. In the latter instance, we may erroneously diagnose the stone as being a retained hepatic duct stone. The recommended treatment for this problem, regardless of whether the stone drops down or rolls up, is the use of careful preventive measure during the first surgical procedure—namely, a complete biliary tract exploration, with removal of all existing calculi. Aird,[1] to avoid the rolling of a common duct stone up into the hepatic ductal system, kept his patient in a reverse Trendelenberg position during surgery. Other surgeons still recommend traditional spooning and probing techniques, as well as copious saline irrigations. This writer recommends the following techniques to help prevent the postoperative occurrence of hepatic or common duct stones that inadvertently roll up or down during the surgical procedure.

Figure 135.   Techniques for hepatic exploration and removal of trapped gallstones.

After the common bile duct has been systemically explored and freed of stones, the common hepatic duct and its major radicles are copiously irrigated with warm saline solution. Spooning and probing in search of possible hepatic duct stones and debris may be employed initially. Through the original choledochotomy stoma, a long, flexible probe determines the sites of ductal resistance. The probe should determine the particular course and direction of each major hepatic duct. Operative cholangiography will assist the final search for hepatic duct calculi and establish the nature of the biliary anatomy (Fig. 135).

Continuous and copious irrigations (1 to 4 liters or more) of the right and left hepatic duct radicles with warm saline solutions using a 50-cc syringe with an adaptor and a 12 Fr rubber catheter will often help dislodge and wash out nonimpacted small hepatic stones and debris. When there is suspected cholangiographic evidence of a hepatic duct stone or stones, the surgeon inserts the small wire helix-shaped extractor instrument (initially shaped as a catheter) into the choledochotomy stoma. The basket was designed by Dormia for extracting or dislodging, trapping, and removing

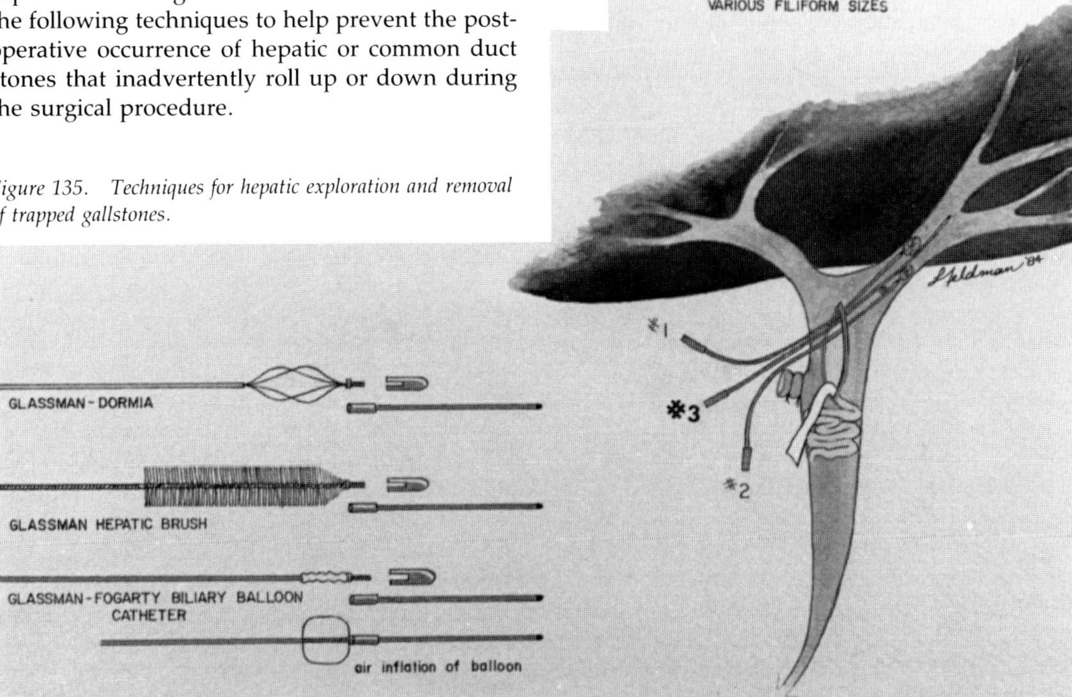

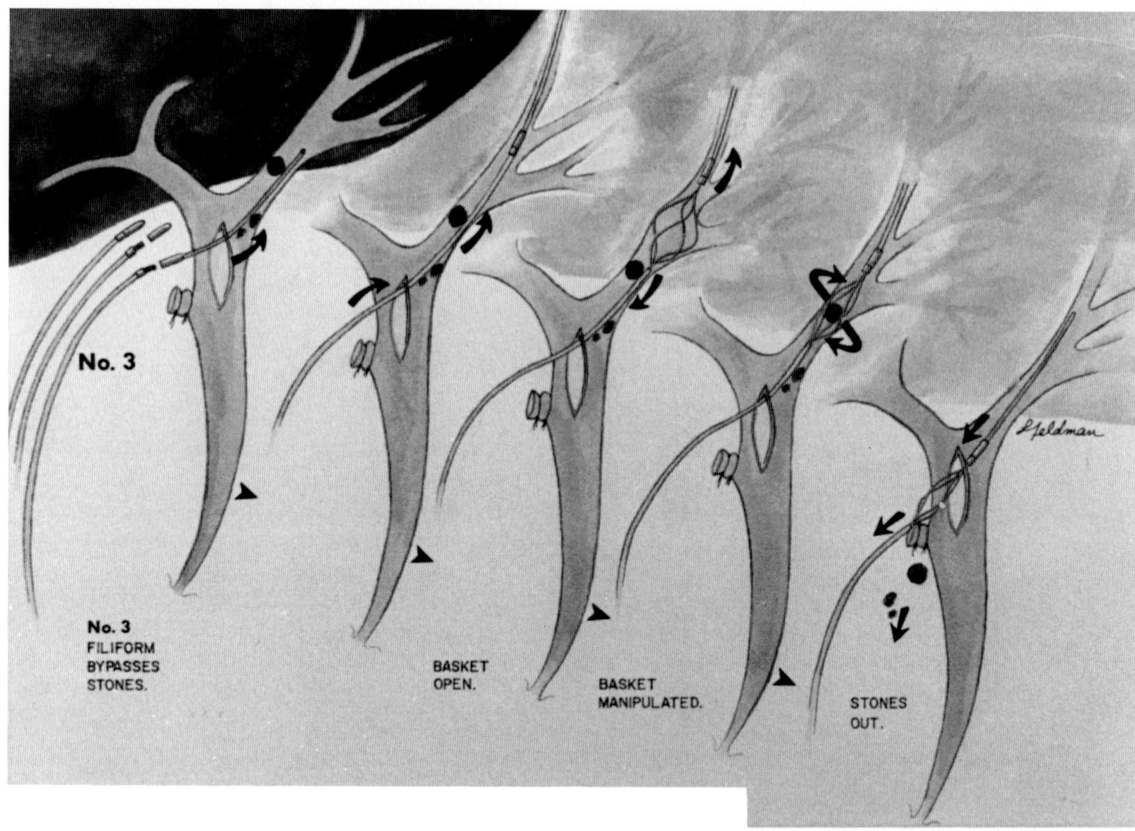

Figure 136. *Hepatic duct exploration with unipolar basket.*

elusive intrahepatic small duct stones. Each instrumentation of the hepatic duct is followed by copious warm saline irrigations (Fig. 136).

The new fine, flexible, bullet-shaped nylon brush was specially designed for intrahepatic duct exploration. It is inserted into the choledochotomy stoma, and its purpose, like that of the helix gallstone basket, is to sweep out elusive or impacted intrahepatic ductal stones. After each brushing, the hepatic ducts are again irrigated with warm saline solution. Figure 136 shows how the new short helix-shaped basket is introduced through the choledochotomy stoma and directed upward into the common hepatic duct. The unopened lead catheter-shaped basket instrument also acts as a catheter or probe; it is inserted and carefully manipulated upward as far as it can go without traumatizing the ductal mucosa. As it is manipulated upward, the collapsed flexible wires are allowed to pass beyond the hepatic stones, and then the fine wire basket is allowed to expand. When the basket catheter attains its highest possible level in the hepatic duct radicle, the helix basket is opened and rotated. The instrument is then manipulated back and forth to

dislodge, disimpact, engage, and finally remove any existing stones. A quick, short, downward pull on the basket instrument (or hepatic duct brush) is the final maneuver that effectively dislodges and traps the resistant hepatic stone. The same procedure may be repeated several times. Repeated saline irrigations should follow each attempted stone extraction. Figure 135 illustrates the small, bullet-shaped, flexible nylon brush extractor instrument designed for sweeping out elusive intrahepatic duct stones and debris. This brush is inserted into the choledochotomy stoma and carefully directed upward as high as it will go without traumatizing the delicate mucosa of the hepatic duct radicle. As the brush bypasses the stones, its bristles bend backward, and when the stones are bypassed, the nylon bristles straighten or realign themselves as before. When the brush instrument has attained its highest level in the hepatic duct radicle, it is rotated and manipulated back and forth to dislodge or disimpact any existing hepatic stones. A quick, short, downward pull on the brush from its highest point is the final maneuver that effectively sweeps out retained debris and hepatic stones. This technique may be repeated several times and should be followed each time with copious saline irrigations (Fig. 137). A final evaluation is carried out with T-tube and X-ray study.

A 12 Fr rubber catheter is passed into the right hepatic duct and then into the left one. In each instance, the duct is copiously but gently irrigated with warm saline solution, using a 50-cc syringe. This irrigation attempts to wash out any remaining adherent or impacted stones, gravel, mud, and debris. It is important to remember that throughout the period of irrigation, a flexible nylon ductal brush or umbilical tape should be kept inside the choledochal stoma to form a plug so that no hepatic duct stone can inadvertently roll down into its lumen (see Fig. 135). After thoroughly irrigating the hepatic duct radicles, the last maneuver consists of lifting out the brush or umbilical plug from the choledochal stoma. There is no assurance that removal of the stones from the intrahepatic duct will offer permanent relief—not even in those cases where cholangiography is negative. Recurrent development of true intrahepatic duct stones cannot be stopped, nor can their migration into the common duct always be avoided. Those surgeons who suspect that small hepatic duct stones roll down into the common bile duct after the operation routinely dilate the sphincter of Oddi with Bakes dilators. The final method to prevent a recurrence of small intrahepatic duct stones and their inevitable drop-down into the common duct, with subsequent impaction and obstruction, seems to be an adequate side-to-side anastomosis between the choledochus and the duodenum. Every effort should first be made to remove all stones from the proximal biliary tree before proceeding with choledochoduodenostomy.

The nylon ductal brush is used to sweep out small stones, sand, and mud, and the copious warm saline irrigations are instituted to clean out the residual debris from the hepatic ducts. The new hepatic duct brush is made of soft nylon and comes in several diameters; it is pointed, with a screw-on tip to glide easily and to accommodate various hepatic duct instruments. This brush is disposable and serves new and important functions. Besides sweeping out the debris from the lumen of the hepatic duct radicles quickly and efficiently, it is used

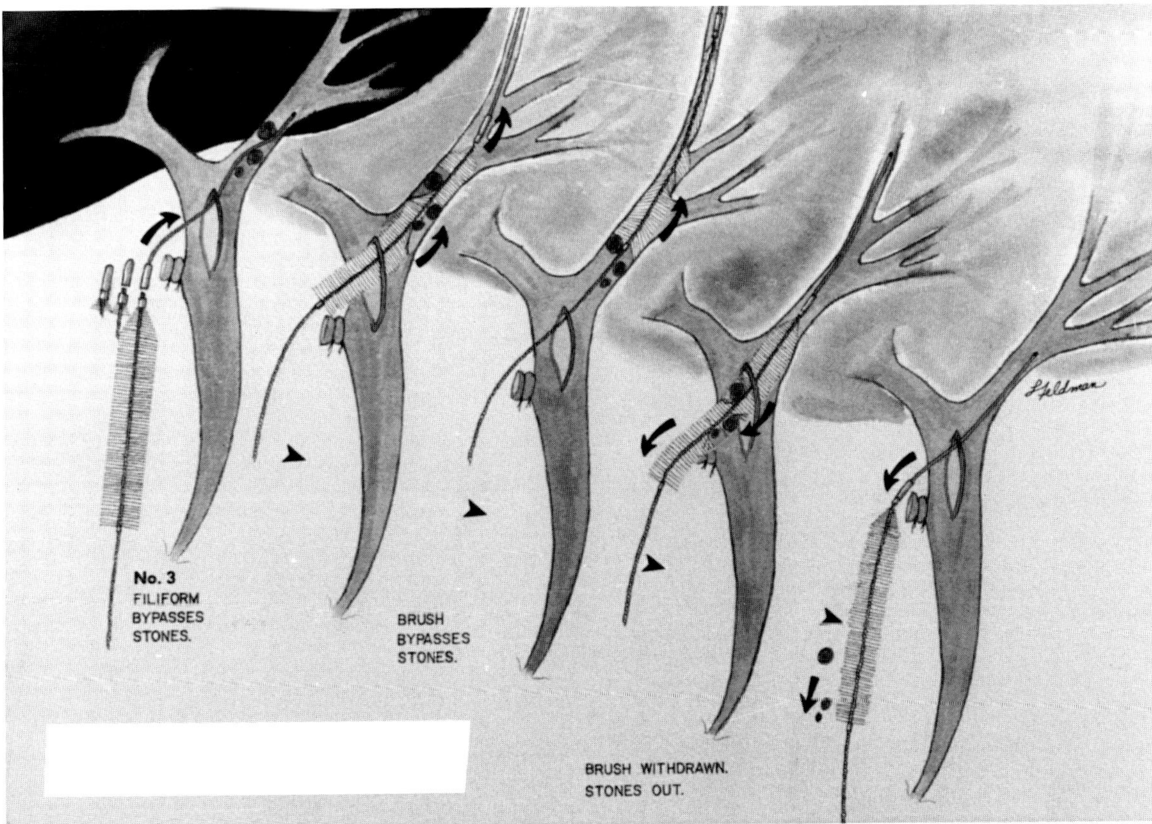

Figure 137.   Cleaning the hepatic duct with brush.

as it was in the common duct, for culture and sensitivity studies, as well as cell block biopsy. The brush, being disposable, is first sent to the department of bacteriology under sterile conditions for culture and sensitivity. It is then sent on to the pathology department, where it is immersed in 25 cc of sterile distilled water and shaken to loosen the attached cells. The fluid is then centrifuged to produce a cell block for possible pathological diagnosis related to the hepatic ducts, i.e., carcinoma of the biliary tract or liver and various liver infestations. This recommended brushing procedure should become routine whenever the common and hepatic ducts are opened and explored (Fig. 136).

LAST-RESORT BILIARY INSTRUMENTS AND RECOMMENDED TECHNIQUES

If, at this point of hepatic duct exploration, all the traditional instruments and techniques have proven to be inadequate in bypassing the impacted gallstone, the writer recommends the use of his newest gallstone extracting instruments and techniques as a last resort.

Through the choledochotomy stoma, a 4-, 6-, or 8-inch fine, flexible filiform probe is inserted upward into the right or left hepatic duct until the gallstone is contacted. The purpose of this maneuver is to manipulate the probe to bypass the stone. If the first probe cannot bypass the stone, it is left in; a second probe is then inserted and manipulated again to bypass the stone. A third, fourth, and fifth probe is inserted until one succeeds in bypassing the stone. If one probe has bypassed the stone, all of the remaining probes are removed. To the female screw-on end portion of the remaining probe the Glassman unipolar basket catheter is attached. The joined instruments are then carefully advanced upward until the collapsed basket portion of the catheter has bypassed the stone. The basket is allowed to open by sliding the sleeve downward. Manipulations such as side to side, up and down, and rotating back-and-forth maneuvers are begun; they are continued until the stone is dislodged or snared by the basket. Withdrawal of the wire basket containing the stone must be gentle. Irrigations with warm saline are in order. If the stone was not snared by the basket, repeat the entire procedure from the beginning. After the stone has been removed, the Glassman nylon bullet-shaped brush is inserted to sweep out the hepatic duct of mud, gravel, and tiny calculi (Fig. 137). This bullet-shaped brush is made up of delicate nylon fibers incapable of traumatizing the biliary mucosa. The hepatic brush is disposable. After it is used to

sweep out the duct, it is sent sterilely to the bacteriology department for culture and sensitivity studies, and then to the pathology laboratory for cell block biopsy (see Fig. 129).

The hepatic nylon brush also has a screw-on male tip which can be attached to the female screw-on portions of the filiform probe. When the basket fails to get the stones out of the hepatic duct, the brush should be tried. First, it is screwed onto the probe; together, the basket and brush are advanced upward as far as they can go. When it is felt that the bristles have completely bypassed the stone, the brush is pulled down sharply. This maneuver is relatively safe because the stone and brush are being withdrawn from a narrower diameter to a larger one. Again, irrigate with warm saline.

If the modified fine unipolar helix basket and the hepatic bullet-shaped brush have failed to remove the hepatic duct stone, the operator should try the writer's double-barreled-biliary balloon catheter (Fig. 138). Though this catheter may appear to resemble Fogarty's biliary balloon catheter, it differs radically from it. The writer's double barreled biliary balloon catheter is guided by the very fine, flexible filiform probe that precedes it in bypassing the calculus. The modified biliary catheter has two channels, while the Fogarty has only one. The modified catheter has a stopcock to hold the 3–5 cc of saline or air injected into the balloon. Fogarty[4] has to hold on to the syringe and plunger, which forces him to operate with one hand. The stopcock allows the operator to use both hands. The new biliary catheter has the advantage of being able to inject a radiopaque dye while the catheter's balloon is in place and distended. This gives the surgeon valuable information regarding the relationship of the inflated balloon to the stone. This extra opening may also be used for local irrigation to make stone removal easier (Figs. 135–138).

Once the new biliary balloon catheter is screwed onto the flexible filiform probe that has bypassed the stone (or stones), the joined instruments are advanced upward until it is felt that the collapsed balloon has bypassed the stone. The balloon is distended with saline (or air) to about 2 or 3 cc and then locked in with the stopcock. This step frees both hands; the stone is now carefully withdrawn until it falls out of the choledochotomy stoma. If the surgeon wishes to check the relationship of the balloon to the stone, he can inject a few cubic centimeters of radiopaque dye (via the blue inlet) and X-ray their positions. Here too, when pulling down the stone and balloon into the common hepatic duct, the surgeon should have no fear because the stone and balloon are passing from a narrow di-

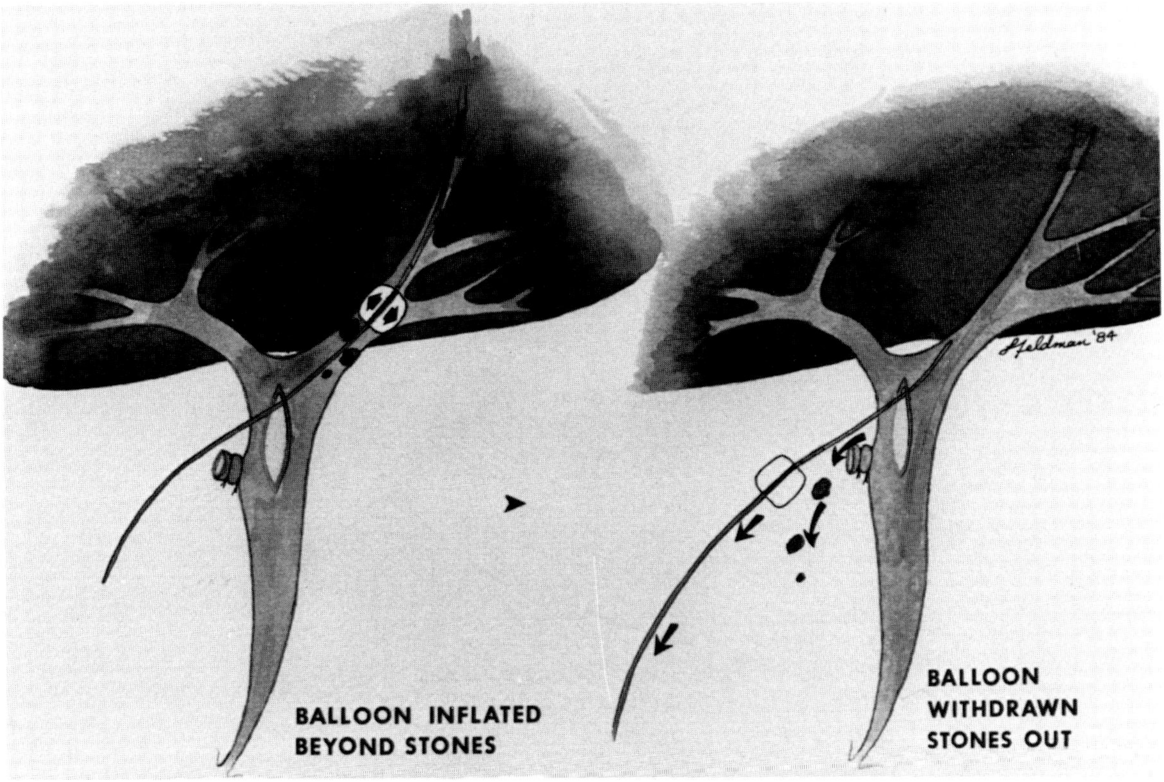

Figure 138.   Illustration of using author's double-barreled biliary balloon catheter. A. Balloon inflated beyond stones. B. Ballon withdrawn; stones are out.

ameter to a wider diameter of the duct. If after trying all techniques recommended above, the stone still remains in place, this writer recommends that the surgeon turn to prophylactic palliative surgery to take care of the patient's future needs. First, gentle dilatation of the sphincter (3–5 mm) of Oddi, employing Bakes dilators, is advised (See Fig. 139). If the stone falls down into the common

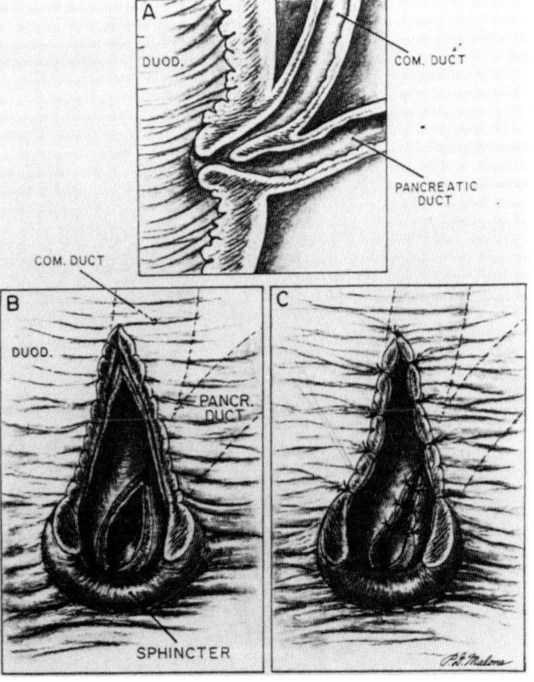

Figure 139.   Sphincterotomy and sphincteroplasty of both the ampulla of Vater and duct of Wirsung. A. Diagrammatic representation of the ampulla of Vater, lateral view. B. Sphincteroplasty with division of septum between common duct and pancreatic duct. The ampulla is divided at about the 11 o'clock position for approximately 2 cm. The septum between the common duct and pancreatic duct is incised. C. The mucosa of the common duct and duodenum is approximated with separate sutures of polyglycolic acid or polyglactin. An apical stitch is placed. The mucosa of the common duct and pancreatic duct can be approximated in similar fashion. (From Bagley FJ, Braasch JW, Taylor RH, et al: Sphincterotomy or sphincteroplasty in the treatment of pathologically mild chronic pancreatitis. Am J Surg, 141:419. 1981; with permission.)

duct at a later date, it will have a reasonable chance of passing out of the dilated sphincter and into the intestinal tract. If the surgeon is loath to do a sphincterotomy or Bakes dilation, he can resort to a prophylactic choledochoduodenostomy (or -jejunostomy).[7] The latter procedure will assure passage of the stones that may later fall down from the hepatic ducts into the common duct. It should be remembered that choledochoduodenostomy (or -jejunostomy) is a last-resort procedure (see Fig. 113).

References

1. Aird, Ian.; "The Surgical Aspects of Intrahepatic Biliary Obstruction": *Ann. Surg.* 1952: 136:27.

2. Glassman JA: Tricks, tactics, and technique for removal of impacted stones from the common duct. *Surg Gynecol Obstet* 151:99, 1980.

3. Glassman JA: Intrahepatic biliary exploration for removal of gallstones. *Int Surg* 68:51, 1983.

4. Glassman JA: Last resort techniques for the removal of impacted stones from the common duct. Presented at the American College of Surgeons Annual Meeting, San Francisco, October 23–28, 1984.

5. Fogerty TJ, Krippahne WW, Dennis DL, et al: Evaluation of an improved operative technique in common duct surgery. *Am J Surg* 116:177, 1967.

6. Berman IR, Pfeffer RB: Technique of extraction of hepatic duct calculi with modified Fogerty catheter on report of a case. *Am J Surg* 114:969, 1967.

7. Hurwitz A, Degenshein GA: The roles of choledochoduodenostomy in common bile duct surgery: Reappraisal. *Surgery* 56:1147, 1964.

12

THE COMMON BILE DUCT

Choledochotomy and Common Bile Duct Exploration

Choledochotomy for choledocholithiasis has indications that are specific and unquestionable. Choledochotomy, or opening up of the common duct to explore for gallstones, must be done in every case where it is indicated. This author does not concede that a routine operative cholangiogram and/or choledochotomy is necessary in every instance where cholecystectomy is performed. In his experience, there are distinct preoperative and operative indications and criteria that show as high a percentage of success in finding gallstones in the common duct as routine cystic duct cholangiograms.

A choledochotomy and common duct exploration is not a small undertaking. This writer believes that it adds to morbidity and mortality. Infection and toxicity from prolonged anesthesia are important factors. Undue traumatic manipulations may contribute to postoperative cholangitis. Not infrequently, cholangiograms return after an undue lapse of time with questionable results (air bubbles, false positives and spasm); repeated X-ray pictures and prolonged waiting are significant factors to contend with, statements to the contrary not withstanding.

In regard to the origin of calculi in the common duct, most surgeons believe that stones originally develop in the gallbladder and then pass on into the common bile duct. We know that it is possible for a stone to pass into the common duct or to fall down until it passes through the ampulla into the duodenum. It must also be assumed that small stones can enter the common duct, fall down to a lower level in the common duct, remain there, and then enlarge without obstructing the duct. Concentric formations develop with time until the stone assumes a form and position that ultimately obstruct the common duct.

Many patients with gallbladder calculi in the ductal system remain asymptomatic; in this case the stone, being nonobstructive, exists without dilating the common duct. This is one of the important reasons why surgeons do routine operative cholangiography: a normal-sized duct is not incontrovertible evidence for absence of a ductal stone. *A gallstone may exist in the common duct without obstruction, and therefore without dilatation of the duct.*

Preoperatively, it is most important to obtain an evaluation of the biliary system. Intravenous cholangiography and ultrasonography are perhaps the best means for obtaining reliable objective preoperative information such as the following: (1) the gallbladder's size and shape, (2) the common duct's size and shape, (3) whether the common duct is patent or strictured, (4) whether there are any obstructions, (5) the existence of biliary anomalies, and (6) whether there are stones in the common or hepatic ducts.

The surgeon who routinely does a cystic duct cholangiogram will have no great need for a complete preliminary preoperative study. *Surgeons who do not believe in routine cystic duct cholangiography look to their complete preoperative workup and the following criteria before preparing a choledochotomy and exploration of the common duct:*

1. The *presence of jaundice* or a history of jaundice are most important factors. *Common duct exploration is mandatory.*
2. *A stone* that can be palpated anywhere along the common bile duct. *Mandatory exploration. Multiple small stones* in the gallbladder with a *large cystic duct diameter.*
3. Whenever the color of the common duct changes from slate blue to gray or white. Strong indication.
4. Whenever the common duct feels thicker than normal; this implies repeated ductal inflammation. Strong indication.
5. When preoperative blood studies reveal elevated bilirubin, high alkaline phospatase, and high lactic dehydrogenase; when stools are acholic and urobilinogen is reduced or absent in the urine and feces. Strong indication.
6. When the gallbladder is contracted, containing stones of assorted sizes with a dilated cystic duct; this implies a chronically inflamed gallbladder that may allow a small stone to pass beyond the cystic duct. *Mandatory exploration.*
7. Patients who are over 60 years of age, with a long history of biliary tract disease, should be considered possible candidates for common duct exploration; that is, they should also require the minimal stated preoperative indications for exploring the common duct. The latter is not to be considered as a routine procedure because of age alone. Serious consideration for exploration.
8. When there is evidence of a *palpable mass in the lower portion of the common duct* and a question of whether there is pancreatic enlargement, ampullary enlargement, or a large impacted stone. For diagnostic reasons, a choledochotomy becomes mandatory. *Mandatory exploration.*

INDICATIONS FOR COMMON DUCT T-TUBE DRAINAGE

There are surgeons who speak adversely about the use of T-tubes after the exploration of the common bile duct. They claim that it is better to close the common duct primarily than to drain it with a T-tube. They further claim that the incidence of cholangitis and fistula formation has been reduced in their hands and that the postoperative period has been less troublesome. They also claim that cholangiography before the termination of the operation should be used to locate all residual stones, rather than resort to postoperative T-tube cholangiography. This writer strongly urges surgeons not to accept this philosophy because once the abdomen has been closed, the surgeon is completely at the mercy of whatever problem develops in the postoperative period, either early or late. *To leave a T-tube in the common bile duct should be a routine procedure, while to close the duct should be routinely avoided.*

The postoperative T-tube and cholangiography in almost every case has revealed findings that were not recognized at the time of surgery, utilizing the same T-tube and the same cholangiography techniques. Therefore, it is imperative that no surgeon accept this so-called modern dogma or recommendation. It is based on a false premise, inexperience, and certainly poor judgment. The use of routine operative cholangiography still is and probably will continue to be a controversial subject. Some surgeons believe that it is not only unreliable but carries with it many false-negative and false-positive results. They add that time is a very serious factor, and in many instances contributes to excess anesthesia toxicity and manipulative shock to the patient.

The trend toward routine operative cholangiography is supposedly based on the fact that the procedure is becoming easier to do, the facilities are more available, the time it takes to do the study is less, and the gallbladder can be removed while waiting for the film to be developed and read. This may be true in some instances, but not in most. One has merely to visit different hospitals and observe. What these advocates write and what is seen when they are observed operating are two entirely different experiences. In the experience of this writer over the past 35 years, cholangiography is reliable in the operating room when choledochotomy and T-tube insertions are considered necessary. Even though T-tube retrograde visualization is the most reliable test at surgery, it is not completely infallible because, on rare occasions, retained or impacted stones are found in the common bile duct a week or two after the surgery has been performed.

This writer contends that every cholecystectomy justifies an operative cholangiography but only when necessary. Every common duct that fails to meet the broad requirements and criteria outlined for common duct exploration should still have the benefit of routine cholangiography if the surgeon continues to remain suspicious of a stone. This writer still believes that this decision must be based on the experience of the individual surgeon who takes on the full responsibility of the case and must answer for all his decisions. If he has nothing but success, there is little reason for him to change. Those surgeons who feel that routine operative cholecystography helps them in evaluating their cases more accurately and reduces the incidence of residual stones postoperatively will use it; they alone will be held responsible. Therefore, nothing in this field should become mandatory except good judgment and the continuation of good technique with good results based on personal experience.

In 1936 Hicken and Best[1] appear to have been among the first to inject radiopaque dye at surgery through a fine needle into the common bile duct. In 1949 Hicken and McAllister[2] reported routine needle cholangiography utilizing a 25-gauge needle to prevent excessive leakage. Subsequent studies and development led to the use of cholangiography through the cystic duct; polyethylene tubes became available, doing away with the need to puncture the common duct. At present, routine operative cholangiography is carried out with a polyethylene tube through the cystic duct just proximal to the common bile duct. An excellent article on the diagnosis of choledocholithiasis, consisting of a review of approximately 15,000 patients who underwent biliary tract surgery during a 5-year period, came from the Departments of Surgery and Radiology, and the Harrison Department of Surgical Research, University of Pennsylvania School of Medicine in Philadelphia.[3]

The authors' conclusions were as follows: Cystic duct cholangiograms were accurate when normal and eliminated many needless common duct explorations. When these cholangiograms were interpreted as abnormal, they did identify pathological conditions in the majority of such patients. Their use was therefore recommended. *However, they were recommended only when other clinical and/or operative indicators of choledocholithiasis were present.* Reliability of the classical indicators of choledocholithiasis was reaffirmed: that is, when there was clinical and operative evidence that no jaundice or history of jaundice existed; when the common duct was approximately 1 cm or less in diameter; when the preoperative intravenous cholangiogram and the sonogram showed a common duct of normal size; when the common duct was thin and of slate blue color; when the cystic duct was small and the stones were large. All of these clinical criteria proved as accurate as routine cystic duct choledochograms at surgery. In the experience of this writer, common duct stones were never found in the presence of most of the named indicators. Accuracy improved as the correlation of the preoperative indicators of common bile duct calculi coincided with the increasing number of intraoperative indicators. Twenty-five percent of 308 patients who had one or more indicators of choledocholithiasis did have stones in the common duct. The incidence of common bile duct stones increased with the correlation of the number of clinical and operative indicators that were present, so that when no indicators were present, no stones were found in the common bile duct of 108 patients. With one indicator present, there was evidence of an 11% incidence of choledocholithiasis. When two or more operative indicators were present in 163 patients clinically and/or at surgery, 42% of the patients who had choledochotomy revealed common bile duct stones. *A combination of preoperative and intraoperative indicators proved more effective than the indicators evaluated separately in predicting the presence of common bile duct stones.*

The author concludes that a T-tube should always be placed in the common duct after exploration of the duct, and that any abnormal findings should be promptly investigated to minimize any possibility of retained stones and secondary surgery. Those who do not leave a T-tube in place and primarily close the common duct deprive the patient and themselves of the following benefits: (1) they cannot do cholangiograms in the postoperative period; (2) they cannot discover an obstructive stenosis or carcinoma that may have been overlooked at surgery; (3) they cannot treat the patient with chemotherapy to dissolve a retained stone; (4) they cannot employ the fistulous tract created by the T-tube for noninvasive removal of stones using the long-arm Dormia basket; (5) they are unable to test the flow of bile (interrupted or uninterrupted) through the ampullary stoma and into the duodenum; (6) and finally, if a secondary surgical procedure is required, the T-tube would simplify the search for the common duct, which is generally most difficult to find. In secondary surgery, the T-tube leads the surgeon directly to the exact site of the common duct and stone.

TECHNIQUE FOR CHOLEDOCHOTOMY AND COMMON DUCT EXPLORATION

Before embarking on a common duct exploration, all of the anatomy must be clearly recognized and proper retraction of all the adjacent structures carried out. In the recommended exploration, this writer does not initially take out the gallbladder; the cystic duct is dissected out and encircled with a (00) chromic catgut and *incompletely ligated* so that, with traction, no cystic duct stones can fall into the common duct during exploratory maneuvers. The gallbladder and the ligature also provide good lateral traction during the common duct exploration; cholecystectomy is left for last.

The popular procedure today is a cystic duct incision in which the tip of a polyethylene tube is inserted; the tube passes through the cystic duct into the common duct, not too far down. A ligature is placed about that portion of the intubated cystic duct to fix and prevent leakage around the plastic tube. A black silk suture (000) is utilized for fixation. The radiopaque dye is injected slowly, and several X-ray films are taken and brought immediately to the X-ray laboratory. Through a direct communication system between the laboratory and the operating room, the roentgenologist can give his expert opinion as to whether a stone or stones are present. When the common duct is found to be clear and evidence shows the dye to have passed easily into the duodenum, the common duct is assumed to be clean and without obstruction. However, if there is evidence of a retained stone in the biliary tree, either intrahepatic or extrahepatic, it is mandatory (if the patient's condition will permit) that the surgeon remove the sewn-in T-tube and continue to reexplore the common duct.

Procedure

The common bile duct should be opened only after all blood vessels traversing the expected linear incision are dealt with by fine suture ligatures or hemostatic clips. The longitudinal incision is made after preliminary needle aspiration has been carried out through the common duct to be sure that bile and not blood is present. The aspirated bile is utilized for culture and sensitivity studies. The longitudinal incision is made into the anterior surface of the common duct and enlarged to about 2 to 2.5 cm when possible. The stoma should be just above the level of the superior border of the duodenum. Hemostasis is secured, and all bile should be aspirated. The color of the bile should be noted, and, as stated before, culture and sensitivity studies as well as cytology should be ordered. The cut edges of the common duct should be held apart either by black silk stay sutures (000) or by two delicate Glassman noncrushing 8-inch modified Allis clamps. Holding the edges apart facilitates the work within the common duct.

A routine procedure for cleansing the common

duct should be instituted immediately. At first, all the bile is aspirated and the common bile duct packed off at all sides so that no leakage of bile can occur around the choledochotomy stoma. Everything that comes out of the opening should be sucked out or removed by spoon or forceps. The common bile duct should then be carefully and tactfully spooned out for more stones. If stones are palpated at a lower level, they should be milked back, using the forefinger and thumb of the left hand. The stones should be gently manipulated all the way up to the stoma and removed. From this point on, in attempting to milk back low-lying stones, a Kocher maneuver should be employed (see "The Kocher Maneuver" in Chapter 11).

The Kocher maneuver involves freeing up the duodenum on its lateral aspect. It exposes the vascular area of the duodenum retroperitoneally. At this point, by blunt dissection, using the finger, the duodenum is carefully lifted out of its bed, with complete hemostasis, and reflected toward the left. More often than not, it will reveal more of the distal common duct as it passes down between the pancreas and duodenum. This step allows better visualization and palpation of the common bile duct. Also, if a low-lying stone exists (not quite as low as the ampulla), it can be milked upward with the aid of the forefinger and thumb toward the choledochotomy stoma and evacuated. If this procedure fails to visualize or remove the impacted stone, the reflection of the duodenum will allow downward traction to straighten out a curved or angulated common duct before other techniques are tried.

The exploration is started with an initial probing of the common duct. A blunt-tip flexible probe or a regular cervical malleable probe is employed to determine if the common duct is patent at the ampullary level and whether there is a stricture; or if the ampulla is impassable due to stone impaction. Depending upon the situation, copious warm saline irrigations of the common duct should be carried out and followed by the introduction of Mazzariello-Caprini forceps into the common duct to see if any stones can be grasped and removed. Spoons of varying sizes may also be tried. If the surgeon feels that the common duct is completely cleared of all stones, a 12 Fr rubber catheter should be passed through the ampulla. This maneuver provides a good sign that the common duct stoma is adequately patent. Another test may also be useful, namely, to withdraw the catheter back into the common duct and then inject saline. If the duodenum distends, it is a good sign that the ampullary stoma is unobstructed.

At this point, we shut off the distal common duct

side with a piece of umbilical tape or gauze, and then proceed to work on the proximal opening of the common hepatic duct and its right and left radicles. The technique is fully described in detail elsewhere (see "A New Technique for the Removal of Resistant Gallstones from the Hepatic Duct" in Chapter 11). After this technique is successfully carried out, the common duct and hepatic duct radicles should be considered completely cleansed. A biopsy of the common duct wall is taken in questionable cases. *The Glassman hepatic and common bile duct nylon brushes should be routinely employed to obtain cytology brushings from the biliary tree. These brushings should be sent to the bacterial laboratory for culture and sensitivity studies, and then on to pathology for cell block studies.*

The common duct is then closed with a T-tube selected to fit the size of the lumen. The nurse brings in an assortment of T-tubes, either rubber or silastic, and the surgeon (not the nurse) selects the most suitable size for the common duct lumen in question, preferably 14 or 16 Fr. The surgeon then patterns the T-tube to the common duct lumen. The T-tube is fastened in place with interrupted black silk sutures (000). The closure is made watertight and tested under pressure with warm saline injections, employing an adaptor and a 50-cc syringe. Any point of leakage is further closed off by placing another interrupted silk suture.

When the closure is hermetically sealed and the T-tube is properly positioned within the common duct, 50% Hypaque dye is instilled into the common bile duct in two stages. The first picture is taken after injecting between 3–5 cc, and then as much as 8 cc is slowly injected into the distal portion of the common duct; for a second x-ray picture; this amount better delineates the stones lying in the distal portion of the duct.

Two or more views of cholangiographic X-ray studies should be taken. The first injection into the tube contains approximately 7–8 cc of 50% diluted Diodrast or Hypaque; it is slowly injected and allowed to gravitate downward; the table can be tilted to have gravity assist the dye in draining downward in small amounts toward the ampulla; this will help to visualize the smaller stones instead of obliterating them. Another film is taken with 15–30 cc of Diodrast or Hypaque injected, so that now the entire biliary system is filled, including all of the hepatic radicles within the liver. One or two films should be taken and viewed as quickly as possible after being developed. The surgeon, being no expert on X-rays, should request the assistance of the X-ray department; either an X-ray resident should be in the operating room to assist the surgeon to evaluate the X-rays, or an intercom system should be present so that the roentgenologist can quickly report his findings. The roentgenologist makes the final determination of whether or not a retained stone or stones are still present.

Cooperation between the surgeon and roentgenologist is not only ethical and medically correct, *it is medicolegally correct.*

DUODENOTOMY, SPHINCTEROTOMY, AND HEPATIC DUCT EXPLORATION

If the duodenum has to be opened (duodenotomy), one may see that the stone is the cause for a bulging ampulla. It is possible to merely incise the bulge and allow the stone to fall out (see "Surgical Sphincterotomy" in Chapters 12, 17). The surgeon should complete the sphincterotomy, which is deemed necessary for several reasons: Stones in the hepatic duct and residual stones in the common duct will ultimately find their way out more easily with the return of bile flow. If there is any oozing or bleeding from the cut sphincterotomy, fine (0000) or (00000) black silk interrupted sutures are utilized to secure hemostasis.

The sphincterotomy incision should be made over the gallstone; its direction should be slightly oblique toward the patient's right so that it does not injure or cut into the main pancreatic duct of Wirsung (see Fig. 139). A duodenotomy incision should not be closed with only one layer of sutures, (a most serious complication is a duodenal fistula). The closure of a duodenotomy should be dealt with in detail and with great care. The technique employed by the writer has been to close the duodenal defect with a chromic catgut (000) suture on an atraumatic needle, using a continuous-lock stitch for the first row. *The second row should be made with interrupted (000) black silk. The closure may be in the horizontal or transverse plane.*

Much depends upon postoperative decompression of the stomach and duodenum, and not upon routine gastrostomy drainage, which, in the writer's opinion, is an abused and undesirable major procedure. The surgeon should employ decompression with a Levin tube carefully placed at surgery, with the anesthetist arranging the tube so that it lies unkinked in the stomach near the pylorus. It should be pulled back to prevent any kinks; finally, the tube should be fixed so that no one can disturb its position.

The surgeon now proceeds to evaluate the common hepatic duct and its radicles. He should start with the same plan that was carried out with the common bile duct. The spoon system, adjusted by flexibility to fit the right and left hepatic duct radicles, should be tried first. All supplemental biliary instruments should be tried; the hepatic duct stones must be dislodged and removed before closing the abdomen.

Once it has been established that there are no air bubbles and no leftover stones in the common duct, the exploratory procedure is ended and the gallbladder may now be removed. The cystic duct is doubly ligated; the sutures held as traction are now doubly tied, and the cystic duct is severed. The cholecystectomy and the common duct exploration are completed.

There are many opinions on how a T-tube should be brought out through a subcostal stab incision. Some believe that a Penrose or Jackson-Pratt suction drain should accompany it; the latter drains Morison's fossa. Some surgeons like to bring the Penrose drain out through a separate stab wound. This writer believes that one stab wound is adequate; this stab wound should be enlarged so that, with little effort, the Penrose drain is brought out first and the arm of the T-tube follows. Both are carefully placed so that they don't intertwine or lock; thus they can easily be removed separately. Closure is carried out only after the operator carefully studies the abdomen again, ensuring that hemostasis is fully secured and that the organs have been properly replaced. The T-tube and Penrose drain are finally adjusted from the inside; when they have been correctly placed, the abdominal incision is closed in layers as described in the procedure for cholecystectomy. The T-tube is immediately connected to a urological plastic bag or rubber glove. The latter are excellent receptacles for immediate bile collection. If a small catheter, i.e. 12 Fr is employed, its best attachment is to intravenous plastic tubing that will drain directly into a bag, glove, or bottle. At this time, it is important to take measures to prevent accidental removal of either the Penrose drain or the T-tube. To avoid such a catastrophic accident, the T-tube is routinely attached to the wound's edge with a silk suture. The Jackson-Pratt suction tube is similarly fixed. A Penrose drain need not be attached; if it is to be anchored, the suture is passed through the gauze wick and fixed to the skin edges.

Closure of the abdomen should be delayed until the last resistant leftover gallstone has been removed. Surgeons must persist in their effort and use every biliary trick, tactic, and technique they are capable of; in addition, they should call for every available supplemental special biliary instrument to further assist them in their efforts. Such instruments include:

1. Fogarty's biliary balloon catheter
2. Mazzariello's long, thin, curved, stone-grasping forceps
3. Storz's *rigid* choledochoscope
4. Machida's *flexible* choledochoscope
5. A fine catheter-optical light for common duct exploration and visualization.

If, despite all the efforts of the surgeon, the left-over stone resists removal, the surgeon should, as a last-resort procedure, use Glassman's gallstone extractor set of baskets and balloons; the recommended techniques were specifically designed for such recalcitrant situations (see the discussion of Glassman extractor instruments and techniques in Chapter 11).

If the stone resists the recommended last-resort instruments and techniques, and the patient's condition still remains stable, a last-resort palliative procedure is recommended: either choledochoduodenostomy or - jejunostomy. These procedures are time proven and relatively safe; they offer high-risk and elderly patients a reasonable alternative, since a secondary surgical operation will probably not be necessary.

OBSTRUCTION OR SPASM OF THE SPHINCTER OF ODDI

When the probe passes easily into the duodenum, and water passes through a catheter distending the duodenum with ease, and subsequent X-rays still show obstruction, one may then consider *spasm* as the causative factor. The spastic process will relax in due time, and the flow of bile will invariably be resumed. The postoperative T-tube study with cholangiography will recognize the progress; this study is most important and accurate, but it is not completely infallible. On occasion, it may fail to show residual stones, especially when the stones are small and high up in the hepatic duct radicles. Hepatic duct stones can and do roll down later into the common bile duct; they are then diagnosed as recurrent stones. On occasion, the spine may overlap and overshadow the stones, or excessive dye may be present. *In the great majority of cases, postoperative T-tube cholangiograms do not overlook stones or abnormalities of the common bile duct.* The T-tube cholangiogram is one of the most reliable tests we have, both inside and outside of the operating room.

At times, the dye will clearly indicate that the common duct is free of stones at the sphincter of Oddi, yet an obstruction is known to exist because the dye does not enter the duodenum. When no evidence of a stone can be detected and no other mechanical factor are suspected, the obstructive feature must be considered to be spasm. Spasm is common in the sphincteric musculature, especially when it is affected by local edema. Irritation during the exploratory procedure may have led to further spasm of the sphincter of Oddi. Therefore, it is important to remember that distal ampullary obstruction may not necessarily be organic. It is possible to relieve the spasm during the surgical procedure. One may employ amyl nitrite or inject magnesium sulfate through the T-tube to relax ampullary spasticity. Some surgeons use intravenous glucagon. It is well known that preoperative morphine sulfate can induce ampullary spasm. One must bear in mind that the ampulla may open spontaneously several hours or days later. In many cases, amyl nitrite, magnesium sulfate, or glucagon administration will successfully open up or relieve the sphincteric spasm, and the next X-ray picture will show good duodenal filling.

On many occasions these relaxing drugs will not work, and one must therefore reconsider whether there is a retained stone or stricture. Surgeons must know their work, and, more importantly, they must have confidence in their technique and judgment. Obviously, further workup is indicated.

POSTOPERATIVE MANAGEMENT OF THE T-TUBE

Weeks after the surgery, a second T-tube cholangiogram may be even more accurate. If a residual stone is discovered postoperatively, the T-tube can serve as an effective guide for the surgeon and roentgenologist to readily locate the common duct and stone. *Before entertaining thoughts of a secondary surgical procedure, surgeons must consider the following noninvasive procedures available to them:*

1. *Conservative attempts* to induce the retained stone to pass out of the common duct. Bile salts administered daily via T-tube for several weeks or months may ultimately dissolve the stone.
2. *Instrumental manipulations via the T-tube* to push the stone out or fracture it into smaller fragments, together with copious irrigations to flush them out. Muscular relaxants, i.e., amyl nitrate, glucagon, and magnesium sulfate, are employed.
3. *Chemotherapy,* namely, chenodeoxycholic acid or derivatives, given systemically and/or locally via the T-tube to dissolve the stone.
4. *Endoscopic retrograde choledochography (ERC);* With this technique, a papillotomy (sphincterotomy)

will allow the stone to pass out. Failing that, the stone can be removed by long-arm retrograde basket or balloon techniques.

5. *Burhenne's technique,* via fistulous tract created by the T-tube, employs a long-arm Dormia basket and balloon catheter, and with the aid of a TV monitor, can trap or fracture the stone and remove it. ERCP may be employed supplementally to remove the fractured fragments.

Through the fistula created by the long arm of the T-tube, one can flush out gravel and small stones, push a stone through the ampulla, or wear the stone down with chemotherapy (see "Dissolution of Gallstones" in Chapter 3).

Failure to remove the impacted stone with any or all of these conservative noninvasive procedures makes a secondary surgical procedure mandatory.

A Rule for Safe Withdrawal of the T-Tube

The rule for final removal of a T-tube is based upon the findings of multiple cholangiograms. All X-rays must indicate that there is no stone anywhere in the biliary tree; that the dye flows freely through an unobstructed common duct and ampulla into the duodenum, producing a good duodenal pattern. Only then is it safe to remove the T-tube. However, before the catheter is finally removed, the conservative first step should be the clamping off of the T-tube. This indicates whether or not the patient remains asymptomatic and can pass all the bile into the gastrointestinal tract without spilling over. If the patient passes 5–7 days of the test in which the long arm of the T-tube has been clamped off without any accompanying signs or symptoms, such as pain, fever, chills, jaundice, and acholic stool, it is safe to remove the T-tube. The T-tube is finally pulled with impunity only after the patient says that he or she feels better and the stool has turned darker in color.

To reiterate, there is no set time for the removal of a T-tube, as many textbooks and articles would have one believe. There is no set routine for removing it after 1, 2, or 3 weeks or longer. *Everything depends upon the condition of the patient.*

EVALUATION OF CHOLANGIOGRAPHY IN THE OPERATING ROOM

Preexploratory cholangiography, by whatever method the surgeon deems best, is being questioned at this time. It is not accepted by all roentgenologists and surgeons. It has been asked whether a routine cystic duct cholangiogram with radiopaque dye provides more information than a routine exploration of the duct after opening it, probing it, irrigating it, viewing it, spooning it, and brushing out the stones or gravel. In preexploratory cholangiography, the surgeon must always be aware of the possibility of false negatives and false positives. Air bubbles are common and, not infrequently, the roentgenologist may be unable to judge the findings, especially when air bubbles enter via the T-tube and give the impression of residual stones. Some argue that only when the technique of cholangiography is improved will it become unanimously accepted as a routine preexploratory procedure.

Shorter operations, with needless procedures eliminated, will help the patient to tolerate the surgery better and reduce the complications that so often attend routine operative cholangiography, i.e., acute pancreatitis, shock, false negatives, and false positives. This writer, when making use of operative cholangiography, never evaluates the X-rays on his own. He has direct communication with the X-ray department, and even though the X-ray films are developed on the same floor within minutes and brought for reading to the surgeon, the final word must be given by the attending roentgenologist. It takes time for the film to go down to the roentgenologist by messenger and then, by a speaker communication system, have the results reported as negative, positive, or questionable. Not infrequently, the roentgenologist must come into the operating room, sterilely dressed, to consult on an X-ray film. Often repeat X-ray films must be taken; this requires additional time, which can be critical to the condition of the anesthetized patient who may also have associated systemic problems and be of advanced age, with poor tolerance of prolonged anesthesia. This question is far from settled; there are still strong advocates on both sides. Those surgeons who report finding a residual stone after routine cholangiography claim the lowest possible figures attainable. Those who do not do preexploratory cholangiography and instead use the aforementioned criteria for opening the common duct have experienced a similar proportion of retained stones (1–3%), depending upon the experience of the reporting surgeon.

Today we have agents for dissolving the gallstone, namely, bile acids and chenodeoxycholic acid, as well as various manipulative means for removing stones by nonoperative methods. Through a fistulous tract created by the T-tube in the X-ray department, a stone can be removed by nonoperative techniques in a high percentage of cases (see Casal's Non-Invasive Techniques, Chap. 5). These new methods have significantly reduced the need for reoperation. The writer has introduced new instruments and techniques that may reduce the incidence of leftover stones at the time of the initial surgery, as well as the need for postoperative noninvasive techniques for the extraction of such stones. *It is the writer's opinion that if all stones are removed at the first operation, there will be no need for all these complicated, time-consuming, and costly noninvasive procedures; we can also eliminate long-term, expensive medical treatments with chenodeoxycholic acid and its derivatives, and, at long last, a second exploratory operation* (see the discussion of Glassman's last-resort gallstone extractor baskets and balloons in Chapter 11).

The surgeon and roentgenologist must be sure to have the correct answer before he or she decides to proceed with the manipulations to extract the stone, or what is interpreted to be a retained stone. An X-ray laboratory on the surgical floor is an important facility and should be installed in all hospitals. The roentgenologist can then appear in the operating room within minutes to consult with the surgeon. It is the writer's opinion that the surgeon should not take it upon himself to make a final decision on the X-ray films and proceed with or without an extraction procedure. This is an era of medicolegal consciousness, and every decision must be made with all the consultatory assistance the surgeon can muster. The writer emphasizes that after a T-tube is positioned in place and sealed off watertight, cholangiography must be done *before* the abdomen is closed. There is still time to make any correction based upon the findings. A reexploration of the common duct, if necessary, must be meticulously carried out with the greatest accuracy. *When surgeons open a common bile duct, they must be dedicated to the clearance of the entire biliary tree, and not to the common duct alone; therefore, every trick, tactic, and technique known to biliary surgery must be put into play.*

REASONS FOR FAILURE OF OPERATIVE CHOLANGIOGRAPHY

In an excellent report entitled "Failure of Operative Cholangiography to Prevent Retained Common Duct Stones," Hall et al.[3] stress the importance of clearing the biliary ducts at the first operation. This principle has been encouraged and taught for the past 30 years by this writer. After evaluating 302 patients who had T-tube cholangiograms before discharge, these authors found that undue reliance was placed on cholangiography. They do not discourage cystic duct cholangiography per se; they

only wish to discourage the unwarranted blind confidence in this technique.

The authors enumerate what they believe to be the pitfalls in T-tube cholangiograms:

1. Contrast material may be too concentrated; if the T-tube cannot be visualized, the calculi cannot be seen.
2. A stone in motion may elude visualization by the dye.
3. Incomplete filling may be overcome by diluting the contrast medium (see the discussion of Foley catheter use in occluding part of the common duct for better visualization in Chapter 11, Figs. 131, 132, 133).
4. The X-ray cassette may not be properly positioned; there may also be a failure to obtain proper exposure.
5. When the common duct is over the spine, rotation of the patient is required; the left side should be elevated 15–20°.
6. Superimposition of ducts requires multiple exposures.
7. The surgeon may fail to consult with or may ignore the advice of the roentgenologist.
8. Even if the cholangiograms appear to be excellent, *the thoroughness of the surgical exploration must not be lessened.*

This writer wishes to remind the surgeon of certain other precautions to be observed when taking cholangiograms:

1. Do not forget to take a preliminary flat film.
2. Eliminate air bubbles in the common duct (see T-tube Techniques by Casal and Martinez in Chapter 6).
3. Before instilling the dye, irrigate the common duct with warm saline.
4. After the T-tube is sewn into place, test for any leakage; leakage will obscure the field.
5. The anesthesiologist must obtain apnea during exposure.
6. Relaxants are acceptable; however, *avoid the use of morphine!*
7. If left-over barium is in the colon, pack off the hepatic flexure from the operative field.

NO-NO'S IN BILIARY SURGERY

There are surgeons who, after exploring the common bile duct, feel so confident that the common duct and hepatic radicles are free of stones, that they proceed to close the choledochotomy stoma primarily without benefit of T-tube drainage. They may also choose not to employ a Penrose or Jackson-Pratt drain. *This judgment and technique are condemned by the writer. No one should take that gamble with the patient's life!* In every case that requires opening of the common bile duct, routine drainage by a T-tube is mandatory. After 1–2 weeks, when postoperative cholangiographic studies have reconfirmed that the biliary tree is free of stones, *then and only then* should the T-tube be withdrawn and spontaneous closure allowed to take place. To close a common bile duct primarily without benefit of a T-tube, particularly when there has been sludge, mud, gravel, and small stones in it, is a reckless act and must be condemned.

Without a T-tube left in the common duct after exploration, the possibilities of postoperative complications are increased. Leakage from cut but unrecognized biliary canaliculi in the liver bed can cause bile peritonitis. *There is no antibiotic for biliary peritonitis!* Postoperative cholangiograms are no longer possible. The only treatment is surgical intervention to drain the bile and close the leaking site. A drain will still have to be employed for external drainage of serum, blood, and bile. Chenodeoxycholic acid and its derivatives employed via the T-tube for possible dissolution of the gallstone is denied the patient; also Burhenne's noninvasive bracket or balloon technique for removal of a retained gallstone via a fistulous tract created by the long arm of the T-tube.

Some surgeons find it convenient to drain the common duct via the cystic duct stoma as an outlet for the long arm of the T-tube. This is not recommended by the author because a 14–16 Fr catheter does not always fit, and the cystic duct does not obliterate so well when the tube is removed. In those instances where a postoperative retained stone is recognized, the cystic duct only serves as an obstruction to the Dormia basket and stone. This writer recommends that all cystic ducts be doubly ligated after they are utilized for cholangiograms, and that only a choledochotomy T-tube drainage be selected as the choice.

The T-tube is carefully placed in the choledochotomy stoma, which is then closed snugly around the long arm of the tube. Interrupted black sutures (000) are employed. *Avoid suturing the T-tube itself!* Suturing the tube itself creates a most serious problem at the time of T-tube withdrawal. Secondary surgery in such instances is a distinct possibility. The surgeon should place the long arm of the T-tube where it is positioned best. *The terminal end portions of the T-tube should not extend into the right hepatic or left hepatic duct or into the cystic duct.* They must be in a free position where they can conveniently drain the entire biliary system without creating mechanical obstruction. From this point on, the choledochotomy stoma must be closed watertight. The closure should be tested with saline under pressure so that any spot leakage can be recognized and closed with an additional interrupted suture or two. Only after a watertight seal is attained should a routine cholangiogram be taken. Leakage of dye will spoil the picture's detail.

In regard to withdrawal of the T-tube, the time for removal must never be reduced to a routine measure. It must always be dealt with as an individual problem. Removal of a T-tube in the postoperative period should always depend upon the original pathology, the surgery performed, and, most of all, the condition of the patient. Some T-tubes may be removed earlier than others—*but no T-tube should ever be removed too soon!* The criteria for T-tube removal are fully discussed under "A Rule for Safe Withdrawal of the T-Tube." (See Post-operative management of the T-tubes.)

References

1. Hicken NF, Best RR, Hunt HB: Cholangiography: Visualization of the gallbladder and bile ducts during and after surgery. *Am Surg* 103:210, 1936.
2. Micken NF, McAllister AJ: Operative cholangiography as an aid in reducing the incidence of "overlooked" common duct stones: A study of 1293 choledocholithotomies. *Surgery* 55:753, 1964.
3. Hall RC, Sakiyalak P, Kim SK, et al: Failure of operative cholangiography to prevent retained common duct stones. *Am J Surg* 125:1, 1951.

MANOMETRY

Operative manometry is predicated on the idea that stones impacted at the distal end of the common duct will partially obstruct the outflow of bile and thereby increase the intrabiliary pressure. This same increase in pressure will follow sphincter spasm or stenosis. Essentially, Caroli's operative manometry is set up by attaching to a manometer a Merriott bottle containing a radiopaque dye which can be adjusted on a track to a set level above the common bile duct. The Merriott bottle can be raised gradually until a continuous bubbling develops, which indicates that the flow has passed into the duodenum. An image intensifier can show the exact point at which the dye enters the duodenal lumen. Those who use manometry during biliary surgery claim that overlooked small stones may be picked up where operative cholangiography may fail. A sphincteric pressure of over 16 cm of water is considered an obstruction to the bile flow.

This writer places more confidence and reliability on the direct findings of intraoperative cholangiography than on the indirect readings of manometry. He also believes that those who employ operative manometry to avoid doing intraoperative cholangiography are putting too much importance and reliability on manometry, and eliminating valuable factual information that is attainable only with direct cholangiography, i.e. anomalous biliary anatomy, stones or lesions in the ampulla of Vater, and intrahepatic pathology.

Manometric techniques, when performed endoscopically, provide a more rational approach to characterizing the dysfunction of motility of the sphincter of Oddi.

Recommended Reading

Van Sonnenberg E, Ferrucci JT Jr, Neff CC, et al: Biliary pressure: Manometric and perfusion studies at percutaneous transhepatic cholangiography and percutaneous biliary drainage. *Radiology* 148:41, 1983.

Greenen JE: Sphincter of Oddi manometry. *Clin Gastroenterol* 12:108, 1983.

Hogan WJ, Greenen JE, Dodds W, et al: Cholecystokinin (CCK-OP) in patients with suspected sphincter of Oddi dysfunction. *Gastroenterology* 12:108, 1983.

Tanaka M, Ikeda S, Nakayama F· Continuous measurement of common duct pressure with an indwelling microtransducer catheter introduced by duodenoscopy: or postcholecystectomy dyskinesia. *Endoscopy* 29:83, 1983.

Gregg JA, Carr-Locke DL: Endoscopic pancreatic and biliary manometry in pancreatic, biliary and papillary disease and sphincteroplasty. *Gut* 11:1247, 1984.

Infections of the Common Bile Duct

CHOLANGITIS (CHOLEDOCHITIS)*

The biliary system is a series of tubules that deliver bile from their origin in the hepatic cells into the common duct, and ultimately through the ampullary opening into the duodenum. This biliary system originates in a vast network of microscopic tubules called *canaliculi*, which are located in the clefts or openings formed by the epithelium of the adjacent hepatic cells. These microscopic tubules drain into bile ductules called *cholangioles*, which are lined with cuboidal cells, and continue to traverse or pass through the hepatic lobule, ultimately joining up with the larger interlobular ducts that are situated within the portal tracts. The latter, consisting of cuboidal or low columnar epithelium,

*(See Sclerosing Choledochitis, page 283).

pass through the hepatic lobule, ultimately join with the interlobular ducts that are situated within the portal tracts, and that have a much wider lumen and are lined with taller epithelial cells.

Larger ducts from the right and left lobes ultimately fuse at the porta hepatis to form the main or common hepatic duct. The common hepatic duct continues down a variable distance before the cystic duct enters it and the union becomes the common bile duct. The latter continues downward between the duodenum and pancreas, enters the wall of the duodenum obliquely, and finally exits via the ampulla of Vater (see Anatomy in Chap. 2). It is not often that the biliary tree system is discussed as a system in which cholangitis is the main feature. An acute or chronic inflammatory process may develop in any portion of the biliary tract, yet despite the continuity of the tree, isolated segmental portions of an inflammatory process may develop. There is an overlapping of the involved areas that may extend into its many communications with the smaller and larger branches. When we refer to *cholangitis*, we usually mean an inflammatory process involving the wall and the lumen of the extrahepatic and/or intrahepatic ducts; *cholangiolitis* refers to a similar inflammatory involvement, but it is mainly of the intralobular bile ductules. Often combinations of this inflammatory process are encountered.

Causes

There are many factors capable of producing a histopathological picture and a possible clinical syndrome that are characteristic of cholangitis. It is well to assume that the diagnosis of cholangitis, when employed, involves the need for further evaluation of the intra- and/or extrahepatic causes of this condition.

BACTERIAL. The majority of suppurative lesions are produced by bacteria that are usually admitted via the biliary tree system secondary to extrahepatic sources. The common organisms are *E. coli, Aerobacter aerogenes, Streptococcus fecalis, and B. proteus.* Bacteria have been known to reach the biliary tract system not only by direct portal tracts but also via the bloodstream and lymphatics.

PARASITES. *Ascaris lumbricoides,* and trematodes such as *Clonorchis sinensis* and *Fasciola hepatica* are parasitic infestations usually found in the Orient. They produce what is commonly known as *cholagiohepatitis.* The worm or parasite and/or their products may produce severe irritation of the bile ducts, as well as desquamation of the epithelium that is often associated with secondary infection. This inflammatory process, so commonly seen in oriental countries, further leads to stricturing of the ductal system at various sites locally or diffusely. Calculus formation is often associated with obstruction, and abscesses, either single or multiple, develop subsequently [see "Asiatic (Oriental) Cholangiohepatitis"].

GEOGRAPHIC CONSIDERATIONS. Where the hygienic conditions of a country are good or superior, parasitic infections are either reduced or rare. The countries of the East, i.e., China, India, Egypt, and others, often have to deal with these parasitic infections, but to date there is no effective plan of therapy for them other than to manage the secondary complications as they are recognized.

What we see more frequently in the Western countries is usually a cholangitis of bacterial origin, usually from a secondary source. These organisms are pyogenic as a rule; they are mentioned above. There is also a condition known as *benign sclerosing cholangitis*. The cause is unknown and is commonly referred to as being *idiopathic*. The pathological process of the extrahepatic biliary system is primarily a sclerosing or narrowing process called *sclerosing cholangitis*. Sclerosing cholangitis may coexist with rarer forms of retroperitoneal fibrosis. It may also coexist with ulcerative colitis and may be associated with neoplastic lesions of the ampulla and ductal walls. Benign sclerosis may involve the entire biliary ductal system at times, or it may involve specific segments for no explainable reason. The sclerosing process involves the entire circumference of the ducts; it therefore infringes upon the lumen, ultimately leading to obstructive signs and symptoms. The latter are indistinguishable from those of a slow-growing carcinoma arising inside or outside the biliary system. Sclerosing cholangitis, though not common, is not uncommon.

This writer cannot recall ever diagnosing sclerosing cholangitis preoperatively; he has often found it at surgery, but then only after cholangiographic studies have revealed it. At present, no specific etiological factor has been mentioned to cover all the benign forms of sclerosing cholangitis, but this writer recalls several cases where common ducts have been strenuously and traumatically explored, especially after impacted stones were removed employing every possible traumatic manipulation. After many years, perhaps 5–10 or even 20 years later, the surgeon sees the same patient with a jaundice simulating neoplasia. In such cases, at surgery, a benign sclerosing cholangitis is found.

Often the pathologist may have difficulty in differentiating a severe case of sclerosing cholangitis from invasive carcinoma of the bile duct wall. Errors have been made in diagnosing a sclerosing carcinoma of the common bile ducts when in fact the disease was actually a benign sclerosing cholangitis. Though we have ideas and theories about the etiological factors producing this disease, benign sclerosing cholangitis still remains a mystery.

Pathology

As previously stated, the diagnosis of benign sclerosing cholangitis is rarely if ever made preoperatively, and, according to this writer, is been recognized at surgery only when the gross picture reveals a severe fibrosis of the common duct—a thickening that involves the lumen, so that a 8-10 Fr T-tube cannot enter. Often dilatation is required to relieve the marked stenosis. The biopsy for a frozen section study usually reveals a sclerotic process characteristic of sclerosing cholangitis.

Not infrequently, the pathologist asks for an additional specimen in order to rule out a sclerosing carcinoma. The Glassman common duct nylon brush (see Chapter 11) may be useful in obtaining cells for cytology. If any glands have been removed, they too should be sent for frozen section; they may help corroborate or rule out further evidence of carcinoma. Much has been learned about the histopathology of sclerosing cholangitis because of liver biopsy. Percutaneous liver biopsy is now a common diagnostic tool, and from these small portions of liver tissue the pathologist can often make an accurate histological diagnosis and demonstrate the histopathological changes characteristic of cholangitis.

In inflammatory suppurative cholangitis, the pathologist will usually find a predominance of inflammatory cells, namely, polymorphonuclear leukocytes; they may be present in and around the duct wall and may be associated with an inflammatory exudate found in the lumen of the biliary tree. Cholangitis is often associated with a marked degree of obstruction of the smaller ductules that result in a centrolobular cholestasis. This is often noted when periportal fibrosis is a contributing feature. The more chronic forms of benign sclerosing cholangitis may be associated with a lymphocytic infiltrate associated with cholestasis and periportal fibrosis. In considering benign sclerosing cholangitis, we should remember that the hepatotoxic drugs such as the phenothiazines, carbon tetrachloride, arsphenamines, halothane anesthetics, and sulfonamides, as well as paraaminosalicylic acid and others. These drugs produce an intrahepatic cholestasis; with an inflammatory process and a predominance of lymphocytes. The lymphocytes usually accumulate around the bile ducts, ductules, canaliculi, and cholangioles.

In primary biliary cirrhosis, there is a marked lymphocytic infiltrate surrounding the smaller biliary radicles similar to that which may be found in other forms of chronic cholangitis. The pathologist is well aware that the clinical picture of drug-induced cholestasis, as differentiated from primary biliary cirrhosis, seldom simulates the acute process of cholangitis. Drugs should always be considered a contributing factor, if not a primary factor, in all cases of cholangitis.

Signs and Symptoms of Benign Sclerosing Cholangitis

Technically, there is an insidious onset of jaundice, which becomes more marked over a period of weeks and months (see the chart "Differential Diagnosis of Jaundice" in Chapter 6). It is a painless jaundice with increasingly intense discoloration; gastrointestinal complaints may develop, especially those similar to the signs and symptoms seen in gallbladder disease. A differential diagnosis is very difficult to make at this time, but must be attempted since time is an important factor. Not infrequently, the patient has been operated on before for common duct stones, where irritation and excessive instrumental manipulation of the common duct may have caused mucosal trauma. Even Whipple once considered this process to be initiated by primary cholecystectomy and cholelithiasis, implying that the common duct was unduly manipulated and irritated in a careless, traumatic manner. This traumatizing exploration initiates a stimulative or irritative process that ultimately induces fibrosis, leading to a sclerotic process within the duct.

This writer, like Whipple, has always felt that an important causative factors is previous cholecystectomy, especially the unduly long scraping of common duct explorations. Glassman's gallstone extractors were developed to prevent prolonged, traumatizing common duct explorations (see Chapter 11).

The signs and symptoms of sclerosing cholangitis are predominantly those of epigastric discomfort, particularly in the right upper quadrant, that strongly simulates gallbladder disease. There might be weight loss and enlargement of the liver on physical examination; the findings are often the same as those encountered in conditions involving obstructive jaundice. The bilirubin becomes elevated beyond 2, 3, or 4 mg%, and often obviates the value of an intravenous cholangiogram or cholecystogram.

Ultrasonography, endoscopic retrograde pancreatography, and percutaneous transhepatic cholangiography can be helpful. The urobilinogen is usually positive; the bile is found in small amounts, and its color may be lighter than golden, possibly yellow. Sclerosing cholangitis is a disease with a jaundice that usually becomes progressively marked or fixed. However, since this is a progressive disease, the ultimate and inevitable pathological change is cirrhosis of the liver; this, not infrequently, becomes terminal.

Diagnosis of Acute Cholangitis

Acute cholangitis is usually an acute suppurative process of the biliary tree system and is associated with fever, chills, and jaundice; the temperature may spike and may be associated with an enlarged, tender liver. Laboratory data in acute cholangitis usually show a polymorphonuclear leukocytosis with a shift to the left and a count as high as 30,000 or more. If there is no intra- or extrahepatic obstruction, the bilirubin level, though elevated, is usually not very high. It may range between 3 mg% and 12 mg%, and a Direct van den Berg is usually a predominant finding. SGOT and SGPT are markedly elevated and can reach levels of 1,000. When the levels are unduly high, one must assume that the inflammatory process has affected the hepatic cellular structure and has possibly produced an associated hepatocellular necrosis (see Chart I, "Differential Diagnosis of Jaundice" in Chapter 6).

Liver biopsies may be attempted, and here a pathological diagnosis will be of great help; one of the biopsy specimens may be utilized for culture and sensitivity studies. If multiple abscess formation is suspected, liver biopsy should not be performed. To detect whether liver abscesses are present, a liver scan can be of great value in explaining a possible elevated diaphragm and/or multiple filling defects in the liver. As stated before, when the bilirubin is over 3, cholangiographic studies fail to show any effective visualization and therefore the surgeon must resort to studies other than X-rays. A computed tomography scan is an effective means of finding and localizing liver abscesses (see "Percutaneous Transhepatic Drainage of Liver Abscess" in Chapter 5).

Whether the tentative diagnosis is acute or chronic cholangitis, exploratory laparotomy may have to be carried out, not only as a diagnostic measure but for the immediate treatment itself.

However, laparotomy should not be resorted to until every proper conservative medical treatment has been attempted. Percutaneous transhepatic cholangiography is considered an excellent method of draining the liver abscess.

The surgeon and the operating room personnel must stand by to operate immediately if any complication, i.e., bile leakage or hemorrhage, develops. Transhepatic cholangiography performed at the time of surgery results in fewer complications. It is better, quicker, and allows more accurate placement of the needle. Also, the surgeon is ready to correct any correctible defect encountered at the time of surgery. A finer long needle has been developed in Japan; it is called the *skinny* or *Chiba* needle. Essentially, it is a long, fine needle with a large-size bore; it is less traumatic, creating fewer complications during liver biopsy or percutaneous transhepatic cholangiography.

Treatment of Cholangitis

A patient with cholangitis has to be carefully evaluted, as well as managed and observed preoperatively. A diagnosis of cholangitis (either acute or chronic), when established, will be found secondary to a suspected mechanical lesion, such as a stone in the common duct, stricture, neoplasm, or a fistula from the gallbladder or common duct. The latter are indications for immediate corrective surgical intervention, the patient having been continuously prepared for the urgent surgery. A percutaneous liver biopsy should help give the precise diagnosis. Another advantage is obtained by having the needle biopsy sent for culture and sensitivity studies to help identify the organism and select the ideal antibiotic for pre- and postoperative treatment.

An antibiotic with the broadest spectrum or a combination of antibiotics should be utilized before, during, and after surgery. One must always be on the lookout for endotoxic shock, which is usually caused by gram-negative and bacteroides organisms. In such instances, the patient is usually seriously ill with a septicemia and its associated signs and symptoms. The proper antibiotic or combination of antibiotics should be used, and in the proper dosage. In the bacterial studies of Salk et al.,[1] the organisms most frequently cultured from the common bile duct were (1) *Escherichia coli*, (2) *Klebsiella*, (3) *Streptococcus*, (4) *Aerobacter*, (5) *Pseudomonas*, (6) *Enterobacter*, (7) *Bacteroides*, (8) *Citrobacter*, (9) *Staphylococcus*, (10) *Clostridia*, and (11) *Proteus*, in that order. Their study was made from 26 out of 28 patients who underwent surgery with

cholangitis; they noted that 16 of the patients gave cultures containing multiple organisms. The high incidence (90% or more) of cultured organisms in the presence of stones in the common duct have been reported by many investigators, and the incidence of positive biliary cultures was definitely related to the severity of the clinical findings.

The preoperative blood culture studies for antibiotics simulated the order in which the frequency of organisms was found in operated cases. Possibly it could be shown that preoperative culture and sensitivity studies may be very significant in reducing morbidity and mortality. It should be noted that in several cases the bacterial flora changed during the course of the antibiotic therapy, and therefore required a change in chemotherapy. Patients with *E. coli* subsequently developed positive cultures for *Candida* and other bacteria; gram-negative organisms were found to change over to *Pseudomonas* and *Bacteroides*. Salk et al., in considering the surgical aspects of this disease, stated that the operative approach to cholangitis has been inconsistent. They stated that operative intervention for decompression of the common duct is mandatory, especially where the patient is becoming moribund. They noted that 50% of the patients operated on survived, whereas two who were not operated on died. Others have also confirmed this experience with their series of studies. In the series reported by Salk et al. 75% of the patients with biliary tract disease underwent surgery, and 28% of this group had cholangitis.

The procedures performed in these cases were variable. Patients treated by decompression after common duct exploration had a much better chance of living than those in whom a cholecystectomy alone or a cholecystoduodenostomy was performed. The latter results can only be attributed to inadequate drainage of the common duct and false reliance upon cholecystostomy. Salk et al. stated that of their patients operated on for biliary tract disease, 23% had common duct exploration, and that of all the patients in whom cholangitis was found, 63% had common duct exploration. Of all the patients who underwent surgery for cholangitis, or developed it subsequently, 82% had common duct exploration; Salk et al. postulated that the figure should be 100%.

Salk et al.[1] concluded that drainage of the gallbladder alone, without prudent visualization of the common duct or patency of the cystic duct, remains an inadequate operation for cholangitis; the writer agrees with this and deplores the time required to do a cholangiographic or cystic duct study. A common duct procedure such as a choledochostomy with warm saline irrigation and T-tube drainage is far more suitable and will be followed with less morbidity and far less mortality. The final conclusions of Salk et al. are as follows:

1. Cholangitis is generally associated with high morbidity and mortality; the mortality may range from 25 to 60% and is related to the severity of the disease.
2. Haupert et al.[2] noted that in their cases the mortality was 13% in the usual patient; it increased to 48% (almost four times) when the signs and symptoms of hypotension and septicemia appeared to coexist. They felt that regardless of the severity of the disease, surgery was mandatory, especially where septicemia and hypotension developed.
3. In the series of Haupert et al.,[2] all patients who were not operated on died of cholangitis associated with septicemia and hypotension. Salk et al. stated further that all patients who developed shock preoperatively and had to be treated for it prior to surgery died preoperatively. The writer feels that Salk et al. were dealing with endotoxic shock. He goes on to state that in the final evaluation, 60% of their patients with hypotension without septicemia survived. Patients who had contraindications to surgery, when given antibiotics, had an immediate response with a satisfactory course and no relapse; those with inoperable malignant disease were spared surgery.

The selection of antibiotics is very important; it may depend primarily upon the blood culture, which can reveal possible specific sensitivity studies. Tetracyclines (Terramycin), cephalosporins (Keflin, Mandol), chloramphenicol (Chloromycetin), and ampicillin have been rather successful in a majority of cases. One broad-spectrum antibiotic is usually adequate; however, two should be utilized when one alone does not give the desired response. Whenever there is a favorable response, surgery can be delayed as long as possible, especially in the presence of contraindications. Delay is appropriate and wise, because the surgery will subsequently be carried out with less morbidity and mortality.

Delayed surgery gives the surgeon an opportunity to correct all early evidence of shock, fluid deficits, and electrolyte imbalances. The tendency toward renal failure may be decreased by administration of mannitol, steroids, and colloid replacement wherever blood is unavailable. One should never forget the important part that hypoglycemia

and diabetes mellitus play in these cases, and one should not hesitate to use hypertonic glucose when evidence of hyperinsulinism and hypoglycemia exists.

In the final analysis, unless contraindications exist, an operative procedure should be considered and an exploration carried out. Most important is the drainage of the common duct. *The writer wishes to emphasize that common duct exploration is most important and that cholecystostomy is rather ineffective, especially when there is pathology within the cystic duct or an obstructing defect at the cystic duct junction with the common duct.* Where conservative management fails to produce a response, operation even in the presence of continued symptoms or aggravated symptoms becomes mandatory. In summary, Salk et al. state the following:

1. The diagnosis must be established as early as possible.
2. The diagnosis should be confirmed by culture and sensitivity studies; if possible, these should include a culture of the urine, blood, and sputum.
3. As early as possible, the proper antibiotic or antibiotics should be administered, especially in elderly and high-risk patients.
4. All conditions that could jeopardize the surgery must be corrected, such as shock and cardiovascular-renal factors, as well as replacement of fluid and electrolytes and the utilization of insulin or glucose, whichever may be necessary.
5. Clotting abnormalities must be evaluated and corrected.
6. The common bile duct must be surgically drained.
7. At surgery, culture of the bile and peritoneal fluid is important.
8. If there is time and the patient is not seriously ill, an operative cholangiogram should be considered; otherwise, it should best be postponed for the postoperative period.
9. It is important to operate as quickly as possible. Postoperative care is very important, including monitoring of the blood pressure, pulse, respiration, urinary output (with a urinometer), and, in certain cases, central venous pressure readings; controlled intravenous feedings are also important.
10. There must be careful and propitious use of antibiotics before, during, and after cholangiography for any traumatic manipulation of the biliary ductal system during the surgery, and for any studies that must be done in the postoperative period.

Of the surgical patients reported by Salk et al., 20 had cholecystectomy, 4 had cholecystostomy, and 23 had common duct exploration; positive findings were obtained in 21 of the common ducts explored. Operative cholangiography was performed in the 23 patients in whom exploration was carried out. A sphincteroplasty was done in three cases, choledochoduodenostomy in three, and cholecystoduodenostomy in one. No surgery was performed in eight cases.

Corticosteroids may be indicated and can help to correct shock. The internist at this point should be cognizant of all the cardiovascular-renal problems that are usually associated with this problem and be prepared to deal effectively with them. Wherever large or multiple small hepatic abscesses are found, they are not usually responsive to antibiotic therapy. Percutaneous transhepatic localization and drainage is an ideal treatment for liver abscess. The pus can be evacuated and the cavity irrigated with the proper antibiotic instillations (see Casal's "Percutaneous Drainage of Liver Abscess," in Chapter 5). It is also possible to remove the products of necrosis and then instill an antibiotic into the lumen of the abscess. Computed tomography scans in follow-up studies show abscess cavities shrunken in size.

Parasitic infestations of the Orient, when recognized, are difficult to treat; in fact, as far as we know, they are incurable. Nevertheless, every attempt should be made to provide palliation and possible cure. When *A. lumbricoides* is found to be the cause, peparazine derivatives may be utilized with the hope of eradication. As far as the treatment of *Cl. sinensis* or *F. hepatica* is concerned, drugs such as chloroquin phosphate and emetine hydrochloride are given as in amoebiasis; the overall results remain questionable to poor [see "Asiatic (Oriental) Cholangiohepatitis"].

Surgery is indicated wherever multiple abscesses develop in the liver, and drainage of the biliary tree is the treatment of choice. These cases often result in multiple surgeries, with ultimate fatality from obstruction and/or infection, i.e., suppurative cholangitis and septicemia. Ultimately, cirrhosis of the liver develops, with precoma and death.

Hemorrhage is not an infrequent occurrence when the liver is badly destroyed; a high prothrombin time and a bleeding tendency are the underlying causes. Often the latter problem is treated with multiple antibiotics and numerous transfusions, but still the prognosis remains grave. The treatment today is ineffective at best; the prognosis remains consistently poor up to the ultimate demise of the patient.

If laparotomy is chosen as the only diagnostic means of approaching suspected benign sclerosing cholangitis, it is imperative that the biliary tree be thoroughly evaluated, and though the gallbladder may or may not contain stones, the immediate evaluation must be of the common bile duct. Here, after careful dissection, visualization of the common duct will reveal, after it is properly denuded, to be a rigid tube that can be rolled between the forefinger and thumb of the left hand and felt as a cord-like structure. The duct at times is so thick that compressibility is not possible, and the small size of the lumen remains a serious question. As previously stated, this sclerosing process may or may not involve the entire biliary ductal system, or any particular portion thereof, and if the entire process is interductal, nothing will be palpated over the surface of the common duct.

The obstruction will often exist within the liver itself. If the common duct is sclerosed concomitantly with the intraductal system, the disease will be more acute in onset and more fulminating in character. It is imperative that when the common duct is opened a small lumen be suspected and watched for, because it is so very easy to injure the opposite wall; when an opening is accomplished and the small lumen is recognized, it is imperative to take a specimen from the wall and send it immediately to pathology for frozen section, culture, and sensitivity studies. Microscopic examination is the most accurate method of establishing a final diagnosis.

Of course, a sclerosing carcinoma of the common duct wall must be ruled out. It is conceivable that the sclerosing process, even though it is benign, may continue until death. At autopsy it will be possible to demonstrate that what was thought to be sclerosing cholangitis was in fact a carcinoma. It should be remembered that at surgery it is most difficult to recognize a carcinoma, especially when it simulates benign sclerosing cholangitis. Usually small-cell carcinoma is not easily identifiable. On several occasions, the pathologist may request another specimen, usually a bigger one. The gallbladder may or may not be involved; if it is, it is usually no different than a cholelithiasis when found as the only existing disease. The gallbladder should be removed, and the common duct opened and drained with a small-size catheter or T-tube that will fit into the small lumen. If necessary, it may be wise to employ a Cattell long-arm T-tube, now modified by this writer at surgery with multiple perforations at the lower end of one arm so as not to obstruct the pancreatic duct. At times, the surgeon may wish to cut away half of the longitudinal tube because only half of the circumference of the tube will fit into the small lumen of the common duct. A small polyethylene tube may have to be employed on occasion.

If in the evaluation of the common duct the gallbladder appears normal, and its cystic and common duct unobstructed, it is wise to preserve the gallbladder and not remove it, because if obstruction develops distal to the cystic duct later on, the gallbladder can still be utilized to short-circuit the bile into the jejunum. The continued medical management of benign sclerosing cholangitis or chronic cholangitis may entail the added use of steroids, i.e., cortisone and prednisone. These drugs must be used cautiously in decreasing dosage; they are used because their antidesmoplastic action may prevent progression of the sclerosing process. Conceivably, they may even cause improvement by softening the ligneous nature of the sclerosis. Steroid use at this stage is certainly worth a try unless there are contraindications to its use. *Steroids have not been as beneficial as was hoped, but they are the only medical treatment available.*

If the pathologist requires more time, a second operation may be necessary at a later date, in which case a bypass procedure may be mandatory. Often during this waiting period when carcinoma may ultimately be discovered, decompression of the liver renders the patient a better candidate for a second-stage definitive surgery. In the final analysis, the surgical procedure will have to await the obvious findings at surgery, so that if the lesion is in the hepatic area and can be resected, it may be possible to do a palliative hepaticojejunostomy.

There are differences of opinion regarding the undue trauma of manipulation to the common duct that ultimately leads to cholangitis. This writer has been teaching and cautioning for years that rough manipulations during common duct exploration and undue, careless dilatation of the sphincter of Oddi are traumatic, unnecessary, and serious. Of definite importance and interest are five patients in the Salk et al. series in whom cholangitis developed after procedures were carried out in the X-ray department. A surgical attempt at extraction of a retained stone with a Dormia basket was also followed by cholangitis.

This writer recently had two patients who, shortly after routine postoperative T-tube cholangiography, developed signs and symptoms of cholangitis. Both of these patients had had prior episodes of cholangitis suggesting instrumentation and increased intracholedochal trauma from a previously explored common bile duct.

Flemma et al.[3] reported 5 of 75 patients who developed cholangitis after transhepatic cholangiogram. They suggested that the surgical trauma of cholangiography can induce irritation with sudden or late obstruction of the bile duct.

Recommended Reading

Chetlin SH, Elliot DW: Biliary bacteremia. *Arch Surg* 102:303, 1971.

Donaldson RM Jr: Normal bacteria populations in the intestine and their relation to intestinal function. *N Engl J Med* 270:994, 1954.

Engstrom J, Helldtrom K, Hogman L, et al: Microbiliary diseases. *Scand J Gastroenterol* 6:177, 1971.

Goswitz JT: Bacteria and biliary tract disease. *Am J Surg* 128:644, 1974.

Gregg JA: Detection of bacterial infection of the pancreatic ducts in patients with pancreatitis and pancreatic cancer during endoscopic cannulation of the pancreatic duct. *Gastroenteroloy* 73:1005, 1977.

Huang T, Bass JA, Williams RD: The significance of biliary pressures in cholangitis. *Arch Surg* 98:629, 1969.

Kalser MH, Cohen R, Arteaga I, et al: Normal viral and bacterial flora of the human small and large intestine. *N Engl J Med* 274:500, 1966.

Lygidakis NJ: Incidence of bile infection in patients with choledocholithiasis. *Am J Gastroenterol* 77:12, 1982.

Lykkegaard NM, Juesten T: Anaerobic and aerobic infections. Bacteriological studies in biliary tract disease. *Scand J Gastroenterol* 11:437, 1976.

Musgrove JE, Grindlay JH, Karlson AG: Intestinal-biliary reflux after anastomosis of common duct to duodenum or jejunum. *Arch Surg* 64:579, 1952.

Rosch W, Burkhardt B, Schmack B, et al: Biological and biochemical analysis of endoscopically aspirated bile. *Endoscopy* 13:33, 1981.

Wiesner RH, La Russo NF, Ludwig J, et al: Comparison of the clinicopathologic features of primary sclerosing cholangitis and primary biliary cirrhosis. *Gastroenterology* 88:108, 1985.

Wood RAB, Cuschieri A: Is sclerosing cholangitis complicating ulcerative colitis a reversible condition? *Lancet* 2:716, 1980.

References

1. Salk RP, Greenberg GA, Farris JM, et al: Spectrum of cholangitis. *Am J Surg* 130:143, 1975.
2. Haupert AP, Carey LC, Evans WE: Acute suppurative cholangitis: Experience with 15 consecutive cases. *Arch Surg* 94:460, 1967.
3. Flemma RJ, Flint LM, Osterhout S, et al: Bacteriologic studies of biliary tract infection. *Ann Surg* 166:563, 1967.

ACUTE SUPPURATIVE CHOLANGITIS

Acute suppurative cholangitis, as the name implies, is a serious acute pyogenic inflammatory process that develops following biliary obstruction (complete or incomplete) and is caused by gallstones, strictures, or neoplastic growths. Suppurative cholangitis may follow foreign bodies in the biliary tree; not infrequently, it may develop via the stoma of a biliary-intestinal anastomosis. What are the mechanisms or pathogenetics that lead to suppurative cholangitis? They are:

1. Inadequate biliary flow through an obstructed or stenotic anastomotic stoma of a choledochodenostomy or choledochojejunostomy. *(An adequate biliary flow rarely causes reflux and inflammatory changes.)*
2. Conceivably by regurgitation via the ampulla of Vater.
3. Conceivably by spread from an infected acute cholecystitis.
4. Conceivably via the ascending lymphatics along the portal vein.
5. Conceivably by bacteremic arterial blood passing into the liver sinusoids and then into the biliary canaliculi.
6. Primary pyogenic cholecystitis may develop without any known underlying cause.
7. Iatrogenic sclerosing cholangitis may be caused by ERCP.

Pathogenetics, Symptoms, and Signs

An acute sclerosing cholangitis implies that a sclerosing process has developed in the biliary tract and that the pus, being under pressure, will regurgitate up into the liver canaliculi, then into the venous sinusoids, and finally will enter the hepatic venous system, producing toxic shock syndrome.

The symptoms and signs usually include fever, chills, jaundice, and right upper quadrant and/or epigastric pain. Mental aberration may complicate the picture. The patient's condition continues to deteriorate as the disease process spreads, and unless emergency measures are taken to decompress the suppurative process within the closed system of the biliary tree, the patient will succumb.

Complications

Leukopenia, thrombocytopenia, hypoprothrombinemia, and hypoglycemia may develop, as well as renal failure. In the latter instance, acute tubular necrosis is a frequent accompaniment.

Treatment

The treatment must depend upon the severity of the patient's condition. If the patient is not seriously ill, the treatment should be aimed at a more definitive diagnosis and an intensive preoperative preparation for probable surgical intervention. The surgical intensive care unit (SICU) is the ideal place to institute intensive management of a seriously ill patient. All systems must be carefully monitored and the following therapy administered: IV fluids—Ringer's lactate, about 2–4 liters; plasma (fresh frozen), if available and needed (2–4 units may be required); vitamin K (Mephyton), 10–20 mg/kg IV, given slowly; antibiotics, i.e., ampicillin, gentamicin, and clindamycin—if necessary, vancomycin or chloramphenicol may be employed. If the blood pressure is dropping or unstable, dopamine may be employed; 2–4 mg/kg/min is given initially and may be increased, if necessary, to 20 mg/kg/min; corticosteroids (methylprednisolone), 30 mg/kg IV may be started at the same time with dopamine.

If necessary, a Swan-Ganz catheter may be employed in the older high-risk patient with a cardiopulmonary problem. Younger patients will probably do well with a central venous line. Urine output should be monitored with an indwelling Foley catheter. Constant nursing care is paramount.

If the Patient's Condition Improves

If possible, surgery should be delayed in order to adequately assess the patient's systems and associated problems, and hopefully to pinpoint the diagnosis. Flat films of the abdomen, ultrasonography, scan, and ERCP may be attempted so long as the patient is deemed capable of tolerating the added burden. If the patient stabilizes and the tentative diagnosis is established, urgent elective surgery should be carried out. The postoperative care should also be carried out in the SICU.

If the Patient's Condition Does Not Improve

If the patient's condition does not get better or if it worsens, the patient should be taken to surgery immediately for emergency decompression of the biliary tree. The surgeon should keep in mind that the primary purpose for operating in this emergency is to decompress and drain the biliary system—not the gallbladder but the common bile duct, with or without a complementary cholecystostomy. The largest possible T-tube that the common duct can accommodate should be employed; the operating room nurse should not bring the surgeon one T-tube. She must bring tubes of all sizes and allow the surgeons to choose the ideal size. Cholecystectomy is not advised at this time unless absolutely indicated. Good judgment must prevail.

Prognosis

The prognosis is fair to poor; morbidity and mortality remain high. The outcome will depend on the time elapsed between disease onset and surgical consultation; the age of the patient and whether associated systemic disease exists; and lastly, the good judgment of the surgeon in determining whether the severely ill patient should go to surgery immediately for decompression, or whether surgery should be delayed in favor of preparing the patient to better tolerate a formidable procedure.

Recommended Reading

Boey JH, Way LW: Acute cholangitis. *Ann Surg* 191:264, 1980.

Carmona RH, Crass RA, Lim RC Jr, et al: Oriental cholangitis. *Am J Surg* 148:117, 1984.

Chock E, Wolfe BM, Matolo NM: Acute suppurative cholangitis. *Surg Clin North Am* 61:885, 1981.

Choi TK, Wong J, Ong GB: Choledochojejunostomy in the treatment of primary cholangitis. *Surg Gynecol Obstet* 155:43, 1982.

Dooley JS, et al: Antibiotics in the treatment of biliary infection. *GVT* 25:988, 1984.

Lam SK: A study of endoscopic sphincterotomy in recurrent pyogenic cholangitis. *Br J Surg* 71:262, 1984.

Lygidakis NJ: Acute suppurative cholangitis; comparison of internal and external biliary drainage. *Am J Surg* 143:304, 1982.

Ostemiller W, Thompson R, Carter R, et al: Acute obstructive cholangitis. *Arch Surg* 90:392, 1965.

Reynolds BM, Dargan EL: Acute obstructive cholangitis. *Ann Surg* 150:299, 1959.

Schwartz SI: Primary sclerosing cholangitis; a disease revisited. *Surg Clin North Am* 53:1161, 1973.

Thompson JE, Tompkins RK, Longmire WP: Factors in the management of acute cholangitis. *Ann Surg* 195:137, 1982.

Tincler L: Primary sclerosing cholangitis. *Postgrad Med* 47:666, 1971.

ASIATIC (ORIENTAL) CHOLANGIOHEPATITIS

Asiatic or Oriental cholangiohepatitis is a recurrent suppurative cholangitis and is found exclusively in the Far East, i.e., China, Hong Kong, and a number of other nearby areas. The writer has seen a few patients who have come from Cuba, but in whom a careful history revealed that they originally came from China. Others who have come from Cuba have given a history of having lived in Hong Kong. The disease has also been found in Japan and Singapore. On occasion, it may be found in Australia and even in the United States. The etiology of Asiatic or Oriental cholangiohepatitis is believed to be the infestation of a fluke known as *Clonorchis sinensis*.

It is most likely that the secondary infection may be pyogenic, and the organisms most often responsible are *B. coli*, *Strep. fecalis*, and *Staphylococcus*. These organisms can be cultured from the bile, as well as from the portal venous blood. On many occasions, reports have appeared in which *Cl. sinensis* (fluke or ova) was not recognized. It is quite possible that those surgeons who have tried to isolate the clonorchis infestation may have failed because the superinfection with *B. coli* and *Strep. fecalis* overshadowed it. It is also possible that the clonorchis organism died and disappeared. Fung[1] in 1961 presented a series of 242 cases, and stated that *Cl. sinensis* ova were discovered in the feces or bile in over 90% of the cases, a finding confirmed at surgery. When this same study was carried out in a surgical population in the Orient, it was found that approximately 45% revealed the clonorchis organism, and then only in the stool. *Cl. sinensis* infestation of the bile ultimately reaches the biliary passages and produces a severe irritation that results in epithelial desquamation, hyperplasia, and stricture formation. A malignant cholangioma was reported by Hou[2] in 1965.

Ascaris lumbricoides has also been reported as a predisposing cause of cholangiohepatitis; these worms have been found in the common duct and the intrahepatic duct radicals, and have resulted in severe hemolysis with a subsequent increase in bilirubin excretion that favored bilirubin deposits in the biliary tree. Intrahepatic changes may occur at various levels in skip areas, and ultimately result in stenosis and puddling of the infection with abscess formations. Fever may appear at intermittent periods and may require high doses of IV antibiotics; this writer has administered penicillin in doses of several million units in order to reduce the infection and the high fever. Chills often accompany the high temperatures, which usually are spiked. In over 50% of the cases jaundice occurs, and even in those cases where jaundice does not appear to be a conspicuous factor, the serum bilirubin is markedly elevated. The total bilirubin may become progressively higher or it may decrease. It is possible that even in the absence of jaundice, the bile ducts may be obstructed or stenosed at several given sites, and that in those strictured areas stones may form, producing further and more complete obstruction associated with infection and multiple abscess formations.

The signs and symptoms of cholangiohepatitis usually consist of high and hectic temperatures associated with chills and rigor. This writer's patients have had intermittent episodes from the time they left the Orient to the time they went to Cuba and then on to America. They had had surgery on several occasions whenever a recurrence of the pathology developed, namely, intrahepatic and extrahepatic obstructions. On each occasion, transfusions, long tube decompression, antibiotics, and continuous IV feeding were required. Although the patients improved and the temperature subsided, the recurrences ultimately were severe enough to result in their death.

An acute attack of cholangiohepatitis consists essentially of fever, tenderness, and jaundice in the majority of cases; the tenderness may result in marked guarding of the right upper quadrant. Most patients that this writer has seen have had their gallbladders removed; therefore, the diagnosis always centered on the common bile duct and the intrahepatic radicles. The main tenderness was in the subcostal area in the right upper quadrant, and if the gallbladder was present, it was usually palpable. It should be added that splenomegaly is not infrequently found, but it is not a specific diagnostic feature.

The laboratory data during an acute attack reveal leukocytosis, commonly as high as 15,000 or over, with a predominance of polymorphonuclear leukocytes with a marked shift to the left. The urine often reveals the presence of bile or bilirubin. The biochemical profile includes liver studies such as alkaline phosphatase, SGOT, lactic dehydrogenase, and prothrombin time, all of which indicate apparent liver damage. Enzyme studies usually show elevation and indicate impairment of liver function.

X-Ray Findings

A scout X-ray film is usually negative but, on occasion, may show evidence of calcific stones in the liver. Occasionally, stones in the gallbladder and/or common duct may be outlined on the scout film. In some instances, there may also be air in the biliary tree. This is not easily accounted for because we are not usually dealing with a biliary-intestinal fistula. Nevertheless, a fistula must be suspected when air is found in the biliary tract. It may be due to the usual pathogenesis of stones in the common duct that ulcerate through the wall of the duct and make their way into the duodenum, producing a choledochoduodenal fistula. We must always consider the possibility of a gas-forming organism that may produce air in the common duct. This is one reason why a culture of the bile or open common duct is so important.

In the presence of jaundice, a good picture with IV cholangiography is unusual, but in those cases where the jaundice is minimal (a bilirubin level of 2 or less), the cholangiogram may indicate stones (filling defects) in the intrahepatic radicals as well as in the common duct. Sonography should offer additional information. A better definition of stones can be seen at surgery during biliary cholangiography; this will give a true picture of the liver and the extrahepatic ducts. It may also show filling defects at given points throughout the liver. These large liver defects may be abscess cavities produced by obstruction and secondary infection.

Pathology

In most cases of Oriental cholangiohepatitis the gallbladder does not appear inflamed, but where an acute process is in progress, dilatation and inflammation or even gangrene may be found near the fundus, where rupture is common. The gallbladder is usually distended with thick, dark bile, and the gallbladder wall is invariably thickened. Stones may be present, but not always. As a rule, the common bile duct is thickened and markedly distended, and is often filled with large, palpable stones; at times, they can be seen through the walls of the common duct. These biliary stones may extend into the liver and smaller biliary radicals. As stated before, a cholangiogram will indicate the sites of obstruction and the lakes of pus behind the stenosis that are found in the biliary tree throughout the liver. Ducts in the liver are constricted at various intervals; at the point behind each obstruction, there are lakes of pus which occupy liver spaces and can be recognized on scans or ultrasonic pictures.

Liver biopsy will often show inflammatory changes in the periductal tissue, as well as evidence of fibrosis and stricture formations which are the result of the body's attempt to heal itself. Stones are usually found behind the strictures. Whether they are formed in the hepatic duct is still questionable, but those who see many of these problems believe that stones, in fact, do form in the biliary radicals but are not structurally the same as the stones in the gallbladder. Their origin may have been a nucleus of the fluke worm itself, and layers of cholesterol, calcium, and bile salts further increase the size of the stones with time.

As time goes on, the infectious condition of the liver and the parenchymatous destruction continue to progress. Ultimately, fibrosis may lead to biliary cirrhosis. Liver biopsy will show hyperplasia of the lining of the ducts accompanied by an extensive desquamation of their cells. There is an inflammatory process of the portal spaces that is often associated with abscess formation, and the septicemia that so often accompanies these processes is responsible for the hectic behavior of the temperature. The latter fluctuations may be caused by the fact that the abscesses erode the capillary walls, allowing bacteria to enter the bloodstream, producing bacteremia and/or septicemia.

The stones, as previously stated, are different from those found in the gallbladder; most likely they are produced by a nidus of bile pigments, desquamated epithelial cells, or other products of inflammation. The nucleus of the stone may also be the *Cl. sinensis* fluke itself or the ova, or it may be *A. lumbricoides*. In this writer's experience, the stones were removed on repeated occasions from the common duct and biliary tree, and cholangiographic studies indicated that stones no longer existed; yet, the patients had to be reoperated because of the rapid reformation of stones in the same places where they had previously been removed. This is certainly a factor in the belief that stones do form in the biliary tract but are not related to the same or usual pathogenesis of gallbladder stones. The few patients whom this writer has dealt with have ultimately become exhausted from intermittent attacks of jaundice, hectic temperatures, weight loss, anemia, and multiple surgeries; their ultimate demise followed collapse and coma.

Diagnosis

The diagnosis of Oriental cholangiohepatitis is first made on the basis of the patient's residence or travel through an endemic area of the Far East. The patient complains of pain, fever, and chills; he suffers an intermittent symptom complex that develops with spontaneous remissions. One must bear in mind that though stones in the common duct can produce this picture, the geographic history must be given credence and not overlooked, especially if the patient is of Oriental origin.

Carcinomas of the liver, biliary tract, or ampulla of Vater are all capable of producing jaundice, but usually a "silent" jaundice, and, not infrequently, an intermittent fever. If the patient is of Asiatic origin—and we know that choledocholithiasis per se, as we see it in Western countries, is rather uncommon in patients of Chinese origin—we must begin to strongly suspect that an Oriental disease such as *Cl. sinensis* or *A. lumbricoides* exists. Amebic abscess of the liver rarely produces jaundice or a distended gallbladder; amebiasis is more related to a gastrointestinal infestation with a complication such as hepatic abscess. Since jaundice does not exist, the diagnosis may be more difficult, but in cases that simulate choledocholithiasis and cholecystolithiasis, the best differentiating factor is an IV cholecystogram. This study will sometimes outline the biliary tree, the stones, and the constrictions and abscess lakes that occur in the liver with fluke infestation. Air in the biliary tree indicates a biliary or duodenal fistula, and though these may occur with cholelithiasis, we know that they are also frequent in the Oriental disease. The clinching factors in the diagnosis are the finding of the offending fluke, *Cl. sinensis*. The ova must be located in the stool or bile; that finding is pathognomonic. Even in endemic areas such as China, Singapore, or Hong Kong, the search for the organism must remain the diagnostic clincher, and at surgery, exploration of the biliary tree ultimately makes the diagnosis certain.

Treatment

The treatment of Oriental cholangiohepatitis is primarily with antibiotics. Chloramphenicol and streptomycin are preferable, and very high doses of penicillin, ampicillin, or cloxacillin are also beneficial. IV therapy is employed to prevent dehydration and correct electrolyte imbalance. The anemia is dealt with by supplying the deficient factor, whether packed red cells or whole blood itself. Aqueous vitamin K_1 (Mephyton) is also an important supplement because of the parenchymatous damage and diminished liver function that occur. Vitamin K deficiency may also be improved by blood transfusions.

In choledocholithiasis with jaundice or jaundice per se, no emergency measures need be undertaken. The preoperative management may often clear up the problem, in which case the offending factor may not turn out to be *Cl. sinensis*. When it is decided that the disease must be evaluated by exploratory laparotomy, the patient is usually in better shape for an extensive surgical exploration and procedure. At the propitious moment, and after the patient has been judged greatly improved during the preoperative conservative period of management, the surgical treatment should provide adequate permanent drainage of the intrahepatic biliary and extrahepatic biliary trees.

If the case is one of advanced cholangiohepatitis, this type of treatment will be extremely difficult to carry out. These cases are considered highly infectious, and wound contamination is very possible. The wound must therefore be protected with towels, laparotomy pads, and incise drape constantly isolating the field of surgery. During closure, the wound should be washed and scrubbed with Phiso-Hex or Betadine. Rubber glove finger drains are employed from the peritoneum up and placed between the sutures that close the wound. If the patient is found to be very ill because of associated cholecystitis, the minimum amount of surgery that will attain adequate drainage is cholecystostomy. However, if the patient is in better condition and has been improved by preoperative measures and the delay, a more definitive procedure may be carried out, such as cholecystectomy and exploration of the common duct. The common duct and the biliary tree must be completely cleansed of all debris, stones, epithelial cells, mud, gravel, and other matter.

Cleaning the common duct should be done with complete walling-off precautions, i.e., the use of lap pads about the choledochostomy stoma as the biliary tree is being copiously irrigated. A (00) chromic catgut suture is routinely used to encircle the cystic duct temporarily so that no bile from the gallbladder pours back into the common duct while it is used for retraction. The latter procedure is not only done for retraction during the surgery; the cystic duct may be ligated for cholecystectomy at the end of the surgery. Stones in the common bile duct and biliary tree are removed as in cases of choledocholithiasis, i.e., with the use of forceps, scoops, brushes, balloons, baskets, a choledochoscope, or whatever may be used to clean out the extra- and intrahepatic ducts.

Bakes dilators or the blunt-tip flexible silver probe and a hepatic brush may be used to probe the right and left hepatic ducts with the intent of dilating the strictures so that stones, bile, and trapped lakes of pus are allowed to drain out. Irrigation with copious amounts of saline is carried out to help dislodge and wash out debris, stones, gravel, pus, and perhaps the flukes. The Glassman biliary nylon brush was devised especially for the hepatic ducts; it is recommended for withdrawing stones from the upper smaller intrahepatic radicals of the biliary tree (see "A New Technique for the Removal of Resistant Gallstones from the Hepatic Duct" in Chapter 11). The Glassman flexible probe may be used to dilate hepatic duct strictures and thereby assist in further draining the more remote sections of the liver. The procedure is concluded after cultures for growth and sensitivity have been taken, and a T-tube is inserted into the common duct for decompression and subsequent cholangiographic studies.

There is no hurry to remove the T-tube because of early recurrences. Recurrences may readily be recognized by repeated cholangiographic studies of the biliary tree. The T-tube may be used therapeutically to sterilely irrigate the biliary tree. The nurse can be taught to do this. This writer notes that as soon as the T-tube is removed, the disease continues to progress and the patient progressively deteriorates; coma and ultimately death usually ensue. In one case, this writer resorted to choledochoduodenostomy with a 2.5-cm opening between the common duct and the duodenum, which allowed easy passage for reforming stones.

The ultimate result was the same, i.e., the patient was in excellent condition for a short period, but signs and symptoms soon redeveloped. Hectic temperature, chills, rigors, and high leukocyte counts ultimately resulted in death. Another surgical procedure, recommended by those who have had greater experience with this disease, is transduodenal sphincterotomy. Here too, the purpose is to allow reformed stones to pass easily into the duodenum. *Unfortunately, the multiple stenotic features high in the biliary tree prevent the easy passage of high-lying stones, which remain trapped behind the strictures.* Only a limited number of smaller stones actually pass through the enlarged opening. Ultimately, the bile itself is obstructed by strictures, and lakes of pus continue to take their toll in parenchymatous destruction. The back pressure that accompanies jaundice and the secondary infection are the cause of chills and fever and, ultimately, the demise of the patient.

Cholecystectomy is the last procedure of the exploratory operation, and since the gallbladder is not typically inflamed, it is still advisable to remove it. There are those who do not believe that the gallbladder is involved in this process and therefore do not do a cholecystectomy. These surgeons ultimately find that a subacute inflammatory process within the gallbladder develops, possibly obstructing the cystic duct. In this case, the gallbladder becomes a closed system and fails to respond to T-tube decompression. This writer feels that although the gallbladder is not the primary site of the disease, and often is not inflamed, it should be removed because the gallbladder can lead to complications in the postoperative period.

Prognosis

The prognosis is always guarded but usually poor to grave. Repeated cholangiograms indicate that even though the biliary tree has been cleansed of all its contents—namely, stones, debris, epithelial cells, and gravel—they recur despite repeated irrigations. Antibiotics help mainly when secondary infections set in but have no effect upon the fluke infestation itself. The disease is progressive. The complications, i.e., multiple abscesses caused by secondary infection that results in hectic fever and inanition, ultimately are responsible for the death of the patient. The only effective treatment to prolong life is surgical, which at present is only palliative. The only known cure for Oriental cholangiohepatitis caused by *Cl. sinensis, A. lumbricoides,* or any other worm infestation is *prophylactic treatment.* This is really a public health matter and must not be in the exclusive domain of the private physician. Public health departments should teach the people that when visiting Asiatic countries or Middle Eastern countries, there is a distinct danger in eating inadequately cooked food, particularly uncooked freshwater fish. Raw fish of any kind is forbidden. Eating snails from Egyptian waters or in any Asiatic country can give rise to bilhariasis, another incurable disease. Prophylactic measures forbid drinking or eating food from infested water. One should avoid food suspected of being contaminated. Finally, the prognosis is poor to fatal; the patients will ultimately succumb to liver failure, toxemia, and at long last, carcinoma of the biliary tree.

Recommended Reading

Faust EC, Khaw OK: Studies on *Clonorchis sinensis* (Cobbold). *Am J Hyg,* monogr ser no 8., 1927.

Hsu HF, Wang LS: Studies on certain problems of *Clonorchis sinensis.* IV. Notes on the resistance of cysts in fish flesh, the migration route, and the morphology of the young worm in the final host. *China Med J* suppl 2:385, 1938.

Kobayashi H: A study of *Clonorchis endemicus* (in Japanese). *Dobuzu Zasshi (J Zool)* no 264, 1910.

Mukoyama T: Experimental studies on the route of migration by *Clonorchis sinensis* in the final host. *Nippon Byori Gakkai Kaishi* 11:443, 1921. (Japanese test with addenda by T. Asada, and German summary, p 124).

Muto M: Studies on the first intermediate host of *Clonorchis sinensis* (in Japanese). *Nippon Igakkai Zasshi* 8:151, 1918.

References

1. Fung JJ, Demetris AJ, Porter KA, et al: Liver fluke infestation and cholangiohepatitis. *Br J Surg* 48:404, 1961.
2. Hou PC: Pathological changes in the intrahepatic bile ducts of cats *(Felis catus)* infested with *Clonorchis sinensis. Pathol Bacteriol* 89:357, 1965.

SCLEROSING CHOLEDOCHITIS

Sclerosing choledochitis is a fibrosing or sclerosing process that affects the entire biliary ductal system. At surgery the common duct is found to be hardened and narrowed, and its wall thickened. When the common duct is incised, the fibrous tissue is found to be hard to cut, and in fact resembles carcinoma. A slow, deliberate incision into the thick common duct wall is essential until one finally enters the small lumen of the duct. A biopsy should be made immediately of the ductal wall; it will help to distinguish ductal fibroplasia from carcinoma of the biliary tract. Carcinoma of the bile duct wall is not common, but neither is it uncommon. The thickening of the bile duct wall may vary in degree, and there are instances where the thickening is so severe that even the smallest catheter will not fit into the lumen. In most instances, the T-tube will have to be small or sectioned longitudinally in view of the occluding process. No one really knows the exact pathogenetic process involved; sometimes it is seen as a primary finding, and at other times it is discovered at a second or third procedure where the continuing underlying pathological process ultimately led to a recognizable sclerosing process.

The clinical picture may be that of an insidious pathological process, or it may be associated with signs and symptoms of chronic cholecystitis and cholelithiasis. It is most often discovered in a secondary procedure where, after a previous common duct exploration, reexploration of the common duct reveals a marked thickening of the wall. The latter may be a form of secondary sclerosing cholangitis. Insidious sclerosing cholangitis is not accompanied by pain, but there may be a slight increase in jaundice, as evidenced by a rising serum bilirubin level and an elevated liver enzyme reading. The digestive complaints may be vague; if anything, they relate to gallbladder dysfunction. As noted previously, more often than not, the disease is an associated finding in patients who have been operated on for cholecystitis and cholelithiasis. In severe cases of sclerosing cholangitis, the liver may be slightly enlarged and there may be evidence of some obstructive jaundice. Because of the presence of jaundice and the finding of a total bilirubin level exceeding 1 or 2, and IV cholangiogram may not visualize the problem. Bile, however, will be found in the stool, as well as urobilinogen.

Sclerosing cholangitis, in the opinion of this writer, is a progressive disease with increasingly marked jaundice. If the disease is left untreated the process sometimes becomes arrested, but usually it proceeds on an intermittent basis. Today there is little hope of reducing the desmoplasia in the biliary wall even with steroid drugs. Steroids have offered relief in some instances, but their lasting value is questionable. They have been given in the postoperative period after common duct exploration, where biopsy revealed a sclerosing cholangitis. They are continued for some time, gradually tapered and finally discontinued.

Adenocarcinoma of the bile ducts is probably the most frequent simulator of sclerosing cholangitis. However, carcinoma of the bile ducts is found on cholangiography and very often is localized, with obvious proximal dilatation of the biliary tree. On occasion, bile duct carcinoma may show evidence of multiple filling defects in the ductal system, and a scirrhous carcinoma can produce a confusing extensive stricture formation which is indistinguishable on X-ray from a true sclerosing cholangitis.

Rogers et al.[1] in 1981 verified cholangiographic studies by other writers on the subject of sclerosing cholangitis and found that one or many strictures of the hepatic duct must be present to entertain a diagnosis of sclerosing cholangitis. In all of their reported cases, the extrahepatic ducts have been involved. The intrahepatic ducts are also presumed to be involved, since there is usually little or no dilatation proximal to the stenosis of a major bile duct. Often there are elongated isolated strictures. A "beaded" appearance is caused by multiple strictures with skip areas; this is probably related to an obliterative process produced by fibrosis. The lack of dilatation of the proximal ductal system makes percutaneous cholangiography more difficult than in the obstructive biliary disease associated with proximal dilatation of the intrahepatic ducts, as in carcinoma and choledocholithiasis.

It should be remembered that a distended gallbladder is a good clue (Courvoisier's law) to an obstructed common duct in a patient with a patent cystic duct and and uninvolved gallbladder. A gallbladder that is empty is also a valid clue to the presence of stenotic hepatic ducts. Rogers et al. reported five cases of sclerosing cholangitis; they believed that four were primary and that one was possibly related to choledocholithiasis. Two patients had ulcerative colitis, one had pancreatitis, and one had retroperitoneal fibrosis. Therefore, these writers felt that involvement of the intrahepatic ducts is an important feature in identifying and differentiating sclerosing cholangitis. This writer stresses that when thickening of the wall simulates carcinoma, it must always be biopsied.

Sometimes a very fine catheter or T-tube has to be used to drain the common duct, since there is no way to stretch it; an 8 or 10 Fr T-tube may sometimes have to be inserted to drain the narrowed common duct. Medical assistance should be sought for whatever benefits it may offer. In the hope of decreasing the fibroplastic or desmoplastic process, we have given adrenocorticotropic hormone or cortisone. Its value is highly questionable.

Surgery

During the laparotomy procedure for which cholecystitis, cholelithiasis, and jaundice have been the presenting signs and symptoms, exploration of the common duct may not be easy, and the duct may be very difficult to recognize. However, palpation with the forefinger and thumb may help one to recognize a cord-like structure that feels thickened and lacks compressibility; usually the common duct can be felt. These findings may serve as clues to the presence of a sclerosing cholangitis. If it is found through biopsy of the common duct and liver that the sclerosing process is diffuse (intra- and extrahepatic), the prognosis is more serious. The gallbladder removed in cases of sclerosing cholangitis may show the same fibrinous thickening commonly associated with cholelithiasis. Therefore, this fibrous thickening of the gallbladder wall should not be considered part of the same pathological process.

The biopsy taken at this time is not only for evaluation of the intensity and degree of the sclerosing process, but primarily to rule out carcinoma of the common bile duct. The microscopic pathological diagnosis is the only sure means of differentiating the two diseases. Another reason for establishing the diagnosis is that if the condition is a sclerosing cholangitis, cholecystectomy can be carried out without fear. However, if it is carcinoma, cholecystostomy may be performed, with the removal of all debris and stones; the gallbladder is left in and drained. Perhaps at a later date, if carcinoma of the biliary tract or the common duct proves to be the ultimate diagnosis, a bypass procedure may be considered. The prognosis in either event is poor, and it should be left to the surgeon to decide whether to allow a partially involved gallbladder to remain for such a future contemplated purpose.

After the common duct is opened and explored with a suitable probe, it is wise to insert an appropriately sized T-tube—perhaps an 8 Fr or possibly even a polyethylene tube. It may be wise to determine the extent of the sclerosing disease by injecting a radiopaque dye at the time of surgery. An operative cholangiogram may give much information on the present status and subsequent outcome of this disease. Of course, a better prognosis can be entertained when it is found that only the common duct is affected by the sclerosing process, and that the intrahepatic portion of the biliary system is totally unaffected. This can be shown by blood studies and liver biopsies that indicate a benign and minimal sclerosing process.

When the liver biopsy indicates that there is an extensive biliary cirrhosis, it implies an advanced form of liver disease with a prognosis that is most serious. Occasionally, a severe localized ductal sclerosis will be found, yet the gallbladder may not contain stones and is not thickened with chronic cholecystic fibrosis. If this is the case, one need not wait for a secondary procedure to help decompress an already obstructing sclerosing cholangitis. If the gallbladder is unaffected, one may proceed with a cholecystojejunostomy to assist better drainage of bile from the liver.

This writer feels that the extremely diffuse forms of sclerosing cholangitis that affect the entire biliary system, including the liver, must not only be considered a surgical problem. With the advent of steroids, it is possible that no further procedure, i.e., transhepatic decompression, need be carried out. The surgical procedures that have been recommended so far are sufficient. The postoperative period should focus on medical management, using steroids.

When the common duct is drained in cases of sclerosing cholangitis, the closure must be watertight, and the Penrose drain should not be near the site of T-tube emergence. Preferably a Penrose drain with wick or a Jackson-Pratt suction drain should be inserted down to Morison's fossa, but on indicated occasions one may bring the drain down to the foramen of Winslow. No drain should lay directly over the site of the sewn-in T-tube because it may permit the withdrawal of serofibrinous plastic exudate that helps to seal the choledochotomy stoma, the anastomotic site, or any other situation in which one expects good sealing off at the sites of increased biliary pressure.

In conclusion, a sclerosing cholangitis involving the entire biliary system may be in various states of occlusive formation in which jaundice may ultimately develop in the same manner as in the gradual process of extrahepatic obstruction. This disease may be local, i.e., confined to the common duct or to one or both hepatic ducts. Alternatively, it may spread, involving the entire biliary system. The prognosis must be guarded; it is more favorable in the early stages, which may or may not be a truly sclerosing process. In those cases where a sclerotic process develops postoperatively, i.e., as

after a previous choledochotomy and duct exploration, the prognosis is usually more favorable. It is the primary sclerotic process that offers a prognosis that should be carefully guarded. It is more serious when the process is found to be diffuse. When biliary cirrhosis develops, the prognosis is ominous. Thus the prognosis of sclerotic cholangitis ranges from guarded to poor to ominous. Whenever infection is associated with this process, antibiotics should, of course, be given. Bile specimens taken at the time of surgery should routinely be sent to the laboratory for culture and sensitivity studies.

Recommended Reading

Cameron JL, et al: Sclerosing cholangitis: Anatomical distribution of obstructive lesions. *Ann Surg* 200:54, 1984.

LaRusso NF, et al: Primary sclerosing cholangitis. *N Engl J Med* 310:899, 1984.

MacCarty RL: Primary sclerosing cholangitis: Findings on cholangiography and pancreatography. *Radiology* 149:39, 1983.

Pitt HA, Thompson HH, Tompkins RK, et al: Primary sclerosing cholangitis: Results of an aggressive surgical approach. *Ann Surg* 196:259, 1982.

Rahn NH III, et al: CT appearance of sclerosing cholan gitis. *Am J Radiology* 141:549, 1983.

Thompson HH Jr, Tompkins RK, Longmire WP Jr, et al: Primary sclerosing cholangitis: A heterogeneous disease. *Ann Surg* 196:127, 1982.

Wiesner RH, La Russo NF, Ludwig J, et al: Comparison of the clinicopathologic features of primary sclerosing cholangitis and primary biliary cirrhosis. *Gastroenterology* 88:108, 1985.

Wood RAB, Cuschieri A: Is sclerosing cholangitis complicating ulcerative colitis a reversible condition? *Lancet* 2:716, 1980.

Reference

1. Rogers CM, Adams JT, Swartz SI, et al: Carcinoma of the extrahepatic bile ducts. *Surgery* 90:596, 1981.

Sclerosing Cholangitis after Surgery of Hepatic Echinococcal Cysts

Primary sclerosing cholangitis may occur as an isolated entity in association with ulcerative colitis, retroperitoneal fibrosis and Riedel's struma. Sclerosing cholangitis may be secondary to common bile duct stones, congenital biliary anomalies, bile duct carcinoma and iatrogenic stenosis.

Sclerosing cholangitis was reported by Teres et

al.[1] of Barcelona, Spain, to have followed surgery on a hepatic echinococcal cyst. The authors described three cases, each occurring within 1 month after surgical removal of echinococcus cyst of the liver. One patient developed jaundice with a bilirubin level of 21 mg. % and an alkaline phosphatase level of 295 (normal, less than 180). Reoperation revealed a thickened common duct with a narrowed lumen of the entire biliary tract.

Reference

1. Teres J, Gomez Moli J, Bruguera M, et al: Sclerosing cholangitis after surgical treatment of hepatic echinococcal cysts: Report of 3 cases. *Am J Surg* 148:694, 1984.

BILIARY PANCREATITIS

The main precipitating factor in producing biliary pancreatitis is an impacted stone in the common duct just below the entrance of the pancreatic duct. Another predisposing factor is spasm of the ampullary sphincter. There is another form of pancreatitis, more severe in character, in which a common duct stone is not a factor. The more severe forms of acalculous pancreatitis will not respond to immediate surgery (24–48 hours), as do those milder forms of gallstone pancreatitis. Many surgeons prefer to delay surgery because they fear a high mortality.

Mercer et al.[1] reported on 134 patients diagnosed as having cholelithiasis with suspect associated pancreatitis. Of these patients, 34 were selected because of a more probable association with pancreatitis. These patients had elevated serum and urinary amylase, as well as intraoperative evidence of pancreatic inflammation, i.e., edematous swelling and areas of mesenteric necrosis. About one-half were operated on within 24 hours and the other half within 48 hours. All patients recovered without any complications.

This writer's experience favors emergency surgery in patients diagnosed as having moderate biliary pancreatitis without a history of alcoholism. However in the severer forms of acute pancreatitis in which a common duct stone cannot be visualized by ultrasonography, computed tomography scan, or PIPIDA*, the treatment should be conservative; this means delaying surgery, improving the patient's condition, and doing more studies to make sure that the patient is improving during this waiting period. If the patient improves, the surgery may be planned electively within 7 to 10 days. If the patient fails to improve or worsens progressively, interventional surgery is indicated.

Today there are two schools of thought regarding the management of biliary pancreatitis. The first school believes in immediate operation (within 48 hours). The diagnosis must be established as biliary pancreatitis, i.e., pancreatitis based upon gallstone obstruction of the pancreatic duct. Alcoholism must be ruled out; otherwise, the diagnosis of pancreatitis must be considered to be related to alcoholism as the primary underlying cause. It is conceivable that gallstone obstruction and a history of alcoholism may coexist. These surgeons do a cholecystectomy, choledochographic studies, common duct exploration if indicated, and T-tube drainage. With immediate surgical intervention, it is believed that pancreatitis is prevented from growing worse, i.e., progressing from edematous to hemorrhagic pancreatitis with necrosis. The early interventionists also claim a shorter hospital stay; and surely Mercer's claim of no morbidity, no mortality, and no late complications in all operated cases is most impressive.

The second school of thought believes in the opposite approach, namely, to treat acalculous biliary pancreatitis more conservatively. Ranson[2] strongly believes in this plan of management. He operated on 22 patients diagnosed as having biliary pancreatitis within 1 week of their attack. He reported a 23% mortality. Four of the patients died within 48 hours. Ranson treated 58 patients conservatively until the pancreatitis subsided and then operated electively. He performed a cholecystectomy, common duct exploration, and cholangiogram when indicated. He reported no mortality. Kelly[3] studied 172 patients with impacted gallstones. He operated on 63% of them within 72 hours, and the mortality was 12%. When Ranson waited 5 to 7 days before operating, only 5% of the patients were found to have an impacted stone. There was no mortality. Fifteen percent of his patients failed to improve and had to be reoperated on.

European literature reports on the successes of ECRP sphincterotomy and percutaneous transhepatic sphincterotomy in freeing the obstructing stone in the common duct. If these modalities prove successful, they will replace interventional surgery and bring about a significant reduction in mortality.

Over a 16-year period, Kelly studied 35 patients who had undergone surgery for biliary (gallstone) pancreatitis. They were treated for retained or recurrent gallstones in the common duct. Recurrent attacks of gallstone pancreatitis the first time oc-

---

*Technetium-99m–labeled hepatobiliary agents, particularly several derivatives of iminodiacetic acid (IDA); also, 99m Tc-IDA.

curred in 92%. The interval ranged from 1 month to 30 years, averaging 2 years. In 83% of the cases, stones were found impacted in the ampulla of Vater. Of the patients who had early surgical intervention, 66% had stones in the ampulla; of those who underwent delayed surgery, only 18% had ampullary stones. The second-time recurrence rate was 2%. Kelly concluded that an absolute clearance of common duct stones at the time of the first recurrence (or first time around), will prevent the need for a second operation.

This writer feels that both schools of thought regarding the ideal treatment of biliary pancreatitis have merit. The surgeon must make a decision that is appropriate to the individual case. In cases of cholelithiasis associated with milder forms of pancreatitis, the best course may be early surgical intervention (within 24 to 48 hours). In instances of acalculous biliary pancreatitis, the individual circumstances will dictate the plan of management. For example, if the pancreatitis is not too severe, it is probably best to institute conservative therapy and preoperative preparation. If the patient responds favorably, he or she is better suited to elective surgery 7 to 10 days later. If the pancreatitis fails to subside and worsens progressively, surgery without delay is indicated; the patient should be improved up to the time of surgery.

Recommended Reading

Gadaez TR, Lillemo K, Zimmer K, et al: Common bile duct complications of pancreatitis: Evaluation and treatment. *Surgery* 93:235, 1983.
Littenberg G, Afroudakis A, Kaplowitz N: Common bile duct stenosis from chronic pancreatitis: A clinical and pathologic spectrum. *Medicine* 58:385, 1979.
Skellenger ME, Patterson D, Foley NT, et al: Cholestasis due to compression of the common bile duct by pancreatic pseudocysts. *Am J Surg* 145:343, 1983.
Wisloff F, Jakobsen J, Osnes M: Stenosis of the common bile duct in chronic pancreatitis. *Br J Surg* 69:52, 1982.
Yadegar J, Williams RA, Passaro E Jr, et al: Common duct stricture from chronic pancreatitis. *Arch Surg* 115:582, 1980.

References

1. Mercer LC, Saltzman FC, Peacock JB, et al: Early surgery for biliary pancreatitis. *Am J Surg*, vol 148, 1984.
2. Ranson JHC: The timing of biliary surgery in acute pancreatitis. *Ann Surg* 189:654, 1979.
3. Kelly TR: Gallstone pancreatitis: The timing of surgery. *Surgery* 88:345, 1980.

SURGICAL TREATMENT FOR NONRESOLVING BILIARY PANCREATITIS

During the period of conservative management, computed tomography scan and ultrasonography can be used to rule out the existence of an impacted gallstone and to determine whether or not the pancreatitis (edema) is subsiding; if the edema fails to subside, surgery should be carried out. The plan of therapy should be carried out as follows:

1. *Drainage*
   a. Sump drains in the lesser peritoneal cavity.
   b. Cholecystostomy tube and T-tube for common duct drainage.
   c. A gastrostomy tube (Hurwitz tube) for gastric drainage and jejunal feeding.
2. *IV Fluids:* about 3 liters of colloid during the first 24 hours. Removal of the toxic waste products at surgery assists recovery. Percutaneous peritoneal lavage may be used. Complications following the surgical treatment are infection with abscess formation (20–40%) and nutritional problems.
3. *Antibiotics* (broad spectrum) to avoid bacterial infection.
4. *Pancreatic resection:* Because the acute fulminating process cannot be contained, and since extensive necrosis is progressive, pancreatectomy (distal or total) must be carried out. The probable mortality will be about 40%. In Whipple's procedure (pancreaticoduodenectomy), the mortality may be above 60%. In more experienced hands this percentage drops.

   To wait 5–8 days before deciding on surgical intervention is beneficial. If pancreatitis develops with a progressing necrotic process, the surgeon can more easily recognize and judge what portion of the necrotic pancreas to resect. In the first 24–48 hours of pancreatitis, diffuse edema rather than a line of necrotic demarcation may exist; to decide on the extent of pancreatic resection at this time is hazardous because the necrotic process may have extended beyond the apparently involved site.
5. *Medical treatments*
   a. *Antibiotics:* Many prefer not to use routine antibiotics because they fear the development of resistant strains and *Candida*.
   b. *Calcium* replacement for hypoglycemia is futile.
   c. *Insulin* for blood glucose levels of 200–300 mg/ml may be administered.
   d. *IV Hyperalimentation (total parenteral nutrition)* is unnecessary unless the disease process is protracted.

e. *Drugs,* i.e., anticholinergics, proteolytic enzyme inhibitors, glucagon to reduce secretions, and prostaglandins to inhibit protein synthesis. Protease-binding proteins and reticuloendothelial stimulants may be given.

f. *Sympathetic block:* heparin, low molecular dextran, and corticosteroids are of questionable benefit.

The Pathogenesis and Sequelae of Choledocholithiasis

The extrahepatic biliary tree begins at the hilus of the liver and starts where the right and left hepatic ducts join to form the common hepatic duct. The common hepatic duct joins the cystic duct at a given point and, from that junction on, the tubular formation comes down to form one common bile duct, which continues donward in a straight, slightly curved, or angular manner. It continues on posteriorly behind the duodenum and, to a lesser extent, pressed into the head of the pancreas, which lies behind the duodenum; it then continues on to curve straight down, piercing the duodenal muscular coat in the posterior wall of the descending duodenum. The common duct continues on obliquely for a short distance through the musculature under the submucosa and finally opens into the duodenal lumen at an apical point known as the ampulla of Vater. The common bile duct, after it is formed by the cystic duct joining the common hepatic duct, is usually of a slate blue color and is relatively thin as it extends downward as a fibrous structure with a minimum· of scattered smooth muscle fibers throughout its wall. Somewhere along its course, before it enters the duodenum, the wall of the common duct thickens, and more musculature is added onto its wall (see "Common Duct Anatomy" in Chapters 2, 5, and 13). The added smooth musculature contributes to the sphincteric action of the lower common bile duct. The additional sphincteric musculature is further reinforced by the stronger contractability of the duodenum as the common duct traverses through its wall.

Somewhere along its course, before it enters the lumen of the duodenum, the common bile duct receives the pancreatic duct of Wirsung approximately 0.5–1.0 cm from its terminal point. This junction may vary, and the pancreatic duct may at times even empty independently into the duodenum, but this is not common. Normally, the pancreatic duct joins the common bile duct just before its terminal point to become a common structure, and therefore the common bile duct may become a little wider as result of the combined diameters of the two structures. Nevertheless, the bile duct narrows down to a very fine opening as it terminates as the ampulla of Vater. This anatomical configuration is readily demonstrated on cholangiographic studies. From the cystic duct down to the duodenum, the common bile duct remains about 1 cm in diameter. From the latter point on, its wall thickens and the lumen narrows, both with fibrous and muscular tissue (see "Practical Anatomical Review of Biliary System" in Chapter 2).

The sudden narrowing at the point where the common bile duct enters the duodenal wall is a common site for the entrapment of gallstones that become either fixed or impacted at that point. This obstructive phenomenon leads to jaundice, with or without infection, a disease known as *cholangitis.* The gallbladder stones are formed primarily in the gallbladder. If they are found in the common bile duct, it is because they were once small enough to pass through the lumen of the cystic duct. It is conceivable that gallstones can roll or be propelled through the cystic duct whenever the latter is large enough. The reason that stones are sometimes found to be unduly large in the common bile duct is because they have enlarged within the common bile duct by forming concentric layers over time. These concentric layers can be easily visualized on cross-sectioning of a stone. The concentric layers are usually formed around a nucleus that most likely served as the primary origin or nidus of the stone.

There are certain Oriental diseases caused by tropical parasites such as *Cl. sinensis.* This parasite or worm is similar to *A. lumbricoides* and can develop in the common duct or be found there, but whether a stone can form in the common bile duct is still questionable. Most investigators believe that all gallstones originate in the gallbladder, except in specific cases where gallbladders have been previously removed and the stones that were found postoperatively were not believed to have been leftover or missed stones in the hepatic duct radicles. At this time, no one can be certain about their true site of origin. The great majority believe that gallstones originate in the gallbladder and migrate in some way into the common duct; they are capable of growing with time; and they become impacted when they reach a narrowed portion of the common duct.

The signs and symptoms produced are directly related to the obstruction, namely, an obstructive phenomenon that causes the reversal of the natural downward flow of bile. Common duct stones may be single or multiple; they may be round or irregular, faceted, or have points as a star-shaped structure. Contoured stones sometimes arrange themselves in the common bile duct so close together that there is almost no room left in the common duct lumen to allow a cholangiographic dye to make its way through the spaces between them. At times there is no visualization at all. It is remarkable how, in some cases, the common duct may be fully impacted with tightly fitting multiple stones, and yet bile is still capable of flowing through the interspaces. In other instances, there may be only one stone, yet obstructive jaundice with all its associated signs and symptoms will develop. It is most difficult to determine the incidence of common bile duct stones in cholelithiasis because it is very variable and dependent upon many factors.

This writer made an extensive study that included the major clinics of the country. He found that the average relationship of cholelithiasis to choledocholithiasis was about 15%; that is, 15% of the patients who came to cholecystectomy for cholelithiasis had stones in the common bile duct. Though this figure varies, it is approximately correct. This incidence may, however, vary from time to time in different geographic areas where the incidence of gallbladder disease (cholelithiasis) is either increased or decreased. In addition, stones often pass through the ampulla into the duodenum under pressure, reducing the true incidence of stones in the common bile duct. The number of stones that pass from the common duct into the duodenum will probably never be known.

In choledocholithiasis the stones or stone may become obstructed, fixed, or impacted in the narrow terminal portion of the duct and give rise to an incomplete or complete obstruction. The clinical picture will depend, in fact, on whether or not the obstruction is complete, caused by an impacted stone, or incomplete, caused by a floating or irregularly faceted stone. When jaundice is produced, the differential diagnosis can become very complex, since fibrotic stenosis of the ampulla, carcinoma, and infestation diseases enter into the clinical picture and must be ruled out. In most cases, however, when a stone reaches the narrowed portion of the common duct, the irritation and edema may produce a spasm of the smooth musculature in the thicker portion of the common duct, as well as in the duodenal wall.

A stone may remain floating in the wide portion of the common duct, making it easier to remove.

Every now and then, a stone may extend down into the narrower, thicker portion of the common duct and become impacted, not only because of its large size but because of its coexistent spasm. Fixation is further induced by an inflammatory reaction. These gallstones become more difficult to remove. When a stone passes further down, beyond the junction of the pancreatic duct of Wirsung with the common bile duct, and impacts at the ampullary end, it becomes quite evident that the bile will reflux into the common duct, and possibly into the pancreas via the pancreatic duct of Wirsung. This is a serious problem because bile entering the pancreas activates pancreatic enzymes that can produce an acute pancreatitis, and possibly a hemorrhagic pancreatitis, which is a most serious complication. Cases of acute pancreatitis can become so catastrophic that the only possible means of relief is emergency surgical intervention for exploration and decompression of the biliary tract.

We know that stones may be present in the common bile duct at a rather low level for many years without giving rise to any signs or symptoms of jaundice, with the blood showing a normal bilirubin and normal liver enzyme levels. Nevertheless, ultimately, the stone can produce a sudden obstruction of the common duct, with all of its attendant complications. If the obstruction develops into the intermittent type, specific signs and symptoms will arise, with their own side effects. The latter disease usually produces an intermittent jaundice associated with chills and fever (a ball-valve effect). The combination of the aforementioned signs and symptoms is commonly known as *Charcot's syndrome* or *Charcot's intermittent fever*.

Choledocholithiasis: Acute and Chronic Obstruction of the Common Bile Duct

When a gallstone makes its way into the common duct and becomes arrested at the point where marked narrowing of the common bile duct occurs, it irritates the mucosa, and a spasm of the common duct musculature and duodenal musculature fixes the stone at this point. A mild or severe inflammation sets in, further increasing the spasm and fixing the stone more firmly in place. Jaundice begins to develop rather soon, usually in about 24 to 72 hours, and clinical evidence can be seen and substantiated by increased blood bilirubin, alkaline phosphatase, and other enzyme studies. The stool begins to show a change in color from brown to light yellow and finally to a clay color. The urine becomes darker.

The obstruction may or may not be complete, depending upon whether the stone completely occludes the lumen. This particular point may be compared with a malignant growth that slowly obstructs the common duct intrinsically or extrinsically. Neoplastic obstructions develop gradually, and the liver, with its entire biliary tree, has the opportunity to adjust slowly to the back pressure created by the slowly stenosing growth. The common duct usually enlarges, as does the cystic duct; lastly, the gallbladder distends. The latter is referred to as a *Courvoisier gallbladder*. Even the biliary radicles in the liver increase in size to absorb the increasing back pressure within the biliary tree. Finally, the pressure rises high enough to destroy the fine distal biliary canaliculi. The ruptured canaliculi allow the bile to pour into the bloodstream of the liver sinuses, producing the clinical picture of obstructive jaundice.

If the stone obstructs but does not become fixed or incarcerated by edema and spasm, the bile will surround it and elevate it out of its obstructing position; this allows the bile to flow through freely as the stone rises. This phenomenon has been referred to as a *ball-valve action;* (charots' intermittant fever and chills). When the jaundice clears, the temperature subsides, the pain disappears, and the stool color changes back to brown. The blood findings begin to improve; the serum bilirubin and liver enzyme levels continue to drop. In summary, acute biliary obstruction is invariably associated with acute signs and symptoms of pain, fever, and jaundice, to be followed by elevated corroborative laboratory findings. Charcot's intermittent fever may be intermittent or recurring.

CHRONIC OBSTRUCTION

Stones in the common bile duct over a long period of time may be referred to as *chronic choledocholithiasis* with incomplete obstruction of the bile ducts. If the obstruction is incomplete, no clinical jaundice develops. In some cases the common bile duct may be full of stones, and yet the bile will make its way out circuitously, around and between the interspaces, without causing clinical jaundice. Contributing factors usually help to create a complete obstruction, and these factors are listed above under "Acute Obstruction" (see Chap. 7, 12). The common bile duct becomes dilated because of the back pressure, and may become stretched more than the normal 10 mm (1 cm) in diameter. It is also possible

for the walls of the duct to become thicker and its color to be changed from slate blue to whitish (see "Choledochotomy and Common Duct Exploration"). Distention takes place proximal to the stone and usually involves the entire common duct proximal to the obstruction. The comparative differences in size continue to become more marked as the distention increases with increasing back pressure. Distention extends into the hepatic ductal system, and once that takes place, the increased pressure spreads in the distal canaliculi of the liver, with ultimate disruption of the biliary canaliculi.

Occasionally, a stone may become strongly impacted in the common bile duct, and the pressure against the walls may become so great that ulceration of the mucosa permits the stone to adhere to and even erode the duct wall. This type of stone is most difficult to remove, and any traumatic efforts to loosen it may lead to wall perforation. A stone may become caught in a diverticulum of the common bile duct and may be seen on IV cholangiogram, yet there may be a free flow of bile into the duodenum without obstruction or jaundice. This, of course, is rare but must be kept in mind. Choledocholithiasis, with or without jaundice, will ultimately lead to a fibrosis of the canaliculi in the liver, which in turn will lead to ultimate biliary cirrhosis, a progressive condition associated with progressive jaundice. This same pathogenesis can be seen where there is a fibrotic stricture of the common bile duct instead of impacted stones. Chronic obstruction of the common bile duct, though it may not produce complete obstruction, can slowly produce late obstructive changes in the liver.

When the impact of biliary back pressure diffusely enlarges the liver and canaliculi become disrupted, thrombi may also develop, with an inflammatory reaction around them. Bile duct proliferation can also be detected, and a fibrotic process around the portal tracts can similarly be visualized. For reversible changes to take place, the obstruction must be removed early; otherwise, the fibrotic process will remain chronic and permanent, accompanied by progressive distention, thrombosis, and inflammation. The last ultimately leads to permanent parenchymatous changes.

PAIN

Gallbladder pain usually begins in the right upper quadrant, but it may also be underneath the right costal margin or the scapular area; it tends to radiate to the back, right shoulder, and/or interscapular area. It may be a constant pain or pressure-like discomfort, and usually is colicky in nature. It may be intermittent but is more likely continuous, with exacerbations from time to time. The pain may be severe enough to require narcotic medication for relief; not infrequently, it is accompanied by nausea and vomiting. The patient usually complains of tenderness in the right subcostal area that is most likely due to an enlarged liver, especially if the obstruction has been of long standing. Not infrequently, rebound tenderness may be elicited.

The gallbladder which has not been involved with chronic cholecystitis usually becomes markedly distended because of the persistent obstructing stone in the common bile duct. Palpation of the abdominal mass can usually be felt in the right upper quadrant; this may represent an enlarged liver but more often will signify a Courvoisier gallbladder. In the majority of cases, a Courvoisier gallbladder does not develop because a chronically thickened, fibrous gallbladder with stones will usually remain small and contracted and will resist distention. The gallbladder may be so thick and fibrotic that the lumen will become completely obliterated. The writer has seen cases where there has been no lumen at all, just a mass of scar tissue representing what was once a gallbladder.

In a chronically obstructed bile duct, such as is often seen in association with malignancy, there is progressive growth with gradual obstruction and, with it, gradual progressive distention of the entire biliary tree, including the gallbladder. These gradual changes in distention are compensatory, adapting to compensate for the extreme back pressure of the bile and serve to delay the ultimate pressure damage that is done to the biliary canaliculi. Therefore, the Courvoisier gallbladder should make one think more of a neoplastic obstruction than of an unusual choledocholithiasis. *It should also be borne in mind that an obstruction by a calculus may be chronically intermittent, and therefore, on occasion may produce a Courvoisier gallbladder; gradual benign obstruction can simulate neoplastic obstruction.*

Jaundice in an acute or chronic case of choledocholithiasis is more often associated with pruritis than the jaundice that develops with carcinoma. The stools become pale, the jaundice may or may not persist, and the urine usually becomes darker as the stool becomes lighter; the urobilinogen diminishes as the obstruction becomes more complete. *The urinary urobilinogen is completely negative in total biliary obstruction; this exists in both the urine and the stool.* The serum reveals elevated bilirubin and elevated liver enzymes; this implies that there has been liver damage. For example, alkaline phosphatase almost invariably becomes elevated when liver damage takes place as a result of obstructive jaundice; so do the SGOT, LDM, and CPK enzymes; this indicates that parenchymatous liver damage and possibly pancreatic injury have occurred (see the chart "Differential Diagnosis by Laboratory Studies of Jaundice" in Chapter 6).

If jaundice has lasted for some time, liver function may be so impaired as to interfere with prothrombin formation and reduce vitamin K production. Increased prothrombin time leads to an excessive bleeding tendency. If the blood deficiency is not adequately dealt with in the preoperative period, severe bleeding requiring multiple transfusions may result during surgery and in the postoperative period. *A low prothrombin time should be looked for and corrected before any surgery is undertaken.* IV and IM vitamin K_1 (aqueous Mephyton) should be given until the prothrombin time begins to approach normal levels; then and only then can one proceed with safe planned surgery.

Occasionally, a jaundice will clear up suddenly; this indicates that, in all probability, neoplasia is not the underlying cause and that a floating stone may be the reason for the clearance of jaundice. A ball-valve action, as described previously, may well be the underlying mechanism. Such a remission may last for days, weeks, or months. Nevertheless, a diagnosis of choledocholithiasis calls for interval elective surgery to remove the stone and reestablish a patent common bile duct. There are instances where carcinoma of the ampulla of Vater will produce a deep jaundice that can suddenly be relieved because the intraductal pressure created causes the neoplasm to slough away sufficiently to release the backed-up bile. There are cases where no symptoms or signs are present, especially in elderly individuals. When painless jaundice sets in, one should first think of neoplasia as the cause. Yet, not infrequently, a stone resides in the common duct for a long time, producing jaundice intermittently, and then finally becoming persistent without pain in an elderly, emaciated patient; carcinoma cannot be dismissed. I have occasionally removed huge single stones (golf-ball size) from the common duct and found no evidence of what appeared to be obvious carcinoma. These patients gained complete relief, and left the hospital.

DIAGNOSIS

Every patient with cholelithiasis may have concomitant choledocholithiasis; therefore, one has to search routinely for the possible causes of obstructive jaundice. In the 40- to 60-year-old patient with a history of marked fatty food dyspepsia associated with right upper quadrant pain and radiation to the interscapular area, cholelithiasis becomes the potential diagnosis. When jaundice develops, whether mild, intermittent, or severe, the diagnosis of obstructive jaundice must be strongly considered (see the chart "Differential Diagnosis by Laboratory Studies of Jaundice" in Chapter 6).

Patients who go to surgery for routine elective cholecystectomy for cholelithiasis should be worked up for the possibility of a gallstone in the common bile duct. This decision should, if possible, be made preoperatively; additional studies at surgery should also be carried out. Preoperative studies should include sonograms, cholangiograms (oral and IV), and computed tomography scan. At surgery, if the criteria are present for catheter cholangiograms via the cystic duct or T-tube studies via the common bile duct, an exploration should be carried out. There will be times when an elusive stone will be missed by IV cholangiography. A good exploration of the common duct at the first operation is most important and should help to eliminate the need for secondary noninvasive techniques. T-tube cholangiography at surgery is probably the most reliable study to determine whether a retained stone is present anywhere in the biliary tree. *We look forward to the routine use of intraoperative sonography of the common bile duct.* (See Intraoperative cholangiography; Chapter 5). One must not consider common duct exploration and cholangiography as a benign procedure without morbidity (see "Choledochotomy and Common Duct Exploration"). An exploration of the common duct involves definite morbidity and, in rare instances, even mortality. Ulceration, false passage, and even perforation can also occur. Cholangitis is not an uncommon postoperative development; it is often the result of a faulty or traumatic exploration of the common duct. Stricture of the common duct may develop years later.

Surgeons may find it more judicious to open the duodenum (duodenotomy), explore the ampulla of Vater, and if necessary, carry out a sphincterotomy to allow the stone to fall out of the duct or permit its extraction from below (see Chapter 17). It is not just a dilated and thickened common duct that is suspected of harboring stones; a more reliable sign is a stone that can actually be palpated within the common duct. On occasion, a sediment in the bile may be aspirated from the common duct; this is enough evidence for a surgeon to proceed with a routine common duct exploration. The exploration is justified even if only mud, gravel, and debris are removed. This latter finding may be associated with complaints similar to those of acute, subacute, or chronic pancreatitis. Those surgeons who consider that mud, gravel and debris can become sufficienty compacted to produce clinical symptoms feel justified in thoroughly exploring and evacuating all the debris found in the common duct (see Fig. 109 (7, 8, 9).

Only the personal experiences of the surgeons can and do dictate their action at surgery; no one can talk away the three objective findings that represent mandatory indications for exploration of the common duct: (1) a strong history or presence of jaundice; (2) a dilated, thickened, and opaque-looking common bile duct; and (3) palpation of stones in the common duct. Others feel that no matter what the history and findings are at surgery, a routine cholangiographic study via the cystic duct is mandatory. This writer feels that routine cystic duct cholangiography takes up extra time and that not every patient tolerates this procedure well because it requires additional operative time, extra manipulations, and possible trauma to the common duct. Reflux of dye into the pancreatic duct with pressure can produce shock to the patient or, more likely, an acute pancreatitis. There have been reported cases where sudden death followed routine cholecystographic dye injections. Cholangiography is not just a harmless routine procedure, as some believe; it must be done with great finesse and speed. Those who have the experience and knowledge of when to stop and when to proceed with an alternative plan of action should employ this procedure. Even among experts, there have been reported cases, where residual stones were discovered after a thorough negative *cholangiographic cystic duct* evaluation of the common duct.

When residual stones in the common duct appear postoperatively, whether they were always in the common duct or fell down from a higher level will always remain in question; but the leftover stone still remains as a distinct problem.

Bartlett and Waddell[1] in 1958 reported a mortality of 0.6% for cholecystectomy alone and 1.8% for cholecystectomy with choledochotomy and exploration. Harvard et al.[2] in 1976 reported that, in his experience, choledochostomy and exploration doubles the operative mortality. One must be constantly aware that the mortality may not be related to the physical exploration itself, but rather to concomitant diseases such as preexisting parenchymatous liver degeneration with faulty production of liver products, i.e., enzyme deficiencies, antibody reduction, lowered prothrombin, and reduced albumin production, as well as the inability to detoxify toxic end products. All of these important factors are often at their lowest level at the

time of choledochostomy. The traumatic exploration of the common duct means additional insult
to an already troubled liver, which can and does
influence morbidity and mortality. The additional
time that is involved during prolonged toxic anesthesia also influences liver degeneration.

Where exploration of the common duct is required, it does not as a rule increase the morbidity
or mortality, according to Colcock et al.[3] *This writer
generally believes that an addition to choledochostomy,
of a common duct exploration among less-experienced
surgeons will significantly increase the operative time,
and with it the morbidity and mortality.* Added to this
is the required increased length of stay in the hospital and the extra cost. In the opinion of this writer,
only when the indications mentioned above for
choledochotomy and exploration are strictly adhered to will a minimum of negative explorations
of the common duct result.

Recommended Reading

Cotton PB: Duodenoscopic placement of biliary prosthesis
to relieve maglinant obstructive jaundice. *Br J Surg*
69:501, 1982.
Ferrucci JT Jr, Mueller PR, Hasbin WP: Advances in the
radiology of jaundice, a symposium and review. *HJR*
141:1, 1983.
Jordan GL Jr: Choledocholithiasis. *Curr Prob Surg* 19:722,
1982.
Rubin JR, Beal JM: Diagnosis of choledocholithiasis. *Surg
Gynecol Obstet* 156:16, 1983.
Way LW, Admirand WH, Dunphy JE: Management of
choledocholithiasis. *Ann Surg* 176:347, 1972.

References

1. Bartlett MK, Waddell WR: Surgery of the biliary tract.
III. Secondary operations on the common duct. *N Engl
J Med* 256:11, 1957.
2. Harvard C, Perry D, et al: Cholecystostomy. *Br J Surg*
63:631, 1976.
3. Colcock BP, McManus JE: Experience with 1356 cases
of cholecystitis and cholelithiasis. *Surg Gynecol Obstet*
101:161, 1955.

Choledochoduodenostomy

Choledochoduodenostomy was first performed by
Redell in 1888 but never achieved much popularity
in the United States. Choledochojejunostomy with
a Roux-en-Y jejunal loop, or with a loop jejunostomy and enteroenterostomy, seemed to be more
popular than choledochoduodenostomy, primarily
because of the fear of ascending cholangitis from
reflux of duodenal content into the common bile
duct. Choledochoduodenostomy was first used at
the Cleveland Clinic by Dr. George Crile after
seeing it performed in Europe. It was used exten-
sively by Dr. Tom Jones and became the preferred
operation for decompression of an obstructed biliary system both by Drs. Crile and Jones.[1] Many
surgeons do not like to do a sphincteroplasty or
sphincterotomy; they prefer to do a choledochoduodenostomy for common duct stenosis. This procedure also has definite applicability to chronic
pancreatitis which obstructs a longer portion of the
distal common duct. Choledochoduodenostomy
has also been used to decompress choledochal cysts
(see "Choledochal Cysts" in Chapters 2 and 6).
Many surgeons employ choledochoduodenostomy
for resectable malignant lesions of the head of the
pancreas and distal common bile duct. This writer
has employed it in patients who suffered recurrent
bile duct stones and in those who had residual intrahepatic or residual common duct stones that
could not be completely removed. This writer has
also employed choledochoduodenostomy in instances where biliary fistulas from the common bile
duct had been created by injuries; the latter were
repaired together with a supplementary choledochoduodenostomy (Fig. 90).

Several series have been reviewed in which choledochoduodenostomy was carried out for unresectable malignant lesions of the distal common bile
duct and common bile duct strictures; the operative
mortality proved to be very low; no deaths were
attributed to the operative procedure itself. A leak
from the operative anastomotic site causing subhepatic sepsis, hepatic abscess, or ascending cholangitis during the postoperative period was rarely
observed. The hospital mortality from advancing
lesions, inanition, and malnutrition was due to the
carcinoma itself not the surgical procedure. Several
series reviewed show an overall hospital mortality
of about 3%; the morbidity of the procedure also
remains low.

Choledochojejunostomies have been strictured
from time to time. The incidence of stricture after
choledochoduodenostomy is about as frequent as
it is after sphincteroplasty and choledochojejunostomy. This writer has not experienced sepsis in his
cases. In the past 10 years, a gradual increase in
choledochoduodenostomy has been taking place;
Madden et al.[2] and Hurwitz et al.[3] have reported
good results and have recommended the procedure
very highly. The main advantages of this procedure

is its availability and simplicity of performance. Hugier et al.,[4] from the University of Paris, studied common duct obstructions in patients over the age of 75 who were treated with choledochoduodenostomy and reported favorable results. They claim that it is safe, with low morbidity and mortality. These surgeons prefer this procedure to the more taxing procedures of T-tube drainage, Roux-en-Y choledochojejunostomy, and sphincterotomy. These surgeons state that choledochoduodenostomy is easier and faster, and that this factor has helped to reduce the mortality in older patients.[3] Hurwitz has written favorably about choledochoduodenostomy and has stressed that the stoma must be made adequate (2.5 cm or more) in order to assure patency and good bile flow into the duodenum.

This writer also tries to obtain pre- and postoperative routine liver function studies. Most of these patients are jaundiced, and if it is possible, after a fluctuating jaundice, for the bilirubin to drop down to 2 mg%, we attempt to do an IV cholangiogram. This is very helpful because an operative procedure is best performed on a duct that is dilated, thick-walled, and can hold a suture well. This writer would not recommend choledochoduodenostomy in a patient with a small duct or even a normal-sized duct with a thin wall. This procedure should be performed only on common ducts that have been obstructed for a period of time, preferably where the duct is dilated and thickened. If the patient is persistently jaundiced and one cannot obtain a cholangiogram by indirect methods, one should use more direct methods namely, ultrasonography, percutaneous transhepatic cholangiogram, ERCP, and computed tomography scan. The latter can be performed the morning of the scheduled operation in a patient who may well require a choledochoduodenostomy or any other necessary surgical biliary decompressive procedure.

In a patient who has had jaundice for a prolonged period of time and has had periods of episodic chills and/or fever, it may be best to give antibiotics starting the morning of surgery, employing an effective dose of a broad-spectrum antibiotic, i.e., Keflin, Cefadyl, Terramycin, or Vibramycin injected IM and/or IV. An operative cholangiogram should be performed at surgery, especially if one had not done preoperative studies.

The duodenum is easily mobilized with a Kocher maneuver and then lifted up to the common duct level to evaluate the approximation of the common duct site to the site on the duodenum (see Fig. 90). If the distal common duct is strictured, an alternative procedure may have to be carried out, namely, a direct end-to-side anastomosis. This writer opens the common bile duct as one does for a routine common duct exploration, i.e., longitudinally; if choledochoduodenostomy is strongly considered, an appropriate site on the common bile duct is selected—not too low and not too high, but one that will be ideal for an easy anastomosis and good bile flow to the duodenum, yet without undue tension, (see the discussion of choledochoduodenostomy Chapters 2, 4, 6, 10, 11, 12). The duodenum may be opened transversely or longitudinally, depending upon the presenting anatomy. This writer prefers to bring the duodenum up to the common duct, while lateral tension sutures convert the longitudinal opening of the common duct into a transverse one (see Fig. 90). After the first posterior interrupted row of sutures has been placed, one continues to use interrupted (000) black silk throughout; the surgeon must make sure that mucosa-to-mucosa approximation is accomplished with the first inner row. In cases where no danger of occlusion or reduction of lumen size exists, it is preferable to employ a two-layered anastomosis. The second interrupted row of silk sutures effectively covers the anastomosis and seals it. On occasion, some surgeons splint the anastomosis with a T-tube. The T-tube simply acts as a splint or conduit for the anastomosis. Frequently, the round T-tube will be sectioned longitudinally, i.e., the back wall is cut away, thereby reducing its size and allowing it to be removed more easily.

It should be emphasized that the size of the anastomotic stoma is most important; if at all possible, it should be approximately 2.5 cm, and if one obtains a good anastomosis, a splint is not required. However, if one must employ a T-tube, one should bring it out through the common bile duct above or below the site of the anastomosis—if desired, through the duodenal wall below the anastomosis—with one arm of the T-tube extending up through the anastomosis into the common bile duct and one arm extending into the duodenum. If one brings out the T-tube through the wall of the duodenum, it is important to fix it with a purse-string suture, (00) chromic catgut, placed around the point of exit; this will help to prevent leakage of duodenal contents.

The anastomosis should be carefully inspected for leakage. Some surgeons, feeling insecure about their surgery, choose to drain the site of anastomosis with a Penrose or Jackson-Pratt drain. This writer has never employed a drain for this purpose and has no regrets to date. His belief is that a drain at the anastomotic site might draw away the serofibrinous exudate which is so effective in initially sealing off the anastomosis. However, if a Penrose drain has to be employed, it is best to place it in Morison's fossa, where bile usually gravitates.

One of the advantages of a choledochoduodenostomy is that an endoscopist can inspect the anastomotic area from time to time. Endoscopic survey (ERCP) is very important in patients who must have their strictures dilated after choledochoduodenostomy. It is possible to dilate the site of anastomosis periodically as required. If one finds that the choledochoduodenostomy stoma is narrowing down over the years, one should either dilate the stoma or do a sphincterotomy. Many endoscopists worldwide are employing ERCP to perform sphincterotomies as well as stone extractions from the common bile duct. So far, they have been able to remove only small and medium-sized stones; they have also been able to dilate an anastomotic stoma and keep it open. Another factor in choledochoduodenostomy is that an upper gastrointestinal series can often detect and evaluate the anastomotic stoma; one can also see the biliary system filling up with barium and/or air. Smith,[5] in England, uses a "Coca-Cola-gram"; he allows his patient to drink a Coca-Cola (Classic), and thus gets a better air study of his choledochoduodenostomy. He states that this allows him to see the size of the biliary system, and on occasion he sees stones in the biliary system nicely outlined by the gas. This writer hasn't tried Smith's method yet—but when he decides to do so, he will probably try Diet-Pepsi.

Recommended Reading

Degenshein GA: Choledochoduodenostomy: An 18-year study of 175 consecutive cases. *Surgery* 76:316, 1974.

Ham JM, Sorby W: Measurement of stoma size following choledochoduodenostomy by transduodenal cholangiography. *Br J Surg* 60:940, 1973.

Lygidakis NH: Choledochoduodenostomy in calculus biliary tract disease. *Br J Surg* 68:762, 1981.

Moesgaard F, Nielsen ML, Pedersen T, et al: Protective choledochoduodenostomy in multiple common duct stones in the aged. *SGO* 154:232, 1982.

Thomas CG, Nicholson CP, Owen J: Effectiveness of choledochoduodenostomy and transduodenal sphincterotomy in the treatment of benign obstruction of the bile duct. *Ann Surg* 173:845, 1971.

References

1. Field, Jones: Cholecystostomy, a safe operation in the aged emergencies. *South Med J.*
2. Madden JL, Chun JY, Kandalaft S, et al: Choleodochoduodenostomy: An unjustly maligned surgical procedure. *Am J Surg* 119:425, 1970.
3. Hurwitz A, et al: The role of choledochoduodenostomy in common duct surgery: Appraisal. 56:1147, 1964.
4. Huguier M, Lacaine F, Houry S, et al: Choledochoduodenostomy for calculous biliary tract disease. *Arch Surg* 120:241, 1985.
5. Smith R: *Surgery of the Gallbladder and Bile Ducts.* Washington DC, Butterworth, 1981.

13

COMMON DUCT STRICTURE

The exact incidence of benign strictures of the common duct is unknown. Because of continued interest in common duct strictures, the Lahey Clinic has accumulated extensive experience with this problem. *The great majority of common duct strictures are iatrogenic, that is, man-made, and therefore preventable.* The suffering, the economic loss, the necessity for reoperations, and the unusually high morbidity and mortality represent one of the great misfortunes in surgery. There are many misconceptions about how strictures occur; some believe that pulling on the cystic duct is the cause; others point to hemorrhage. Still others believe that by avulsing the cystic duct, a stricture is formed. The hepatic and common ducts are usually strictured by applying crushing clamps indiscriminately, and this writer believes this to be one of the main causes. Perhaps the greatest cause is the lack of knowledge about biliary tract anatomy and anomalies, as well as a lack of appreciation of the proper technique for cholecystectomy. *There is no such thing as a simple cholecystectomy!* When the patient has left the hospital and returns 3–4 months later without signs or symptoms only then can one say that it was a simple procedure.

Of course, some cases are simpler than others, but no cholecystectomy should ever be undertaken without identifying four anatomic structures: (1) the supraduodenal portion of the common duct, (2) the common hepatic duct and the right lateral aspect of the common bile duct, (3) the cystic artery arising from the right or common hepatic artery, and (4) the junction of the cystic duct with the common duct.

If hemorrhage occurs during the procedure, the surgeon must have one assistant use a retractor and the other aspirate. The surgeon is now free to act. He should first compress the cystic or hepatic artery to control the hemorrhage. Then, by releasing the pressure intermittently, the surgeon can identify the exact site of the hemorrhage. One should not apply a crushing clamp blindly to stop the hemorrhage. It should be controlled with a silk suture ligature under direct vision. The surgeon must demonstrate a calm and controlled attitude.

The only acceptable treatment of common duct strictures is prevention. One way of preventing biliary strictures is making the proper incision. Kenneth Warren,[1] formerly chief of staff at the Lahey Clinic, has analyzed gallbladder incisions for years, and many of his patients had multiple operations. If a vertical incision was used, in general it was too short, too low, or too lateral. If a subcostal incision was used, it was too short, too oblique, or too laterally placed. *Adequate, properly placed exposure is very important.* Warren stressed that the recognition of anatomical variations as well as normal anatomic structures, careful control of hemostasis, and the precise identification of all ligated and cut structures are the essentials of a successful cholecystectomy.

The author has taught that an abdominal incision must always be large enough and must be located over the site of the pathology; if a mistake is made, the incision should be larger rather than smaller. A large incision, properly made and properly closed, will not result in a postoperative herniation; however, a small incision, improperly made, will result in a large postoperative herniation. A larger incision will allow better visualization and more certain identification of anatomical structure, and the operation will be less time-consuming. A smaller incision will invariably make surgery more difficult and time-consuming, and will expose the surgeon to possible serious errors.

One of the tragedies of biliary strictures is that two-thirds of the cuts or tears are not recognized at the time of surgery. If a surgeon does recognize a kink or tear at the time of surgery, it is mandatory to attempt to repair it on the spot.

Too often, after the patient develops a biliary fistula, the surgeon blames it on an anatomical anomaly or claims that a ligature must have slipped off the cystic duct. Most small biliary fistulae draining a small amount of bile will usually close spontaneously. However, a persistent postoperative fistula usually means that a stricture of the common duct exists. Warren warns that the surgeon who produced a stricture should not attempt to repair it. The repair of a stricture is a highly sophisticated surgical problem, and the surgeon must recognize that with every reoperation there is progressive attrition of the patient. Strictures are very difficult to repair, but even after six or seven operations, correction is still worthwhile. Sometimes the third operation may be more satisfactory than the first, depending upon how long the patient had been free from recurrent cholangitis. Warren[2] states that the experience at the Lahey Clinic with common duct strictures exceeds 1,500 cases; the majority of them occurred secondary to cholecystectomy and common duct explorations. The usual causes of strictures were related to undue manipulation and trauma.

Pancreatitis and hemorrhage during surgery have been considered by some to be a leading cause of stricture, yet Warren[3] states that in almost 1,000 cases, only 28 strictures developed. On occasion, one may see a common duct stricture secondary to a subtotal gastric resection. In postgastric resections, a different type of stricture develops; when the duct of Santorini and the duct of Wirsung are inadvertently divided a stricture may occur. Warren stresses that the tragedy of strictures is that the patient is often admitted with subhepatic and subdiaphragmatic abscesses, bile collections, hematomas, pancreatitis, pancreatic abscess, damage to the pancreatic ducts, liver abscess, and bronchobiliary fistula. Warren states that fistulae are a kind of a blessing in that they help to decompress the biliary tract for a while, but never sufficiently to give a lasting result.

External fistulae tend to minimize liver damage, as well as dilatation of the bile ducts. Dilatation of the bile ducts may be a prime consideration in selecting the type of repair, i.e., whether or not a stent will be required.

Mortality is related to the type of ductal injury and to whether or not a myocardial infarction has occurred. Warren found that death in older patients was commonly due to vascular accidents; pneumonia was also a serious cause of postoperative death. Pancreatitis is a devastating postoperative complication, but fortunately is rare. Warren states that the mortality following stricture repair depends on whether or not the original surgeon makes the first or second attempt. It also depends upon the other associated complications and on whether or not there is adequate biliary ductal structure to work with. Mortality for the first operation, according to Warren, is 4–6%. The cause is cirrhosis, with or without portal hypertension.

The location of the stricture is important. Most strictures are high, often located above the cystic duct junction. Some strictures are even higher. Not infrequently, a division involves both hepatic ducts. Warren states that repair is very simple if the ductal division is in the supraduodenal portion of the common duct. High strictures require a different type of anastomosis and splinting. Warren emphasizes the importance of obtaining immediate bacteriological studies at operation, especially anaerobic cultures. He recommends broad-spectrum antibiotics; a combination of of an aminoglycoside (gentamicin) and chloramphenicol (Chloromycetin) may be given a few hours before surgery, and if the operation is prolonged, Chloromycetin may be repeated during the surgery. Most often, gram-negative and anaerobic organisms will be cultured out.

Dr. Richard Cattell[4] developed a Y-tube for high strictures. Warren has modified the Cattell Y-tube by attaching an external solid core limb that is not in communication with the lumen of the Y-tube. The purpose of the long, solid arm is to remove the Y-tube without resorting to another operative procedure. Warren stresses that no one really knows when to remove it. In the past, he used the loop of the jejunum for many biliary reconstructions; he does not advocate choledochoduodenostomy. Warren still employs the Cattel Y-tube in many instances for his anastomosis. He recommends dissecting away the scar tissue and some liver at the hilus in order to get exposure a little higher. His results with this type of repair have been satisfactory, but he states that the length of time the Y-tube remains in place is important. The longer it remains in place without cholangitis, the better the result. Warren reported that his Y-tube has remained in for as long as 3 years without producing signs or symptoms. The tubes were ultimately removed when cholangitis developed.

Warren's results were 80–85% good. A stricture secondary to gastric resection leaves a longer segment of duct, which makes it easier to anastomose to the duodenum or jejunum (see "Management of Benign Biliary Stricture").

Endoscopic retrograde pancreatography (ERCP) is a procedure that can localize the site of obstruction with a minimum of complications. An alternative diagnostic procedure is percutaneous cholangiography. Where a cholangiolytic type of jaundice exists and ERCP is unsuccessful, Warren recommends percutaneous transhepatic cholangiography. In the latter instance, surgery should first be scheduled and carried out immediately after the test results are evaluated. Preoperative broad-spectrum antibiotics should be started prophylactically.

References

1. Warren K, Poulantzas JK: Use of a Y-tube splint in the repair of biliary strictures. *Surg Gynecol Obstet* 122:785 1966.
2. Warren K, Mountain JC, Midell AI: Management of strictures of the biliary tree. *Surg Clin North Am* 5:711 1971.
3. Warren K, Christophi C, Armanariz R: The evolution of current perspectives of the treatment of benign bile duct strictures: A review. *Surg Gastroenterol* 1:141 1982.
4. Cattell R, Braasch JW: Primary repair of benign strictures of the bile duct. *Surg Gynecol Obstet* 109:531; 1959.

Diagnosis and Treatment of Extrabiliary Strictures

Common or hepatic duct injury recognized at surgery should be dealt with immediately and by the most ideal method, such as end-to-end anastomosis, or splinting with a T-tube that is brought out through a choledochostomy stoma. Stenotic lesions that occur in the postoperative period can occur soon thereafter or even months or years later by a slow stenosing process. Stenotic lesions that occur in the immediate postoperative period are usually due to retained impacted stones that lead to obstructive jaundice. Strictures can be recognized by jaundice; the latter is often attributed to retained stones or transfusion reactions. If jaundice is believed to be caused by a stenotic lesion created at surgery, it should be operated on immediately. The possibility of a ligature accidentally placed around the common duct has been reported on several occasions.

If the common duct stenosis is due to actual damage of tissue, repair should be done immediately by one of the techniques described by Braasch et al.[1] Inadvertent injuries to the common duct during surgery that resulted only in incomplete blockage will ultimately produce complete stenosis after months or years. It is believed that a partial injury is frequently followed by a fibrotic process (desmoplasia) that continues over time to stenose the lumen of the extrabiliary duct. It is also possible that, in the same period of time, repeated incidents of cholangitis may develop, accompanied by progressive parenchymatous liver damage.

The signs and symptoms may include intermittent fever, chills, and jaundice; they suggest ductal stenosis. However, the possibility of retained or impacted stones must also be considered. It should be kept in mind that one or more conditions may coexist.

On physical examination, the liver may be enlarged and tender, and an external fistula may exist. In some instances, the liver may not be enlarged. IV cholangiography has proven of little value and cannot be used to demonstrate a stricture or stone in the bile duct, particularly because of existing jaundice and liver damage.

We must consider the possible use of percutaneous intrahepatic cholangiography and computed tomography (CT) scan. Other liver tests offer indirect information, while intrahepatic cholangiography offers a direct, objective finding and a diagnosis. One should keep in mind the consequences of percutaneous intrahepatic cholangiography, namely, the possibility of bile leakage and/or blood loss into the free peritoneal cavity. The surgeon must inform the operating room personnel to stand by and be ready to operate in the event of a serious extravasation of blood or bile that not infrequently takes place during or after the test. This has been discussed elsewhere, but in view of the fact that it has to be repeated here, the writer wishes to emphasize the importance as well as the seriousness of the percutaneous transhepatic cholangiographic study. A CT scan may offer a diagnosis when other methods fail. (See Chapter 5).

ACTIVE TREATMENT OF BILIARY DUCT INJURIES

Preoperative treatment is most important in the active treatment of biliary duct stenosis because patients who have developed fistulae as a result of early postoperative complications have lost electrolytes and have developed serious electrolyte deficiencies. Electrolytes must be replaced and balanced to the point where a deficiency no longer exists. In these individuals, we also find concomitant liver damage; it is important to fortify the liver with a high-carbohydrate, high-protein, low-fat diet. Feedings may be administered by hyperalimentation via the subclavian vein through a central venous pressure (CVP) line. The supplemental agents that are added are vitamin B complex, vitamin C, and Aquamephyton, or vitamin K. Vitamins will help raise the prothrombin level, which can serve as an indicator of liver damage repair. When the prothrombin level is corrected, the patient comes closer to the time for safer surgery. If any evidence of anemia or a bleeding tendency develops, blood transfusions should be given to correct the deficiencies. The bleeding tendency should be studied further so that the causes can be identified and corrected with calcium, platelets, fibrinogen, red blood cells, plasma, whole blood, or any special plasma factor.

Where portal hypertension exists with concomitant esophageal varices and hypersplenism, surgery for stenosis should be delayed as long as possible until a procedure to relieve portal hypertension is carried out, i.e., a portocaval, or splenorenal shunt. *The surgery for stenosis should be carried out last.*

PRINCIPLES OF SURGICAL TECHNIQUE IN THE REPAIR OF BILIARY TRACT STRICTURES

Extrahepatic injury to the biliary tree at the time of surgery (inadvertently lacerated or perforated) should be repaired immediately. The repair must be anatomical, i.e., the ampullary mechanism should be preserved and an end-to-end repair carried out. The anastomosis may be splinted by a T-tube that comes out through a separate opening either above or below the line of anastomosis. The long arm of the T-tube is brought out through a subcostal stab wound laterally placed.

If it is impossible to make an end-to-end anastomosis on the spot or at the time the laceration is created, the second best procedure is to utilize the proximal bile duct (hepatic or common bile duct) and anastomose it to the most readily available structure, preferably the jejunum. An end-to-side or Roux-Y (end-to-end) anastomosis is acceptable; the latter is a choledochojejunostomy, either end-to-end or end-to-side. The possibility of mobilizing the duodenum upward must also be considered, since this is the second best procedure, especially if that anatomical relationship is best suited to the procedure.

Another principle to be kept in mind is the anastomotic technique—preferably, as stated above, an end-to-end anastomosis without tension. A (0000) or (00000) interrupted silk suture with an atraumatic needle is ideal for bile duct repair. A good anastomosis can be performed utilizing one row of sutures. The principle of utilizing the patient's own anatomy, that is, no prosthesis, is always preferable.

Longmire's[2] operation is hepaticojejunostomy, i.e., anastomosing the end open portion of the liver to the side of the jejunum. The procedure is not easy to perform; the surgeon should be sure that the right and left hepatic ducts are in communication with one another. Unfortunately, the postoperative results are not too good.

Before attempting the repair of a common or hepatic duct tear laceration, or stricture, it is advisable to obtain the best possible dissection about the target anatomy. The operator must try not to jeopardize the portal vein, the hepatic artery, or their branches before and during the repair. At present, we have no ideal prosthesis for replacing the loss of substance of the common duct. Various rubber, plastic, silicone, intestine, and vein materials have been tried, but to date, the ideal procedure remains direct anastomosis between the patient's own biliary tree and the intestine.

SURGICAL REPAIR OF BILIARY TRACT STRICTURE

The choice treatment, as mentioned elsewhere, is prophylactic, that is, to prevent the initial injury and thus prevent late stricturing of the biliary tract. If the latter is not possible and the actual damage to the common duct has already taken place, the next procedure is the immediate repair of the defect. The surgeon may resort to multiple procedures; for example, a two-stage repair may be considered acceptable for bile duct stricture because the patient is at high risk, overaged, and with concomitant disease problems that must be attended to first;

these drawbacks, if not considered, will be responsible for the ultimate demise of the patient.

It is necessary, therefore, in dealing with high-risk patients, to know exactly what the accompanying problems are. Patients may have suppurative cholangitis and ball-valve problems accompanied by chills and fever, diabetes mellitus, and other conditions capable of reducing hepatic and renal function. Patients with stricture require an urgent repair of their lesion, but they must be initially improved preoperatively and given the maximum time to do so without being jeopardized. The ideal time to intercede surgically is when the patient's condition warrants an operative procedure; it is necessary to evaluate the extent of the procedure, i.e., the length of time and the manipulations required, to prevent shock from entering the picture. Therefore, a simple silastic tube placed into the hepatic duct after it is found may prove to be all that is necessary (see Figs. 140 to 143). This latter short technique can be compared with a cholecystostomy performed for a difficult case of cholecystitis and lithiasis.

A hepaticostomy, in which a multiply perforated tube is placed in the common hepatic duct, directed into the right or left lobe of the liver, and brought out through a subcostal stab wound, may itself be a lifesaving procedure (see "Management of Benign Biliary Stricture"). The liver will improve, the jaundice will disappear, and the infection will subside. The improved patient may then be ready for a definitive second-stage primary reparative procedure.

Regardless of the time required (even several weeks), a second-stage procedure can be undertaken only at the propitious moment. If the end portion of the hepatic duct cannot be easily found or dissected out, it may be necessary to employ a metallic tube or a Y-shaped silastic or rubber tube (see the previous discussion of Warren's bile duct Y-tube repair). The latter prosthesis may effectively drain the liver through a splinted hepaticojejunostomy. This, of course, assures adequate decompression of the liver, reduces liver enzymes, and ultimately improves all of the depleted liver functions. Eventually, regenerative processes will take place until such time as a definitive procedure may be considered.

Vitalium tubes were pioneered at the Lahey Clinic by Cattell et al.,[3] who found that the Y-tube, when necessary, can be left in situ for months or years. These surgeons also found that Vitalium is no substitute for the mucosa of the biliary tree, and that mud and gravel gradually accumulate and obstruct the lumen of the prosthesis. It may be nec-

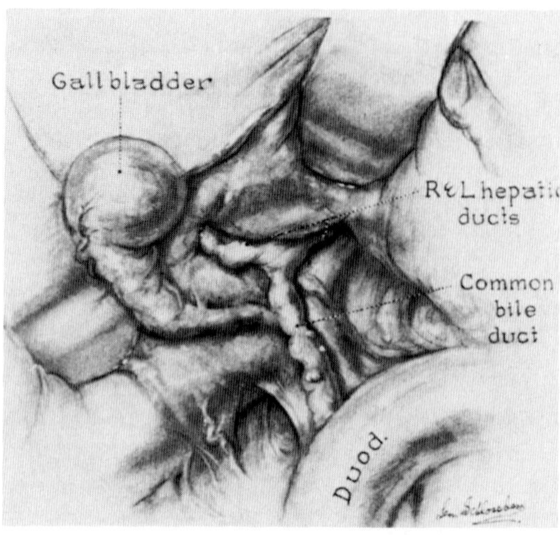

Figure 140.   Cameron et al. used silastic transhepatic stents in benign and malignant strictures (Am J Surg 196 (4); 412; 1982). They found that the most restrictive obstructing lesion was usually at the bifurcation of the hepatic ducts. The bifurcation of the hepatic ducts was resected, and bilateral hepaticojejunostomies were performed using transhepatic biliary silastic stents.

essary to do a third-stage procedure to remove the Y-tube and either repair whatever is left without a metallic prostheses or reinsert a new one. The results, of course, are variable, depending upon who operates.

The condition of the patient, the timing, and the selection of the surgical procedure are most important. The surgeon must recognize that this surgery deals with the most difficult anatomy and that good vision with good exposure is essential to the required meticulous technique and the ultimate successful outcome. A large incision should be made in the vertical plane so that lateral retraction may be attained in any direction. In certain individuals, i.e., the very obese, transverse incisions may be required; a good exposure is the *fish mouth* exposure. When the abdomen is opened and the abdominal cavity is found to contain many adhesions, it is necessary to start in the abdominal cavity, where the anatomy is recognizable and the dissection carried out from the known to the unknown; in this way, the most superficial adhesions are dealt with first and the dissection continues deeper into the abdominal cavity until the target zone is reached and identified.

The incision made, the adhesions are recognized, severed, and separated, working from the normal to the abnormal anatomy. The more abnormal the anatomy, the slower must be the technique, because precise technique is required. Tearing can produce catastrophic results. Not infrequently, the antrum, pylorus, and duodenum are fixed under the porta hepatis with firm adhesions, and must be dealt with by sharp dissection carried out slowly and carefully. The hepatic flexure of the colon frequently finds its way under the liver and is situated

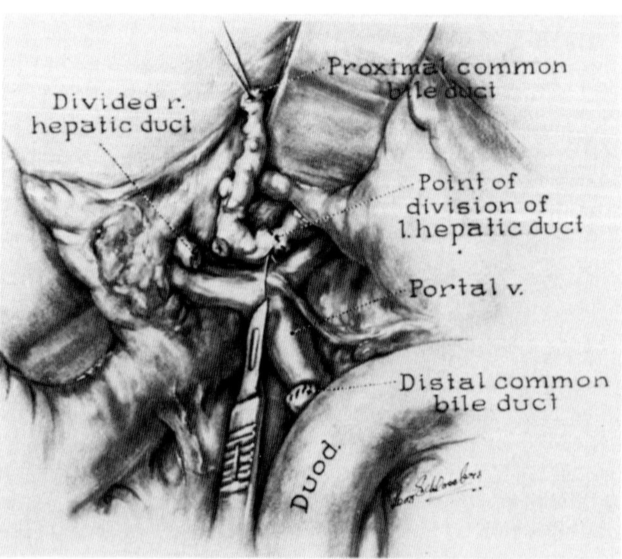

Figure 141.   The common duct is being excised from the point of hepatic division. Initially the common duct is cut distally and elevated. This maneuver assists in isolating the hepatic bifurcation. Each cut hepatic duct has a catheter inserted to assist in identifying them.

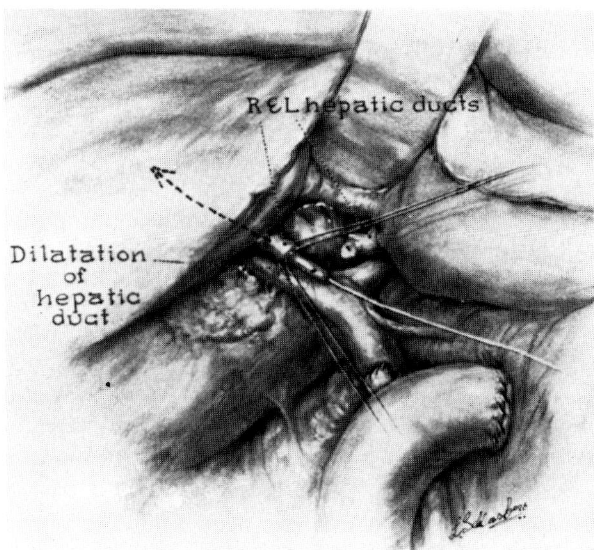

Figure 142. Bakes dilators are used to dilate the hepatic ducts before stents are placed in both ductal systems.

particularly close to the porta hepatis; this, too, must be carefully dissected and retracted downward. The antrum and pylorus are particularly difficult to dissect because their blood supply can be easily infringed upon. The right gastric artery is vulnerable, and the hepatic artery can also be injured. Therefore, it is imperative that slow, delicate dissection be carried out throughout the procedure.

The surgeon must be ready at any moment for a calamitous error, whether inadvertent or careless. The fistulous tract that may exist between the common hepatic or common bile duct and the duodenum, when freed from the hilar area, may result in cutting across the fistulous tract. If this happens, the leakage is immediately dealt with as follows: The duodenum, if small, can be closed with a purse string suture of (0000) black silk with an atraumatic needle. A second row of interrupted silk sutures is recommended. The hepatic or common bile duct should be evaluated for continuity, size, and thickness.

A flexible probe is utilized to probe the remaining

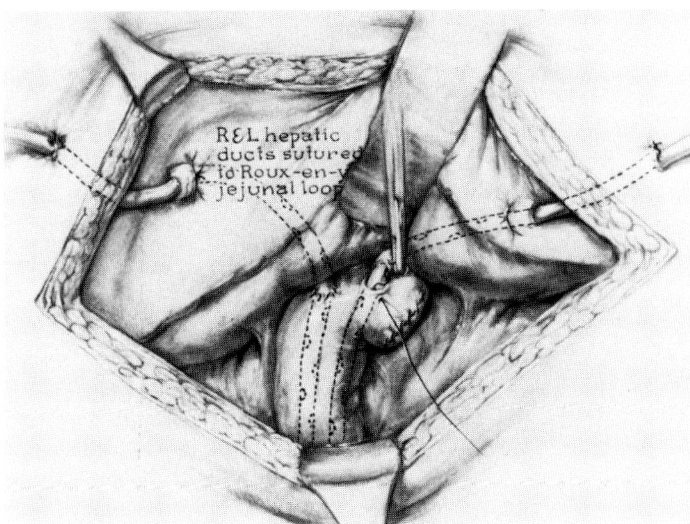

Figure 143. Roux-en-Y-hepaticojejunostomies are completed. The ends of the silastic stents come out from the top of the liver. Stab wounds allow each stent to be brought out through the abdominal wall.

proximal duct in order to determine if the right and left ducts are patent or obstructed. The distal portion of the involved duct is then checked to see if the probe will pass through the ampullary stoma and if it can be dilated. The operator should evaluate and determine if there is patency and if the distal portion of the duct can be utilized. If the stoma is strictured, it should be dilated with a Bakes dilator. The rest of the common or hepatic duct should be checked to see whether the size is adequate and whether the repair can be done immediately. Black silk sutures (0000–00000) with an atraumatic needle are interruptedly placed, through and through, and splinted by a new opening made in the common or hepatic duct above or below the suture line. Splinting can be done with an ordinary T-tube or a long-end Cattell T-tube. A Cattell tube is a long-arm T-tube that allows the long arm of the tube to pass through the ampullary stoma into the duodenum. There have been many objections to this tube; it was modified by Glassman, who perforated the distal half of the long arm so that as it passed through the common duct into the duodenum, it did not obstruct the flow of pancreatic juices; this reduces the fear of complications, i.e., pancreatic obstruction with pancreatitis. The long, straight arm of the T-tube is brought out through a subcostal stab wound laterally placed. The Penrose drain with wick is preferably brought out through the same stab wound; the Penrose or Jackson-Pratt drain is placed in Morison's fossa.

Richard Cattell,* Ken Warren, and John Braasch have been pioneers in the field of common and hepatic duct strictures; they have perhaps repaired more postoperative strictures of the common and hepatic ducts than anyone in the world. Their method has always attempted to preserve the ampullary mechanism by performing an end-to-end anastomosis, where possible, and splinting the common or hepatic duct with a T-tube above or below the site of anastomosis. In their experienced hands, the percentage of successes has been the best attainable anywhere. Therefore, the final results of biliary duct repair must depend upon the wide experience of the operator, the condition of the patient, preexisting concomitant conditions, and preoperative and postoperative management. Warren has wisely recommended that another surgeon be selected to do a secondary biliary repair—preferably a more experienced surgeon.

Occasionally, during the dissection for exposure of the hepatic duct, bleeding may occur. This type of bleeding may often, though not always, be the remnant of the cystic artery; it should be carefully ligated and dissected off the hepatic duct to prevent interference with the subsequent anastomosis, whatever type repair is chosen. One must, however, be certain that the right hepatic artery is not inadvertently ligated.

BALLOON DILATATION OF BILE DUCT STRICTURES

Hutson,[5] of the University of Miami School of Medicine, writing on bile duct strictures, proposes a nonoperative stomatization procedure for recurring stricture formation in such procedures as choledochoduodenostomy, choledochojejunostomy, and hepaticojejunostomy. This stomatization procedure is also recommended in sclerosing cholangitis.

This writer feels that this noninvasive procedure can be utilized for such conditions as recurring malignant strictures, sclerosing cholangitis, and other forms of intractable stricturing. It is conceivable that this new balloon procedure, because it requires exteriorization of the proximal jejunal loop, can be conducive to ascending cholangitis with liver cirrhosis and abscess formation. This procedure should be reserved for the more intractable cases. The writer reemphasizes that a postoperative biliary stricture should ideally be repaired by surgery and is best repaired on the spot (see "Management of Benign Stricture" and "Intubation Techniques in Biliary Tract Surgery").

Cameron et al.,[4] in their study of 29 patients, reported that only when the stenotic disease was mainly confined to the extrahepatic biliary tree did they attempt reconstructive surgery. They found that even though a diffuse sclerosing process existed, the most restricting obstructive lesion was usually found to be at the hepatic duct bifurcation. Cameron et al. devised an operative procedure that consisted of excision of the bifurcation of the hepatic duct, dilatation of the intrahepatic biliary tree with Bakes dilators, insertion of bilateral silicone transparent stents (Silastic), and a bilateral hepaticojejunostomy. In late inoperable cases, a liver transplantation was suggested (see "Liver Transplantation and Biliary Atresia" by Starzl, Chap. 4). Cameron et al. believe that their surgery for sclerosing cholangitis is only a palliative procedure and is best employed where a large duct obstruction is the major contributor to progressive liver disease. (See - Figs. 140–143).

*Deceased.

Recommended Reading

Beinart C, Sniderman KW, Tamura S, et al: Biliary pressure measurement: An aid in the management of patients on internal biliary drainage. *Invest Radiol* 17:356, 1982.

Blumgart LH, Kelley CJ, Benjamin IS: Benign bile duct stricture following cholecystectomy: Critical factors in management. *Br J Surg* 71:836, 1984.

Burhenne HJ: Dilatation of biliary tract strictures: A new roentgenologic technique. *Radiol Clin* 44:153, 1975.

Burhenne HJ, Morris DC: Biliary stricture dilatation: Use of the Gruntzig balloon catheter. *J Can Assoc Radiol* 31:196, 1980.

Centola CAP, Jander HP, Stauffer A, et al: Balloon dilatation of the ampulla of Vater to allow biliary stone passage. *AJR* 136:613, 1981.

Cole WH, Ireneus C, Reynolds JT: Strictures of the common duct. *Ann Surg* 133:683, 1951.

Fernandez M: Treatment of benign strictures of the bile ducts. *World J Surg* 4:479, 1980.

Fretheim B: Operative biliary tract injuries: Secondary reparative operations. *Chir Gastroenterol* 11:451, 1977.

Gallacher DJ, Kadir S, Kaufman SL, et al: Nonoperative management of benign postoperative biliary strictures. *Radiology* 156:625, 1985.

Glenn F: Postoperative stricture of the extrahepatic bile ducts. *Surg Gynecol Obstet* 120:560, 1965.

Glenn F: Iatrogenic injuries to the biliary ductal system. *Surg Gynecol Obstet* 146:430, 1978.

Hermann BE: Diagnosis and management of bile duct strictures. *Am J Surg* 130:519, 1973.

Martin EC, Fankuchen EI, Laffey KJ, et al: Percutaneous management of benign biliary disease. *Gastrointest Radiol* 9:207, 1984.

Martin EC, Fankuchen EI, Schultz RW, et al: Percutaneous dilatation in primary sclerosing cholangitis: Two experiences. *AJR* 137:603, 1981.

Martin EC, Karlson KB, Fankuchen EI, et al: Percutaneous transhepatic dilatation of intrahepatic biliary strictures. *AJR* 135:837, 1980.

May GR, Bender CE, LaRusso NF, et al: Nonoperative dilatation of dominant strictures in primary sclerosing cholangitis. *AJR* 145:1061, 1985.

McAllister AJ, Kicken NF: Biliary stricture: A continuing study. *Am J Surg* 132:567, 1976.

Molnar W, Stockum AE: Transhepatic dilatation of choledochoenterostomy strictures. *Radiology* 129:59, 1978.

Oleaga JA, McLean GK, Freiman OB, et al: Interventional biliary radiology, in Ring EJ, McLean GK (eds): *International Radiology: Principles and Techniques*. Boston, Little, Brown, 1981, pp 245–378.

Pellegrini CA, Thomas MJ, Way LW: Recurrent biliary stricture: Patterns of recurrence and outcome of surgical therapy. *Am J Surg* 147:175, 1984.

Pitt HA, Miyamoto T, Parapatis SK, et al: Factors influencing outcome in patients with postoperative biliary strictures. *Am J Surg* 144:14, 1982.

Saber K, El-Manialawi M: Repair of bile duct injuries. *World J Surg* 1:82, 1984.

Salomonowitz E, Castaneda-Zuniga WR, Lund G, et al: Balloon dilatation of benign biliary strictures. *Radiology* 151:613, 1984.

Teplick SK, Wolferth CC Jr, Hayes MF Jr, et al: Balloon dilatation of benign postsurgical biliary enteric-anastomotic strictures. *Gastrointest Radiol* 7:307, 1982.

Vogel SB, Howard RJ, Caridi J, et al: Evaluation of percutaneous transhepatic balloon dilatation of benign biliary strictures in high-risk patients. *Am J Surg* 149:73, 1985.

Wheeler ES, Longmire WP Jr: Repair of benign stricture of the common bile duct by jejunal interposition: Choledochoduodenostomy. *Surg Gynecol Obstet* 146:260, 1978.

Zeman RK, Burrell MI, Dobbins J, et al: Postcholecystectomy syndrome: Evaluation using biliary scintigraphy and endoscopic retrograde cholangiopancreatography. *Radiology* 156:787, 1985.

References

1. Braasch JW, Bolton JS, Rossi RL: A technique of biliary reconstruction with complete follow-up in 44 consecutive cases. *Am Surg* 194:635, 1981.
2. Longmire WP Jr: Early management of injury to the extrahepatic biliary tract. *JAMA* 195, 111; 1966.
3. Cattell R, Warren K, Braasch J: General considerations in the management of benign strictures of the bile duct. *N Engl J Med* 261:929, 1959.
4. Cameron JL, Broe P, Zuidema GD: The use of silastic transhepatic stents in benign and malignant strictures. *Am Surg* 188:552, 1978.
5. Hutson DG, Russell E, Schiff E, et al: Balloon dilatation of biliary strictures through a choledochojejuno-cutaneous fistula. *Ann Surg* 199:6, 1984.

Causes of Postoperative Biliary Duct Strictures

In the majority of cases (over 75%), postoperative benign strictures result from cholecystectomy for calculous or acalculous cholecystitis. Five percent of bile duct strictures follow exploration of the biliary passages and are caused by undue handling of tissues. Partial or subtotal gastrectomy is often an underlying cause of bile duct stricture at that level. Other causes are penetrating duodenal ulcer or any attempt to excise a diverticulum of the second portion of the duodenum. Still other causes of postoperative stricture of the bile duct are fibrosis of the sphincter of Oddi and choledochoduodenal fistula formation. Stricture may accompany a congenital choledochal cyst and may be produced by sclerosing cholangitis. Even after good gallbladder surgery, a postoperative stricture of the bile duct may occur for unknown reasons (idiopathic).

Approximately one-third or more of the cases of postoperative strictures of the bile duct are iatrogenic. Today the occurrence of postoperative stricture of the bile duct has been greatly reduced, most likely as a result of better surgical training programs and greater improvement in surgical techniques. Today, when a postoperative stricture of the bile duct occurs, it is a catastrophic event to patient and surgeon alike. Depending on the extent of the disease and its underlying cause, approximately 50% of strictures are curable by reconstructive surgery. This depends greatly on the expertise of the surgeon and on the extent and site of the biliary stricture. Porter[1] in 1960 reported 1,000 cholecystectomies, with two patients developing a bile duct injury—an incidence of 0.2%. Private clinics have reported much higher incidences. Some believe that the incidence of strictures of the common duct is on the increase. This author cannot concur with this finding, because better surgeons and better techniques are now available; unquestionably, more cautious surgery is being performed today.

The *best treatment and the most important consideration in the treatment of biliary duct strictures is prophylaxis.* Prevention depends on continued surgical teaching programs on how to prevent common duct injury by applying greater attention to technical skill.

In terms of prophylaxis, this writer advises the following precautions:

1. Adequate operative exposure employing a large rather than a small incision. For gallbladder surgery, a right paramedian or midline incision is sufficient. However, there are instances where oblique or subcostal incisions should be utilized, especially when the habitus of the patient demands it. An obese person with a wide-angled costal margin usually requires a right transverse or bilateral transverse incision. Transverse incisions are ideal in short people with very obese abdomens. In some extremely obese patients, as much as one-half the circumference of the abdomen may be utilized for the incision; it will simulate a fish mouth exposure.
2. Good muscular relaxation, which means excellent anesthesia and preoperative preparation of the patient.
3. Trained assistants. Even paramedical personnel can be extremely valuable. Self-retaining retractors have been greatly improved, but they should be used only in small community hospitals where the staff is inadequate.
4. Good cephalic retraction* with adequate exposure of the operative field. The operative site should be evaluated carefully, and surgery should not be started until the situation is fully surveyed and understood, the pathology has been identified, and all facilities are available. The latter includes good light, the newest instruments, and, of course, a qualified surgeon with trained assistants.
5. A thorough, routine (round-the-clock) exploration of the abdomen before definitive surgery is undertaken. The purpose is to evaluate and determine the critical areas that may alter the outcome of the operation. For example, the cystic artery and the right hepatic artery should be identified and anomalies of the biliary system recognized. There is still much discussion about how liver necrosis or death of the patient may follow inadvertent ligation of the right hepatic artery or the common hepatic artery. This writer believes this to be a very serious matter. To ligate these arteries may in fact cause dire consequences, but there have been many reports stating that the main hepatic or right hepatic artery has been ligated with impunity. Thay may be so, but this writer has experienced both outcomes: consequences following one ligation and death of the patient in another. This writer therefore concludes that the integrity of these important arteries should not be jeopardized at any time. In either event, the surgical procedure must be carried to its conclusion. It is believed that in a number of instances a collateral circulation may exist between the right and left hepatic arteries intrahepatically. The extensive communication between the portal venous system and the hepatic arterial system within the liver probably plays the most important role in the survival of the liver when either hepatic artery has been ligated.
6. It is imperative that so-called biliary surgery never be underestimated; complete hemostasis, with good light and trained assistants, is always mandatory. The cystic artery should preferably be ligated (not clamped) somewhat close to the common duct, about one-fourth inch. It is imperative not to infringe upon the common duct wall. It is better to ligate the cystic artery close to or on the gallbladder wall in order to stay away from any anomalous, short, or aberrant

---

Cephalic retraction is a term that Dr. Raymond W. McNealy (chief surgeon at Cook County Hospital in Chicago and my former preceptor) used to demand "retraction while using one's brain."

right hepatic artery. This precaution is essential; often, with a little lateral traction and fine blunt dissection, an anomalous anatomical situation is often revealed that, if left unrecognized, would have resulted in a calamitous situation.

7. It should be remembered that the cystic duct lies on top of the cystic artery in most instances. However, when the cystic artery lies on top of the cystic duct, the cystic artery must be ligated first; it is most fortunate when this situation exists. Better visualization invariably means safer surgery. The opposite, however, is usually the case, i.e., the cystic duct usually overlies the cystic artery, so that the cystic duct must be ligated first and severed. The clamped cystic duct is then reflected to the right; only then can the cystic artery be properly visualized and doubly ligated. This routine is most important if inadvertent ligation of the right hepatic artery is to be averted. This writer does not use electrocautery or coagulation for smaller bleeding vessels in this area; rather, he uses ligatures, metal clips, pressure, warm packs, Surgicel, Avitene, and Gelfoam, assisted by a little pressure with a warm-wet lap pad. Some surgeons believe that electrocoagulation of anatomy during cholecystectomy may itself be a possible cause of late stricture of the bile duct. Avoid it near or on the common duct.

8. When this writer speaks of the cystic artery and its anomalies, and of faulty dissection in unsuspected situations, he implies that the result may be a serious cystic artery hemorrhage. In such an instance, it is essential for the surgeon not to panic. He should aspirate the blood and compress the bleeder with wet lap pads until the site and cause of the bleeding are established. Blood should be readily available for transfusion if necessary. An excellent light should be adjusted so that when the wet lap pad is removed, the surgeon can quickly see the source of the bleeding. If the bleeding is recognized, a fine metallic clip may be carefully applied; this may be all that is required. If the source of the bleeding is not precisely localized, the surgeon should employ the forefinger and thumb of the left hand to carefully grasp the porta hepatis (all three structures) and compress them to stop the bleeding. By intermittently opening and closing his fingers, he will be able to localize the exact site of bleeding and suture or clip the bleeding site. When a short hepatic artery exists and is closely adherent to the gallbladder wall because of earlier inflammation,

the cystic artery may not be visualized too well. Here is where a thorough knowledge of anatomy, careful dissection, delicacy in handling tissue, and meticulous suturing or clipping pays off. Here, too, is where careless and thoughtless application of a crushing clamp can involve the right hepatic artery, the common bile duct, and even the portal vein. The result is either immediate obstruction or late stricture formation of the common duct.

9. It is not uncommon for a cystic or hepatic artery, when inadvertently cut, to retract behind the porta hepatic structures. It is wise, therefore, to learn how to rotate the biliary structures, employing a delicate, noncrushing clamp to reflect the anterior surface of the hepatic or common duct to the left in order to reveal the underside and the exact site of bleeding. It is most important to know that the portal vein is a possible site for injury and serious bleeding. When injured, the portal vein causes severe hemorrhage, which can be disastrous if it is not found and repaired. In the presence of active bleeding during gallbladder surgery, there must be no panic and certainly no blind clamping at the site of bleeding. Clamping must be pinpointed precisely over the site of bleeding, which is intermittently controlled with the forefinger and thumb (compressed and released) under good light, with the aid of reliable assistance. With proper retraction and good relaxation, the surgeon should be able, using an Adson or thinnose Mixter clamp, to grasp the exact site of bleeding without traumatizing important structures close by. *The surgeon should not clamp a bleeder blindly; clamping must be done under proper light and by careful direct application of a clamp or clip to the exact site.*

10. Unfortunately, another common cause of strictures to the extrahepatic biliary tree is a sad lack of anatomical knowledge. This is primarily a reference to the normal anatomy. Most cases will be within normal limits, with only slight variations from the norm. However, by knowing the norm, the surgeon can easily recognize an abnormal or anomalous structure. If the surgeon cannot establish a normal relationship between the biliary system and the arterial and venous blood supplies, he should immediately *stop. He must move slowly and think fast!* He must "de-booby trap" the area by slowing the tempo of his dissection; he must recheck the operative field by improving his light, assistants, and exposure. He must move slowly and deliberately,

with the utmost delicacy. The surgeon must repeatedly reevaluate the specific anatomy of the patient. If the anatomy is not cleared as normal, it must be considered anomalous. With a new and better understanding, a more definitive surgical approach can be carried out. It makes no difference where the cystic artery originates from—whether it comes from the right hepatic artery, common hepatic artery, or gastroduodenal artery; so long as the ligation of the cystic artery takes place on or into the wall of the gallbladder, there is nothing to fear. The cystic artery supplies the gallbladder and enters the gallbladder wall; safe ligation of the cystic artery must take place as close to or in the gallbladder wall.

11. Not infrequently, a gallbladder has no cystic duct at all, but merely joins up with the common duct; in this instance, the initial surgery may entail applying the ligature too close to the common duct, creating a site for future fibrosis and stenosis. In other words, a stricture will ultimately develop at that level. It is this writer's strong feeling that at the time of cystic duct ligation, the surgeon who employs a crushing clamp instead of an encircling ligature stands a greater chance of infringing upon the circumference of the common duct; an iatrogenic stenosis or stricture of the common bile duct is most likely to follow.

    An unfortunate situation exists when a young surgeon brags about how little time it takes him to do a gallbladder operation. As this surgeon matures, he will discover (after sad experiences) that there is no simple or "easy" gallbladder operation. The only gallbladder surgery that can be called simple is the one that finally turns out to be easy. Never say "It's going to be easy." The young surgeon who tries to see how fast the surgery can be done will often apply undue traction on the common duct and then clamp a short cystic duct—and possibly no cystic duct—but the common bile duct. Gallbladder surgery must be considered a complex operation, and all facilities and assistants must be available for a long and complicated procedure. In this writer's opinion, it must be considered to be one of the most difficult operative procedures in existence because it is so variable and unpredictable. It is invariably loaded with anomalous arrangements, either in the arteries or in the biliary tree. The gallbladder and biliary tract frequently have their anatomical relationship seriously altered by previous disease or surgery. One cannot predict what one will find or what one will have to contend with when the abdomen is opened. Only after the surgery is completed can the surgeon say, "It *was* easy" or "It *was* difficult." This writer has encountered difficult gallbladder cases despite normal anatomy, but in which a high-lying gallbladder was found under the ribs of obese patients with a high-lying, small liver. In such instances, the gallbladder is invariably found where the liver is, with the ribs unrelenting and difficult to retract. The surgeon often has to "stand on his ear," so to speak, in order to be able to visualize and deal with a so-called normal gallbladder. It is here usually, in these so-called normal anatomical situations, with a normal gallbladder in a deep, high-lying position, poor light, and mediocre assistants, that one is led to commit grievous errors.

12. When surgeons enter an abdomen that has been operated on before, they must expect to encounter distortions caused by multiple dense adhesions. Experienced surgeons will invariably play it safe; even their mistakes must benefit rather than harm the patient. As stated earlier, *the surgeon must move slowly and think fast.* No procedure should ever be carried out blindly. Proper dissection, excellent visualization, and anatomical recognition are the key criteria to the correct surgical approach. An experienced surgeon knows he can always come back at a later date and fight a new battle on his own terms; one example is a cholecystostomy rather than a cholecystectomy in a blind field full of adhesions and distortions produced by previous repeated inflammations of the gallbladder. When Napoleon was asked "How is it that you win all your battles?" he answered, "Because I never enter into a battle without first planning a line of retreat. When I return the battle is fought on my terms and at the time I choose."

13. Another common cause of stricture of the common or hepatic duct is chemical irritation by the bile itself. Bile that leaks out in a given area and accumulates at a given point, if not properly drained off, may affect the wall of the common duct; an irritative desmoplasia (or a dense fibrous reaction) will develop, with subsequent contraction of the area, resulting in thickening, stenosis, and obstruction. Bile is an irritating agent, and can externally affect the very anatomy that houses it. It is important to drain the biliary system properly with a T-tube

and employ a Penrose-wick drain or Jackson-Pratt suction drain at the proper site to prevent a collection of bile.

14. Another unsuspected cause of stricture of the common bile duct is undue blind traumatic probing of this duct. In the probing process, it is essential to employ a firm, flexible, yet delicate instrument, such as a blunt tip flexible probe or a flexible uterine probe. Even though these metallic probes have dull tips, improper or rough handling can predispose to tears or perforation. The scoops or spoons can also be damaging if allowed to scrape unduly along the inside of the common duct in a manner that ulcerates the mucosa. The healing scar that forms will ultimately result in a stricture. The smaller scoops are usually thinner and sharper, and careless handling of these instruments can easily produce an erosion or perforation of the duct.

The key to proper exploration of the common bile duct is the utilization of proper instruments with love and attention; no strong arm is called for here. As soon as any difficulty is encountered, *stop!* There are alternative techniques that can be employed, such as a transduodenal approach, in order to establish better visualization and manipulation from below.

A commonly discussed cause of stenosis of the common bile duct is the stricture that follows an antrectomy, or subtotal gastric resection; the surgery, as well as the intractible and penetrating duodenal ulcer, are usually the direct causes. Deeply penetrating ulcers should not be dealt with by resection, in this writer's opinion. They should preferably be left alone. Nothing will stop the penetrating ulcer from healing if the food and gastric juices are diverted away from this pathological site. It is recommended that the ulcer not be dissected or resected from the pancreas; to excise a chronic peptic ulcer out of the pancreas is tedious and unrewarding because it results in undue trauma and bleeding and often leads to postoperative complications. It is wiser to deal immediately with the stomach proximal to the pylorus and to do a diverting Bancroft operation. A Bancroft procedure preserves a section of the uninvolved antrum that is not edematous or inflamed, with its antral mucosa removed so that no gastrin will be secreted. In the writer's experience, the antrum, when properly closed with three layers of silk, is far safer than attempting to close an inflamed, edematous, and traumatized duodenum. The penetrating ulcer is now completely bypassed and free from continued irritation by acid and digestive juices. A subtotal gastric resection now follows with an antecolic gastrojejunostomy. Because this writer likes to make sure that no reflux of content backs up into the duodenum where the ulcer still exists, he performs an enteroenterostomy to direct the acid flow into the distal loop of jejunum and away from the duodenum. The Bancroft exclusion or diverting operation has proven to be very effective and is recommended by the writer. Common duct strictures that take place after antrectomy or routine subtotal gastrectomy are unquestionably iatrogenic.

Iatrogenic biliary strictures usually occur when the surgeon accidentally nicks the duct with his knife, crushes it with his clamp, traumatizes it with probes, or carelessly ligates or coagulates it.

Reference

1. Porter AJ: Cholangiographic morphology as a guide to the demonstration of the bile duct by ultrasound. *Clin Radiol* 25:1, 1981.

Management of Benign Biliary Stricture

John W. Braasch, M.D., F.A.C.S.

Since the first repair of a biliary stricture by Lahey in 1919, continued interest in this problem has resulted in extensive experience with management of strictures. Previous reports have detailed the causes and prevention of bile duct injuries and described methods of repair. Over the years, modifications of our approach to this problem have evolved, with improved operative results. A description of our present techniques forms the basis for this report.

In our experience, more than 90% of benign biliary strictures are related to previous operative trauma.* Although the vast majority of these strictures occur secondary to cholecystectomy, they may also follow choledochostomy, pancreatoduodenectomy, or gastrectomy, particularly for posterior penetrating duodenal ulcer. Nontrau-

From Bolton JS, Braasch JW, Rossi RL: Management of benign biliary stricture. *Surg Clin North Am* 60:, 1980. With permission of Dr. John W. Braasch.

*This percentage varies with different authors. This writer's experience agrees with Braasch's 90%.

310

matic stricture of the bile ducts, while less common, may ensue from erosion of a gallstone into the extrahepatic biliary tree, pericholedochal infection (subhepatic abscess), recurrent cholangitis, or severe pancreatitis surrounding the intrapancreatic portion of the common bile duct (see Figs. 144, 145).

DIAGNOSIS

The diagnosis of benign biliary stricture can usually be made on clinical grounds. The onset of jaundice in the 24 to 48 hours after cholecystectomy is a telltale sign. Alternatively, an external fistula may develop, in which case jaundice may be low grade or absent or may develop only when drainage from the fistula abates. As drainage from the fistula

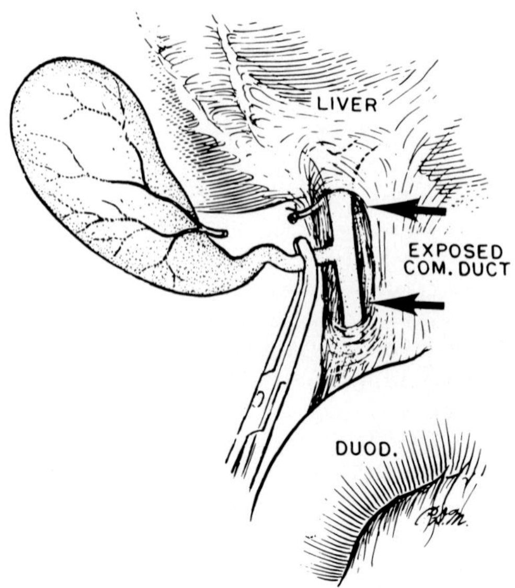

Figure 145.   Anatomy to be demonstrated during cholecystectomy.

slows, chills and fever may develop. However, if an internal fistula develops, these symptoms might be less severe.

Less often, some patients present with intermittent chills, fever, and jaundice years after an apparently uneventful cholecystectomy. In this situation, differentiation from choledocholithiasis on purely clinical grounds is difficult, although careful questioning may reveal a history of prolonged biliary drainage after the initial operation. The typical finding in these patients is that of low-grade stenosis or of complete obstruction, with an internal biliary fistula decompressing the proximal obstructed ducts.

Examination of these patients reveals a variable degree of jaundice, depending on whether an external or internal biliary fistula is present. An enlarged, firm liver is common. The presence of ascites, splenomegaly, or venous collaterals is an ominous sign, pointing to long-standing obstruction with cirrhosis and portal hypertension. The feces will be acholic if the obstruction or the external fistula is complete.

Laboratory tests will usually confirm the presence of conjugated bilirubin in the urine, and levels of serum bilirubin and alkaline phosphatase are typically elevated to a variable degree. Reversal of the albumin:globulin ration indicates that the obstruction is long standing.

Although intravenous cholangiography is rarely useful, fistulography through an external fistula might visualize the obstructed duct. In patients in

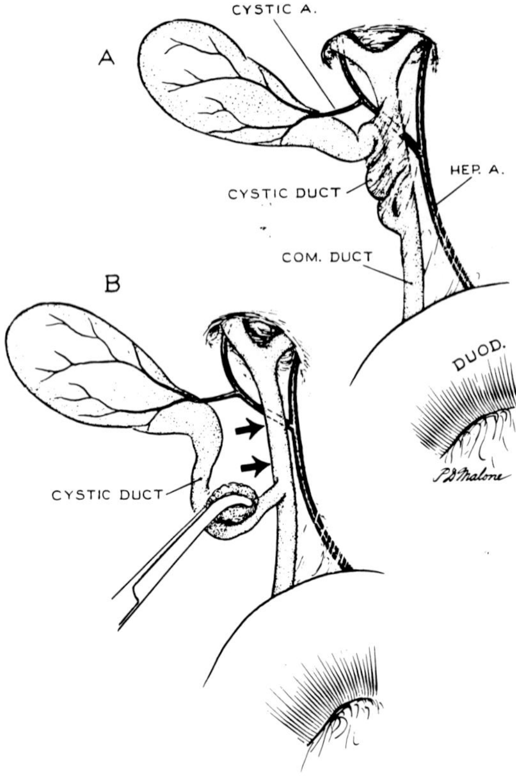

Figure 144.   A. Anatomy to be demonstrated at cholecystectomy. The precise point of the junction of the cystic duct with the common hepatic duct must be demonstrated. Division of connective tissue between these two structures releases a longer length of cystic duct than is usually anticipated. Early division of the cystic artery allows easy dissection of this area and less danger of inadvertant tearing of the vessel by manipulation. B. Arrows indicate a common point of injury of the common hepatic duct. (From Warren KW, and McDonald WM: Facts and fiction regarding strictures of the extrahepatic bile ducts. Ann Surg 159:1001, 1964.)

whom radiologic confirmation is necessary pre-operatively, the most useful examination is percutaneous transhepatic cholangiography using a Chiba needle. This procedure confirms the diagnosis, delineates the proximal extent of the stricture, and provides information about the quality of the proximal ducts. Endoscopic retrograde cholangiography is of lesser value and is not performed routinely. When a patient has previously undergone choledochoduodenostomy or choledochojejunostomy, a barium gastrointestinal study employing maneuvers to reflux contrast material into the biliary tree is often helpful. In general, the diagnosis is secure without elaborate radiologic localization and recognition and is based on a careful history, accurate notes of the previous operation, and appropriate laboratory blood tests.

PREOPERATIVE CARE

Intensive preoperative preparation often circumvents postoperative problems, particularly in the patient suffering from long-standing obstruction and intermittent cholangitis. Blood volume is replaced preoperatively, and prothrombin time is studied routinely as a guide to parenteral replacement of vitamin K. If accessible, bile samples are cultured, and all patients should start receiving broad-spectrum parenteral antibiotics 24 to 48 hours preoperatively. An aminoglycoside is included in the antibiotic regimen to provide optimal coverage against gram-negative aerobes. Nutritional status is assessed carefully, and enteral or intravenous nutritional support is provided when indicated. Inhalation therapy is employed effectively in patients at risk for pulmonary complications. Additional medical problems, when present, are stabilized preoperatively to minimize their effect on the postoperative outcome.

OPERATIVE PREPARATION

Certain situations that demand a two-stage operative approach deserve mention. A number of these patients present with life-threatening variceal hemorrhage as a result of biliary cirrhosis with portal hypertension. Alternatively, extensive varices in the porta hepatis may make operative exposure of the obstructed duct extremely hazardous. In these patients, a portasystemic shunt, preferably of the splenorenal variety, is performed initially, and definitive bile duct repair is delayed until a later date. A second group of patients, those with a preoperative bilirubin level of 20 mg per 100 ml or higher, have an increased mortality because of

the hepatorenal syndrome or hepatic failure. These patients can best be managed with percutaneous catheter drainage of the biliary tree until jaundice has subsided. If percutaneous drainage is unsuccessful, simple tube hepaticostomy can be performed as a first-stage procedure followed by definitive repair several weeks later as determined by the bilirubin level and the overall status of the patient. Third, subhepatic abscesses, which might prevent a satisfactory repair when adjacent to the obstructed duct, can be drained in conjunction with a tube hepaticostomy as a first-stage procedure.

OPERATIVE APPROACH

The approach to and location of the obstructed proximal duct entail a predictable set of maneuvers. A right paramedian incision provides the best exposure. The peritoneal cavity is entered through the upper aspect of the incision, since this area is most likely to be free from adherent loops of bowel. The small bowel, omentum, and stomach are released from the attachment to the left side of the anterior abdominal wall and the undersurface of the liver. Careful dissection is required to avoid entering either the capsule of the liver or the colon (see Fig. 146).

Adhesions between the duodenum and stomach and the undersurface of the left lobe of the liver and anterior surface of the hepatoduodenal liga-

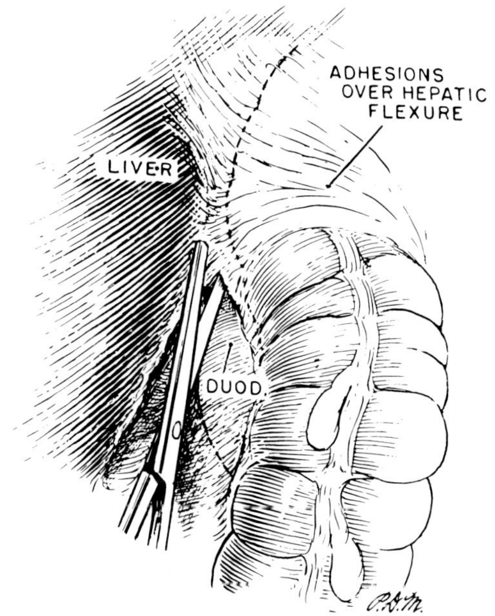

Figure 146.   Release of adhesions between the hepatic flexure of the colon and the undersurface of the liver.

312

ment are encountered next and should be released in stepwise fashion. As a first step, the stomach is mobilized, followed by a Kocher maneuver to mobilize the third and fourth portions of the duodenum. This allows clear visualization and easy dissection of the superolateral margin of the second and third portions of the duodenum as it adheres to the anterior surface of the porta hepatis and the hilus of the liver. After these adhesions are released, the Kocher maneuver is completed to mobilize fully the duodenum, pancreas, and lower end of the bile duct, the foramen of Winslow is opened to permit finger occlusion of the hepatic artery and portal vein (Pringle maneuver), should this be necessary at any point (see Figs. 147, 148).

Attention is next turned to identification of the bile duct. The hepatic artery is located by palpation, and the area of the expected location of the duct lateral to the artery is carefully inspected and palpated for any telltale clues to the location of the duct. At times, a persistent suture or clip, inadvertently placed on the duct in an attempt to control hemorrhage from the porta hepatis during the previous cholecystectomy, will lead to the duct. At other times, an internal biliary fistula divided during initial mobilization of the colon, stomach, or duodenum can be traced to its junction with the obstructed proximal duct. Often, a small area of dense fibrous tissue in the region of the course of the duct is the only clue to its location. When this is the case, the scar tissue must be transected with a knife, keeping in mind at all times the anterolateral position of the duct in the porta hepatis relative to the portal vein and the hepatic artery. Needle aspiration may be helpful in locating the duct and in avoiding inadvertent injury to the hepatic artery or portal vein (see Figs. 149, 150).

Once the duct has been located, a bile specimen is obtained for bacterial culture and sensitivity testing. Scoops and saline solution irrigations are used to clear the proximal duct of stones, if present. A small Foley catheter is inserted, and operative cholangiography is performed to demonstrate that all segments of the liver are drained. Should cholangiography fail to visualize one of the main hepatic ducts or one of the segmental branches of the right lobe, further search in the hilus of the liver is made for the missing duct, using the technique outlined. Occasionally, dissection of the bed of the gallbladder may disclose a posterior segmental duct of the right lobe, or left lateral subsegmentectomy may provide access to the left hepatic duct. In a few patients, chronic obstruction of the duct has so enlarged the liver as to cause an extrahepatic duct to become intrahepatic, and hilar dissection

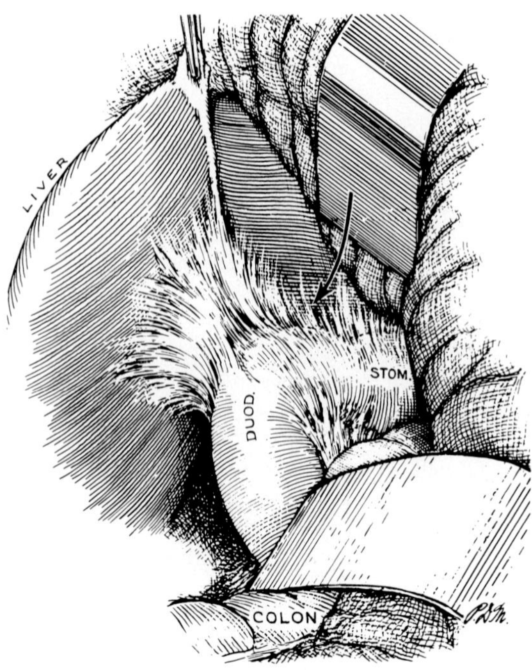

Figure 147. Adhesions between the duodenum and stomach and the undersurface of the left lobe of the liver and anterior surface of the hepatico-duodenal ligament.

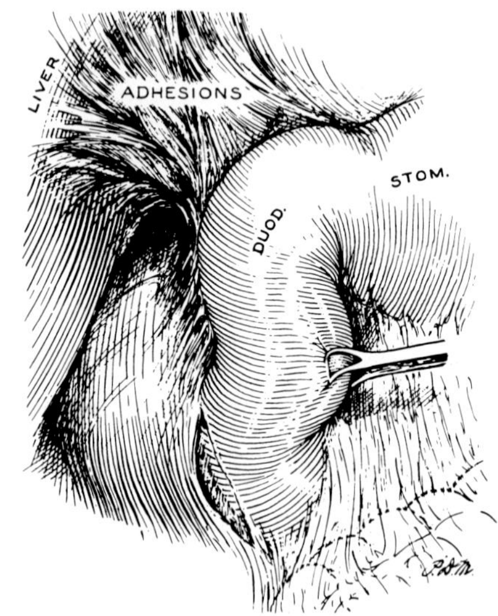

Figure 148. The duodenum is mobilized by the Kocher maneuver.

may fail to reveal any extrahepatic duct. When this occurs, dissection in the plane between the left and right lobes of the liver may reveal the stump of the common hepatic duct and allow an anastomosis.

Occasionally a patient at exploratory laparotomy will be found to have marked atrophy of one lobe of the liver, with a proportional increase in size of the opposite lobe. Subsequent hilar dissection may reveal stenosis of the duct draining the hypertrophied lobe, while the duct from the atrophied lobe will either not be found at all or, if found, will be

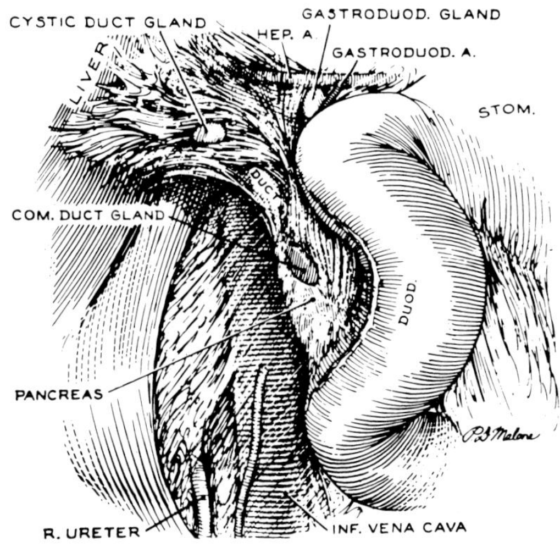

Figure 149.   The completed Kocher maneuver. (From Braasch JW, and Rossi RL: Liver, gallbladder, biliary tract, pancreas, and spleen. In Beahrs OH, and Beart RW Jr. (eds.): Therapy Update Service: General Surgery. Boston, Houghton Mifflin Professional Publishers, 1979.)

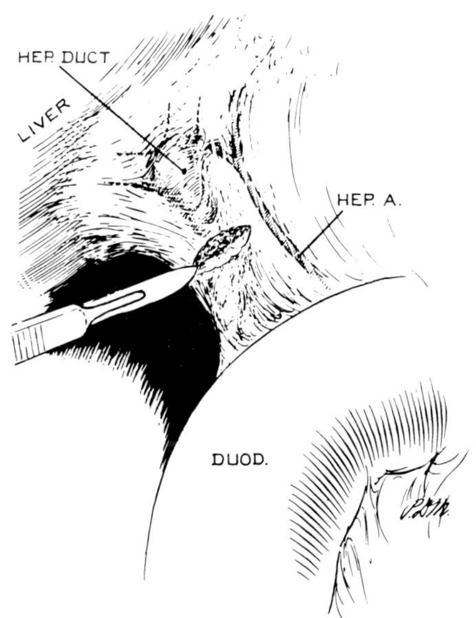

Figure 150.   Scar tissue at the site of the common bile duct stricture to be transected. (From Braasch JW: Part II. Reconstruction of biliary tract. In Nora PF (ed.): Operative Surgery: Principles and Techniques, 2nd ed. Philadelphia, Lea & Febiger, 1979.)

obstructed completely. Surgical correction of the stenosis only need be achieved without wasting time searching for and reanastomosing the duct from the atrophied side. Lobar or segmental atrophy of the liver as a long-term consequence of complete obstruction in the absence of infection of the duct draining that segment or lobe has been observed experimentally and clinically and may be well tolerated unless an added insult (sepsis, hepatitis, ductal stricture, congestive heart failure) has compromised the remaining portion of the liver.

PREPARATION OF THE DUCT

We have long believed that the quality of the proximal duct is the most important factor in determining the outcome of stricture repair, and efforts to secure as nearly normal a proximal duct as possible for the anastomosis are worthwhile. The scar tissue in the immediate vicinity of the stricture is trimmed away until relatively normal ductal mucosa is reached (see Figs. 151, 152). In some patients, the proximal biliary duct has been made so friable by cholangitis that it will not hold a stitch securely. In these instances, preliminary hepaticostomy, as alluded to previously, should be performed as an initial procedure. Definitive repair should be delayed for 3 to 6 weeks.

Important information regarding the blood supply of the biliary ducts has surfaced recently. Using resin casts in human cadavers, Northover and Terblanche demonstrated that the arterial supply to the supraduodenal duct (common hepatic and upper common bile ducts) is axial, with the main vessels being located at the three o'clock and nine o'clock positions along the lateral and medial borders of the duct (see Fig. 152). Clearly, these vessels

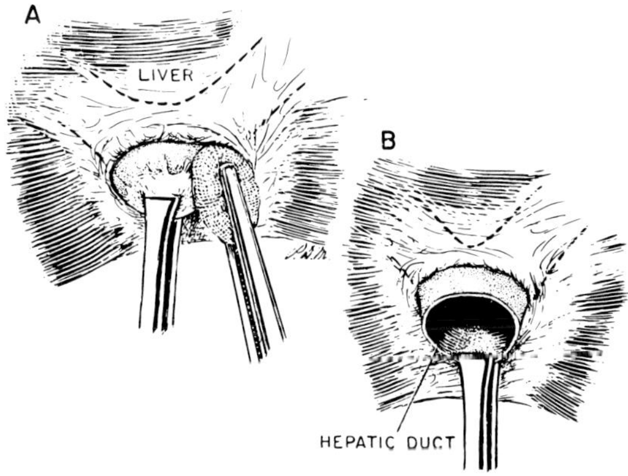

Figure 151.   A and B. Securing normal duct above the level of the stricture.

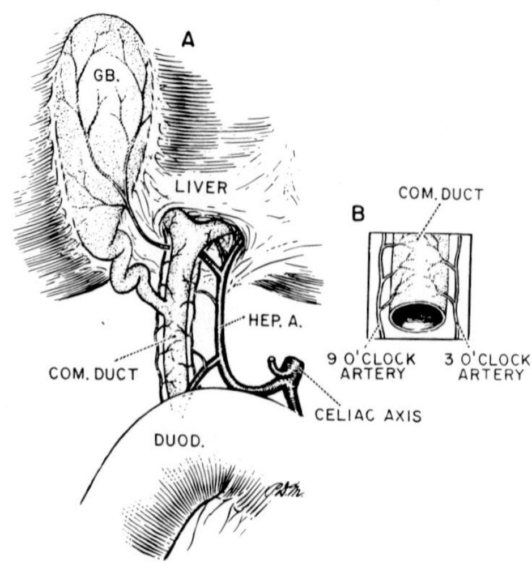

Figure 152.   A and B. Blood supply to the supraduodenal bile duct.

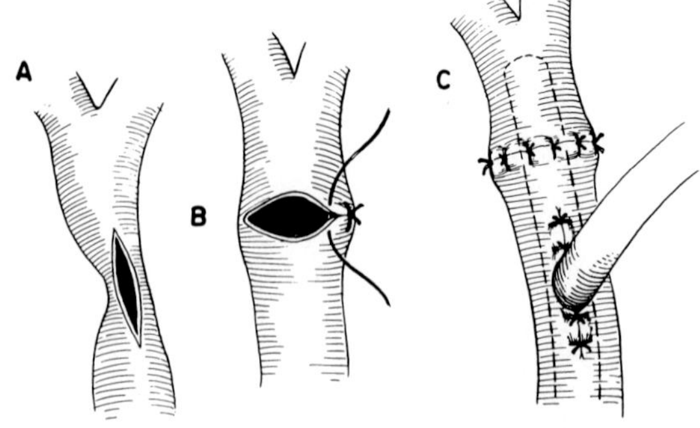

Figure 153.   A–C. Choledochoplasty (Heineke-Mikulicz) stented with a T-tube. (From Braasch JW: Part II. Reconstruction of biliary tract. In Nora PF (ed.): Operative Surgery: Principles and Techniques, 2nd ed. Philadelphia, Lea & Febiger, 1979.)

can be damaged easily by overzealous mobilization of the duct, and ischemia of the duct has been implicated in the formation of biliary strictures. We regard this information as highly important and, on the basis of this, now mobilize the duct only minimally to protect its blood supply.

TECHNIQUE OF REPAIR

Since the technique of repair is of great importance in determining the final outcome, it must be tailored to the conditions encountered at the operating table. As stated, certain patients are best treated initially by hepaticostomy. This includes an occasional patient in whom excessive hemorrhage or a serious degree of shock or cardiac dysfunction occurs intraoperatively and in whom rapid termination of the operative procedure is desirable. Hepaticostomy is accomplished most simply by placing a large catheter in the proximal duct and securing it in place with a single stitch in the scar tissue surrounding the duct. This subhepatic space is drained to remove the bile, which inevitably leaks around the hepaticostomy tube.

Symptomatic strictures of minimal extent may be treated by a choledochoplasty of the Heineke-Mikulicz type. The choledochoplasty should be stented by a T-tube, the external limb of which is brought out above or below the suture line (see Fig. 153). Only minimal strictures, generally not more than 4 mm in length with an internal diameter of not less than 1.5 to 2 mm, can be handled in this fashion. Such strictures are unusual. An occasional right hepatic duct stricture with a residual lumen located within the liver substance and

therefore relatively inaccessible can be dilated and splinted with a T-tube for a minimum of 9 months. Dilation should be carried out by a Bakes dilator, at least 5- or 6-mm. Again, such situations are unusual, as most strictures are accessible to a definitive reconstruction.

Our procedure of choice for most strictures is hepaticojejunostomy to a simple jejunal loop with enteroenterostomy between the afferent and efferent limbs. Use of a Roux-en-Y loop is equally acceptable but slightly more involved. The biliary anastomosis is performed in one layer, using six to eight interrupted 3-0 or 4-0 catgut sutures in such a fashion as to provide an onlay of jejunal mucosa (see Fig. 154). In some patients, "fishmouthing" the ductal opening will allow a larger anastomosis (see Fig. 155). The jejunal loop is attached to the hilus of the liver with several silk sutures to avoid tension on the suture line. The anastomosis is performed over a stent, usually consisting of a rubber tube in the T-tube or modified Y-tube configuration. The stent should fit loosely within the anastomosis, and the external limb is brought out through a separate stab incision in the proximal bile duct if possible. An external limb brought out through a stab wound in the jejunal loop is likely to be dislodged by peristalsis at an early date. We try to avoid transhepatic stents, as the complications of hemorrhage or leakage of bile with resultant subphrenic abscess in our experience are somewhat greater than generally appreciated. Strictures that include bifurcation of the common hepatic duct require a separate right and left hepaticojejunostomy over individual stents (see Fig. 156).

Hepaticoduodenostomy is considered an alternative to hepaticojejunostomy only in patients with a previous Billroth II gastric resection. We are prej-

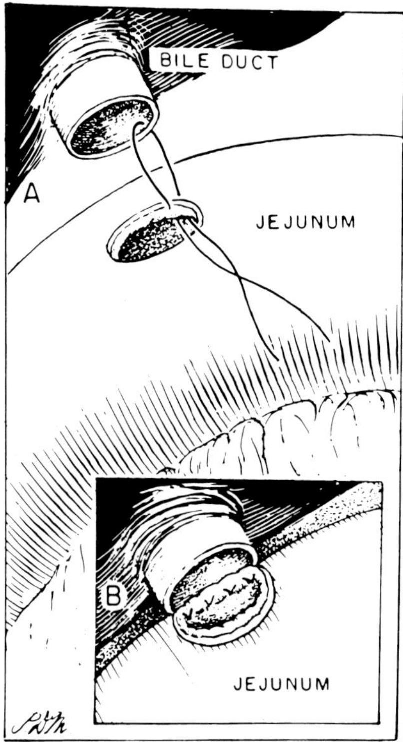

Figure 154.   A and B. Hepaticojejunostomy.

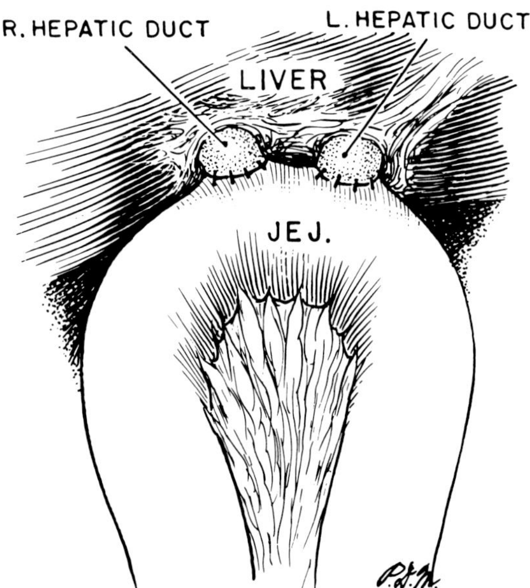

Figure 156.   Double hepaticojejunostomy.

udiced in favor of hepaticojejunostomy for most patients because of the relative seriousness of a fistula arising from hepaticoduodenostomy as compared with that from hepaticojejunostomy and the ease in locating the hepaticojejunostomy should stricture recur and reoperation be necessary. Although end-to-end choledochocholedochostomy remains useful in selected patients, more often than not, the distal duct is of insufficient caliber or its mobilization entails such injury to its blood supply that end-to-end anastomosis is not frequently employed at this clinic (see Fig. 157).

In only an occasional patient is the stricture so high that a directly sutured anastomosis is not fea-

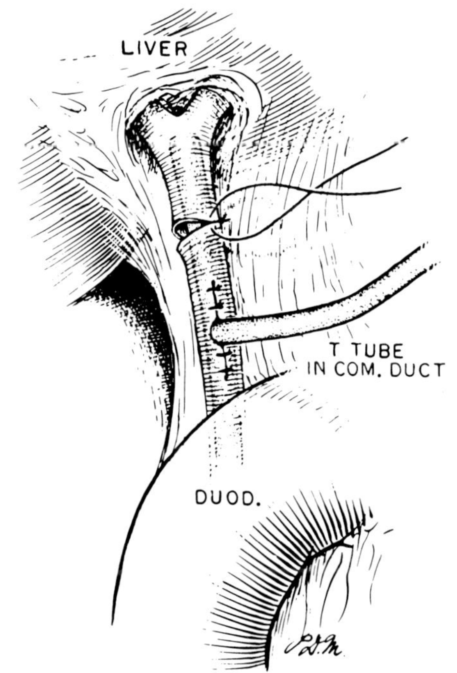

Figure 157.   End-to-end repair.

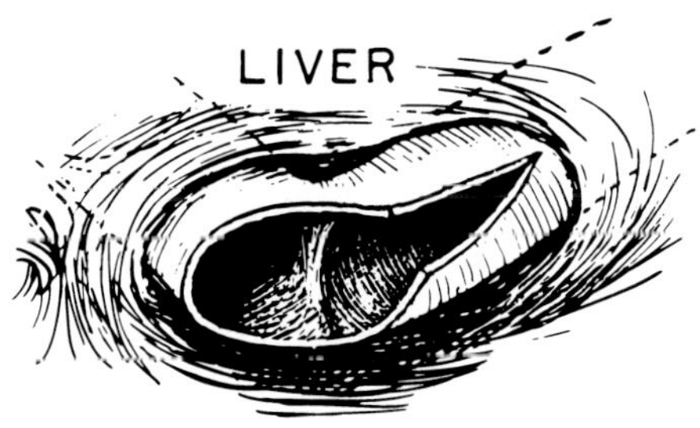

Figure 155.   "Fishmouthing" the ductal opening to enlarge the anastomosis.

sible. In such situations, a mucosal pull-through procedure employing a transhepatic stent, as popularized by Wexler and Smith, is used (see Fig. 158). We have not adopted this technique in all strictures, as advocated by Smith, believing that a sutured mucosa-to-mucosa anastomosis is both

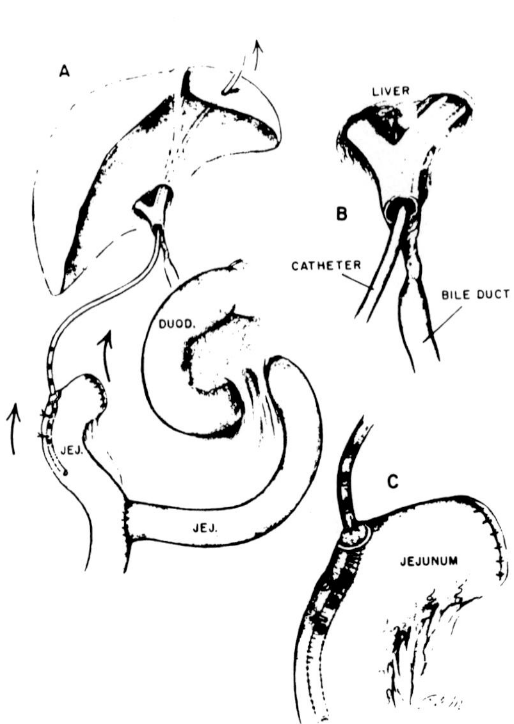

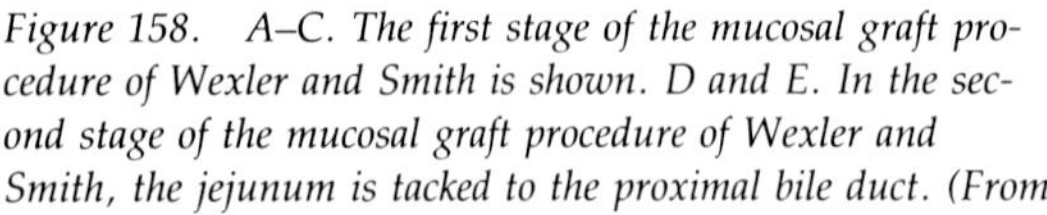

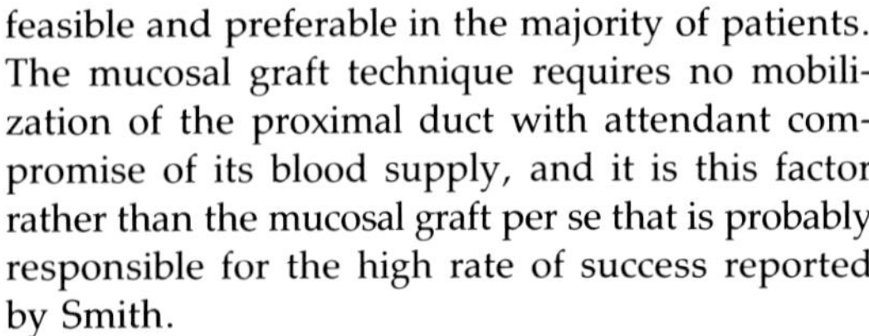

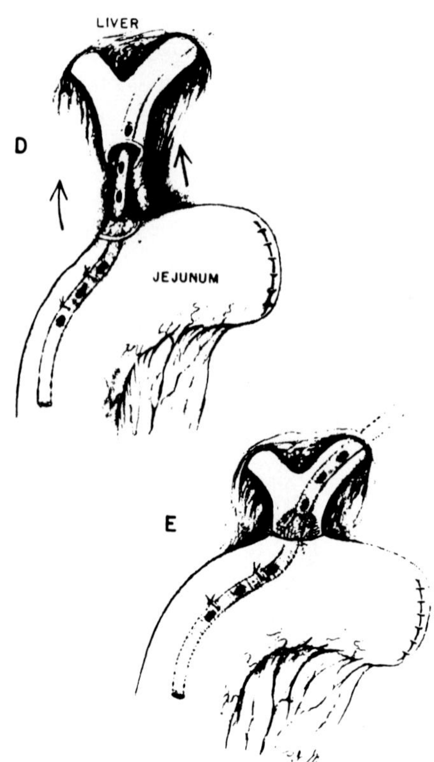

Figure 158.   A–C. The first stage of the mucosal graft procedure of Wexler and Smith is shown. D and E. In the second stage of the mucosal graft procedure of Wexler and Smith, the jejunum is tacked to the proximal bile duct. (From Braasch JW: Part II. Reconstruction of biliary tract. In Nora PF (ed.): Operative Surgery: Principles and Techniques. 2nd ed. Philadelphia, Lea & Febiger, 1979.)

feasible and preferable in the majority of patients. The mucosal graft technique requires no mobilization of the proximal duct with attendant compromise of its blood supply, and it is this factor rather than the mucosal graft per se that is probably responsible for the high rate of success reported by Smith.

At the completion of the biliary reconstruction, wide drainage of the subhepatic space with sump drains is employed. Although minor biliary fistulas are common, almost all close within 3 weeks of operation and do not pose severe clinical problems as long as adequate drainage is provided. When transhepatic stents are used, sump drainage of the subphrenic space should also be employed.

POSTOPERATIVE CARE

Postoperative infection is the commonest hazard and may run the gamut from overwhelming septicemia secondary to cholangitis in the early postoperative period to subphrenic or subhepatic abscesses and superficial wound infections. Antibiotics begun preoperatively are continued for

several days into the postoperative period, and bile taken at operation is cultured to ensure that antibiotic coverage is adequate. Fever persisting into the second week postoperatively may indicate subphrenic or subhepatic infection, and if an air-fluid level is demonstrated on upright abdominal radiographs in these patients, surgical drainage is necessary.

Bleeding from the operative site is occasionally a problem and can usually be managed conservatively with transfusion and parenteral vitamin K in the expectation that it will stop spontaneously. Massive bleeding may indicate hemorrhage from the hepatic or gastroduodenal artery and requires reexploration and ligation of the bleeding point. Upper gastrointestinal tract hemorrhage is a serious threat and may originate from varices, stress ulceration, or associated duodenal or gastric ulcer disease. Initial management should be conservative, including the use of the Sengstaken-Blakemore tube when indicated.

We are currently leaving anastomotic stents in place for at least 6 months after operation until the early phase of scar maturation at the anastomotic site is complete (see Fig. 159). When this procedure is applicable, patients are taught to irrigate the stent daily to avoid buildup of sludge, which might obstruct the lumen of the tube. We have not found oral administration of bile salts to be helpful in this regard. Episodes of cholangitis occurring with the anastomotic stent in place usually resolve with removal of the stent. After removal of the stent, however, recurrent cholangitis is an indication of recurrent stricture and demands reexploration with revision of the anastomosis.

RESULTS

Our prior experience indicates that a minimum follow-up period of 3 years after removal of the anastomotic stent is necessary to evaluate results accurately. While recurrent strictures do occur after this length of time, they are rare in patients who have had no evidence of cholangitis for this duration. Our recent experience has been that 85% of these patients will have a successful long-term result after repair of biliary stricture. Of the remaining 15% with less than satisfactory results, one-third of the failures will not be from recurrent biliary stricture but from either established, irreversible biliary cirrhosis or from secondary sclerosing cholangitis of the intrahepatic ducts present at the time of stricture repair. Earlier referral and repair are necessary to salvage these patients. Thus, 10% of patients will have unsatisfactory results because of recurrent biliary stricture. In these patients recurrent stricture is usually heralded by reappearance of attacks of cholangitis. Should a patient suffer more than two mild attacks of cholangitis per year, reoperation should be undertaken, as the long-term outlook depends on the establishment of unobstructed biliary drainage.

Recommended Reading

Braasch JW, Preble HE: Unilateral hepatic duct obstruction. *Ann Surg* 158:17, 1963.

Braasch JW, Warren KW, Blevins PK: Progress in biliary stricture repair. *Am J Surg* 129:34, 1975.

Braasch JW, Whitcomb FF Jr, Watkins E Jr, et al: Segmental obstruction of the bile duct. *Surg Gynecol Obstet* 134:915, 1972.

Cameron GR, Hou CT: An experimental study of stricture of the common bile duct in the guinea pig. *J Pathol Bacteriol* 83:265, 1962.

Carlson E, Zukoski CF, Campbell J, et al: Morphologic, biophysical, and biochemical consequences of ligation ·of the common bile duct in the dog. *Am J Pathol* 86:301, 1977.

Cattell RB, Braasch JW: Long-term follow-up after repair of bile duct strictures. *Lahey Clin Bull* 10:194, 1958.

Cattell RB, Braasch JW: General considerations in the management of benign strictures of the bile duct. *N Engl J Med* 261:929, 1959.

Lahey FH: External and internal biliary fistulae following cholecystectomy. *Ann Surg* 92:649, 1930.

Lahey FH: Strictures of the common and hepatic ducts. *Ann Surg* 105:765, 1937.

Lahey FH, Pyrtek LJ: Experience with operative management of 280 strictures of bile ducts, with description of new method and complete follow-up study of end results in 229 of the cases. *Surg Gynecol Obstet* 91:25, 1950.

Longmire WP Jr, Sanford MC: Intrahepatic cholangiojejunostomy for biliary obstruction—further studies; report of 4 cases. *Ann Surg* 130:455, 1949.

Longmire WP Jr, Tompkins RK: Lesions of the segmental and lobar hepatic ducts. *Ann Surg* 182:478, 1975.

Nakayama T, Ikeda A, Okuda K: Percutaneous transhepatic drainage of the biliary tract: Technique and results in 104 cases. *Gastroenterology* 74:554, 1978.

Northover JM, Terblanche J: A new look at the arterial supply of the bile duct in man and its surgical implications. *Br J Surg* 66:379, 1979.

Sedgwick CE, Hume A: Management of bile duct strictures with associated portal hypertension. *Surg Gynecol Obstet* 108:627, 1959.

Smith R: Obstructions of the bile duct. *Br J Surg* 66:69, 1979.

Templeton JY III, Dodd GD: Anatomical separation of the right and left lobes of the liver for intrahepatic anastomosis of the biliary ducts. *Ann Surg* 157:287, 1963.

Waddell WR: Exposure of transhepatic bile ducts through interlobar fissure. *Surg Gynecol Obstet* 124:491, 1967.

Warren KW, Braasch JW: The selection of an operative procedure for benign stricture of the bile duct. *Surg Clin North Am* 44:717, 1964.

Warren KW, Braasch JW: Repair of benign strictures of the bile ducts. *Surg Clin North Am* 45:617, 1965.

Warren KW, Jefferson MF: Prevention and repair of stric-

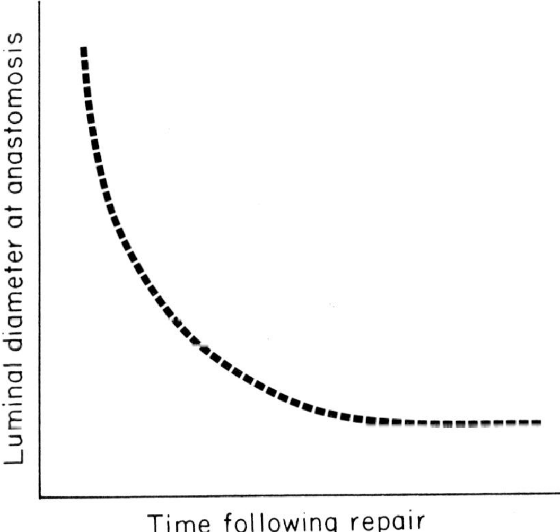

Figure 159. Effect of scar contracture on diameter of anastomosis.

tures of the extrahepatic bile ducts. *Surg Clin North Am* 53:1169, 1973.

Warren KW, McDonald WM: Facts and fiction regarding strictures of the extrahepatic bile ducts. *Ann Surg* 159:996, 1964.

Wexler MJ, Smith R: Jejunal mucosal graft: A sutureless technic for repair of high bile duct strictures. *Am J Surg* 129:204, 1975.

Intubation Techniques in Biliary Tract Surgery

John W. Braasch, M.D., F.A.C.S.

Tubes in the biliary tree are used routinely after surgery of the common duct to stent anastomoses of the biliary tree, to achieve decompression and palliation from obstructing primary or secondary malignant tumors of the biliary tree, to allow formation of a tract that can later be used for external instrumentation, and as a first-stage procedure in decompressing the biliary tree to improve liver function and the general status of the patient before definitive operation for obstructive jaundice.

Biliary tubes have been constructed of Vitallium, Latex, sand polymeric silicone (Silastic) in different forms and in different diameters to adapt to the technical procedure, the anatomic variations of the biliary tree, and the objective of placement of the catheter. The most frequently used material is Latex. Although Silastic theoretically should have the advantage of inducing less precipitation of bile pigment and less fibrosis, in clinical use these advantages have been difficult to prove. When a tract is desired, Silastic appears to require a longer waiting period for formation of an adequate sinus.

The objective of the tube determines the length of time it is left in place. When used for palliation in the presence of malignant disease it should be left until it occludes; then it should be kept in place for at least six months. The tube should be left in for approximately 6 weeks when an adequate tract is required for instrumental manipulation of the biliary tract or for 7 to 10 days after routine exploration of the common bile duct.

When tubes are to remain in place for more than 4 weeks, special care is necessary. Tubes with an external limb should be irrigated daily with 5 to 10 ml of sterile saline solution to decrease incrustation

From Rossi RL, Gordon M, Braasch JW: Intubation techniques in biliary tract surgery. *Surg Clin North Am* 60: 1980. With permission of Dr. John W. Braasch.

by bile pigments and to prolong patency. The skin at the exit site of the drain should be cleaned daily with a disinfectant solution to decrease the local inflammatory reaction and formation of granulation tissue. In general, patients can perform this care themselves and should be instructed in these techniques before being discharged from the hospital. For occlusion of tubes that are to remain closed most of the day, disposable plastic "plugs" (PRN Adapter) are preferred to clamps. These are the same as the plugs used for occlusion of intravenous or arterial lines; they fit to the end of the tube and are lighter and less bulky than the previously used metal clamps.

Patients should be told that the occurrence of chills, fever, jaundice, and change in the color of stool or urine can be secondary to obstruction of the tube or biliary tree and should be reported immediately to the physician. If cholangiography demonstrates occlusion of the tube, the stent should be removed or changed.

T-TUBE

The T-tube is the drain most frequently used in the biliary tree. With few exceptions, most surgeons routinely place a T-tube in the common bile duct on completion of common duct exploration. The horizontal limb of the T-tube should not fit tightly in the duct. When possible, a No. 14 or larger T-tube should be used to obtain a sinus tract of sufficient diameter to allow later instrumental manipulation of the biliary tree in patients with common duct calculi. At present, tubes are available that have a vertical external limb of a larger diameter than the intraductal or horizontal limb. Thus, formation of a tract of adequate size is achieved using a smaller intraluminal tube size, avoiding the possibility of stricture formation. A large-size regular T-tube should be brought out in a straight line, avoiding curves that can make difficult the later instrumentation of the biliary tree through the formed tract.

T-tubes are also useful when end-to-end repair of the common bile duct is performed at the time of iatrogenic injury (see Fig. 160). An end-to-end mucosal anastomosis is performed using a T-tube as a stent, bringing the external limb of the T-tube out through a counterincision in the proximal or distal duct. The external limb of a T-tube should never be brought out through the suture line of the anastomosis, as this increases the incidence of formation of a stricture.

A T-tube can be used as a stent in a hepatico-

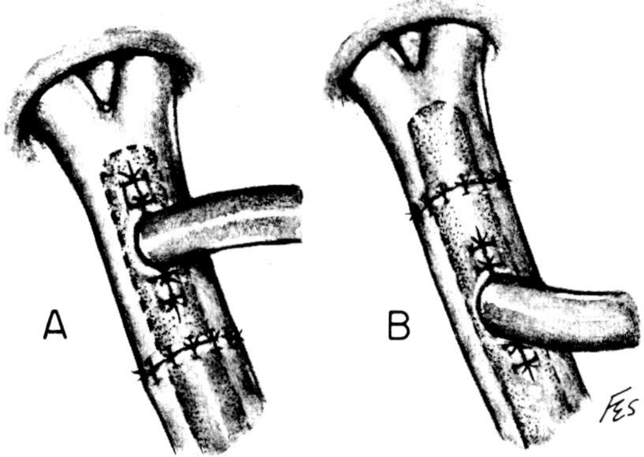

Figure 160.   A and B. End-to-end reconstruction of the hepatic duct stented with a T-tube brought out at a distance from the anastomosis.

jejunostomy in which the suture line is distal to the bifurcation of the hepatic duct. The external limb of the T-tube can be brought out through the proximal aspect of the hepatic duct or, when this is not possible, through an opening in the left hepatic duct (see Figs. 161, 162). When the T-tube is brought out through the bowel wall, the chance of the catheter migrating out of the biliary tree increases.

T-tubes are also used for palliation when tumors high in the biliary tract are not resectable. After the hepatic duct is dilated, the long limb of a T-tube placed in the common bile duct is threaded proximal to the tumor in order to decompress the liver and to avoid or delay compression from the tumor (see Fig. 163). Although this procedure can improve jaundice and pruritis, it will not prevent cholangitis when the other hepatic system not drained is infected.

A clear advantage of T-tubes over tubes without an exterior limb is that cholangiography and daily irrigations of the tube can be performed. New

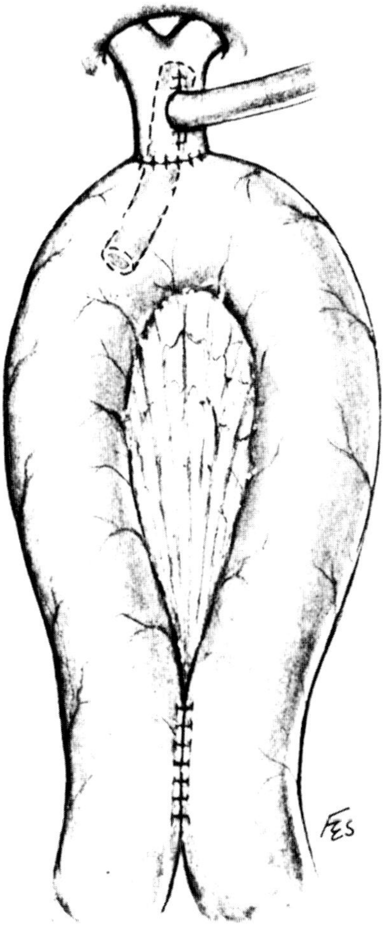

Figure 161.   End-to-side Hepaticojejunostomy. The external limb of a T-tube is brought out through the main hepatic duct.

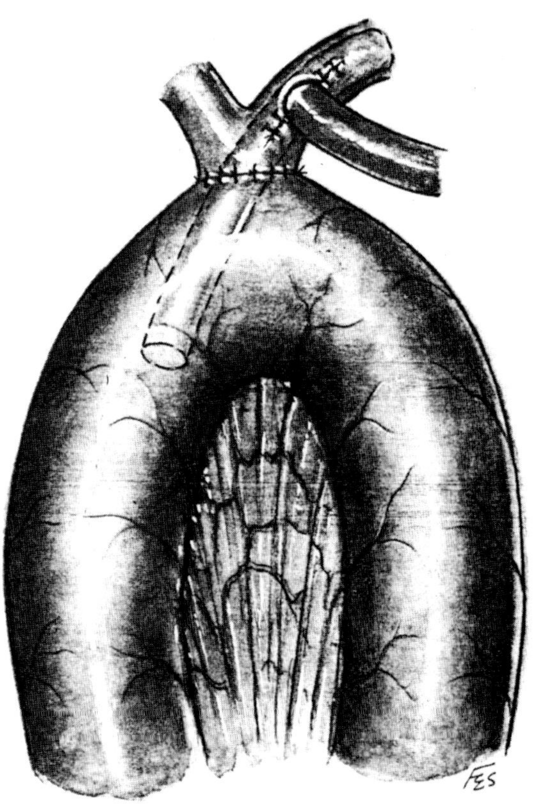

Figure 162.   End-to-side high hepaticojejunostomy. The T-tube is brought out through the left hepatic duct.

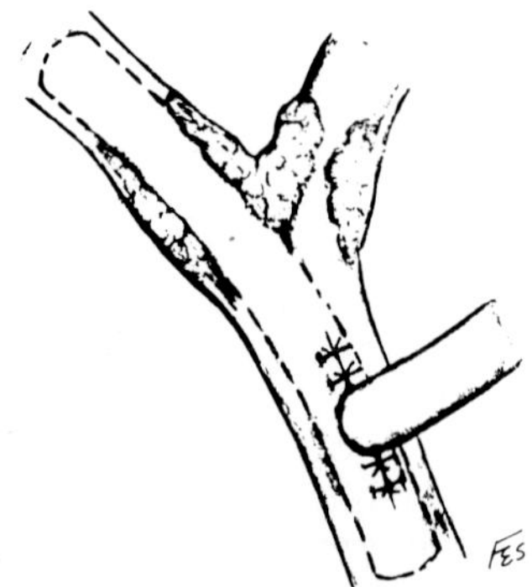

Figure 163.   A T-tube is used to decompress the right hepatic duct, which is obstructed by a carcinoma. After the duct has been dilated, the long arm of the T-tube is passed into the right hepatic duct proximal to the tumor.

techniques make it possible to change T-tubes over guidewires.

MODIFIED Y-TUBE

The original Latex Y-tube used in our clinic by Cattell and Braasch[1,2] was developed to manage proximal lesions close to the hepatic duct bifurcation, but it had no external pull-out limb, and when obstruction developed, reexploration was required for removal of the tube. Warren's modification[3,4] of this tube has an external solid limb that allows removal of the tube and avoids laparotomy. For proximal strictures or malignant lesions at the level of the bifurcation, the Y-tube achieves adequate stenting of both hepatic ducts. Distinct disadvantages of the Y-tube are that cholangiography cannot be performed through the solid external limb and the tube cannot be replaced by nonoperative means.

After the posterior wall of the anastomosis of the jejunal loop to the duct is completed in a single layer with absorbable material, the Y-tube is inserted, and the external limb is brought out through an opening in the anterior wall of the bowel not far from the site of the anastomosis. On occasion it is possible to bring it out through the more proximal ducts. The anterior suture line of the anastomosis is then completed, and the site of exit of the external limb is secured with an absorbable suture to avoid leakage (see Fig. 164).

TRANSHEPATIC TUBES

Transhepatic tubes were also developed as a way of dealing with lesions of the proximal hepatic duct. They are used to splint biliodigestive anastomoses or to achieve drainage in the presence of the tumors causing stenosis. When transhepatic tubes are

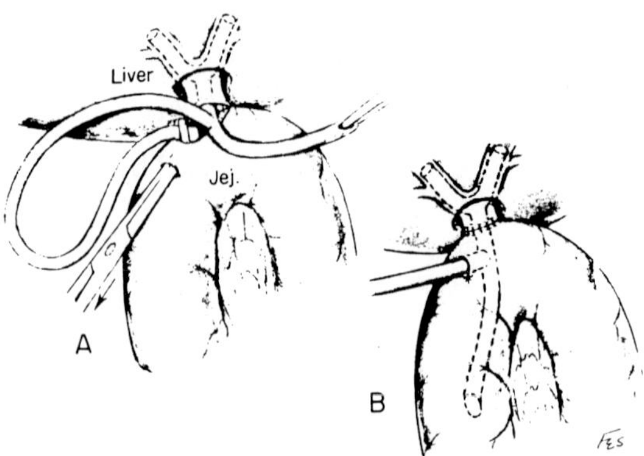

Figure 164.   Insertion of a modified Y-tube. A. After the posterior wall of the hepaticojejunostomy has been completed, the Y-tube is placed in the biliary tree. The external limb is brought out through the jejunum close to the anastomosis (1.5 to 2 cm). B. The distal limb of the Y-tube is placed in the jejunum, and the anterior wall of the anastomosis is completed. The site of exit of the external limb is closed with absorbable sutures.

placed, we prefer to use a uterine probe (hysterometer) because it has more rigidity, is easier to handle, and has a longer stem than the biliary dilators or stone forceps. If a single tube is to be used, we prefer to place the tube in the hepatic system to avoid the inconvenience presented by the costal margin on the right side.

The uterine probe is passed into the biliary system as distally as possible and brought out through the liver substance anteriorly to avoid injury to the major hepatic veins. The catheter to be used (a red rubber catheter, Argyle nasogastric tube, or Silastic tube) is threaded onto the distal end of the uterine probe and fixed in position with a tie (see Fig. 165). Lateral perforations are made in the intrahepatic and intrajejunal portions of the catheter, and the tube is tested for strength. The uterine probe is retracted, and the tube is thereby pulled through the liver substance into the biliary system and hepatic duct. It is positioned so that no tube perforations are outside the liver. The external limb of the transhepatic tube is brought out through the skin through a counter-incision where it is positioned comfortably to avoid kinking. Angulations are difficult to avoid when tubes are placed in the right biliary system because of the presence of the costal margin. The tube is secured to the parietal peritoneum with an absorbable suture. Two chromic catgut sutures are placed in the liver at the site of exit of the catheter to decrease leakage of bile or blood. The hepaticojejunostomy is completed (see Fig. 166).

Adequate drainage of the right hepatic duct

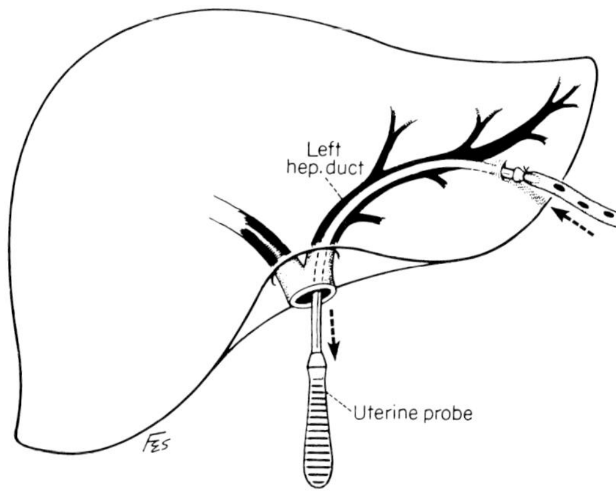

Figure 165. *Insertion of the transhepatic tube. The uterine probe is passed distally into the left hepatic duct and brought out anteriorly. The end of the tube is secured to the end of the probe with a tie. The uterine probe is retracted, achieving placement of the catheter.*

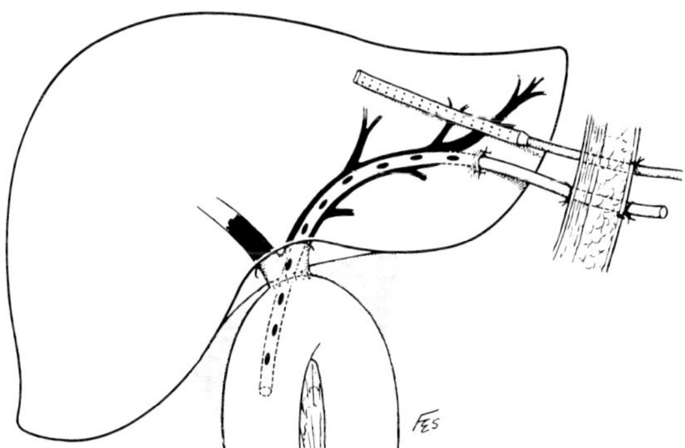

Figure 166. *The hepaticojejunostomy has been completed, and two catgut sutures are placed on the liver at the site of exit of the tube. The tube has been secured to the peritoneum and skin. The subphrenic space and subhepatic space are drained.*

should be ensured by avoiding a tight-fitting tube at the level of the anastomosis or by making side holes in the tube at the level of the right duct. A sump drain placed in the subphrenic space drains any bile and blood from the tract of the transhepatic tube. Another drain is placed in the subhepatic space to drain the anastomosis. When transhepatic tubes are employed for palliation of proximal malignant tumors, the distal end of the catheter can be left in the distal portion of the common bile duct and the choledochotomy closed (see Fig. 167). These tubes drain externally for at least 10 days, and thereafter cholangiography can be performed to rule out any leakage of bile. At this stage and if no leaks are evident, the tubes can be clamped and internal drainage is achieved. The tubes should be irrigated daily with normal saline solution. They

can also be changed when necessary at fluoroscopy, using a guidewire.

Two variations of this technique require description. In the use of a U-tube, as popularized by Terblanche et al., the internal limb of the transhepatic tube is threaded through the anastomosis, brought out through the jejunum, and passed through the abdominal wall (see Fig. 168). This variation allows

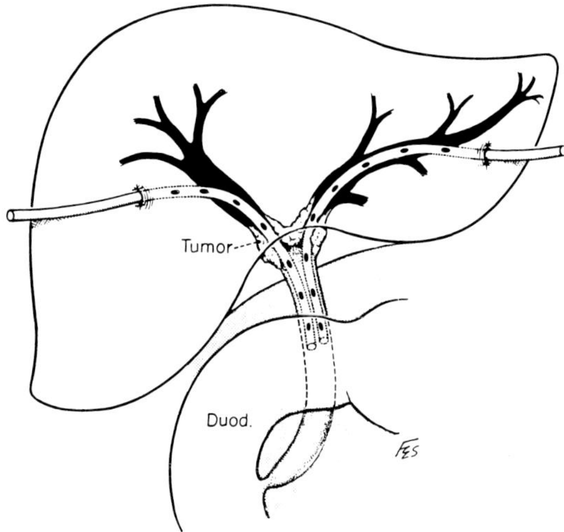

Figure 167. *Transhepatic tubes are placed in both the right and left hepatic ductal system for palliation of an obstructing proximal tumor. The internal ends of the tubes are left in the distal common bile duct, and the choledochotomy is closed.*

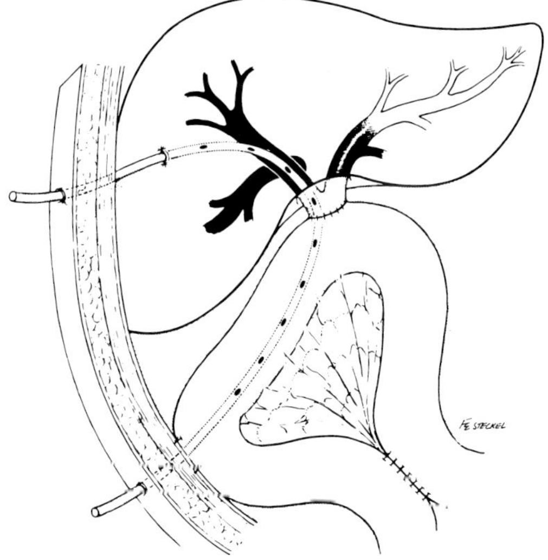

Figure 168. *The internal limb of the transhepatic U-tube is passed into the jejunum and brought out through the bowel and abdominal wall. The enterostomy at the site of exit of the tube is closed with an absorbable suture, and the bowel is secured to the parietal peritonium.*

replacement of the tube by tying a new tube to the one already present and removing the old tube, which achieves placement of a new stent. This technique is employed mainly for palliation of carcinoma and when the guidewire technique of replacement is not available. A disadvantage is that the patient's discomfort increases with the number of exit wounds for tubes.

The other modification of this procedure is that used by Wexler and Smith[5] in the repair of proximal strictures. After the transhepatic tube has been placed, a small opening is made in the seromuscular layer of the jejunal loop, and a cone of mucosa is allowed to evert at this level (see Fig. 169). The stent is introduced through a small opening in the dome of this mucosal cone and is threaded into the distal limb of the jejunal loop. The stent is secured to the jejunal loop with two separate sutures of chromic catgut. By putting traction on the transhepatic tubes, the jejunum with its jejunal mucosa are pulled up to the proximal bile duct (see Fig. 170). This loop is secured to the undersurface of the liver with separate sutures of catgut. All anastomoses should be drained.

One complication with this procedure is the high incidence of subphrenic abscess, approaching 10%. Although transhepatic tubes are used in patients with difficult technical problems associated with a high morbidity and mortality, placement of a drain through the substance of the liver can produce leakage of bile or blood into the subphrenic space. Hematobilia and massive bleeding from the liver

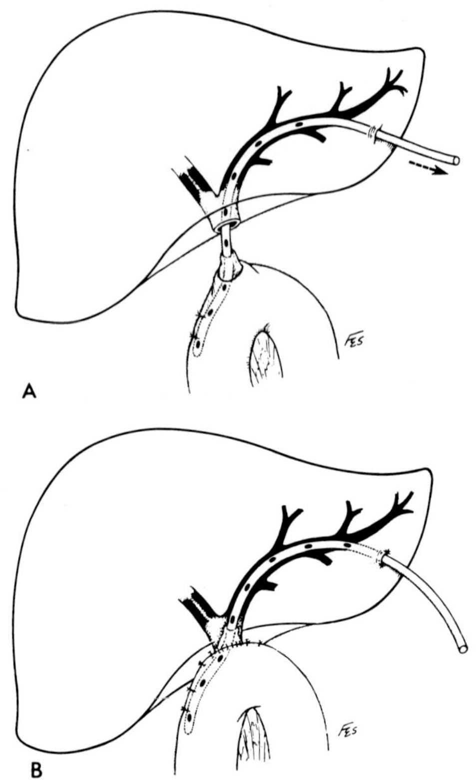

Figure 170. *The jejunal mucosal graft. A. The internal limb of the transhepatic tube is placed into the jejunal loop through the opening in the cone of the mucosa. The tube is secured to the bowel wall with two sutures of chromic catgut. An additional fine catgut suture can be placed from the apex of the cone of mucosa to the tube. A side hole in the tube should be close to the apex of the mucosa to ensure drainage of the right hepatic duct. Traction is applied to the external end of the catheter, carrying the jejunal mucosa and loop into the hilum of the liver, B. The jenunum is secured to the scarred undersurface of the liver with separate absorbable sutures.*

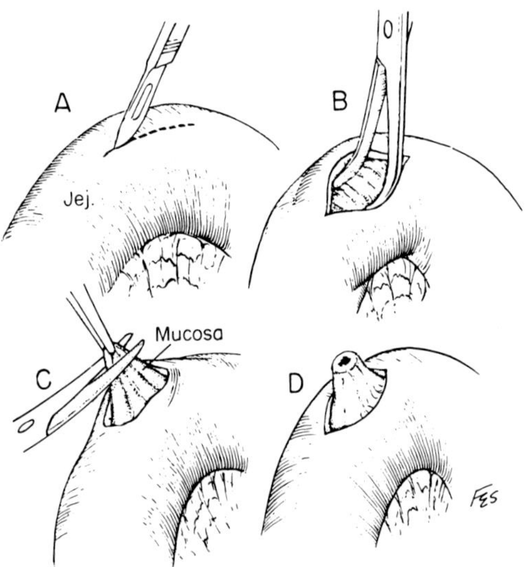

Figure 169. *The mucosal graft. A. The seromuscular layer of the jeunum is incised. B. The muscular layer is separated from the mucosa. C. A cone of mucosa protrudes spontaneously. D. A small opening is made in the apex of the mucosal cone.*

occur with this procedure and are more commonly found in the presence of a firm fibrotic liver, a situation that partially contraindicates the use of this method.

PERCUTANEOUS TRANSHEPATIC TUBES

The technique of percutaneous placement of transhepatic tubes has recently become available in the management of patients with an obstructed biliary system. The biliary system is outlined radiographically using a Chiba needle as described by Okuda et al.[6] in 1974 (see Fig. 171a). A segmental duct is selected, and with use of biplane fluoroscopy or lateral filming, a stylet with a sheath of polyethylene over the needle is passed into the bile duct (see Fig. 174b). The sheath is exchanged for

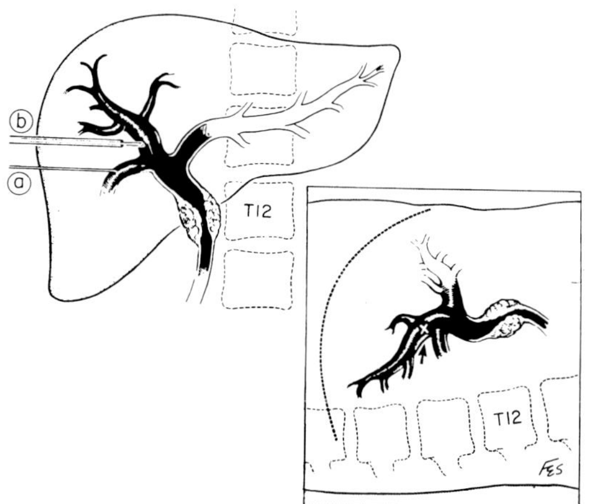

Figure 171.   Percutaneous transhepatic tubes. a. The biliary system is outlined radiographically using a Chiba needle. b. A stylet with a plastic sheath is passed into the biliary tree. The sheath is exchanged for a pigtail catheter.

a pigtail catheter with multiple side holes. This catheter can be left in place for external decompression or passed through the area of obstruction into the duodenum for internal drainage. Many of these catheters can be placed to drain different lobes or segments of the liver. The lumen of these catheters is small, requiring frequent changes every 3 to 4 weeks.

This method can be used in the palliation of patients with an inoperable tumor that is obstructing the biliary tree. It can also be used as a first-stage external drainage procedure in patients with benign strictures or operable tumors who have bilirubin levels greater than 20 mg per 100 ml. Decompression of the liver allows improvement of liver function, control of infection, and lowering of the complication rate after the subsequent definitive operation. These methods are not free from complications; bleeding and sepsis occur, and antibiotic prophylaxis is advised. The reported complication rate is about 5%.

SOME ASPECTS OF THE LAHEY CLINIC EXPERIENCE

We have reviewed our experience with 214 patients with benign strictures and 95 patients with carcinoma of the bile duct who were treated at the Lahey Clinic between 1969 and 1976. These 214 patients with benign strictures underwent a total of 306 procedures to reconstruct the biliary tract, and in all but 18 of them some type of tube was inserted to stent the repair. On 27 occasions, one or two transhepatic tubes (either straight or U-tube) were used, whereas in the remaining 261 procedures,

regular tubes (Y-tubes, modified Y-tubes, or T-tubes) were used. This group of 27 patients with transhepatic tubes was compared with another group of 173 patients with high hepaticojejunostomy in whom regular tubes were used. The overall postoperative complication rates were 55 and 27%, respectively, a difference that was statistically significant. Detailed examination of the different complications revealed the transhepatic tubes were more often associated with biliary fistulas (32% versus 9%) and intra-abdominal sepsis (13% versus 3%) than were regular tubes. In one instance, a transhepatic tube placed through a fibrotic liver produced fatal bleeding.

Of the patients with carcinoma of the bile ducts, 64 had placement of regular tubes and 20 had placement of transhepatic tubes. Intra-abdominal abscesses developed in 10% of patients in whom transhepatic tubes were used and in none of those who had regular tubes placed.

Transhepatic tubes are a useful means of hepatic intubation, but, although this study was retrospective and can be biased by patient selection, the possibility of a higher complication rate with this procedure has to be considered.

References

1. Cattell RB, Braasch JW: General considerations in the management of benign strictures of the bile duct. *N Engl J Med* 261:929, 1959.
2. Cattell RB, Braasch JW: Primary repair of benign strictures of the bile duct. *Surg Gynecol Obstet* 109:531, 1959.
3. Warren KW, Poulantzas JK, Kune GA: Use of a Y-tube splint in the repair of biliary strictures. *Surg Gynecol Obstet* 122:785, 1966.
4. Warren KW, Mountain JC, Midell AI: Management of strictures of the biliary tree. *Surg Clin North Am* 51:711, 1971.
5. Wexler MJ, Smith R: Jejunal mucosal graft: A sutureless technic for repair of high bile duct strictures. *Am J Surg* 129:204, 1975.
6. Okuda K, Tanikawa K, Emura T, et al: Nonsurgical, percutaneous transhepatic cholangiography—diagnostic significance in medical problems of the liver. *Am J Digest Dis* 19:21, 1974.

Percutaneous Balloon Dilatation of Strictures in the Biliary Tree

In *Radiology* in July 1986, an article entitled "Biliary Stricture Dilatation: Chronic Management of 73 Patients" appeared; the authors were P.R. Mueller, J.T. Ferrucci Jr., R.J. Butch, R.A. Malt, E. van Sonnenberg, P.J. Weyman, and H.J. Burhenne.* The combined experiences of these six radiologists and one surgeon in balloon dilatations on 73 patients are presented. Essentially, three types of strictures were treated: anastomotic strictures, iatrogenic strictures, and sclerosing cholangitis.

The majority of strictures (44) were in the *anastomotic stricture* group; there were 28 *Iatrogenic strictures* and 17 cases of *sclerosing cholangitis*. The *anastomotic strictures* occurred in 44 patients who had had choledochojejunostomy and hepatojejunostomy. Forty-three of 73 patients in the benign stricture category had undergone at least one previous attempt at surgical repair.

The results of balloon dilatations were as follows: The overall patency rate for all patients was 67% (49 of 73); for the anastomotic strictures, 67%; and for the sclerosing cholangitis strictures, 42%. Of the 25 patients who suffered stricture recurrence, 16 were treated by repeated percutaneous dilatation; 9 patients required surgical intervention. The overall recurrence rate was 33% over a 3-year period. Pelligrini et al.[1] reported a recurrence rate of 24% in patients who were initially treated with surgery for recurrent biliary stricture (Figs. 172–174).

Surgical repair has been the mainstay of common duct strictures and in experienced hands has had a good record of successes. Warren et al.[1] reported on 987 patients who underwent surgical repair of biliary stricture. They claimed a 78% success rate (22% recurrence rate). Pelligrini et al.[2] and Pitt et al.[3] confirmed Warren's results. The literature on repair of strictures reports a general recurrence rate that varies from 20 to 30%. The writers believe that their combined reported 33% recurrence rate compares favorably with the traditional surgical repair rate. This statement is challenged by the author, who still believes that surgical repair, when feasible and available, is superior to ballooning. In 73 cases reported by the multiple authors, the morbidity rate was considered low; they concluded that despite their 33% recurrence rate, when compared to surgery, the percutaneous balloon dilatation approach is justifiable. (According to this writer that is not so!)

The *complications* of percutaneous balloon dilatations included fever, septicemia, hypotension,

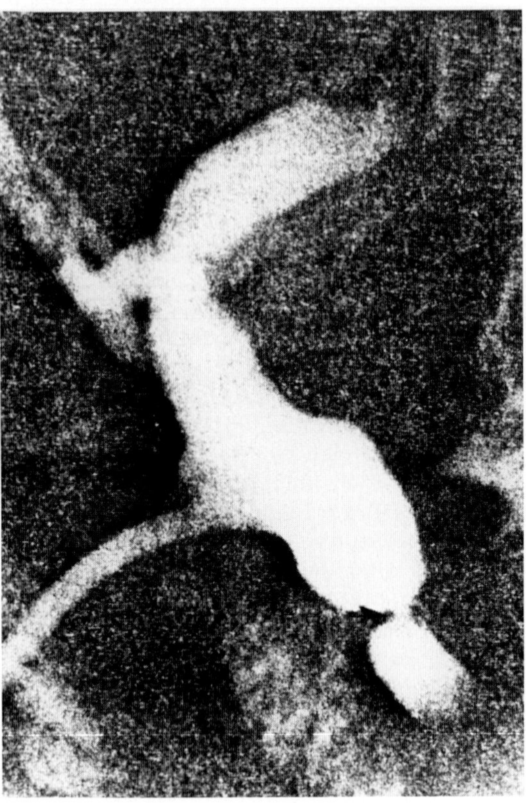

Figure 172. Common duct stricture before balloon treatment.

and pain during the dilating procedure. This pain required anesthesia in 10 patients.

Sclerosing cholangitis had the highest recurrence rate (58%). This disease is progressive and usually presents multisegmental strictures. The writers feel that the percutaneous approach is less serious than surgery, and therefore worthwhile. The writer concurs with the multiple authors regarding balloon dilatations for sclerosing cholangitis. It is understandable that any attempt at surgical repair of a diffuse, multisegmental, and progressively sclerosing process would be less desirable and less likely to succeed.

In regard to specific forms of stricture such as carcinoma and pancreatitis, the percutaneous balloon dilatation technique offers fewer benefits. These patients were treated with an internal/external catheter over a long period of time. Carcinoma recurs when the catheter is removed. Balloon dilatation may be helpful at first to dilate the tract through the liver or through the tumor in order to better place a larger drainage catheter. Like carcinoma of the common duct, pancreatitis does not respond well to balloon dilatation.

*P.R. Mueller, J.T. Ferrucci Jr., R.J. Butch, Department of Radiology, and R.A. Malt, Department of Surgery, Massachusetts General Hospital, Boston, and Harvard Medical School; P.J. Weyman, University of California Medical Center, San Diego; Eric van Sonnenberg, Mallinckrodt Institute of Radiology, St. Louis; and H.J. Burhenne, University of British Columbia, Vancouver.

The diagnosis of stricture in all patients was established by direct cholangiography via percutaneous transhepatic cholangiography or T-tube cholangiography. A quantitative evaluation of the stricture was obtained by manometric measurement. Preoperative clinical evaluation included bilirubin (direct and indirect) studies, and alkaline phosphatase determinations. Further significant studies included ultrasound and CT scan. It is important to integrate the radiological studies with the clinical symptoms because on several occasions balloon dilatations were carried out on normal-caliber hepatic ducts.

Long-term stenting has been employed, but with variable success. Warren et al. stressed long-term stenting postoperatively. They believed that inflammatory fibrosis at the site of repair can stabilize with time. Pelligrini et al. felt that there was no correlation between a successful result and prolonged stenting. There is a legitimate question regarding prolonged stenting: If prolonged stenting by an indwelling catheter can effect a stabilized dilatation of the stricture, what is the reason for balloon dilatations? Some surgeons believe that stents should remain indwelling for a minimal of 6 months.

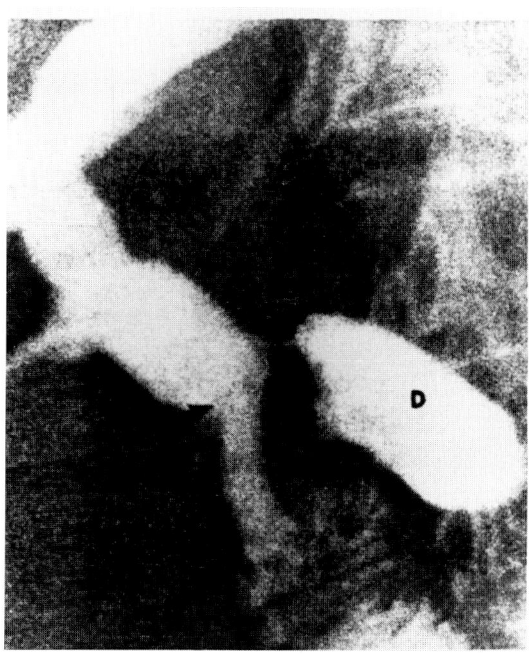

Figure 174. Arrow points toward improvement of stricture site.

COMMENT

This writer believes that there is no substitute for elective surgical repair under good light, direct vision, and in competent hands. If the patient can tolerate surgery, an open surgical correction of the stricture is preferable. This writer is in full agreement with Warren et al. and Braasch that if the first surgeon fails to correct the biliary injury at the time of original surgery, he should seek another surgeon or a center that is familiar with secondary stricture repairs. A surgeon who repairs an occasional biliary stricture should not do a secondary repair, and should refer the case to a center where biliary repairs are not uncommon. As for percutaneous T-tube and fistulous tract balloon dilatations, this writer feels that these techniques are useful but should be reserved for high-risk surgical patients and those with sclerosing cholangitis.

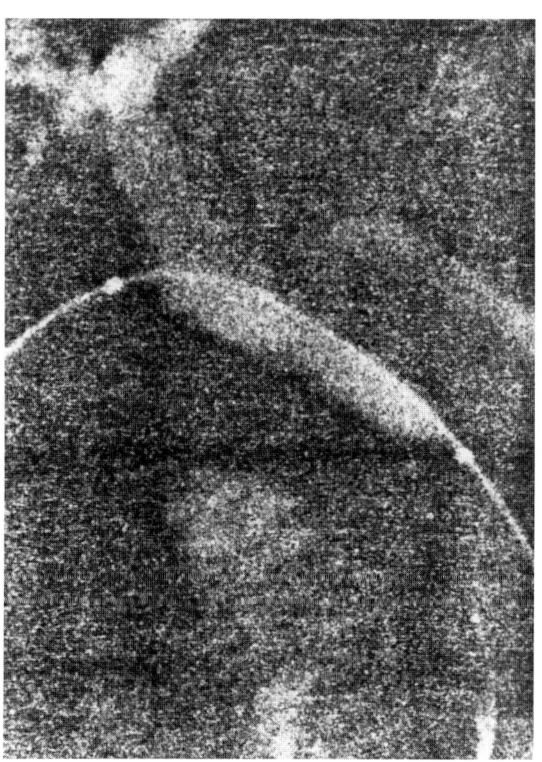

Figure 173. Balloon distending common duct stricture.

Recommended Reading

Beinart C, Sniderman KW, Tamura S, et al: Biliary pressure measurement: An aid in the management of patients on internal biliary drainage. *Invest Radiol* 17:356, 1982.

Blumgart LH, Kelley CJ, Benjamin IS: Benign bile duct

stricture following cholecystectomy: Critical factors in management. *Br J Surg* 71:836, 1984.

Burhenne HJ: Dilatation of biliary tract strictures: A new roentgenologic technique. *Radiol Clin* 44:153, 1975.

Burhenne HJ, Morris DC: Biliary stricture dilatation: Use of the Gruntzig balloon catheter. *J Can Assoc Radiol* 31:196, 1980.

Centola CAP, Jander HP, Stauffer A, et al: Balloon dilatation of the ampulla of Vater to allow biliary stone passage. *AJR* 136:613, 1981.

Cole WH, Ireneus C, Reynolds JT: Strictures of the common duct. *Ann Surg* 133:683, 1951.

Fernandez M: Treatment of benign strictures of the bile ducts. *World J Surg* 4:479, 1980.

Fretheim B: Operative biliary tract injuries: Secondary reparative operations. *Chir Gastroenterol* 11:451, 1977.

Gallacher DJ, Kadir S, Kaufman SL, et al: Nonoperative management of benign postoperative biliary strictures. *Radiology* 156:625, 1985.

Glenn F: Iatrogenic injuries to the biliary ductal system. *Surg Gynecol Obstet* 146:430, 1978.

Glenn F: Postoperative stricture of the extrahepatic bile ducts. *Surg Gynecol and Obstet* 120:560, 1965.

Martin EC, Fankuchen EI, Laffey KJ, et al: Percutaneous management of benign biliary disease. *Gastrointest Radiol* 9:207, 1984.

Martin EC, Fankuchen EI, Schultz RW, et al: Percutaneous dilatation in primary sclerosing cholangitis: two experiences. *AJR* 137:603, 1981.

Martin EC, Karlson KB, Fankuchen EI, et al: Percutaneous transhepatic dilatation of intrahepatic biliary strictures. *AJR* 135:837, 1980.

May GR, Bender CE, LaRusso NF, et al: Nonoperative dilatation of dominant strictures in primary sclerosing cholangitis. *AJR* 145:1061, 1985.

McAllister AJ, Kicken NF: Biliary stricture: A continuing study. *Am J Surg* 132:567, 1976.

Molnar W, Stockum AE: Transhepatic dilatation of choledochoenterostomy strictures. *Radiology* 129:59, 1978.

Oleaga JA, McLean GK, Freiman OB, et al: Interventional biliary radiology, in Ring EJ, McLean GK (eds): *Interventional Radiology: Principles and Techniques.* Boston, Little, Brown, 1981, pp 245–378.

Saber K, El-Manialawi M: Repair of bile injuries. *World J Surg* 1:82, 1984.

Salomonowitz E, Castaneda-Zuniga WR, Lund G, et al: Balloon dilatation of benign biliary strictures. *Radiology* 151:613, 1984.

Teplick SK, Wolferth CC Jr, Hayes MF Jr, et al: Balloon dilatation of benign-postsurgical biliary enteric-anastomotic strictures. *Gastrointest Radiol* 7:307, 1982.

Vogel SB, Howard RJ, Caridi J, et al: Evaluation of percutaneous transhepatic balloon dilatation of benign biliary strictures in high-risk patients. *Am J Surg* 149:73, 1985.

Wheeler ES, Longmire WP Jr: Repair of benign stricture of the common bile duct by jejunal interposition: Choledochoduodenostomy. *Surg Gynecol Obstet* 146:260, 1978.

Zeman RK, Burrell MI, Dobbins J, et al: Postcholecystectomy syndrome: Evaluation using biliary scintigraphy and endoscopic retrograde cholangiopancreatography. *Radiology* 156:787, 1985.

References

1. Warren K, Mountain JE, Midell AI: Management of strictures of biliary tree. *Surg Clin North Am* 51:711, 1971.
2. Pelligrini, CA, Thomas MJ, Way LW: Recurrent biliary strictures: Patterns of recurrence and outcome of surgical therapy. *Am J Surg* 147:175, 1984.
3. Pitt HA, Miyamoto T, Parapatis SK, et al: Factors influencing outcome in patients with postoperative biliary strictures. *Am J Surg* 144:14, 1982.

Biliary Tract Obstruction Related to Duodenal Diverticulum

Wolfson and Miller[1] studied 96 postmortem specimens and found six duodenal diverticula situated in the second portion of the duodenum. In each instance, the common duct terminated in the diverticulum adjacent to its neck. On two occasions, the pancreatic duct of Wirsung emptied into the diverticulum.

A true congenital diverticulum is rare and contains all the layers of the duodenum. Acquired diverticulum is classified as primary or secondary. A primary diverticulum is a protrusion or outpouching of the mucosa and is the most common form of diverticulum. The pathogenetics may resemble those of the colonic diverticulum, i.e., they may be related to the vascular openings in the duodenal wall. A secondary diverticulum is found in the first portion of the duodenum and is attributed to traction by peptic ulcer disease and possibly cholecystic disease. The majority of these diverticula do not cause symptoms and therefore require no treatment. This writer feels that diverticula do in fact produce signs and symptoms and that biliary and pancreatic obstructions do occur.

Bile stasis may be one factor in obstruction, but a more probable cause is diverticular distention and compression of the intraduodenal portion of the common duct. The latter type of intermittent obstruction may be an etiological factor in postcholecystectomy syndrome. Of the various diagnostic methods mentioned, a word of caution is in order regarding the use of ERCP. This examination may be hazardous because of the difficulty of entering a distorted ampulla of Vater and because the thinned-out, distorted anatomy may be easily perforated.

Because congenital diverticulum is still a controversial clinical entity, more definite criteria must be established for surgical intervention in which

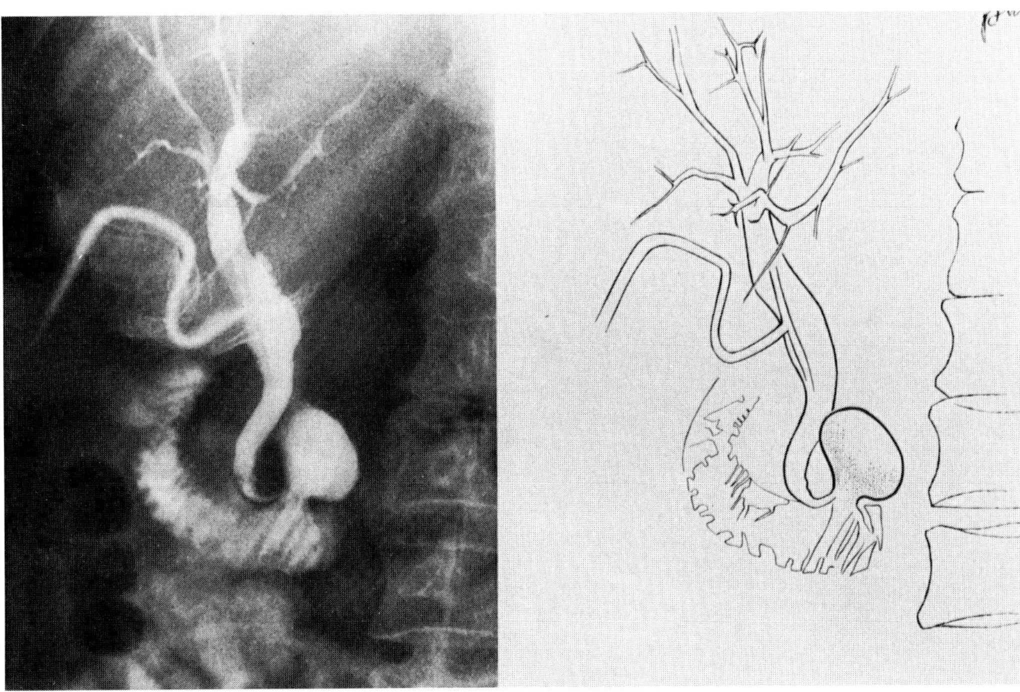

Figure 175.   A postoperative T-tube cholangiogram demonstrates an enlarged common bile duct with a normal caliber intramural terminal segment that empties into a duodenal di-

verticulum. Fluoroscopic examination revealed the opaque material entering the diverticulum and, as it filled, the material passed into the lumen of the duodenum.

excision of the diverticulum must be considered. Though surgical intervention is highly questionable, this writer feels that there are instances where it may be indicated. In still other cases, though removal is indicated, there may be certain coexisting medical contraindications, i.e., systemic disease, advanced age, and cardiopulmonary-vascular-renal problems. There are instances where the jaundice and pain appear to be related to a duodenal diverticulum near the ampulla of Vater, yet may not be related to the diverticulum per se. Coexisting unrecognized pathology may in fact be the real cause. Repeated inflammation and edema at the stoma site of the diverticulum will obstruct the ampullary opening by extrinsic pressure, causing intermittent attacks of pain and jaundice. The jaundice will invariably clear up in a few days with conservative management.

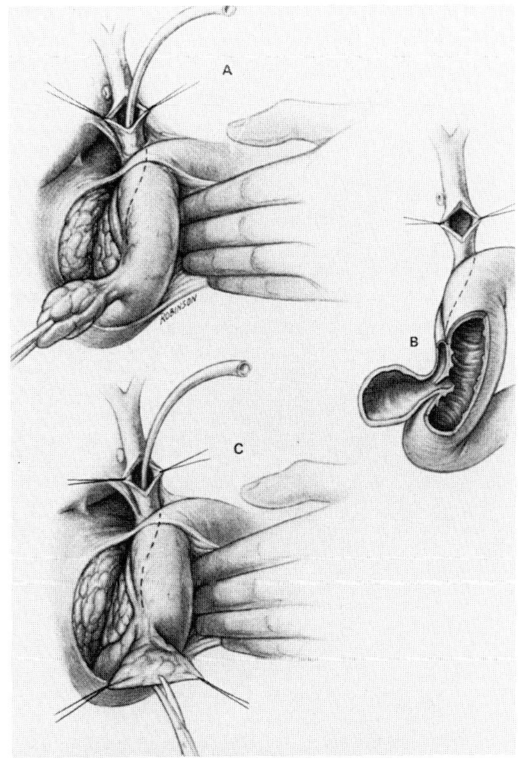

Figure 176.   A. The duodenum has been reflected medially to locate the stalk of the diverticulum arising from the lesser curvature of its second portion. A bougie catheter has been inserted into the common bile duct. B. Terminal portion of the common bile duct opens into the diverticulum. C. Slight tension is maintained with traction sutures to reveal the diverticulum. The fundus is incised to enter the lumen.

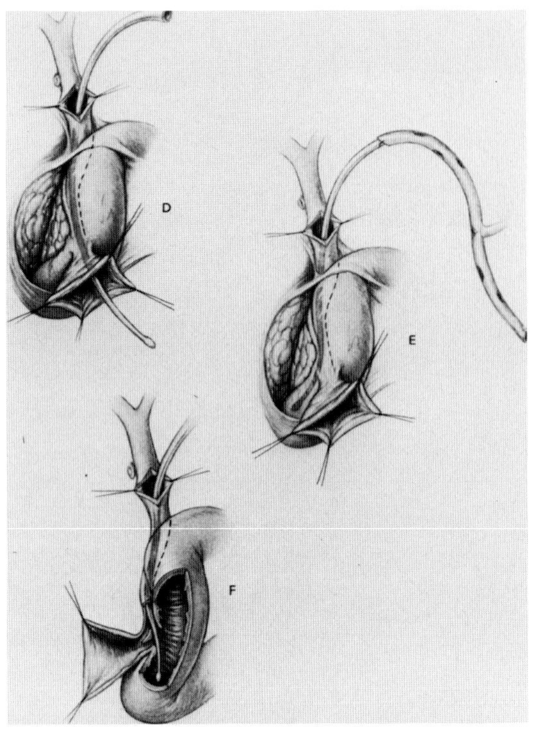

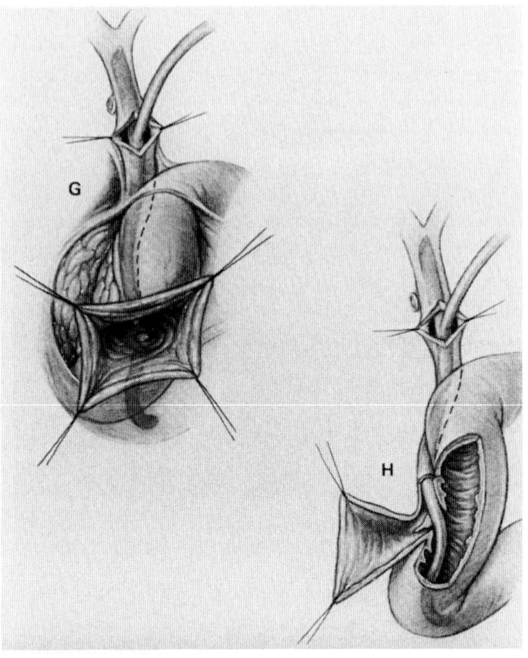

Figure 177. D. The bougie catheter extends through the ampulla of Vater into the diverticulum. E. The long arm of a T-tube is drawn through the distal portion of the common bile duct and into the lumen of the duodenum by securing it to the bougie with a silk suture. F. Bougie pierces the duodenal mucosa to enter the lumen directly.

Figure 178. The T-tube is in place with the long arm extending a few centimeters beyond the newly created choledochoduodenal orifice. H. Position of distal limb of the T-tube prior to excision of the diverticulum.

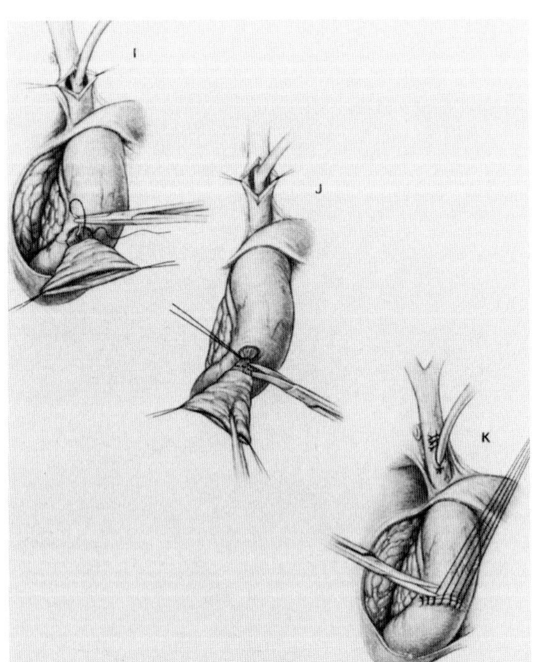

Figure 179. I. The neck of the diverticulum has been incised to expose the muscularis mucosae. The lumen is obliterated by a purse-string suture of No. 000 chromic catgut. J. The diverticulum is transected close to the purse-string suture. K. The obliterated neck of the diverticulum is inverted by a series of fine silk sutures. The choledochotomy has been closed around the T-tube.

When jaundice occurs and no biliary stone can be identified, a diverticulectomy may be considered. This writer's patient was an 84-year-old female, frail and with serious cardiovascular problems. Her internist and surgeon recommended surgery because her jaundice and pain appeared to be persistent. This writer decided to treat the patient conservatively. She was put on absolute bed rest, IV fluids, nothing by mouth, an antibiotic, and smooth muscle relaxants. She recovered after several days and left the hospital with a recommended strict liquid and soft diet. The patient is now 94 years of age and still follows the same diet and routine. Where the jaundiced patient reveals biliary stones and is suspected of having diverticulitis, surgical intervention is indeed indicated. A cholecystectomy and choledochotomy may be performed, but where the ampulla opens into the diverticulum and a stone is discovered, it should be removed and the diverticulum preferably left undisturbed (see Figs. 175–179).

Recommended Reading

McSherry CK, Glenn F: Biliary tract obstruction and duodenal diverticula. *Surg Gynecol Obstet* 130:829, 1970.

Pinotti HW, Tacla M, Pontes JF, et al: Surgical procedures upon juxta-ampullar duodenal diverticula. *Surg Gynecol Obstet* 135:11, 1972.

Willox GL, Costopoulos LB: Entry of common bile and pancreatic ducts into a duodenal diverticulum. *Arch Surg* 98:447, 1969.

Reference

1. Wolfson NS, Miller FB: Anatomic relationship of insertion of the common bile duct into primary duodenal diverticula. *Surg Gynecol Obstet* 146:628, 1978.

14

TRAUMA TO THE BILIARY TRACT:
Operative and Postoperative Complications

Penetrating and Nonpenetrating External Injuries to the Gallbladder and Biliary Tree

Dunn[1] reported a series of 5,670 cases of penetrating and nonpenetrating injuries of the abdomen collected from the medical literature and indicated that there were 109 cases of actual gallbladder injuries; this would imply an incidence of approximately 2%.

Penetrating injuries of the gallbladder may be due to gunshot wounds, stabs, and even penetration by blunt instruments. It is now definitely established that injuries to the gallbladder and/or biliary tree resulting from external trauma are affected more by penetrating than nonpenetrating injuries. There are, of course, iatrogenic causes of injury to the gallbladder wall resulting in some form of laceration that occurs during biopsy or percutaneous intrahepatic cholangiography.

Percutaneous intrahepatic cholangiography should not be performed when the blood quality is questionable, as in certain blood dyscrasias (leukemias, purpuras) and in patients who have a high prothrombin time, due either to liver damage or to the use of anticoagulant drugs. Faulty percutaneous intrahepatic cholangiography may result in a laceration, tear, or perforation, which may result in hemorrhage or escape of bile into the peritoneal cavity. The operating room and the surgeon must be scheduled to stand by whenever percutaneous intrahepatic cholangiography is performed. An X-ray will indicate how the dye outlines the biliary tree; in cases of marked dilatation based on distal obstruction, immediate surgery may or may not be decided upon, depending upon whether the obstruction is caused by a stone or carcinoma.

In penetrating injuries, the gallbladder may be lacerated or cut in any manner, but the total injury may be more extensive; a complete abdominal exploration must be carried out (see the discussion of the around-the-clock abdominal exploration in Chapter 12). *Nonpenetrating injuries* of the gallbladder may rupture the organ but may also result in additional types of lacerations. Therefore, whenever a blow produces such an effect, a complete abdominal exploration is indicated because one cannot afford to miss any area of the bowel or pancreas that has inadvertently been lacerated. It must be remembered that a correction of the gallbladder problem per se may still result in death from an unrecognized intestinal or visceral laceration.

Dunn reported that the organs most commonly avulsed in recognized gallbladder injuries were the liver (72% of cases), small intestine (36%), and colon (32%). Other types of injuries encountered with gallbladder trauma were contusion of the gallbladder, avulsion of the gallbladder, rupture of the gallbladder, and traumatic cholecystitis. In contusion of the gallbladder by a penetrating or nonpenetrating injury, there may be only a bruise or hemorrhagic appearance of the wall, with no evidence of perforation or laceration to the viscus. Avulsion of the gallbladder indicates that there has been a partial or total tear of the gallbladder from its liver bed. Even when the gallbladder is only incompletely avulsed, it has still been torn from its liver bed and hangs, so to speak, more freely in the peritoneal cavity, yet remains attached to the cystic duct, common duct, and cystic artery.

A gallbladder that lies freely in the peritoneal cavity should be removed; otherwise, the possibility of complications is great. Total avulsion, of course, implies that the gallbladder has been completely torn from its liver bed and blood supply, including its ductal connection to the common duct. This requires immediate laparotomy with evacuation of all damaged tissue found in the abdomen, i.e., damaged gallbladder, bile, and blood. Immediate control of the bleeding and replacement of blood loss is essential. The degree of bile leakage depends upon where the tear and laceration occurred; most likely it will be at the cystic duct junction with the common bile duct or somewhere beyond. Here, of course, more than one laceration may take place, and it is imperative that after all visible sites are repaired, drainage from other sites be instituted to prevent an unexpected bile peritonitis in the postoperative period. The mortality in total avulsion obviously would be much higher than in partial avulsion of the gallbladder.

In case of rupture of the gallbladder, the picture is more likely to be that of acute cholecystitis; the gallbladder is ruptured, and the cystic artery and/or duct may or may not also be involved. If the latter are involved, a cholecystectomy is mandatory. In those instances where the cystic artery has been damaged and hemorrhage is a significant part of the picture, the bleeding must be stopped; here again, care must be taken to attain a clear field in order to clamp and suture the exact site of bleeding. If the right hepatic artery is involved, it must be ligated or the patient will bleed to death. Gangrene of the liver or necrosis of a portion of it is a possibility, but the surgeon has no alternative in this emergency. He must stop the bleeding. In most instances, the extrahepatic and intrahepatic collateral circulations between the right and left hepatic arteries will more than suffice to maintain the integrity of the right lobe of the liver.

Where there is an accumulation of blood within the gallbladder, the blood or hematoma is subject to infection, with possible empyema of the gallbladder. Surgery, of course, becomes the only alternative; the gallbladder must be removed or drained. The blood that accumulates in the gallbladder may even pass beyond, through the cystic duct and into the common duct, giving rise to signs of upper and lower gastrointestinal bleeding, or possibly melena. When the blood in the common duct coagulates, it may produce an obstruction simulating an obstructing stone. Here, then, we have an obstructive jaundice caused by coagulated blood in the common duct (hemobilia). The picture will be recognized only at surgery unless the clot had passed first.

In traumatic cholecystitis, bile may escape from the perforation or laceration into the abdominal cavity, resulting in bile peritonitis. Bile peritonitis may give rise to further changes, such as ascites, when the bile becomes loculated. In either event, there is no treatment for bile in the abdomen other than to remove and drain this highly irritative material from the abdomen. If this is neglected, infection will surely follow, and the patient will die from a bacterial peritonitis accompanied by severe toxemia and endotoxic shock.

In conclusion, treatment entails a policy of high suspicion and routine complete abdominal evaluation, particularly in the right upper quadrant. If the abdomen is opened and abdominal exploration is carried out, it should be routine to make a complete search for possible unsuspected associated injuries. A gallbladder injury that is so severe as to result in shock requires emergency surgery; but one must be sure to first treat the patient for shock. Only when the patient's condition has definitely improved should a surgical procedure be undertaken. One should not wait for jaundice to occur because that is a late finding, usually occurring after the third or fourth day. In this case, surgery is too late. The delay invites biliary peritonitis and subsequent death. *The writer is not an advocate of needling the abdominal cavity because negative findings are not indicative of the absence of gallbladder injury.*

The history and clinical picture are the outstanding factors in the decision to intervene surgically. This writer concludes that cholecystectomy, when possible, is the safest procedure, particularly when the contusion was severe and the chances of per-

foration or laceration are high. This decision is not just advisable, it is mandatory! *One word of caution: The finding of a pathological gallbladder as a result of the trauma should not prevent the operator from continuing with his routine around-the-clock exploration of the abdomen; to overlook an unsuspecting intestinal laceration spells doom for the patient.*

In regard to *penetrating wounds* to the extrahepatic biliary system, most cases of trauma are caused by stab and gunshot wounds; even blunt instruments are capable of penetrating the abdominal wall. In the great majority of cases, there will be concomitant injuries to other abdominal viscera. One must look for injuries to the pancreas, stomach, colon, intestine, and diaphragm. Flat scout films taken immediately will offer helpful clues in diagnosing the injuries; free air found under the diaphragm is pathognomonic for perforation of a hollow viscus. Fluid seen above the diaphragm indicates definite penetration and bleeding above the diaphragmatic level. Hemothorax, if present, will indicate the extent of the injury that must be further examined. In injuries such as stabs, gunshot wounds, and wounds made by other sharp, penetrating instruments, it is mandatory that the abdominal cavity be opened and thoroughly explored. One cannot omit this procedure.

Unquestionably, the most common associated finding in penetrating injuries is shock, and before the patient can be treated surgically, the management of shock must precede all other forms of therapy. The treatment of shock provides an opportunity to improve the patient's condition before surgery by offering the necessary fluids, blood or blood substitutes, electrolytes, nasogastric suction, steroids, and antibiotics. *When the patient is out of shock and his condition becomes more stable, surgery may be undertaken.* However, surgery will still depend on the age and condition of the patient. Probing the wound is not an infallible procedure; the history, the condition of the patient, and the surgeon's experience should take precedence over whether or not the exploratory probe extends into the abdomen. Reported injuries to the extrahepatic biliary system may range from small perforations to extensive tears and as far as complete severance of the common or hepatic ducts. Though the latter injury is rare, lesser injuries to the gallbladder are not uncommon. It is very important to stress early exploration because any delay in repairing extrahepatic biliary tears, severance, or perforation will allow the development of chemical peritonitis, which ultimately will lead to bacterial peritonitis, endotoxic shock, and death. *It is imperative that the differential diagnosis of penetrating or nonpenetrating injury to the abdomen be made as soon as possible, and if surgery is indicated, time must not be lost in procrastination!*

SURGICAL TREATMENT

The abdomen is carefully explored (see the discussion of round-the-clock exploration in Chapter 12) through a right upper paramedian, midline, or oblique Kocher subcostal incision, depending on the habitus of the patient. The penetrating wound itself should be completely excised as the incision is made. If bile and blood are found in the abdomen, they should be completely aspirated and their source searched out. The round-the-clock search technique is the safest and most methodical of all laparotomy searches.

The primary pathology must be found and corrected in the best possible manner. If bile is in the abdomen and all tissue have stained green, but the gallbladder is not traumatized or lacerated in any way, the surgeon must continue the search for damage to the extrahepatic biliary tract. The search should be directed to the common bile duct or the cystic duct junction with the common duct, after which the entire common duct should be carefully explored. If nothing is found in the latter search, one must proceed to search out the hepatic ductal system.

A meticulous search must be conducted under the finest light and exposure possible in order to search out a small tear, laceration, or perforation. If necessary, one must dissect out the right and left hepatic ducts. To explore the common duct more thoroughly, it may be necessary to perform a Kocher maneuver (see "The Kocher Maneuver" in Chapter 11). With better visualization and more determination, the surgeon should explore the lower portion of the common duct and the head of the pancreas. Here one may discover a perforation in the posterior wall of the duodenum, as well as injury to the head of the pancreas.

If a retroperitoneal hematoma is found, it should be evacuated immediately and a search made for the source of the bleeding. The latter suggests a possible perforation of the duodenum and/or the common bile duct. If after a thorough search one finds that the common bile duct has been severed or the common hepatic duct transected, the best way to handle it is to trim the edges of the ends and perform an end-to-end anastomosis, utilizing very fine (0000) or (00000) interrupted black silk sutures. A T-tube, of course, should be inserted above or below the line of anastomosis, not only to drain the bile but to splint the site of anastomosis as well. When all this is accomplished, a further complete reexploration must be carried out, and if no other injury has been revealed, drainage should be employed. Drainage should be as elsewhere, namely, wherever leakage or bleeding may restart and infection develop. A Penrose (wick) drain should be placed in Morison's fossa, one in the foramen of Winslow, and, on specific occasions, one subdiaphragmatically. Jackson-Pratt suction drains may be employed instead of Penrose (wick) drains.

Recommended Reading

Wiener I, Watson LC, Wolma FJ: Perforation of the gallbladder due to blunt abdominal trauma. *Arch Surg* 117:805, 1982.

Schwartz SI, Adams JT, Cockett ATK, et al: Blunt trauma to the upper abdomen. *Surg Annu* 3:273, 1971.

Barnes JP, Diamonon JS: Traumatic rupture of the gallbladder due to nonpenetrating injury. *Tex State J Med* 59:785, 1963.

Brickley HD, Kaplan A, Freeark RJ, et al: Immediate and delayed rupture of the extrahepatic biliary tract following blunt abdominal trauma. *Am J Surg* 100:107, 1960.

Divicenti FC, Rives JD, Laborde EJ, et al: Blunt abdominal trauma. *J Trauma* 8:1004, 1968.

Evans JP: Traumatic rupture of a gallbladder in a three year old boy. *J Pediatr Surg* 11:1033, 1976.

Fielding JWL, Strachan CJL: Jaundice as a sign of delayed gallbladder perforation following blunt abdominal trauma. *Injury* 7:66, 1975.

Fletcher WS: Nonpenetrating trauma to the gallbladder and extrahepatic bile ducts. *Surg Clin North Am* 52:711, 1972.

Frank DJ, Pereiras R, Souza-Lima MS, et al: Traumatic rupture of the gallbladder with massive biliary ascites. *JAMA* 240:252, 1978.

Hall ER, Howard JM, Jordan GL, et al: Traumatic injuries of the gallbladder. *Arch Surg* 72:520, 1956.

Hogue RJ, Munnele ER: Traumatic rupture of the gallbladder. *Surgery* 29:155, 1963.

Isch JH, Finneran JC, Nahrwald DL: Perforation of the gallbladder. *Am J Gastroenterol* 55:451, 1971.

McCarthy J, Picazo J: Bile peritonitis: Diagnosis and course. *J Surg* 116:664, 1968.

Mentzer SH: Bile peritonitis. *Arch Surg* 29:227, 1934.

Olson WR, Redman HC, Hildrath DH: Quantitative peritoneal lavage in blunt abdominal trauma. *Arch Surg* 104:536, 1972.

Pen I: Injuries to the gallbladder. *Br J Surg* 49:636, 1962.

Perry JR, DeMeules JE, Root HD: Diagnostic peritoneal lavage in blunt abdominal trauma. *Surg Gynecol Obstet* 131:742, 1970.

Root HD, Hauser CW, McKinley CR, et al: Diagnostic peritoneal lavage. *Surgery* 57:633, 1965.

Schechter DS: Solitary wounding of the gallbladder from blunt abdominal trauma. *NY State J Med* 69:2895, 1969.

Songsanad P, Croff DB: Treatment of gallbladder rupture in an infant. *Am Surg* 38:335, 1972.

Sparkman RS, Jernigan CR: Visualization of gallbladder and bile ducts following trauma. *Surgery* 41:595, 1957.

Wangensteen OH: On the significance of the escape of sterile bile into the peritoneal cavity. *Ann Surg* 84:691, 1926.

Reference

1. Dunn EL, Moore EE, Moore JB, et al: Penetrating abdominal trauma index. *J Trauma* 21:439, 1981.

Hemobilia

Hemobilia refers to hemorrhage in or through the biliary tract. It takes place when trauma (accidental or operative) and disease (tumors, aneurysms, gallstones, and inflammation) permit the blood vessels to communicate with the biliary tree. The blood and bile mixture enters the duodenum and intestine. The bleeding may be occult and insignificant or massive. It can lead to exsanguination and death. The usual signs and symptoms of hemobilia are pallor and, if allowed to go on, severe anemia. In such instances, where a deficiency of coagulating factors exists, the bleeding may become more severe. The bleeding may originate intrahepatically or extrahepatically, i.e., in the biliary tract, blood vessels, and pancreas. The blood may coagulate within the biliary tree and cause obstruction, with signs and symptoms of jaundice and severe colic.

In his excellent monograph *Hemobilia*, Philip Sandbloom,[1] from the University of Lund, Sweden, successfully traces the earliest report describing hemobilia. Sandbloom believes that Francis Glisson (1597–1677) gave the first detailed description of liver anatomy and made further significant observations on liver pathology (hemobilia). In 1948, Sandbloom published a report[2] on nine cases in which massive hemorrhage into the biliary tract took place after liver trauma; he named this condition *traumatic hemobilia*. Hemobilia is a rare condition, and there is a general unawareness of its development. In order to diagnose rare conditions, one must constantly be on the alert for their development or presence.

PATHOGENETICS

Sandbloom believes that disruption of liver parenchyma, bile ducts, and thin-walled blood vessels accounts for the accumulation of devitalized tissue, blood, and bile within a closed space. Usually the products are resorbed, and healing takes place with scar formation. However, when the material remains unresolved, a bile cyst or liver abscess follows. Necrosis within the closed wound may permit the sequestered products to erupt into a bile duct, creating a hemorrhage that flows into the gastrointestinal tract, and out through the rectum as melena.

TRAUMATIC HEMOBILIA

Though considered a primary complication, hemobilia may also develop as a later complication.

Case 1[3]

A 22-year-old black male received a blunt abdominal injury. At laparotomy multiple liver lacerations were found, as was rupture of Glisson's capsule and spleen. Hemostasis was secured and a splenectomy carried out. Hemostasis was attained with duly placed deep sutures on a Gelfoam sponge. The patient was discharged. Ten days later, the patient reported gross hematuria associated with right flank colic. In the hospital the patient became asymptomatic. The diagnosis was renal aneurysm with late renal colic due to the passage of clots. The patient was readmitted because of occult blood in the stool. On examination, right upper quadrant (RUQ) tenderness was found. Since his previous admission, his blood count had dropped 5 points. Though the alkaline phosphatase was elevated, as was the bilirubin level, no jaundice was observed. Throughout his hospital stay, the patient had persistent occult gastrointestinal bleeding. On the 29th day after the accident, the patient suffered a biliary colic, which was dramatically relieved. Despite blood transfusions, the blood count dropped. Repeated attacks of colic continued. Latent hemobilia was suspected. An oral cholecystogram demonstrated filling defects within the gallbladder; this suggested blood clots rather than gallstones. In view of the fact that the patient was a healthy young male, persistent hemobilia and colic appeared to be more consistent with a latent hemobilia. At surgery the sutured liver laceration was incised and a 3 × 7 cm cavity was found. In this cavity, a single large hepatic vein was in communication with several bile ducts. The content of the cavity was soft clot and fresh blood. The extent of the laceration included an almost complete severance of the lateral segment of the left lobe of the liver. The lateral segment that contained the site of the venous-biliary communication area was resected. The gallbladder was distended with blood clots but was left alone.

Postoperatively, the alkaline phosphatase and lactic dehydrogenase gradually returned to normal levels. An oral cholecystogram 4.5 months later was negative. The patient fully recovered.

Case 2[4]

A 22-year-old black man was brought into the emergency room suffering from an abdominal stab wound. IV fluids and antibiotics were started, and the patient taken to the operating room for abdominal exploration. There was a small amount of blood in the abdominal cavity. The injury appeared to be a single stab wound of the liver. The wound was closed with deep chromic catgut sutures, and the right subhepatic space was drained. Recovery was uneventful until the eighth postoperative day, when the patient complained of RUQ pain. There were no physical findings. The patient vomited blood and blood clots, and the hematocrit fell 10 points. Five units of whole blood were given to raise the blood count back to 30%. Surgery was considered, and after another bout of hematemesis the patient was explored. The gallbladder and common bile ducts were filled with blood and clots. The common duct alone was explored and a T-tube inserted. After 5 hours in the recovery room, the T-tube spilled a massive amount of bright red blood and the patient became hypotensive. After several rapid transfusions, the patient was returned to the operating room. This time the liver wound was cut into its depth and explored. Deep inside (about 12 cm), a 2 × 2 cm hematoma was recognized, and in the center was an actively bleeding divided artery. Both arterial ends were ligated with chromic catgut. The T-tube was irrigated to free it of clots. The defect in the liver was drained by a Penrose drain. Throughout the procedure, the patient received fluids and antibiotics. The postoperative course was uneventful. The T-tube was removed 3 weeks later. The patient was discharged on the 30th day.

Diagnosis

A *history* of abdominal or thoracoabdominal trauma associated with RUQ pain and gastrointestinal hemorrhage should evoke a suspicion of hemobilia. Laboratory studies will show increasing levels of alkaline phosphatase, transaminase and bilirubin; there will be nonvisualization on the cholecystogram. Liver scan studies and a CT scan may be of help before surgery; eudoserpic examination may

also be effective. The constant clinical features associated with hemobilia are:

1. *Liver trauma*–sharp or blunt.
2. *A variable time interval* of pain, colic and hematemesis.
3. *Episodic bleeding*, usually arterial, which may or may not stop.
4. *Intrahepatic necrosis* (or hematoma) that is distinct at the site of bleeding.

The presumptive pathogenesis is that arterial bleeding continues in a closed hepatic compartment until the increased intrahepatic pressure results in necrosis and ultimate erosion into the biliary tract. The necrotic material is lysed by liver enzymes, creating recurrent bleeding into the biliary tract (hemobilia). Temporary control of the bleeding at surgery can be established by digital occlusion of the hepatic artery. Once control of bleeding is assured, other diagnostic tests can be carried out, i.e., direct visualization and probing of the right and left hepatic ducts, direct hepatic arteriograms, and actual intrahepatic exploration may be employed to search out the precise location and source of hemobilia.

Treatment

Effective treatment will depend on the following:

1. *Exploration and evacuation of necrotic material and clot, with T-tube drainage of the biliary tree to decompress or reduce the biliary pressure.*
2. *Debridement of devitalized tissue* and abdominal drainage.
3. *Effective control of the bleeding vessel,* which may involve specific intrahepatic ligation of the artery or vein; lobectomy, segmentectomy, or hepatic artery ligation.
4. *Supportive therapy,* including whole blood transfusions, antibiotics, fluid volume and electrolyte replacement, Vitamin K (Mephyton), and avoidance of hypoxia and hypotension.

HEPATIC LOBAR INJURIES

When hemobilia is confined to a single lobe, it can be treated effectively by specific arterial ligation, segmentectomy, or total lobectomy. Left lobectomy is not too difficult, but right lobectomy is a last-resort procedure because of the associated high mortality. Complications following total lobectomy are shock, emboli, and hemorrhage.

CENTRAL HEPATIC INJURIES

Hemobilia from both the right and left hepatic lobes poses a difficult problem. Massive hepatic hemorrhage carries a forbidding mortality; therefore, hemobilia of central hepatic origin is best dealt with by debridement of all necrotic tissue, with ligatures applied to the traumatized blood vessels. All necrotic material should be evacuated and the common duct drained with a T-tube. The abdominal cavity must also be drained. If this measure fails to stop the bleeding, a common hepatic artery ligation should be tried as a last resort measure.

COMMON HEPATIC ARTERY LIGATION

Where there is intractable bleeding, one is readily tempted to ligate the hepatic artery, but there remains a persistent fear of compromising the entire liver parenchyma. There are two schools of thought on this question. One group believes that the right and left hepatic arteries are end arteries and have no collaterals between them. Another group states that in over 50% of cases the right and left hepatic arteries do have intrahepatic collateral anastomosis. This writer believes the latter group to be correct. *When ligation of the hepatic artery becomes the last resort to save a life, it should be tried.* In principle, three sites may be selected: (1) the common hepatic artery, (2) the hepatic artery proper, and (3) one of its branches, i.e., lobar or segmental. After ligation of the common hepatic artery, the gastroduodenal artery becomes the main collateral. The intrahepatic blood pressure is markedly affected, which can lead to stoppage of the bleed. In the last analysis, one must be aware of the admixture of arterial and venous blood that exists within the liver parenchyma. The liver may survive, but with a marked degree of hypoxia. Arteriolar collaterals may come from the gastroduodenal and diaphragmatic blood vessels; also from possible intrahepatic collateral anastomosis between right and left hepatic branches.

Case 3[5,6]

A 50-year-old woman was admitted to the hospital with a diagnosis of calculous cholecystitis. Choleystectomy was performed, and the common bile duct was opened and drained with a T-tube.

On the second day postoperatively, the patient was found in shock, vomiting blood, and bleeding through the T-tube. She was given 3 units of whole blood and taken to the operating room. At surgery when the T-tube was removed, blood was noted seeping out of the choledochostomy. The porta hepatis was completely clamped off, and in a dry field a good-sized hole in the posterior wall of the common duct was found communicating with the portal vein. The hole in the portal vein was closed, and after the clamps were released, no further bleeding was noted. The T-tube was reinserted, and the wound was drained with a Penrose drain. The patient made an uneventful recovery. Hakami et al. urge a minimum of handling to avoid such complications and cautions, *"do enough to help and less to hurt the patient."*

Case 4[6]

A 56-year-old Iranian male was admitted to the hospital with epigastric pain of 3 days' standing. The pain radiated to the right shoulder; friends of the family added that there was fainting, cold extremities, and air hunger. Several hours later, the patient moved his bowels with blood. On admission, the patient had yellow conjunctivae. On examination the essential findings were tenderness in epigastrium and RUQ pain, and no palpable mass. The red blood cell count was 2,850,000 despite transfusions of whole blood, the blood pressure dropped to 90/60, and the the blood cell count fell further to 2,200,000. A cholangiogram revealed nonvisualization of the gallbladder. On the fifth day, because of continued bleeding, the patient was taken to the operating room. At exploration the gallbladder was markedly distended with blood. The gallbladder was opened to remove a large stone and to evacuate the bloody bile. On the left side of the gallbladder was a nut-sized tumor that pulsated. On careful inspection, a jet of blood spurted out of the tumor. The hepatic pedicle was clamped and the bleeding stopped. Careful dissection revealed aneurysm of the cystic artery. The aneurysm was clamped and ligated. The clamp on the porta hepatis was released and the gallbladder removed. Because the common duct was filled with blood and clots, it was opened. The common duct and Morison's fossa were drained, and the patient made an uneventful recovery. *The final pathological diagnosis was rupture of a cystic artery aneurysm into the gallbladder. A selective hepatic arteriogram at surgery made the diagnosis.*

Hemobilia is also a potential complication of needle biopsy of the liver. In such instances, when the clinical features include colicky pain and periodic gastrointestinal hemorrhage (hematemesis or melena) with jaundice, hemobilia must be suspected. The onset of colicky pain about 3 days after the needling usually precedes the gastrointestinal bleeding. After hematemesis, the pain subsides, most likely due to release of intrabiliary pressure. Jaundice appears periodically and is related to an obstructive biliary tract.

Angiography has proved most useful as a diagnostic tool and is especially valuable in localizing the site of bleeding; also valuable is its ability to guide the surgeon when he must decide to resect the liver. Other diagnostic tests include radioisotope scan and splenography. In those cases where bleeding does not stop spontaneously, a partial lobectomy may be the treatment of choice. The procedure is exposure of the bleeding site and the bleeder. Ligation of the hepatic artery *may become necessary*, but this has not always proved effective.

Case 5

In 1935, a 74-year-old female was treated for acute cholecystitis; 8 years later, after three intermittent attacks, she was admitted to the hospital with cholecystitis and jaundice. The jaundice was accompanied by increasing anemia and melena. Two weeks later, the jaundice increased and the patient suffered hematemesis and melena. Despite repeated transfusions, she went into shock. A preoperative diagnosis of hemobilia was made. At exploratory surgery, no blood was found in the abdominal cavity. The duodenum was filled with blood. The cystic duct was opened, and bleeding was seen coming from the gallbladder. Ligation of the cystic artery terminated the hemorrhage. The common duct was opened, and blood and clots were evacuated. A T-tube was inserted and the operation completed. The patient had an uneventful recovery.

This report illustrates that a neglected or untreated case of cholelithiasis can lead to complications such as carcinoma, fistula formation, gallstone ileus, obstructive jaundice, pancreatitis, and, finally, erosion of the adjacent artery with resultant hemobilia.

Other rarer causes of hemobilia are:

1. *Tumors* of the gallbladder that grow into and erode the blood vessel wall.
2. *Vascular disorders* such as aneurysms, vascular disorders associated with hypertension, and varicosities associated with the portal vein.

The writer wishes to alert the internist, gastroenterologist, and surgeons to the remote possibility of hemobilia in those cases where blood is found in the stool. Failure to consider hemobilia as a possibility in cases of blunt and sharp abdominal trauma, cholelithiasis associated with hematemesis and/or melena, angiographic findings of cystic and hepatic artery aneurysms with anemia, and incidental findings of neoplasms of the gallbladder can result in an avoidable fatality.

Recommended Reading

Bismuth H: Hemobilia. *N Engl J Med* 288:617, 1973.

Druy EM: Hepatic artery-biliary fistula following percutaneous transhepatic biliary drainage. *Radiology* 141:369, 1981.

Dunnick NR, Doppman JL, Brereton HD: Balloon occlusion of segmental hepatic arteries—control of biopsy-induced hemobilia. *JAMA* 238:2524, 1977.

Franklin RH, Bloom WF, Schoffstall RO: Angiographic embolization as the definitive treatment of posttraumatic hemobilia. *J Trauma* 20(8):702, 1980.

Goodnight JE, Blaisdell FW: Hemobilia. *Surg Clin North Am* 61:973, 1981.

Kaplan RB, Kaplan L, Panish J.: Hemobilia, endoscopic diagnosis and association with pancreatitis. *Dig Dis Sci* 25:140, 1980.

Wilkinson GM, Mikkelsen WP, Berne CJ: The treatment of posttraumatic hemobilia by ligation of the common hepatic artery. *Surg Clin North Am* 48:1337, 1968.

References

1. Sandbloom P: *Hemobilia.* Homewood, IL, Charles C Thomas, 1972.
2. Sandbloom P: Hemorrhage into the biliary tract following trauma: Traumatic hemobilia. *Surgery* 42:571, 1948.
3. Wright PW, Orloff MJ: Traumatic hemobilia. *Ann Surg* 160:42, 1964.
4. Rheinhardt G,F, Hubay CA: Surgical management of traumatic hemobilia. *Am J Surg* 121:328, 1971.
5. Hakami M, Beheshti G, Amirhan A: Hemobilia caused by a rupture of cystic artery aneurysm. *Am J Proctol* 27(4):56, 1976.
6. Hakami M, Beheshti G, Amirhan A: Report of a case of hemobilia. *Am J Proctol*, vol 27, no 4, 1976.

15

THE PROPHYLACTIC AND THERAPEUTIC USE OF ANTIBIOTICS IN BILIARY TRACT SURGERY

The availability of many potent antibiotics has had a profound effect on every branch of surgery. Antibiotics have vastly improved our results in the field of biliary tract surgery, especially where complications were so frequently encountered. The use of antibiotics prophylactically in elective cholecystectomy cases still remains a controversial subject. Because the antibiotic must preferably be selected before a biliary procedure is carried out, and bacterial cultures are not always available, a knowledge of antibiotics becomes mandatory. The surgeon must be aware of the antibiotic's specific effectiveness and toxicity; he must also know of its capability of being excreted into the bile and tissues in high concentrations.

Prophylactic antibiotics can prevent infection in certain surgical patients, but not without some disadvantage and/or risk. Some of the risks are toxic or allergic drug reactions; other potential risks are fungal and bacterial superinfections. It is conceivable that the hospital environment can be altered to favor bacterial strains that are resistant to the antibiotic. An effective prophylactic antibiotic program need not be active against all suspected organisms, because the antibiotic that decreases the total number of organisms can permit the patient's own immune defense system to resist the active organisms. The effective use of prophylactic antibiotics depends on the time of administration. *Antibiotics should be started before surgery—preferably (1) hour before going to OR. This is the time required to reach a therapeutic level throughout the surgical procedure.* The antibiotic therapy should be continued for as short a period as possible, preferably 24 to 72 hours. Antibiotic prophylaxis in biliary tract surgery is justified only in those cases where an increased risk of infection exists. Patients considered ideally suited for routine antibiotic prophylaxis are those over 70 years, those with acute cholecystitis, suppurative cholangitis, and all forms of suspected biliary obstruction, and all patients with obstructive jaundice caused by gallstones. A routine elective cholecystectomy procedure in a young or middle-aged patient in good general health is not a good choice for antibiotic prophylaxis. However, if the surgeon expects the elective cholecystectomy to include a common duct exploration, the use of antibiotic prophylaxis is considered good judgment.

A.A. Gunn[1] in 1976 conducted a controlled study on the prophylactic use of antibiotics in cases of common duct dilatation believed to be caused by stones. He chose seven criteria for selecting his cases for prophylactic antibiotics:

1. Age of over 50
2. History of jaundice
3. Empyema of the gallbladder
4. Elevated liver enzymes
5. Dilated common bile duct
6. Ductal obstruction (stone or stricture)

Gunn employed prophylactic antibiotics when three or more of the above criteria were present. His conclusion was that there was a significant reduction in wound infections and septicemia.

What should be done in those instances where extenuating circumstances exist, i.e., chronic bronchitis, emphysema, diabetes mellitus, and chronic obstructive pulmonary disease? A patient with an uncomplicated diabetes should be considered like any other patient in regard to susceptibility to infection. So far, it has not been shown that a controlled diabetic's defense mechanism is significantly impaired. Kidney transplant surgery has shown that controlled diabetics fare just as well as nondiabetic patients where postoperative infections are concerned; in such cases, the diabetic patient does not receive routine antibiotics prophylactically and does just as well as the nondiabetic. In patients with chronic pulmonary disease, antibiotic prophylaxis need not be considered unless, of course, the patient has a suspicion of active lung infection. In instances where coexisting immune depression or decreasing immune host resistance exists, i.e., malnutrition and cachexia, systemic antibiotics are justified and should be given before, during, and after surgery. In instances where neoplastic obstructions of the common duct exist, i.e., biliary or pancreatic carcinoma, we must assume that the bile is infected; if stones are the cause, the bile will certainly be infected. In other coexisting problem cases, preoperative antibiotic use is considered good judgment. If an IV choledochogram reveals a nonobstructing stone in the common duct, antibiotics should still be given preoperatively. This writer believes that age is a significant factor and that patients 65 years old or more should be considered as having bacteria in their bile; in these patients, antibiotic prophylaxis is justifiably indicated even in an apparently uncomplicated cholecystectomy. In patients with chronic bronchitis, the supplemental use of ampicillin or penicillin may be beneficial. When a perforated viscus, i.e., stomach, appendix, or gallbladder, is suspected or diagnosed, the surgery must be considered "dirty"; therefore, postoperative infection is to be anticipated. Instead of employing preoperative prophylactic antibiotic therapy, we immediately institute *active therapy;* this involves a higher antibiotic dosage, and the therapy must be carried out for a longer period of time postoperatively. The use of two antibiotics may be more desirable, depending on the situation.

The choice of antibiotics must depend upon the site of the surgery and should cover the widest spectrum possible. In patients who are questionably allergic to penicillin and cephalosporins, certain antibiotics may be judiciously employed; cefamandole (Mandol) and cefoxitin (Mefoxin) are presently considered to be more effective than cephalothin (Keflin) because they supposedly possess a broader spectrum of activity. Whether they are more effective prophylactically remains to be seen. In the meantime, for routine use, Keflin has proven to be quite adequate.

The finding of anaerobic organisms in common bile duct cultures is increasing in frequency. Bacteria that are isolated from an uninfected biliary system are distinctly different from those recovered from an infected biliary tract. Most surgeons recognize that organisms from the gastrointestinal tract are directly related to the bacteria cultured from the bile and that most likely these organisms travel via the portal vein and are excreted by the liver into the bile. Antibiotic selection must depend on the isolated organisms and their sensitivity responses. Cephalosporins, aminoglycosides, and penicillins are the most commonly employed antibiotics, either singly or in combination. *Klebsiella* organisms may prove resistant to ampicillin, but when this antibiotic is combined with aminoglycoside, i.e., kanamycin, tobramycin, or gentamicin, the combination proves to be very effective. One should constantly keep in mind that tetracyclines can be hepatotoxic, and that chloramphenicol is known to be toxic to the bone marrow; and that aminoglycosides are nephrotoxic. Chetlin and Elliott[2-4] reported that when the bile was infected, the chances of development of septic complications were 40 times greater.

The biliary tract is usually sterile, but certain groups of patients frequently have positive bile cultures. A positive operative bile culture will most often yield *Escherichia coli, Klebsiella,* and enterococci. Anaerobic organisms are not infrequently isolated from the biliary tract. Bacterial isolates from wound infections developing after biliary tract operations are usually identical to those found in intraoperative bile cultures.

With biliary tract procedures, most studies show a reduction in the infection rate when antimicrobial groups are compared to control groups. Agents found effective in reducing the rate of postoperative wound infection in biliary tract surgery include cefazolin, trimethoprim-sulfamethoxazole, gentamicin, cephaloridine, cefuroxime, rifamide, and cefamandole.

In one study, cefamandole was compared with cephalothin in high-risk patients undergoing cholecystectomy; both agents were administered preoperatively and continued for 48 hours postoperatively. Wound infections occurred in the cephalothin group; none occurred in the cefamandole group.

One factor often discussed in relation to antibiotics and biliary tract procedures is bile penetration. Cefamandole produces bile concentrations higher than those produced by most other cephalosporins. The importance of bile penetration is not completely understood, since Gentamicin had a minimal biliary tract excretion and significantly reduced infection rates in two studies. Rifamide, an agent with high biliary excretion, significantly reduced the infection rate when compared with a placebo. Biliary tract penetration should not be the primary factor in choosing an agent for prophylaxis of infection in biliary tract operations.

Clindamycin, an agent with good activity against *Bacteroides fragilis,* significantly reduced the infection rate. The author believes that anaerobic coverage will prove to be important in the prevention of wound infection by bacteroides.

In a patient diagnosed as having *acute cholangitis,* most surgeons agree that antibiotics should not only precede surgery but should also be continued into the postoperative period. In fulminating cases of acute cholangitis, i.e., suppurative cholangitis, the proper use of antibiotics can be lifesaving. It is not uncommon to see an acute cholangitis subside with antibiotics alone and without surgical interference; however, since most cases of acute cholangitis are associated with gallstones, it is probably best to provide relief sooner and thus prevent later recurrences. One must make certain of the diagnosis; that is, viral hepatitis must be ruled out. Patients with suppurative cholangitis associated with obstruction will not respond to any therapy other than a drainage procedure. Decompression with a nasogastric tube is recommended, and antibiotics should be instituted immediately. The writer prefers IV tetracycline or a cephalosporin, and on occasion, depending on the severity of the disease and the resistance of the organism, one of the aminoglycosides will be added. Other surgeons employ a combination of IV aqueous penicillin, 1 million units, and gentamicin, 1 mg/kg, both every 6 or 8 hours. In severe cases of cholangitis, the writer prefers Keflin alone; if the patient fails to respond within 24 hours, he adds gentamicin or clindamycin (cleocin) as indicated.

Antibiotic use reduces the infectious process, allows time to improve the patient generally, and, finally, permits the patient to be operated on at the most propitious moment with the hope that all complications related to the infection will have been averted. *This writer believes that all acute infectious diseases of the biliary tract should be treated preoperatively with suitable antibiotics before proceeding with surgery.* When the first antibiotic employed does not contain the infectious process, some surgeons, instead of adding another supplemental antibiotic, switch to an entirely new one. It should be remembered that a suppurative process usually does not respond immediately to any antibiotic, and that it will respond best to a drainage procedure. This writer uses Keflin, 1 g IV, preoperatively, followed by 1 g IV at surgery, and then continues to use it in the postoperative period on a 4-hour schedule, depending upon the severity of the disease process. Some surgeons prefer to employ penicillin in a high dosage, i.e., 10–12 million units daily, and Keflin, 8–12 g daily, depending upon the severity of the infectious process and the response of the patient.

Blood culture studies are important and should be carried out routinely in all severe infectious cases. Cultures taken preoperatively and at surgery are helpful. Preoperative cultures reveal the predominant organism and therefore help the surgeon to select the best antimicrobial agent. Unfortunately, blood culture results arrive long after the surgery has been performed. This makes it mandatory to employ antibiotics that deal effectively with the known spectrum of pathogens common to the biliary tract. An appropriate antibiotic can be chosen before culture in over 90% of the cases. The most significant cultures, of course, are taken from the actual bile of the common bile duct. This may be accomplished by needling or opening the common duct. If the common duct is not opened, a culture from the cystic duct is considered adequate. Some surgeons believe that a culture is best taken from the gallbladder mucosa. Penicillin is still a very effective drug against anaerobic bacteria, except bacteroides. The cephalosporins can also be effective against anaerobic organisms. *Liver* abscess is a serious complication, and should be suspected and looked for in instances where suppurative cholangitis is being considered. Liver abscess can most often be picked up by gallium scans, technetium-99m scans, and chest X-rays that reveal an elevated diaphragm with a fluid level. Angiogra-

phy, either preoperatively or at surgery, can also be helpful in localizing a liver abscess. Where there are multiple liver abscesses, a scan is of little or no help. Angiography, however, may prove valuable here. Incision and drainage of a large intrahepatic liver abscess is mandatory. Antibiotics should be continued into the postoperative period. Percutaneous transhepatic catheter drainage where indicated has been successfully carried out. (see Chapter 5).

In the average case of *acute cholecystitis,* conservative treatment is recommended, i.e., hospitalization, IV, fluids, gastric decompression and antibiotics such as Keflin, penicillin, or tetracycline. If the patient responds within 2 or 3 days, the antibiotics are discontinued, oral feedings are gradually instituted, and IV fluids are phased out. The patient should preferably be operated on an elective basis, i.e., 4 to 6 weeks later. If, however, there are good reasons why the patient cannot be available for elective cholecystectomy, the writer recommends elective surgery 1 or 2 weeks later. Preoperatively, the patient may have antibiotics 1 day before surgery, at surgery, and 1 or 2 days postoperatively. Some surgeons do not employ antibiotics at all in this case. The writer respects both views but follows the former practice. Some surgeons consider fever and elevated white blood cell count to be indications of infection. Others feel that a chemical biliary inflammation can also produce the same result, and therefore they do not necessarily call for antibiotics. Here again, the writer prefers to employ antibiotics because a chemical inflammation in the presence of bacteria can easily be converted to a bacterial infection. Therefore, the writer prefers the use of antibiotics pre- and postoperatively, as well as during surgery. There is evidence that antibiotics used as stated above will significantly reduce the incidence of postoperative wound infections.

In an uncomplicated case of acute cholecystitis, the recommended procedure should be conservative, i.e., to employ antibiotics and wait for the inflammatory process to subside. During the 4- to 6-week wait for an elective cholecystectomy, the patient should be worked up more carefully. A cholecystogram, IV choledochogram, ultrasonic study, and IV pyelogram, as well as any necessary cardiopulmonary studies, can be performed. Not uncommonly, a so-called typical attack of cholecystitis turns out to be no more than a right kidney stone, or an unresolved basilar pneumonia, or even a myocardial infarction with anginal pain. (See Differential Diagnosis of R.U.Q. pain). As it happens, the antibiotics administered during the acute attack are most likely to have a beneficial effect upon the patient. During an acute attack of cholecystitis, antibiotics are given. If after 24 hours the fever has not subsided and the patient still has pain and tenderness, the dosage may be increased for another 24 hours. If after 48 hours the pain and tenderness still persist and no mass can be palpated in a patient who is not worsening clinically, the writer supplements a cephalosporin with an aminoglycoside for another 24 hours. If the patient still fails to respond and appears clinically worse, it is then felt that the infection has been given an adequate chance to subside, and immediate surgery is recommended. To treat a nonresponsive acute cholecystitis with antibiotics for more than 72 hours is to gamble. Most antibiotics act similarly against the usual biliary organisms and therefore, to change to new antibiotics and delay for an additional 24 hours of medical treatment merely endangers the patient by going beyond the ideal time for surgical intervention.

Glenn and Jaffee[5] studied 266 patients who underwent cholecystectomy for benign biliary tract disease. They concluded that not all patients undergoing biliary surgery should be placed on antibiotics because of the possible development of resistant strains. They believe that the patients at risk are those with acute cholecystitis, choledocholithiasis, a history of jaundice, cholangitis, a recent bout of acute cholecystitis, and those over 60 years of age. They state that diabetes mellitus is still an equivocal risk factor and is subject to the surgeon's judgment. (See-Cholecystitis in the Diabetic.) All the above-listed situations call for prophylactic antibiotics. The major bacteria found in infected bile are *Escherichia coli*, enterococcus, and *Streptococcus viridans*. First-generation cephalosporins are a sound first choice in prophylaxis. In septic patients, antibiotics should cover every organism cultured.

The incidence of cholecystectomy wound infections among Glenn and Jaffee's 266 patients was 3.4%; in acute cholecystitis it was 8%; in chronic cholecystitis it was 2.5%; where the common duct was opened and explored, it rose to 5.7%. When Glenn and Jaffee studied the cholecystectomy patients who received antibiotics, they referred to five different studies: Keighley et al[6,7] reported 21% wound infections without antibiotics; Chetlin and Elliott[3,4] reported 11%; Stone et al[8-11] reported 11%; Strachan et al[12] reported 17%; and Halsall et al[13] reported 5%.

The same researchers reported on similar types of cholecystectomy patients who received prophylactic antibiotics. Keighley et al, who used gentamicin, reported 6% wound infections; Chetlin et al who used cephaloridine, reported 4% wound infections; Stone et al who used cefazolin, reported 2% wound infections; Strachan et al, who used cefazolin, reported 4% wound infections; and Halsall et al, who used metronidazole, reported 7% wound infections.

The presence of bacteria within the biliary tract determines the risk of postoperative infections and the complications that ensue. As a rule, the normal biliary tract is sterile, but in cholecystectomy patients in whom bile studies were carried out, bacteria were isolated in 20–50%. In acute cholecystitis, bacteria were found in the bile in 50–74%. Where common bile duct exploration was carried out, the bacterial cultures showed positive in 58–90%. In a group of 70-year-old patients, bacteria in the bile (bacteriobilia) was found in 50–72%. In patients below 60 years of age who had chronic cholecystitis, the incidence of bacteriobilia was 18%.

Patients in whom anaerobic organisms were found comprised up to two-thirds of the total. *Proteus* and *Pseudomonas* species were commonly found. As anaerobic culturing improved, a greater number of anaerobic organisms were found. Older studies had revealed 0–16% anaerobes; more recent studies have increased this finding to 21–39%. Glenn and Jaffee recommend an antibiotic that covers the organisms commonly found in the bile of cholecystectomy patients, i.e., cephalosporins, ampicillin, mezlocillin, and piperacillin; aminoglycosides, though excreted slowly, have been used successfully. There is an increased incidence of bacteria in the draining bile where choledochotomy and T-tube placement are carried out despite the use of antibiotics. *This suggests that antibiotics that will give a higher blood serum level are more important in preventing bacterial growth.* Stone et al believes that a single dose of a third-generation cephalosporin, i.e., cefoperazone, moxalactam, or cefotaxime, is useful for prophylaxis in abdominal and gynecological cases.

This author again emphasizes that, in his experience, the preoperative (IM or IV) administration of an appropriate antibiotic and its continued employment during surgery and for 24–48 hours postoperatively has reduced infections in the urinary bladder, lung, and operative wound.

Liver

In liver injuries, this writer finds it safer to administer antibiotics preoperatively. It is conceivable that in blunt and sharp injuries to the abdomen, more than liver laceration may occur. It is possible that bowel, duodenum, and/or part of the biliary tract are concomitantly involved, and the surgeon would be remiss not to institute antibiotics preoperatively. If during an exploration of the abdomen the liver alone is found to be injured, the antibiotic should be administered for at least 1 additional day before being discontinued. Where bleeding from the liver is severe and the hepatic artery requires ligation, it is much safer to administer selected antibiotics in order to prevent possible infection in an ischemic and necrotic liver. Numerous investigators have reported ligation of the hepatic artery without antibiotic use and without infection; fortunately, there are more conservative surgeons who prefer to employ antibiotics prophylactically. This writer feels that it is much safer and more prudent to continue with antibiotics once they are started before surgery.

In regard to penetrating wounds of the abdomen, immediate preoperative administration of a selected antibiotic is mandatory. Some surgeons make a distinction between blunt and penetrating injury and give a preoperative antibiotic only for penetrating wounds. In blunt injuries, they choose not to give routine antibiotics because they may not be necessary. *This writer gives all patients with injuries (blunt and penetrating) in whom laparotomy appears to be indicated a select antibiotic. If at surgery the bowel or biliary tract is found to be lacerated, an additional antibiotic is given and continued into the postoperative period.* In other words, if a patient requires early surgical intervention (as a result of blunt or sharp injury), this writer routinely starts antibiotics preoperatively; and if at surgery no hollow organ is involved, he discontinues the antibiotic after 1 day.

If subdiaphragmatic free air is found on the flat plate, an antibiotic is started immediately and continued into the postoperative period. There should be no guesswork preoperatively as to whether the gastrointestinal tract is secondarily involved; *the diagnosis must be positively established or ruled out at surgery.*

In those instances where blunt injury has occurred and no surgery is indicated, antibiotics need not be started. If during the observation period the patient's condition worsens and disruption of a hollow organ (duodenum, intestine, or colon) is suspected or recognized, and no antibiotic was given before surgery, an appropriate antibiotic should be ordered immediately and given by IV push. *Late administration of antibiotic therapy is not ideal, but it is better than no antibiotic at all;* a maximal dosage is advised in late-start situations and should be carried into the postoperative period.

Most patients with lacerations or capsular disruptions develop intraperitoneal hemorrhage and require surgical intervention. *There are a number of less significant liver injuries, such as small capsular tears or subcapsular hematomas, that do not necessarily require immediate surgery. These cases can usually be identified with radioisotope liver scans and treated conservatively.* These patients may require blood transfusion, first aid treatment of associated wounds, bed rest, IV fluids with electrolytes, nasogastric decompression, and *broad-spectrum antibiotics as a prophylactic measure.*

This writer has had good results with antibiotics prophylactically placed directly into the skin wound and has never regretted inserting antibiotics into a local site of infection. In instances of acute cholecystitis where no spillage of bile has occurred, this writer still prefers the systemic use of antibiotics. Where spillage of contaminated bile takes place in the liver bed, local use of antibiotics has proven beneficial. Irrigations with saline solution alone have not impressed this writer. *There are instances of excessive spillage within the retroduodenal area that call for effective irrigation, but a ritual of routine irrigation at the close of surgery is not considered beneficial and therefore not recommended.* The writer warns against the local use of irrigations in which aminoglycosides, i.e., gentamicin or amikacin, are employed. There is a real danger of neuromuscular blockage. If aminoglycosides are indicated, the systemic route is recommended.

Drainage in Cholecystectomy

Most surgeons still debate the pros and cons of routine drainage after cholecystectomy without considering the most important reason for this procedure. Some surgeons reason that spillage of infected bile during surgery calls for drainage; others fear the continued bile leakage that may take place postoperatively from the numerous unseen but opened biliary canaliculi in the liver bed. Infected bile may be a source of postoperative infection complicated by subdiaphragmatic and/or subhepatic abscesses. *This writer emphasizes that bile leakage from the liver bed, cystic duct stump, or choledochoduodenostomy site—whether or not infected—may create a chemical peritonitis resistant to all antibiotics; only proper drainage will do. This is the main reason for routinely draining the liver bed (Morison's fossa).* To do a cholecystectomy without drainage is mere grandstanding; it offers no benefit and encourages potential postoperative complications and possible disaster. In his 40 years of surgical experience, this writer has dealt with the question of drainage over and over again. He has seen it buried and exhumed, only to be properly buried once more. It is time to bury it peacefully again. There are surgeons, who instead of using a Penrose drain in the right upper quadrant, prefer to use closed drainage; they employ a constant suction like a sump drain, or a Jackson-Pratt continuous drainage. There are hard and semihard sump drains, soft silicone drains, and various forms of suction drains. This writer prefers a Penrose drain with a wick, but feels that whatever drain is used is of little consequence. *What is important is that a drain be routinely employed after every biliary procedure—for safety considerations.*

When selecting the antibiotic best suited to gallbladder microorganisms, should one choose the antibiotic most effective against the bacterial flora per se, or should one be more concerned with the one that produces a higher concentration in the bile and tissues? *This writer feels that the most important consideration is the blood concentration of the antibiotic; whether it has a higher concentration in the bile is probably less important.* It would seem that the effective distribution of the antibiotic throughout the body tissues should be of greater importance. The ideal antibiotic should therefore be the one that is best suited to the microorganisms common to the biliary and gastrointestinal tracts and that gives the highest blood level and the greatest possible concentration in the bile. And, while considering the antibiotic concentration in the wound, let us not forget that 40 years ago, without the aid of antibiotics and sulfa drugs, we attained clean wounds and a surprisingly low level of postoperative infections. We attributed our excellent results to definitive and fast but fastidious surgery, a minimum of crush to the tissues, and strict aseptic technique. We have an unwritten rule, which is, "Don't paw the skin"—or "Hands off—unless needed." Here is where I recommend the use of the incise drape.

It should be clear that the employment of prophylactic antibiotics in surgery is no substitute for good anatomical surgical technique. One must not forget that in the preantibiotic period, good surgical technique, noncrushing instrumentation, minimal wound exposure, gentle handling of tissues, and respect for tissue vascularity successfully concluded many operations without postoperative infections. *It is therefore imperative that we not abandon the hardlearned surgical principles and lessons of the past 75 years and employ antibiotics only as a supplement to good* *sound surgical judgment and fastidious surgical technique.*

Recommended Reading

England DM, Rosenblatt JE: Anaerobes in human biliary tracts. *J Clin Microbiol* 6:494, 1977.

Finegold SM: Anaerobes in biliary tract infection. *Arch Intern Med* 139:1338, 1979.

Fukunaga FH: Gallbladder bacteriology, histology, and gallstones. *Arch Surg* 106:169, 1973.

Hinchey EJ, Couper CE: Acute obstructive suppurative cholangitis. *Am J Surg* 117:62, 1969.

Longmire WP: Suppurative cholangitis, in Hardy JD (ed): *Critical Surgical Illness*. Philadelphia, WB Saunders Co, 1971, pp 397–424.

Lou MA, Mandal AK, Alexander JL, et al: Bacteriology of the human biliary tract and the duodenum. *Arch Surg* 112:965, 1977.

Lykkegard-Nielsen M, Justesen T: Anaerobic and aerobic bacteriological studies in biliary tract disease. *Scand J Gastroenterol* 11:437, 1976.

Maddocks AC, Hilson GRF, Taylor R: The bacteriology of the obstructed biliary tree. *Ann R Coll Surg Engl* 52:316, 1973.

Mason GR: Bacteriology and antibiotic selection in biliary surgery. *Arch Surg* 97:533, 1968.

Paul MG, Jaffee SN: Bacteria in the biliary tract. *Contemp Surg* 27: 1985.

Pitt HA, Postier RG, Cameron JL: Biliary bacteria: Significance and alterations after antibiotic therapy. *Arch Surg* 117:445, 1982.

Reynolds BM, Dargan EL: Acute obstructive cholangitis, a distinct clinical syndrome. *Ann Surg* 150:299, 1959.

Welch JP, Donaldson GA: The urgency of diagnosis and surgical treatment of acute suppurative cholangitis. *Am J Surg* 131:527, 1976.

References

1. Gunn AA: Prophylactic use of antibiotics in common duct dilatations. *Br Med J Surg* 13:248, 1976.
2. Chetlin SH: Bacteriology of calculous cholecystitis. *Int J Surg* 58:169, 1973.
3. Chetlin SH, Elliott DW: Biliary bacteremia. *Arch Surg* 102:303, 1971.
4. Chetlin SH, Elliott DW: Preoperative antibiotics in biliary surgery. *Arch Surg* 107:319, 1973.
5. Glenn PM, Jaffee SN: Bacteria in biliary surgery. *Contemp Surg* 27:1, 1985.
6. Keighley MRB, Drysdale RB, Quoraishi AH, et al: Antibiotic treatment of biliary sepsis. *Surg Clin North Am* 55:1379, 1975.
7. Keighley MRB, McLeish AR, Bishop HM, et al: Identification of the presence and type of biliary microflora by immediate gram stains. *Surgery* 81:469, 1977.
8. Stone HH, Hooper CA, Kolb LD, et al: Antibiotic prophylaxis in gastric, biliary and colonic surgery. *Ann Surg* 63:528, 1976.
9. Stone HH: Basic principles in the use of prophylactic antibiotics. *J Antimicrob Chemother* suppl B, p 33, 1986.

10. Stone HH, Haney BB, Kolb LD, et al: Prophylactic and preventive antibiotic therapy. *Ann Surg* 189(6):691, 1979.
11. Stone HH, et al: Reliability of criteria for predicting persistent or recurrent sepsis. *Arch Surg* 120:17, 1985.
12. Strachan CJL, Black J, Powis SJA, et al: Prophylactic use of cephazolin against wound sepsis after cholecystectomy. *Br Med J* 1:1254, 1976.
13. Halsall AK, Welsh CL, Craven JL, et al: Prophylactic use of metronidazole in preventing wound sepsis after elective cholecystectomy. *Br J Surg* 67:551, 1980.
14. Wilson et al: Comparison of prophylactic use of cephalosporin versus cefotetan. *Surg Gynecol Obstet* 1987.
15. Ratzen KR: Chief, Dept of Infectious Disease, Mt Sinai Medical Center, Miami Beach, Fla., personal communication.
16. Condon RE: Most frequently isolated hospital-acquired bacteria on a surgical service. *Surgical Practice News* 1986.

When to Discontinue the Use of Antibiotics

Stone[1] reviewed 2,567 patients who were on antibiotic therapy for various surgical infections. Special attention was given to the patient's red blood cell count, kidney and liver function tests, arterial blood gases, and clotting factors at the end of IV therapy on the date of discharge. After the antibiotics were discontinued, sepsis recurred in 19% of the patients who still had a normal rectal temperature; in 3% of these patients the temperature and white blood cell count were normal. None of the patients with a normal temperature and normal white blood cell count had a granulocyte count of less than 73% and an immature cell count of less than 3%.

It is well known that heavy dosages of antibiotics can lower the temperature to normal, yet have no effect on the white blood cell count or the infection. Surgeons undoubtedly have employed the criteria of normal temperature and normal white blood count before discontinuing antibiotic therapy. In view of Stone's research, this author strongly recommends that a drop in the granulocyte count, as well as in the immature cell count, should also be looked for before discontinuing antibiotics and discharging the patient.

References

1. Stone HH: Reliability of criteria for predicting persistent or recurrent sepsis. *Arch Surg* 120:17, 1985.

2. Stone HH: Basic principles in the use of prophylactic and preventative antibiotic therapy. *Ann Surg* 189:691, 1979.

Economic Considerations in Comparing the Cost Effectiveness of Antibiotics

Wilson et al.[1] in March 1987 compared the prophylactic preoperative use of cefamandole (a second-generation cephalosporin) with cefotetan (a third-generation cephalosporin) in biliary cases. Antibiotics were given at the induction of anesthesia and repeated 3 hours later. Two groups of patients were studied.

The most prevalent bacteria isolated from aerobic and anaerobic cultures made from bile and gallbladder wall were *E. coli*, *Streptococcus*, and *Klebsiella*. The incidence of bactibilia from either culture was 75% in cancer, 69% in patients 65 years of age and over, 33% in jaundice, 58% in pancreatitis, 60% in common bile duct exploration, and 22% in cholecystitis.

Microbiological agar diffusion assays of tissue from the wall of the gallbladder, subcutaneous fat, rectus muscle, and samples of bile and serum 30 minutes after the second dose of antibiotic showed a substantially significant greater concentration of cefamandole in the gallbladder wall. Otherwise there was no difference. Wound infections, urinary infections, hospital stay, intensive care unit stay, and readmissions after 1 month showed no special advantage of one antibiotic over the other. *Wilson et al. concluded that the more expensive cefotaxime provided no advantage in biliary surgical prophylaxis when compared with the less expensive cefamandole.* Obviously the savings over a period of time can be considerable.

Kenneth R. Ratzen,[2] chief of the Division of Infectious Diseases at the Mount Sinai Medical Center in Miami Beach, Florida, reporting on the antimicrobial sensitivity patterns of most organisms responsible for hospital-acquired infections, stated that the strains of *Enterobacter*, *E. coli*, *Klebsiella*, *Proteus*, *Pseudomonas*, and *Serratia* continue to be sensitive to tobramycin and gentamicin. In these infections, Ratzen recommends the exclusive use of gentamicin because it is far cheaper than tobramycin and results in a considerable financial saving. When Ratzen compared the relative costs of tobramycin, 80 mg, given three times daily at a cost of $0.23 per dose, with gentamicin, 80 mg, given three times daily at a cost of $5.22 per dose, he found that after 10 days of hospital therapy, the cost was $182.40 for tobramycin compared to $32.70 for gentamicin—a difference of over 500%.

Recommended Reading

England DM, Rosenblatt JE: Anaerobes in human biliary tracts. *J Clin Microbiol* 6:494, 1977.

Finegold SM: Anaerobes in biliary tract infection. *Arch Intern Med* 139:1338, 1979.

Fukunaga FH: Gallbladder bacteriology, histology, and gallstones. *Arch Surg* 106:169, 1973.

Hinchey EJ, Couper CE: Acute obstructive suppurative cholangitis. *Am J Surg* 117:62, 1969.

Longmire WP: Suppurative cholangitis, in Hardy JD (ed): *Critical Surgical Illness.* Philadelphia, WB Saunders Co, 1971, pp 397–424.

Lou MA, Mandal AK, Alexander JL, et al: Bacteriology of the human biliary tract and the duodenum. *Arch Surg* 112:965, 1977.

Lykkegard-Nielsen M, Justesen T: Anaerobic and aerobic bacteriological studies in biliary tract disease. *Scand J Gastroenterol* 11:437, 1976.

Maddocks AC, Hilson GRF, Taylor R: The bacteriology of the obstructed biliary tree. *Ann R Coll Surg Engl* 52:316, 1973.

Mason GR: Bacteriology and antibiotic selection in biliary surgery. *Arch Surg* 97:533, 1968.

Paul MG, Jaffee SN: Bacteria in the biliary tract. *Contemp Surg* 27: 1985.

Pitt HA, Postier RG, Cameron JL: Biliary bacteria: Significance and alterations after antibiotic therapy. *Arch Surg* 117:445, 1982.

Reynolds BM, Dargan EL: Acute obstructive cholangitis, a distinct clinical syndrome. *Ann Surg* 150:299, 1959.

Welch JP, Donaldson GA: The urgency of diagnosis and surgical treatment of acute suppurative cholangitis. *Am J Surg* 131:527, 1976.

References

1. Wilson, Comparison of prophylactic use of cephalosporin versus cefatamine. *Surg Gynecol Obstet* 1987.

2. Ratzen KR: Personal Communication.

3. Condon RE: Activity of selected antibiotics against the most common surgical pathogens. *Surg Pract News,* Nov 1986.

Author's Routine Antibiotic Schedule

Nature of Surgery	Suspected Organisms	Recommended Antibiotic	Preoperative Dosage
Biliary tract (patients with suspect contamination)	Enteric gram-negative bacilli	Cephalosporins, ie: Cefoxitin, (Mefoxin)	1 g q6h
	Group D streptococci	Ampicillin	1 g q4h
		Gentamicin (Garamicin)	1.5 mg/kg q8h IM
Biliary–Intestinal Anastomotic Procedures	Enteric gram-negative bacilli, anaerobic bacteria, group D streptococci	Cephalosporin (Mandol, Mefoxin, Cefotan)	1 g q4–8h IV and IM
		Ampicillin	1 g q4h IV
		Gentamicin (Garamicin)	1.5 mg/kg q8h IM
		Cleomycin (for anaerobic organisms, i.e. *Bacteroides*)	600 mg q8h IV
		Chloramphenicol (Chloromycetin) when absolutely indicated	50 mg/kg daily IV—not IM. May be increased in resistant cases to 100 mg/kg daily, then reduced rapidly. *Stop* if leukocyte count drops
		Recommended daily complete blood count	
Gallbladder perforation or rupture	Same	Same	Same

Activity of Selected Antibiotics Against the Most Common Surgical Pathogens

	S. aureus	E. coli	Enterococci	Klebsiella	Pseudomonas	Serratia	Anaerobes
Cephalosporins							
First Generation							
Cephalothin							
(Keflin, Seffin)	2	1	0	1	0	0	0
Cefazolin							
(Ancef, Kefzol)	2	1	0	1	0	0	0
Second Generation							
Cefamandole							
(Mandol)	1	2	0	2	0	0	CV
Cefonicid (Monocid)	1	2	0	2	0	0	CV
Ceforanide (Precef)	1	2	0	2	0	0	CV
Cefuroxime (Zinacef, Kefurox)	1	2	0	2	0	0	CV
Cefoxitin (Mefoxin)	1	1	0	1	0	0	2
Cefotetan (Cefotan)	1	1	0	1	0	0	2
Third Generation							
Cefotaxime (Claforan)	1	3	0	3	2/1	2/1	CV
Ceftizoxime (Cefizox)	1	3	0	3	2/1	2/1	CV
Ceftriaxone (Rocephin)	1	3	0	3	2/1	2/1	CV
Cefoperazone (Cefobid)	1	2	0	2	2/1	2/1	CV
Ceftazidime (Fortaz,							
Tazidime, Tazicef)	1	3	0	3	2/3	2/3	CV
Moxalactam (Moxam)	1	3	0	3	1/2	1/2	2
Antipseudomonal penicillins							
Azlocillin (Azlin)	1	2	2	1	3	1	2
Carbenicillin (Geopen)	1	2	0	1	2	2	2
Mezlocillin (Mezlin)	1	2	2	2	2	2	2
Piperacillin (Pipracil)	1	2	2	2	3	2	2
Ticarcillin (Ticar)	1	2	0	0	2	2	2
Antipseudomonal pencillins with beta-lactamase inhibitors							
Amoxicillin/K clavulanate							
(Augmentin)	2	2	3	2	0	0	0
Ticarcillin/K clavulanate							
(Timentin)	1	2	0	2	2	2	2
Monobactam							
Aztreonam (Azactam)*	0	2	0	2	2	2	0
Carbapenem							
Imipenem/cilastatin							
(Primaxin)®	2	2	0	2	2	2	2

*Released in 1987.

Source: Robert E. Condon, M.D., M.S., F.A.C.S.

Most Frequently Isolated Hospital-Acquired Bacteria on Surgical Services (14,596 isolates)

Pathogen	Incidence (%)	Pathogen	Incidence (%)
E. coli	16.2	Candida spp.	4.9
P. aeruginosa	13.0	Serratia spp.	2.0
Enterococci	10.5	Other fungi	1.5
S. aureus	10.4	Citrobacter spp.	1.5
Enterobacter spp.	7.5	Bacteroides spp.	1.4
Klebsiella spp.	6.9	Group B streptococci	0.5
Coagulase-negative staphylococci	6.1	Other anaerobes	0.9
Proteus spp.	5.4	All other	10.4

Data obtained from 51 reporting hospitals: 20 nonteaching, both small and large (39%), 18 small (less than 500 beds) teaching hospitals (35%), 13 large teaching hospitals (26%).

16

NEOPLASMS OF THE BILIARY TRACT

Carcinoma of the Gallbladder

INCIDENCE

Cancer of the biliary tract system is relatively uncommon, but when it does occur, it is most serious and carries with it a high mortality. Carcinoma of the gallbladder usually occurs in the middle and later age groups. The incidence of neoplasia of the biliary tract system in patients under 50 is approximately 0.5%, rising in patients over this age. The surgeon must remain alert to the fact that carcinoma in older patients is a distinct possibility that must not be overlooked. The commonest site for carcinoma in the biliary system is the gallbladder, followed by the biliary tree. Carcinoma of the biliary tract system is usually found at the sites of bifurcation and, more commonly, at the hepatic duct bifurcation or cystic duct junction with the common duct. Another not infrequent site is where the head of the pancreas joins with the duodenum. The frequency of gallbladder disease is distinctly greater in women than in men (about 3:1), as is the incidence of carcinoma. In the writer's experience and that of others, gallstones are present in about 80–90% of the gallbladders with carcinoma. It is only natural to say that stones appear to be the precursor to neoplasia of the gallbladder, yet others believe that the coexistence of cholelithiasis and carcinoma is merely coincidental. Most likely there is a relationship between the long-standing chronic irritation of gallstones and neoplasia of the gallbladder. This writer has often found stones associated with carcinoma of the gallbladder where the stones were unduly sharp (star-shaped with sharp points), suggesting continuous irritation. Race and demographic factors are also involved in the incidence of cholecystitis, cholelithiasis, and carcinoma of the gallbladder.

In 1970, Arminski's[1] collective study of 46,480 biliary operations revealed carcinoma of the gallbladder in 569, an incidence of 1.12%. Gallbladder carcinoma in the United States is ranked as the fifth most frequent carcinoma of the gastrointestinal tract. In a 10-year study (1958–68), Arminski reported that out of 4,000 cholecystectomies, 41 cases of carcinoma of the gallbladder were discovered, an incidence of 1%.

There is a high incidence of carcinoma of the gallbladder in women over 60, especially in American women and in Mexican and Japanese women who have lived in America.

Carcinoma of the gallbladder is extremely rare in the Banti population. In the southwestern American Indian tribes, the incidence of cholelithiasis is extremely high, and carcinoma of the gallbladder has been found to be the most frequent malignancy at autopsy.

The All India Institute of Medical Sciences in New Delhi[2] reported that there is a greater frequency of gallbladder disease in northern India. Bainton[3] reports that cholecystectomy is on the increase in England, being outnumbered only by appendectomy.

As the number of cases of cholelithiasis rises geographically, it is conceivable, based on comparative statistics, that carcinoma of the gallbladder will rise with it.

SIGNS AND SYMPTOMS

The signs and symptoms of gallbladder cancer may range from none whatsoever (completely silent) to recognizable signs and symptoms that vary in degree and are suggestive of cholecystitis and cholelithiasis. A careful history usually reveals that the signs and symptoms of gallbladder disease have existed for a longer period of time than was thought. One should also remember that the duration of signs and symptoms does not usually indicate the type of tumor present, nor does it always suggest the degree of involvement. Nevertheless, the common symptoms in carcinoma of the gallbladder are pain, jaundice (usually silent), and unexplained weight loss. Gallbladder disease associated with jaundice must always be considered most serious; therefore, carcinoma must first be considered and ruled out in the differential diagnosis. When painless jaundice is present and only carcinoma of the gallbladder can be found, the jaundice usually remains the one strong sign that contraindicates operability. One must keep in mind that where cholelithiasis and carcinoma coexist, stones in the common duct may still be responsible for the jaundice. Therefore, every case must be carefully evaluated on its own merits, and only after a complete evaluation at laparotomy can one venture a final diagnosis and treatment.

Pack et al.[4] reported operating on a patient with carcinoma of the cystic duct that caused cystic duct obstruction with consequent huge enlargement of the gallbladder to 24 × 13 × 11 cm in diameter, weighing 2,050 g (hydrops of the gallbladder). Clinically, this case revealed symptoms of complete and incomplete obstruction for about 2 years. Pathologically, the tumor consisted of columnar epithelium that invaded the muscle wall, but there was no evidence of metastasis. Pack et al. felt that since the tumor was well differentiated and slowly progressive, a good prognosis could be anticipated.

Carcinoma of the cystic duct remnant has previously been reported. In each instance, carcinoma developed years after a diagnosis of gallbladder disease was made. For this reason, the earliest possible cholecystectomy is recommended, with a word of warning: Be sure that the entire gallbladder is removed without leaving gallbladder remnants or an unduly long cystic duct stump.

DIAGNOSIS

As a rule, carcinoma of the gallbladder is usually diagnosed at surgery. Every now and then, one may come across a suggestive picture in the cholecystogram, sonogram, or the IV cholangiogram, but the only factual findings of neoplasm in the gallbladder are discovered at surgery when the surgeon can see, feel, and biopsy the lesion. Signs and symptoms on physical examination, together with the laboratory studies, may indicate nothing more than cholecystitis and cholelithiasis. Many carcinomas of the gallbladder originate in the fundus and body, and, not infrequently, metastasis has occurred earlier and insidiously. By the time gallbladder carcinoma is recognized by the signs, symptoms, and X-ray, significant spread to the liver has already taken place (see Fig. 180). *The carcinoma of the gallbladder is usually removed when cholecystectomy is performed for cholelithiasis; the accidental finding of concomitant carcinoma remains the earliest possible means of discovering its existence. The diagnosis that is essential for a possible cure of carcinoma of the gallbladder is chronic cholelithiasis; therefore, cholecystectomy re-*

mains the most important prophylactic measure available. Therefore, all patients with diagnosed cholelithiasis (silent or symptomatic) should have an elective cholecystectomy, which not only prevents possible jaundice and recurrent acute attacks but remains the only effective means of preventing the development or further growth of carcinoma of the gallbladder. The author is well aware of his radical judgment, and he is also aware that most internists and many surgeons recommend cholecystectomy only when the gallbladder becomes symptomatic with recurrent attacks of pain or colic. Most carcinomas of the gallbladder are adenocarcinomas and, to a lesser extent, anaplastic carcinomas; other types of neoplasms are squamous carcinoma, carcinoid, leiomyosarcoma, and melanoma.

PROGNOSIS

Dr. John W. Braasch,[5] chief of surgery at the Lahey Clinic, at the 1973 spring meeting of the American College of Surgeons, stated that when carcinoma of the gallbladder has not yet invaded the muscularis propria, one can expect a 75% 5-year survival. When a true carcinoma is confined to the mucosa and submucosa, one can expect a 100% 5-year survival. Braasch felt that in most instances of carcinoma of the gallbladder in the aged, the disease is usually advanced, with jaundice, pain, and intrahepatic involvement; in addition, spread to other regions renders surgical therapy hopeless. *When a carcinoma is minimal in its development, such as when discovered accidentally during routine chole-*

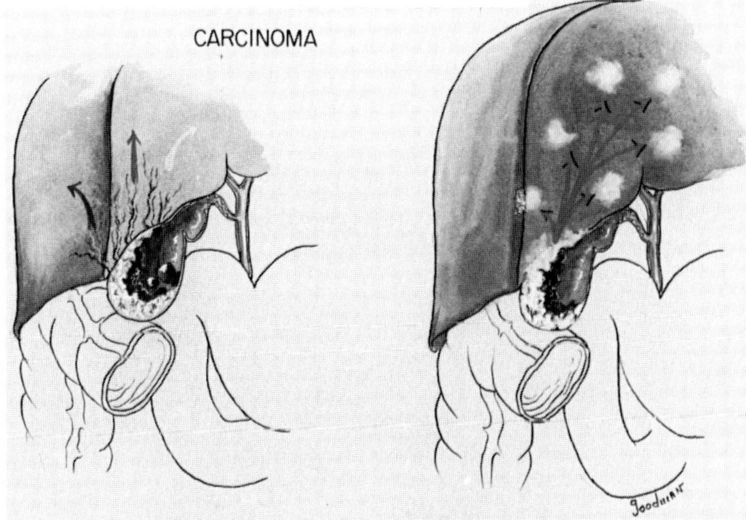

Figure 180. "Silent gallstones in gallbladder with carcinoma. Sequelae: 1. Direct (contiguous) invasion of gallbladder carcinoma into liver. 2. Direct (lymphatic) invasion of gallbladder carcinoma into liver. 3. Direct (venous) invasion of gallbladder carcinoma throughout liver.*

cystectomy, a complete cholecystectomy with removal of an adjacent liver wedge is the procedure of choice today. Braasch was of the opinion that this surgical approach offers a minimal 5-year survival rate. *In advanced carcinoma of the gallbladder, even when treated with cholecystectomy and right hepatic lobectomy, the outlook is bleak.* Braasch has stated, "When considering radical right hepatectomy combined with node dissection, we must recognize that the postoperative mortality and morbidity of these procedures are significant and might outweigh the benefits accrued by this extensive procedure."

J. E. Berk, writing in *Bockus' Gastroenterology,* stresses the statistics of Piehler and Critchlow[6] on survival rates in carcinoma of the gallbladder: 1-year survival, 11.8%; 5-year survival, 2.9%; 262 patients had palliative surgery; survival rate, 0.4%.

TREATMENT

Treatment of carcinoma of the gallbladder is primarily and ideally prophylactic. That is, to prevent clinical carcinoma of the gallbladder is the only cure we know of. Once surgery is undertaken for diagnosed carcinoma of the gallbladder, even in its supposedly early stages, a cure is improbable and, more likely, impossible. *Therefore, the only remaining effective cure for carcinoma of the gallbladder today is an early, complete cholecystectomy in all cases of diagnosed cholecystitis and cholelithiasis. The active treatment of gallbladder carcinoma falls into three classes: (1) Cholecystectomy is routinely performed and a carcinoma is accidentally discovered. This may give the best possible long-term result and the only probability for cure; (2) Carcinoma is suspected and found but early involvement is recognized, i.e., early liver invasion. Here it is possible to consider a cholecystectomy with a reasonable wedge resection of the affected underlying liver.* The possibility of surgically encompassing the whole carcinoma that has already invaded the liver does not exist. The more aggressive surgeon may undertake to establish a cure in the presence of what he may interpret as an early invasive lesion by doing a right lobectomy of the liver. *This writer feels that this procedure is too extensive, and that even though in expert hands it carries with it a reasonably low operative morbidity and mortality, it still provides little possibility of cure or even extended life. This writer feels that in the majority of cases where cholecystectomy is performed, the surgeons, though usually well trained and competent, are not really prepared to proceed with an occasional right hepatic lobectomy. For the more extensive and formidable techniques in advanced liver diseases, the reader is referred to the publications of Thomas Starzl, John Braasch, and Seymour Schwartz, all authorities in this field.*

Therefore, for all practical purposes, cholecystectomy, in which an adequate wedge resection from the contiguous right lobe of the liver is removed, is the best procedure. The patient will most likely benefit, with the least morbidity and mortality and the best possible prognosis. (3) Carcinoma invades the duodenum, pylorus, pancreas, and common bile duct, bringing about gradual but progressive obstructive, painless jaundice. In those instances where no previous gallbladder disease existed and where there is no evidence of a dilated gallbladder, the surgeon should know at once that the gallbladder has not been previously involved with an inflammatory process (see Fig. 181). This type of distended gallbladder (Courvoisier) may be used to bridge over to the jejunum by performing a cholecystojejunostomy and thus relieve the symptoms of obstructive jaundice. The latter procedure is palliative at best; it may, however, provide additional time and comfort to the patient. The writer recommends that this procedure be carried out where feasible and acceptable.

All patients in whom gallbladder disease is suspected, including acalculous gallbladder, where the signs, symptoms, and general appearance of the patient point to cholecystic disease, should receive an exploratory cholecystectomy if confirmed. This is the only positive preventive measure against carcinoma of the gallbladder today. This recommendation is particularly germane to patients over 50 years of age.

References

1. Arminski: Coll. study 46,000 cases (1.12%)
2. All Indian Institute of Medical Science, New Delhi, India
3. Bainton D, Davies GT, Evans KT, et al: Gallbladder disease prevalence in a South Wales industrial town. *N Engl J Med,* vol 294, no 21, 1976.
4. Pack GT, Miller TR, Brasefield RD: Total right hepatic lobectomy for cancer of the gallbladder: report of three cases. *Ann Surg* 142:6, 1955.
5. Braasch JW: Carcinoma of the bile cut. *Surg Clin North Am* 53:1217, 1973.
6. Piehler JM, Critchlow RW: Primary carcinoma of the gallbladder. *Surg Gynecol Obstet* 147:929, 1978.

Treatment of Tumors of the Biliary Tract

The great majority of high-lying carcinomas of the biliary duct system are incurable, and the tumors that are recognized are usually inoperable (or non-

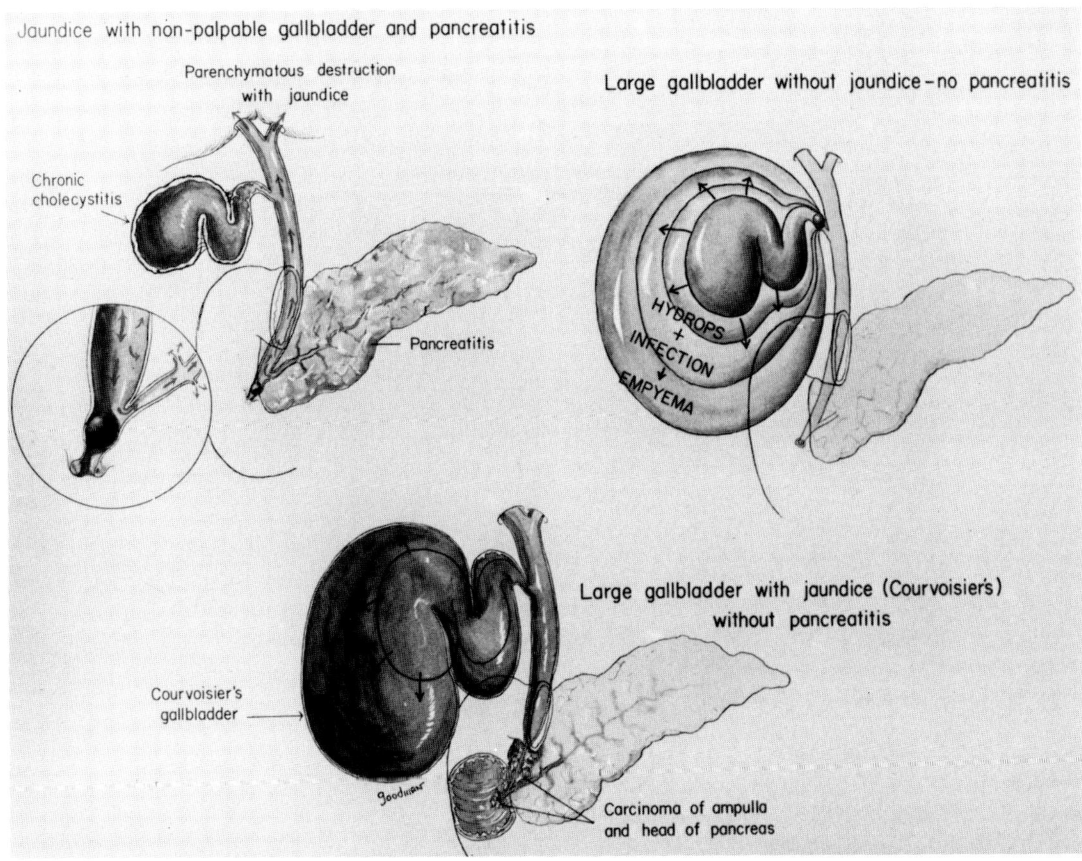

Figure 181.   Demonstrated in these illustrations are three distinct pathological-physiological entities: 1. A stone arrested at the ampulla below the outlet of the duct of Wirsung leads to reflux of bile into the pancreas and subsequent pancreatitis, also possible jaundice. 2. An enlarged gallbladder without jaundice, with or without pain, usually implies cystic duct obstruction, possibly infection and empyema. 3. An enlarged gallbladder with jaundice "silent," usually implies carcinoma of the head of the pancreas (Courvoisier's gallbladder).

resectable). Evaluation of these cancers usually reveal that there is local invasion, sometimes extensive, and often systemic dissemination. Where it is possible to do a hemihepatectomy (right or left), only those with the widest experience in this specialized field should be selected to carry out the surgery. *For the more extensive and formidable techniques in advanced liver diseases, the reader is directed to the publications of Thomas Starzl, John Braasch, and Seymour Schwartz, all authorities in this field.* The inexperienced surgeon, by contrast, must do whatever is safely palliative. If the surgeon feels that a hepatectomy is necessary, he should have someone standing by who can assist him, or take over if necessary and proceed to carry out this formidable procedure, with its well-known high mortality. The resectability rate of carcinomas of the biliary tract is usually 20% or less in expert hands.

The majority of lesions are found in the distal portion of the common bile duct. Here either a limited procedure can be done, such as an end-to-end anastomosis, or, when feasible, a complete pancreaticoduodenectomy (Whipple procedure) can be carried out. This very extensive procedure, which carries a high mortality, should also be done by an experienced surgeon. A relatively low mortality is obtainable only by the most experienced operators. As stated previously, malignancies usually involve the junction sites of the biliary anatomy; at times, it is possible to recognize a small lesion that is totally resectable at the cystic duct level with the common or hepatic duct. When possible, priority should be given to an end-to-end anastomosis and splinting with a T-tube that is brought out either above or below the line of suture. Fig. 182 Parts (1), (2), (3), (4). Otherwise, hepaticojejunostomy should be performed. Any low-lying, resectable tumor of the common duct without evidence of metastasis should be treated with a Whipple procedure.

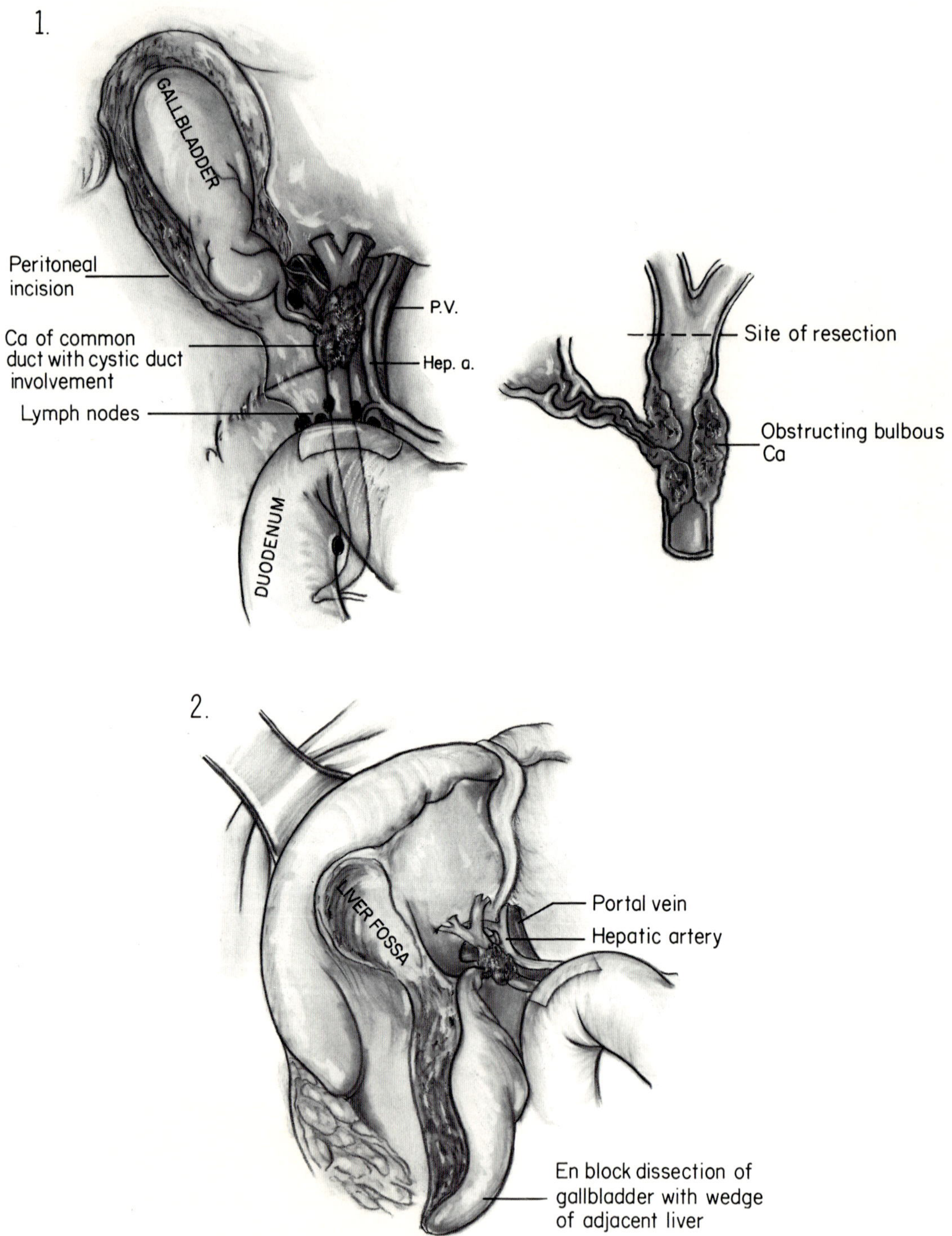

Figure 182.   Part 1: The following diagrams illustrate the technique of dealing with carcinoma of the common bile duct that has invaded the cystic duct. The cross-sectional diagram shows the extent of carcinomatous involvement. The junctional sites of the common duct are most frequently involved with carcinomatous development. Part 2: En-block dissection of gallbladder with wedge of adjacent liver. This diagram shows how the gallbladder is dealt with first. The dissection is carried down to the freed cystic duct. Note that a wedge section of liver was taken down with the gallbladder (an en-bloc dissection). The carcinoma at the cystic junction was widely dissected, taking great care not to infringe upon or damage the Portal vein and Hepatic artery.

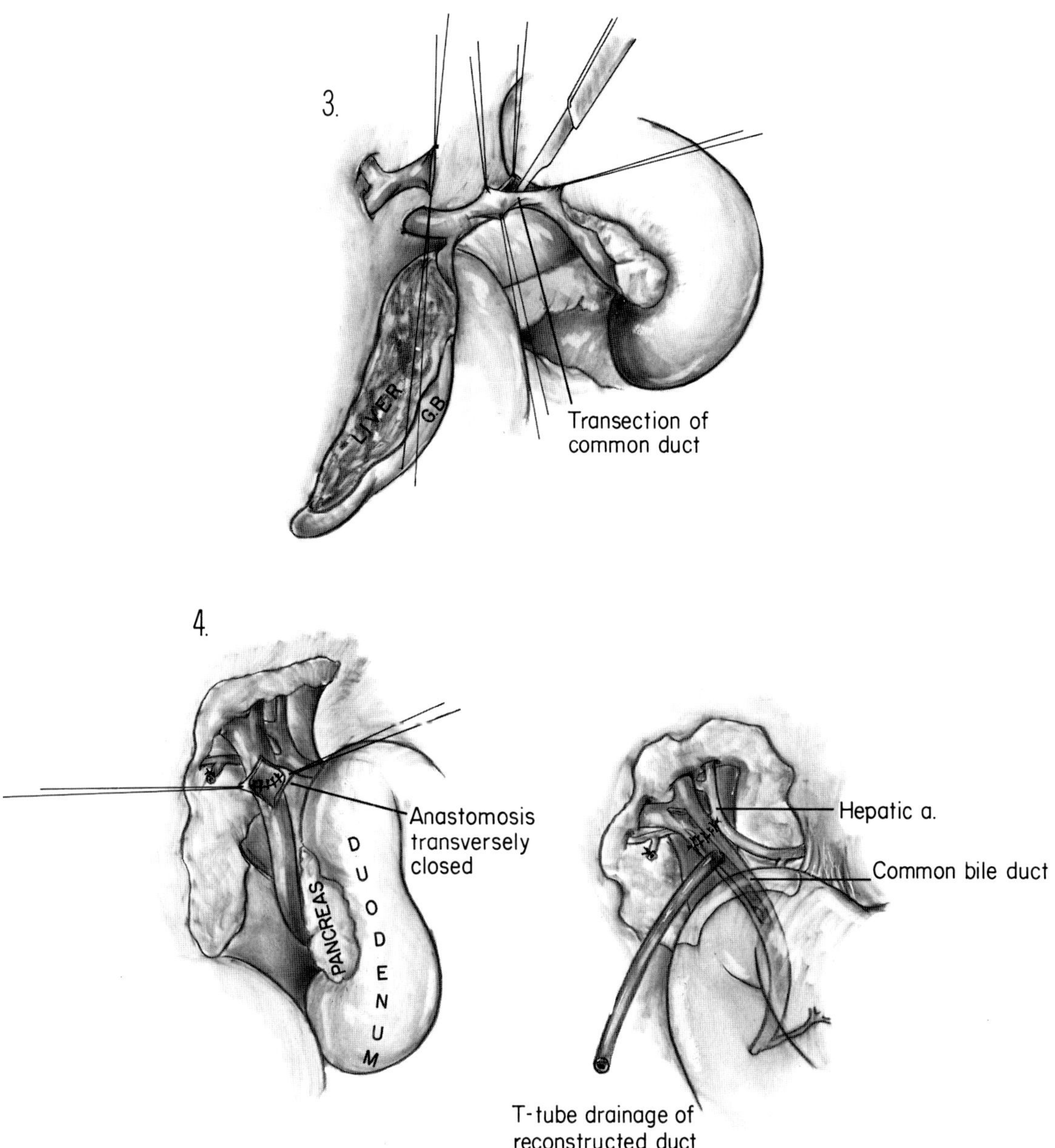

Figure 182.   Part 3: This diagram illustrates the meticulous dissection of the common duct as far down as the normal duct. If there is enough uninvolved common duct, an end-to-end anastomosis can be contemplated. If the common bile duct requires almost complete excision, a choledocho- or hepaticojejunostomy (Roux-en-Y) may be contemplated. Part 4:

An end-to-end anastomosis is performed. The posterior layer is sewn first with interrupted black (4—0) black silk sutures. The T-tube is inserted and brought out through a separate incision below the site of the end-to-end anastomosis. (See Choledochojejunostomy (Roux-en-Y), Chapters 13 and 16.)

PALLIATIVE SURGERY

The surgery required for carcinoma of the biliary tract is too extensive for the occasional surgeon; he should not undertake the procedure on a curative basis. This will only result in an unfortunate complication or mortality. The procedures available for palliation are usually related to the relief of the intense jaundice and its associated itching. As in other places (the esophagus), a tube or stent may be passed through a tumorous area to decompress the biliary system. Permanent decompression, utilizing a T-tube or a catheter properly sewn in place, can serve as a lasting procedure. One should not consider resecting a lobe or a portion of a lobe with a cholecystectomy as a curative operation, since cures in such instances are rare. Therefore, extensive surgery should also be considered palliative. The relief that these patients obtain is worth the effort because these biliary neoplasms are usually slow-growing, and with concomitant therapy (chemotherapy), where indicated and where possible, the rate of tumor growth can be kept to a minimum. The relief of jaundice, of course, is the outstanding feature, because the severe pruritis is maddening. There are surgeons who go so far as to drain the liver with a catheter for palliation; if they can enter one of the dilated biliary radicles, they drain the liver.

At present, this is a philosophical issue; it should be left up to the surgeon, utilizing his experience and judgment in each case. Some surgeons use the long-arm T-tube where there is extensive involvement of the common duct near the pancreas; they first test to see if they can gently dilate the stoma with a probe. They employ a large, long-end T-tube for its palliative value. All procedures requiring hepaticojejunostomy anastomosis, Roux-en-Y, or end-to-side technique, are palliative—not curative. (Figs. 182, 183, 184, 185).

MORBIDITY AND MORTALITY WITH EXTENSIVE BILIARY SURGERY

The results of surgery for biliary tract cancer are generally poor; only a few patients have survived the more extensive procedures. The morbidity and mortality are very high, especially in the radical procedures that involve hepatic lobectomy and pancreaticoduodenectomy. It is possible to reduce this mortality (and it has been reduced), but only when these procedures are carried out by the most experienced surgeons. The widest experience and ideal facilities, together with expert assistance, are

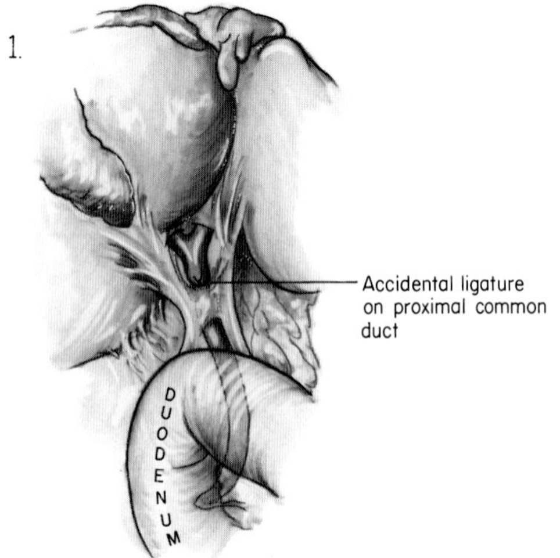

Figure 183. Part 1: When an obstruction results from an inadvertantly placed suture around the common bile duct, the best treatment would be its earliest removal if possible, and the restoration of patency. Where the stitch cannot be removed, the strictured site must be resected and an end-to-end anastomosis carried out. If the inadvertantly placed stitch was placed high up on the common duct, the resection of the strictured site would necessitate a high repair such as a choledochojejunostomy (Roux-en-Y) is illustrated in Figures 185 and 186.

required for the best results. Only when these conditions occur will the mortality and morbidity be significantly reduced. *This writer directs the reader to the publications in advanced and formidable surgical techniques for advanced liver diseases to such authorities as Thomas Starzl, John Braasch, and Seymour Schwartz—all authorities in this field.*

The Lahey Clinic has reported less than a 25% mortality in pancreaticoduodenectomy for carcinoma of the lower portion of the common duct; the New York Hospital has reported an approximately 14% mortality in resectable lesions of the common bile duct (see "The Whipple Operation" and "Modified Whipple Procedures" later in this chapter). There are many pancreaticoduodenectomy patients who survive for 1 to 2 years; some surgeons have even reported 5- and 10-year survivals. Chemotherapy and radiotherapy have thus far been of questionable value, especially in advanced cases. Some claim that with chemotherapy and radiotherapy, definite results have been obtained, but the majority agree that chemotherapy to date has not been the answer to the problem. Chemotherapy via the hepatic duct artery (liver infusion) has also proved to be of limited value.

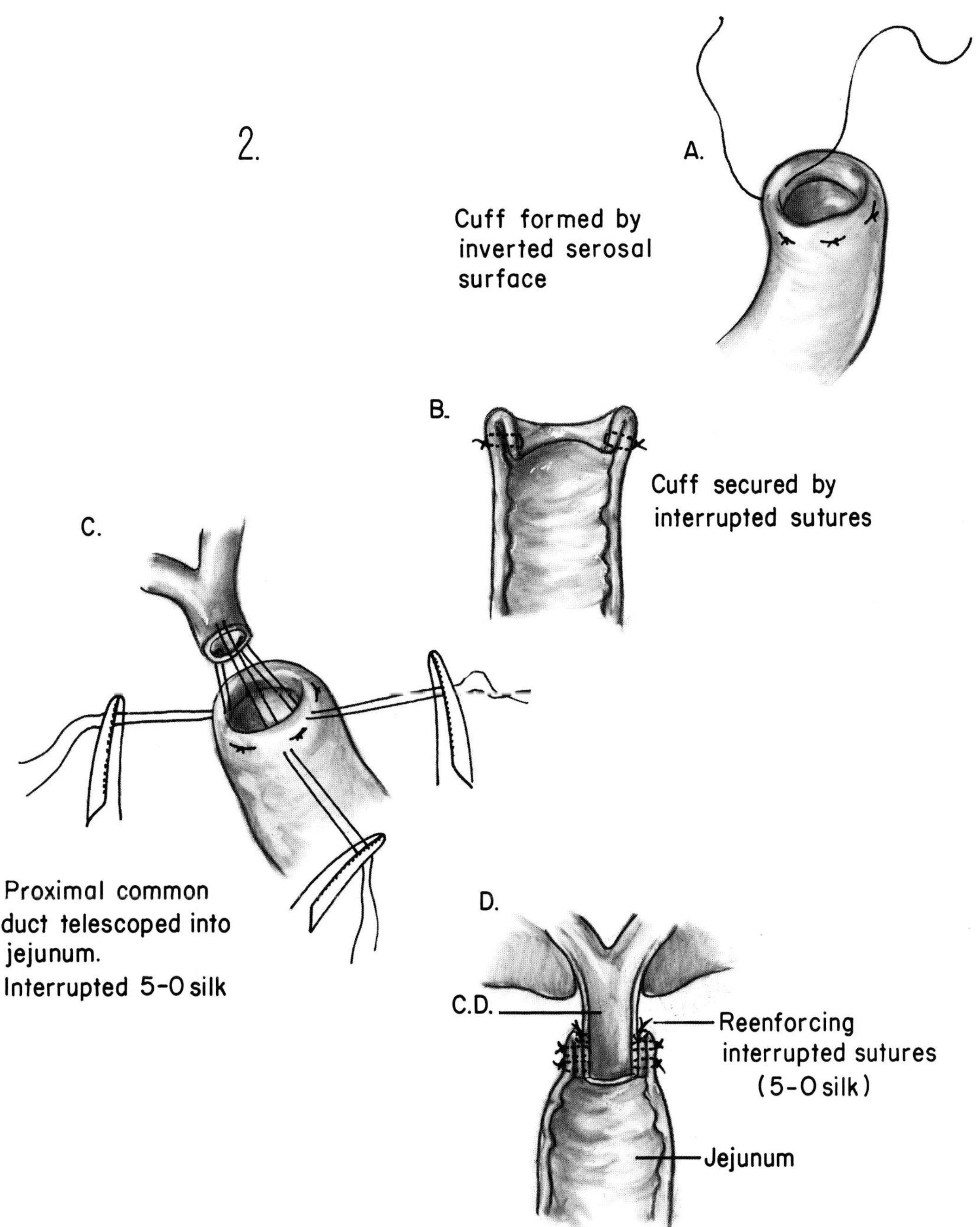

Figure 184.   Part 2: This diagram illustrates the separate steps taken to perform a workable anastomosis between the common hepatic ducts and the jejunum (end-to-end).

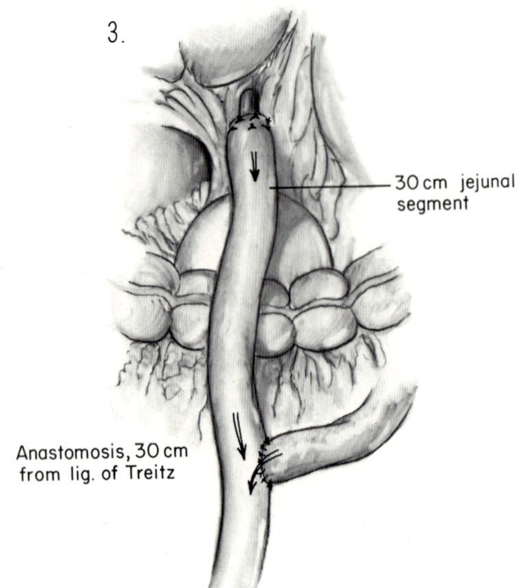

Figure 185. Part 3: The Roux-en-Y Hepaticojejunostomy is completed. This procedure was carried out antecolic.

Recommended Reading

Chandler JJ, Fletcher WS: A clinical study of primary carcinoma of the gallbladder. *Surg Gynecol Obstet* 117:297, 1963.

Donaldson LA, Busuttil A: A clinicopathological review of 68 carcinomas of the gallbladder. *Br J Surg* 62:26, 1974.

Dowdy GS, Olin WG, Shelton EL Jr: Tumors of the extrahepatic bile duct. *Arch Surg* 85:503, 1962.

Gerst PH: Primary carcinoma of the gallbladder, a thirty-year summary. *Am Surg* 153:369, 1961.

Hardy MA, Volk H: Primary carcinoma of the gallbladder. A ten year review. *Am J Surg* 120:800, 1970.

Longmire WP Jr, McArthur MS, Bastounis EA, et al: Carcinoma of the extrahepatic biliary tract. *Ann Surg* 178:333, 1973.

Pemberton LB, Diffenbaugh WF, Strohl EL: The surgical significance of carcinoma of the gallbladder. *Am J Surg* 122:381, 1971.

Ross AP, Braasch JW, Warren KW: Carcinoma of the proximal bile ducts. *Surg Gynecol Obstet* 126:923, 1973.

Sawyer KC: The unrecognized significance of papillomas, polyps and adenomas of the gallbladder. *Am J Surg* 120:570, 1970.

Solan MJ, Jackson BT: Carcinoma of the gall-bladder. A clinical appraisal and review of 57 cases. *Br J Surg* 58:593, 1971.

Strauch GO: Primary carcinoma of the gall bladder. Presentation of seventy cases from the Rhode Island Hospital and a cumulative review of the last ten years of American literature. *Surgery* 47:368, 1960.

Vaittinen E: Carcinoma of the gallbladder. A study of 390 cases diagnosed in Finland, 1953–1967. *Ann Chir Gynecol Fenn* 59(suppl):168, 1970.

Warren KW, Hardy KJ, O'Rourke MGE: Primary neoplasia of the gallbladder. *Surg Gynecol Obstet* 126:1036, 1968.

Weckert A, Roberton B: The natural course of gallstone disease. Eleven-year-review of 781 nonoperated cases. *Gastroenterology* 50:376, 1966.

Carcinoma of the Ampulla of Vater

Carcinoma in the ampullary region of the common bile duct or in the ampulla itself is usually of a medullary or infiltrating type. The most conspicuous manifestation of carcinoma of the ampulla of Vater is a progressively silent jaundice, but this does not always occur. There are cases where pain is also part of the symptom complex. A Courvoisier (dilated) gallbladder does not always accompany ampullary carcinoma or carcinoma of the head of the pancreas, producing biliary obstruction. *Whether a Courvoisier gallbladder develops will depend upon whether or not the gallbladder has been previously inflamed (cholecystitis) with gallstones (cholelithiasis). Failure of the gallbladder to distend usually depends upon a concomitant finding of chronic cholecystitis associated with a thickened, fibrotic gallbladder wall that cannot distend under back pressure. Only the uninvolved or thin, distensible gallbladder can dilate under the gradual back pressure caused by an obstruction at the ampullary site.* In about one-third of the cases, we can expect to find a Courvoisier gallbladder that is large enough to be palpable under the right costal margin. If this is present in association with a silent jaundice, with no reason to suspect the presence of stones, the primary suspicion must be carcinoma of the head of the pancreas or ampulla until this diagnosis is definitely ruled out. This diagnosis can be ruled out either preoperatively, or at surgery.

A very important point is whether the carcinoma arises primarily in the ampulla of Vater or originates in the head of the pancreas, with invasion into the duodenum. The prognosis is much more favorable in carcinoma of the head of the pancreas that invades the lower end of the common bile duct. The diagnosis of the two causes for obstructive jaundice is difficult, but the differentiation should be made, if possible. Cholecystitis and cholelithiasis are often associated with ampullary carcinoma; the latter occurs more frequently in females than in males, but there is a greater frequency of carcinoma of the ampulla of Vater in males.

SIGNS AND SYMPTOMS

Ampullary carcinoma is a very difficult diagnosis to establish in its early stage because of its silent, insidious jaundice, unexplained weight loss, and mild to no gastrointestinal signs or symptoms. If jaundice is intermittent, it may be more difficult to evalute; when pain is present, that too can complicate the early recognition of ampullary carcinoma.

The jaundice becomes progressively intense with time. Under great pressure, the ampulla may necrose and allow the back pressure to overwhelm the lesion, producing a complete release of the bile with sudden relief of the intense jaundice. The relief of sudden jaundice can mislead the surgeon to believe that the stone has passed. The disappearance of intense jaundice must not be interpreted as a positive sign until it has been shown to be unrelated to carcinoma.

Another sign is bleeding from the ampullary tumor. This may be discovered either grossly or on chemical study of the stool. Another sign is unexplained weight loss, which is definitely related to anorexia and the malnutrition that follows. The latter results from poor absorption, since the involvement of the pancreatic duct leads to poor enzymatic digestion. One should look for signs of diabetes because, not infrequently in ampullary carcinoma, there is invasion that involves the pancreatic duct of Wirsung and the back pressure causes pancreatic necrosis, resulting in malfunction of the islets of Langerhan.

So far, the most significant findings are silent jaundice, enlarged (Courvoisier) gallbladder, and an enlarged, palpable liver. Laboratory studies are not very helpful; cholangiography, either orally or by the IV method, is of little value because of the deep jaundice. The pancreatic enzymes may show variations that may cause some suspicion of primary or secondary pancreatic involvement. Upper gastrointestinal studies are sometimes helpful in those cases where the roentgenologist can point out abnormal findings in the duodenal sweep.

Some patients have no fever or chills because cholangitis is not a common accompaniment. However, it may occur, and although it may not be related to the presence of a stone, it is definitely related to the obstructive jaundice at the level of the ampulla. Elevation of enzymes such as alkaline phosphate, lactic dehydrogenase, creatine phosphokinase, lipase, and amylase indicates that there is bile obstruction with associated liver damage, but these tests do not differentiate the type of obstruction or pinpoint the location (see the chart "Differential Diagnosis of Jaundice" in Chapter 6).

Fortunately, today we have additional diagnostic armamentaria which can be used with some benefit. Microscopic studies after duodenal aspiration may indicate that malignant cells are present at the level of the ampulla. A direct biopsy can be taken through a gastroduodenoscope, but this requires a trained endoscopist. The last resort is percutaneous transhepatic cholangiography, which will establish a diagnosis; but when this is done, the surgeon and the operating room personnel must be ready to operate immediately. If bleeding or biliary leakage is suspected, the patient should be explored stat.

PATHOLOGICAL BEHAVIOR

A carcinoma of the ampulla may arise from its own epithelium or, in a few cases, from the duodenal epithelium. Eventually, the lesions appear papillary, involving the entire ampulla of Vater. This lesion usually invades the duodenum, the common duct, and the head of the pancreas. It may also metastasize to the nearby pancreatic nodes. Autopsy figures indicate that this is a slowly metastasizing tumor. This is one of the reasons why radical surgery is more appropriate in carcinoma of the ampulla than in carcinoma of the head of the pancreas. For this reason, this writer prefers to do a radical procedure (Whipple) instead of a local excisional procedure. The radical procedure will offer a higher chance for survival, with a lower percentage of morbidity and mortality. Cattell[1] of the Lahey Clinic found that in about 25% of his cases there was evidence of metastasis. Cohen and Colp of Mount Sinai Hospital in New York reported four cases with no extension of the tumor beyond the borderlines of the lesion. The latter was demonstrated at postmortem. Hirschbaum et al. reported a series of cases of carcinoma of the extrahepatic duct; of 62 cases, 14 were without metastases. A 13% mortality had been reported in their series with bile duct injuries; the complications following surgery were approximately 25%. The main causes of postoperative morbidity were infection, biliary fistulae, and intraperitoneal bleeding.

The commonest causes of death were hepatic failure and ascending cholangitis. The commonest cause of late complications was biliary cirrhosis with liver failure. There were also late cases of portal hypertension associated with esophageal hemorrhage and hepatorenal syndrome with coma. In high-risk patients, mortality rates were based on concomitant preexisting problems, namely, myocardial infarction, renal failure, and cerebrovascular accidents. The very late results of bile duct injury and repair can be evaluated after 2 or 3 years have elapsed. Most surgical failures that develop soon after surgery are commonly related to stenosis of the anastomosis. Whenever end-to-end or end-to-side anastomosis between biliary and intestinal anatomy is carried out, stenosis of the lumen may occur. When biliary stenosis occurs, it is recognized by an ascending cholangitis that soon results in chills and fever, with recurrent bouts of jaundice.

In the first 2 years, the signs and symptoms of jaundice represent the development of a progressive stenosis at the site of anastomosis. As stated before, when a condition seems to be stable and the patient does well for approximately 4 or 5 years, the chance of a very late complication is unusual.

THE WHIPPLE OPERATION: EARLY AND LATER POSTOPERATIVE COMPLICATIONS

Complications that *immediately* follow the Whipple operation are pancreatic fistula and postoperative bleeding (intra- or retroperitoneal). Hemorrhage may also develop at the site of anastomosis, either from the pancreaticojejunostomy or from the choledochojejunostomy.

The *late* complications include postoperative marginal ulceration, especially after an inadequate gastric resection, particularly in those patients with a history of ulcer. Another complication is pancreatic insufficiency based on malabsorption. This condition responds to insulin and pancreatic enzyme supplements. Some surgeons close off the pancreatic duct to prevent the complications that accompany a pancreaticojejunostomy. The latter technique is subject to retention and/or pancreatic pseudocysts, which have to be dealt with at a later stage. Anastomosis of the pancreatic segment with the jejunum will prevent pancreatic insufficiency as well as cyst formation. This writer prefers to do the pancreaticojejunostomy end-to-end; three rows of interrupted (000) or (0000) black silk are used to imbricate or force the pancreatic end portion farther into the mouth of the jejunum. A piece of omentum may be used to help serosalize or seal off the anastomotic site. The complications most often seen by this writer have been retroperitoneal hemorrhage and, less frequently, pancreatic fistula. With the advent of the metal clips, it is now possible to close off many of the small, deep bleeding sites which cannot be reached by clamp or ligature. Clipping has materially decreased the frequency of deep-seated bleeding, especially from the small branches of the superior mesenteric artery that supply the first portion of jejunum.

TREATMENT

Prophylactic Treatment

There is no prophylactic treatment per se for the prevention of ampullary carcinoma. Wherever possible, a routine duodendenotomy should be performed when a suspicious mass is felt in the duodenum. An obstruction of the ampulla of Vater or a mass suggests an impacted stone in the ampulla of Vater or a neoplasm suspicious of ampullary obstruction. The only prophylactic measure is the awareness that carcinoma of the ampulla can behave like a stone. If this is kept in mind, the lesion will most likely be found in its earliest stage, and a radical procedure will then give the best result with the highest percentage of survival.

Active Treatment

The Whipple operation will be described in detail in the next section. It is a pancreaticoduodenal operative procedure which can be accomplished in many ways, depending upon the presenting anatomy, the preferences of the surgeon, and the extent of the pathology. The Whipple operation is the most beneficial palliative measure available. Palliation most often must be accepted because of the local spread of the disease process and the existent metastases. Where a Courvoisier gallbladder is present in a late case, a cholecystojejunostomy bypass is performed to reduce the jaundice and intense itching, as well as to improve the general condition of the patient.

Where it is foreseeable that the growth will in time obstruct the duodenum, it may be wise to perform a gastrojejunostomy as well. Vagotomy may be done at the surgeon's discretion. Because a gastrojejunostomy may lead to marginal ulcerations and hemorrhage, it becomes imperative that every patient be treated postoperatively with cimetidine (Tagamet) antacids, and supplemental enzymes; blood replacement may be required to maintain the longest possible survival.

This writer hesitates to recommend a selective ampullary resection because it is a tedious procedure, fraught with possible error, and gives poor results. Very few cures have ever been reported for localized resection of carcinoma of the ampulla. With morbidity and mortality statistics improving each year, the best procedure, when indicated, is still the Whipple procedure. The earlier the disease process is recognized, the more radical the procedure should be if a cure is to be attained. *The decision to employ local excision of the ampullary lesion should be based on age, condition of the patient, and whether the malignant lesion is localized or invasive.*

PROGNOSIS

The mortality rate for the Whipple procedure throughout the surgical world is 25–35%. The survival rate is far higher when this procedure is performed for early carcinoma of the ampulla of Vater. Patients who survive for 5 years or longer require daily supplemental therapy, of which pancreatic enzyme supplementation is the most important. In cases where enough pancreas exists to supply its own enzymes, supplements are not necessary. Nevertheless, this writer recommends that pancreatic supplements be given routinely in all cases. The presence of diabetes mellitus means that a deficiency of the islets of Langerhan exists, which will vary in severity depending upon how much pancreatic tissue was resected. Insulin may have to be given to the patient who develops diabetes mellitus, possibly for life. Patients who have undergone one or, at most, two reparative procedures attain the best results. Those who have to undergo more than two procedures are more likely to have a diminishing chance of achieving a good result. The success rate declines with the need for multiple surgery. The ideal treatment for postoperative biliary duct stenosis or stricture is the prophylactic surgical skill exercised by a well-trained surgeon. If an accidental biliary injury occurs at operation, the expert surgeon should, under good light, with good assistance and ideal exposure, repair it immediately to attain the best possible result.

MORTALITY

At one time the mortality was 50% or higher, depending upon who did the surgery. Over the years the mortality rate dropped, but mostly in the hands of those who had skill and experience with this operative procedure and complex anatomy. The mortality is well below 15% in certain hands and even lower (5%) in selective cases. Carcinoma of the ampulla has several advantages over carcinoma of the head of the pancreas. Carcinoma of the ampulla, found early, is easier to remove because it is not too invasive and allows easier pancreaticoduodenectomy.

Recommended Reading

Chiappetta A, Sperti C, Bonadenami B, et al: Surgical experience with adenocarcinoma of the ampulla of Vater. *Am Surg* 52:603, 1986.

Reference

1. Cattell, R. Premalignant Lesions of the Ampulla of Vater: Surg., Gynec., Obst. 90:21, 1950

The Whipple Operation

The Whipple operation (total pancreaticoduodenectomy) is a formidable procedure that is reserved for (1) carcinoma of the head of the pancreas, (2) carcinoma of the ampulla of Vater, (3) carcinoma of the lower (duodenal) portion of the common bile duct, (4) carcinoma or fibrosarcoma of the duodenum involving the periampullary area, and (5) certain intractable chronic (alcoholic) pancreatitis.

Many variations of the Whipple operation have been devised, but for the writer, Whipple's one-stage pancreaticoduodenectomy has proven to be most satisfactory. However, there may be certain anatomical variations that will dictate a slight or even more major departure from Whipple's standardized technique (see Fig. 186).

The Whipple technique is as follows:

1. A long midline incision is made from the xiphoid to beyond the umbilicus; it may be enlarged if necessary.

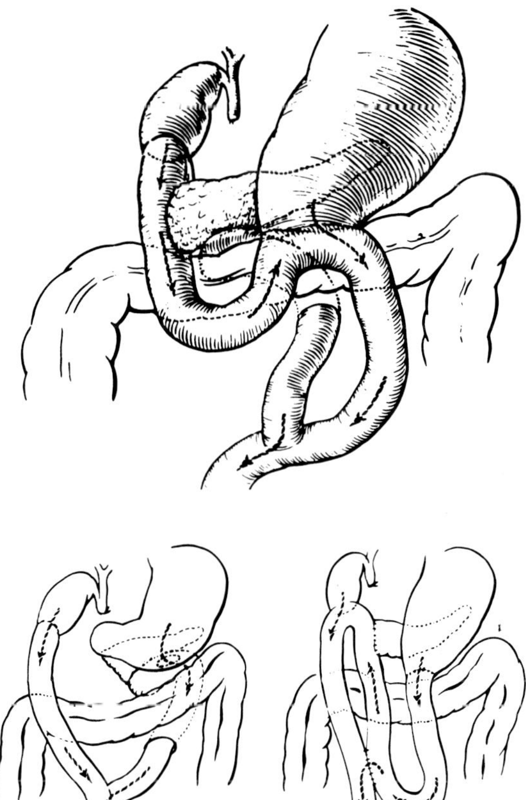

Figure 186. Several common variations of the radical one-stage pancreaticoduodenectomy (Whipple procedure). (With permission from Prestow's CB Surgery of the Biliary Tract, Pancreas and Spleen, Chicago, Year Book Publishers, 1953.)

2. Abdominal exploration is performed (see the discussion of the round-the-clock abdominal exploration in Chapter 10).

3. One must check first for signs of metastasis. Inspect the liver, stomach, spleen, and pancreas. Search for suspected metastatic involvement of the lymph glands; also, check the paravertebral areas and the porta hepatis. Biopsy suspicious tissue and lymph glands. If the pathology report reveals carcinoma without any other evidence of metastasis, the total Whipple procedure may be undertaken. If lymph glands are involved or metastases are recognized, the surgeon must decide against a total pancreaticoduodenectomy and perform a less formidable palliative procedure, such as choledochoduodenostomy (or -jejunostomy). If total resection is feasible, proceed as follows:

4. The gastrocolic omentum is divided between clamps along the distal two-thirds of the stomach; the posterior stomach wall is freed from the underlying pancreas. The Kocher maneuver frees and lifts up the second and third portions of the duodenum by blunt finger dissection. These portions of the duodenum and the head of the pancreas are then mobilized.

5. The first portion of duodenum is freed by dividing the gastrohepatic ligament and ligating the gastroduodenal artery.

6. The common bile duct is ligated distally.

7. The pyloric portion of the stomach is doubly clamped (3 or more inches) proximal to the pyloric sphincter. The duodenum is further dissected distally toward the ligament of Treitz. *The superior mesenteric artery and vein are carefully dissected and elevated from the fourth portion of the duodenum.*

8. Finger dissect the 4th portion of the duodenum as far left as possible.

9. Lift up transverse colon, and locate the ligamentum of Treitz. Pack off the transverse colon and all intestines to clearly expose the duodenojejunal juncture. Now continue the duodenal dissection until it is freed of all its attachments.

10. Check the jejunum and select a site for division several inches distal to the ligamentum of Treitz; also, check the mesentery length that will accommodate elevation of the severed jejunal segment. Suture the open end of the proximal jejunum. To mobilize the proximal jejunal segment completely, divide the mesentery parallel to the bowel. At this point, the duodenum and jejunum are withdrawn from underneath the mesenteric vessels and brought above the transverse mesocolon. Carefully inspect the area for small bleeders, and ligate or clip them.

11. Elevate the stomach and expose the anterior surface of the pancreas. *Elevate the head of the pancreas and carefully dissect it free of the superior mesenteric vessels, portal vein, and splenic vein. Avoid undue rough handling!* The posterior pancreas is mobilized a few inches beyond the intended site of resection.

12. The body of the pancreas is sharply divided, freeing the head and the neck of the pancreas, the entire duodenum and distal common bile duct, the jejunal segment, and the distal portion of the stomach.

13. The covered cut end of the distal jejunum is passed through an opening in the transverse mesocolon and anastomosed to the distal (fresh-cut) end of the common bile duct. Two rows should be used: the first row of continuous fine catgut, the second row of interrupted, nonabsorbable sutures.

14. The cut end of the pancreas is anastomosed to the side of the jejunum about 4 inches distal to the choledochojejunal suture line. Before proceeding with the anastomosis:

   a. Check the patency of the duct of Wirsung with a probe.
   b. The cut end of the body of the pancreas is sewn with interrupted mattress sutures; the stoma of the duct of Wirsung is kept open.
   c. The posterior pancreatic capsule is sutured seromuscularly to the selected site on the jejunum with interrupted nonabsorbable sutures; the duct remains open.
   d. The cut end of the duct of Wirsung is now sewn to an equivalent-sized opening made in the jejunal mucosa. The first layer is of a continuous, fine catgut suture; the second row is of interrupted, fine, nonabsorbable sutures. As a precaution, one end of a fine rubber tube is inserted into the duct of Wirsung and the other into the jejunal lumen. The pancreatic capsule is circumferentially sewn to the seromusculature of the jejunum, using interrupted, nonabsorbable sutures.

15. The divided end of the stomach is now anastomosed to the jejunum at a site distal to the choledochojejunal anastomosis.

16. The gallbladder, if uninvolved, is allowed to remain in case of late stricture formation, when a bypass may be required.

Modified Whipple Procedures

Some acceptable variations in the Whipple procedure will now be discussed.

MODIFICATION 1

1. The cut end of the common bile duct is anastomosed to the cut end of the jejunum, end-to end.
2. The pancreatic cut end is anastomosed to the jejunum at a site distal to the choledochojejunostomy.
3. The retrocolic gastrojejunostomy is placed distal to the pancreatic entrance into the jejunum.

MODIFICATION 2

1. The cut end of the common bile duct is anastomosed to the side of a loop of jejunum brought up anteriorly, end-to-side.
2. The cut end of the pancreas is anastomosed to the same loop of jejunum distal to the choledochojejunostomy.
3. The cut end of the stomach is anastomosed to the same loop of jejunum, but distal to the pancreaticojejunostomy.
4. The distal cut end of the jejunum is closed.

MODIFICATION 3

1. The cut end of the common bile duct is anastomosed to the side of a loop of jejunum brought up anteriorly, end-to-side.
2. The cut end of the pancreas is anastomosed directly to the cut-end of the jejunum, end-to-end.
3. The cut end of the stomach is anastomosed to the side of the jejunum, antecolic.

Because of the reported high incidence of postoperative marginal peptic ulcerations, truncal vagotomy has become an important adjunct to the Whipple procedure.

Villous Adenoma

Benign villous adenoma is far less common than carcinoma of the ampulla of Vater. The former is a rare lesion and is known to undergo malignant changes in about 30% of the cases. Endoscopic examinations can contribute greatly to the early diagnosis of benign adenoma by including routine biopsy of all suspicious lesions. The persistence of a radiological abnormality in the ampullary area despite negative endoscopic findings should make a transduodenal exploration and biopsy mandatory. Direct examination and definitive biopsy will decide the diagnosis and the surgical judgment.

In approximately 30% of diagnosed ampullary villous adenomas, a malignant transformation may be discovered. If the surgeon can recognize these degenerative changes early, the operative survival will certainly be longer. In a review of 45 cases of villous adenoma, Sobol and Cooperman[1] reported carcinoma in 26%. Kozuka, et al.[2] reviewed the microscopic findings in 22 cases of carcinoma of the ampulla of Vater and identified adenomatous residue in 82%. This finding is highly suggestive of carcinoma developing from preexisting adenoma.

With the wider use of ERCP, more benign lesions of the ampulla of Vater will be discovered and dealt with surgically. Management of diagnosed villous adenomas may require local or radical surgery, depending upon the histological findings and the extent of the lesion. An early, small, benign lesion may be dealt with local excision; however, a diagnosis of invasive carcinoma is best dealt with by a more radical procedure, i.e., the Whipple procedure (pancreaticoduodenectomy) (see "The Whipple Operation"). The late Richard Cattell[3] preferred and advocated this procedure. Conservative surgeons advocated wide submucosal excision and a sphincteroplasty when treating polyps of the ampulla, especially where microscopic findings of carcinoma could not be established.

Because villous adenoma is usually a slow-growing neoplasm, and because its location favors earlier diagnosis, the prognosis becomes more favorable. X-ray and ERCP favor an earlier diagnosis; together with prompt surgical intervention, they will prolong the patient's survival.

Recommended Reading

Archie J, Murray H: Benign polypoid adenoma of the ampulla of Vater. *Arch Surg* 113:180, 1978.
Starling J, Turner J: Villous adenoma involving the ampulla of Vater. Treatment by submucosal resection and double sphincteroplasty. *Am Surg* 48:188, 1982.

References

1. Sobol S, Cooperman A: Villous adenoma of the ampulla of Vater. *Gastroenterology* 75:107, 1978.
2. Kozuka S, Tsubone M, Yamaguchi, et al: Adenomatous residue in cancerous papilla of Vater. *Gut* 22:1031, 1981.
3. Cattell R, Pyrtek L: Premalignant lesions of the ampulla of Vater. *Surg Gynecol Obstet* 90:21, 1950.

17

ENDOSCOPIC RETROGRADE CHOLEDOCHOPANCREATOGRAPHY

Endoscopic retrograde choledochopancreatography (ERCP) is a fairly recent addition to the diagnostic armamentarium. It has become an important supplemental modality for evaluating difficult or undiagnosed conditions. Its most important contribution is its ability to differentiate a medical jaundice from a surgical jaundice in the high-risk patient.

With the advent of the fiberoptic duodenoscope, a new diagnostic field opened preoperatively for visualization of the duodenum, cannulation of the ampulla of Vater, and ERCP. Very favorable reports have appeared on the effectiveness of this new diagnostic instrument in visualizing duodenal disorders as well as disorders of the pancreas, common bile duct, and ampulla of Vater. Reports by Vennes[1,2] of the University of Minnesota and Satake et al.[3] of the University of Osaka Medical School in Japan have indicated that very favorable results and very effective diagnoses can be established prior to operative procedures. The duodenoscope is a flexible fiberoptic instrument made by the manufacturers of the Olympus, the American Cystoscope Makers, and others. All have developed a side-viewing instrument through which cannulation procedures can be satisfactorily performed. The details of the technique for this procedure must be obtained elsewhere.

Block et al.[4] reported on ERCP and presented their conclusions based on their experience with 41 patients who had biliary tract problems; in 10 cases, difficulties arose that prevented them from making a diagnosis. Incomplete dye filling of bile ducts, which usually signifies organic obstruction, was found not to be completely true. The specific origin or histological character of the lesion causing a bile duct obstruction was not completely delineated by retrograde endoscopic cholangiography. Also, with this method, small or minute stones were not recognized. Confusing anatomical variations contributed to the difficulty of diagnosis. There were also limitations in defining the status of recurrent strictures. Block et al. concluded that inflammatory changes in the papilla of Vater can simulate carcinoma, and vice versa. Inflammatory changes cannot be definitely diagnosed solely by endoscopic study. A normal pancreatogram does not always rule out the presence of carcinoma of the ampulla. A biopsy of the ampulla by endoscopy must be considered unreliable, and as usual, a negative biopsy is not acceptable.

It should be mentioned that Block et al. were early pioneers, reporting their ERCP results in 1956. Nevertheless, despite great advances in the use of this modality both diagnostically and therapeutically, the precautions, drawbacks, and advice given by Block et al. should be heeded, especially by beginners in the field of ERCP. More recently, Kune and Sali[5] have listed some of the hazards attributed to ERCP; they include preexisting pathology, the contrast medium, irradiation, and instrumentation. These factors can account for 3% of the complications incurred during ERCP. Filling a pancreatic cyst with contrast medium can predispose to septic cholangitis, abscess formation, and possible death. Kune and Sali stated that 10% of their patients died of cholangitic sepsis and 20% died of infected pseudocyst. Routine antibiotics given pre- and postoperatively are advised by most endoscopists. Ampicillin, aminoglycosides (gentamicin), and cephalosporins (Keflin, Mandol) are commonly used. Chloramphenicol (Chloromycetin) and vancomycin should be tried in the more resistant infections that fail to respond to the usual antibiotics (see "Antibiotics" in Chapter 15).

The patients in whom ERCP is particularly indicated and most helpful fall into four categories: (1) A nonjaundiced patient with a history of biliary surgery and suffering from unexplained symptoms may now be finally diagnosed by ERCP. (2) A jaundiced patient, with or without symptoms, in whom intra- or extrahepatic involvement is suspected may benefit from ERCP. (3) When existing studies fail to reveal the source of biliary pathology, ERCP may reveal the site and precise diagnosis. (4) If a postoperative high-risk patient is suffering from a retained common duct stone, ERCP is certainly preferable to a second-stage surgical procedure. ERCP is useful particularly because it offers reliable information. According to Vennes, it reveals the site of pathology and its cause in over 94% of his patients; in addition, it offers specific therapeutic answers (Figs. 187–192 show endoscopic x-ray studies). Sphincterotomy for stenosis of the ampulla of Vater may be accomplished, with or without the intention of freeing a retained gallstone. A long-term Dormia basket or balloon may be employed to trap and remove a leftover resistant stone from the common duct. This has now become an accepted routine procedure in most hospitals around the world.

ERCP in Choledocholithiasis

According to Vennes, stones in the common duct after surgery may remain and grow or pass out spontaneously; about 50% of the remaining stones will become symptomatic within 5 years. Often after an attack of gallstone colic, cholangiography

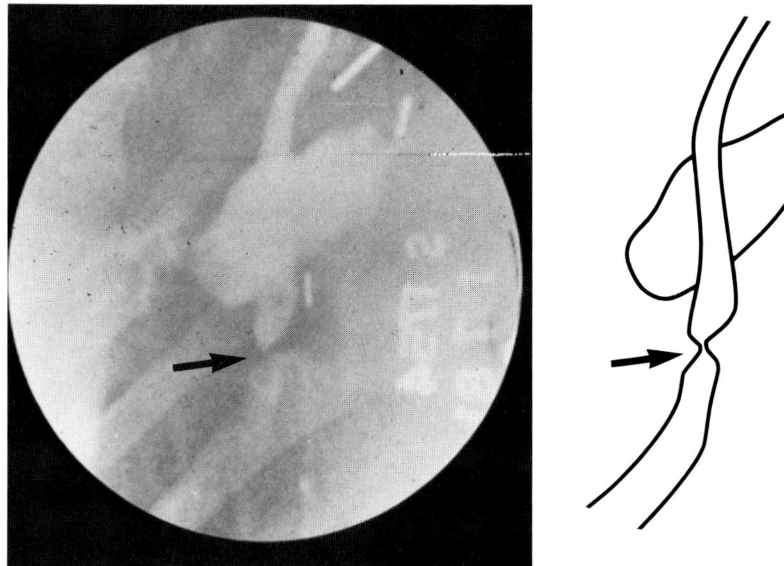

Figure 187.   Retrograde endoscopic X-ray of common bile duct showing stricture. Treatment: surgical repair; end-to-end anastomosis. (The writer is grateful to Dr. Dennis Neuhart, Endoscopist for Mt. Sinai and St. Francis Hospitals, Miami Beach, Florida, for supplying the excellent diagnostic endoscopic X-ray studies shown in Figures 188—193.)

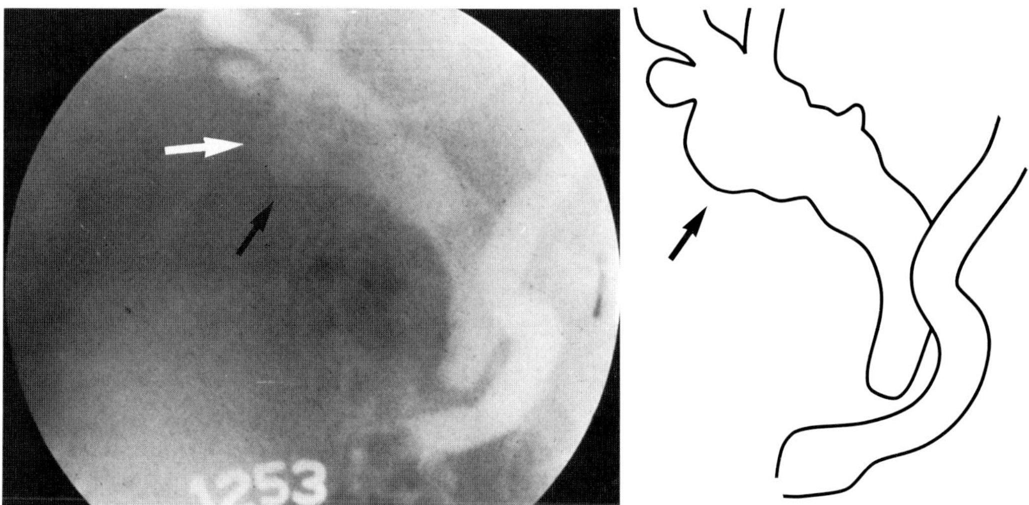

Figure 188.   Retrograde endoscopic X-ray of the common bile duct showing carcinoma of the gallbladder. Treatment: cholecystectomy with wedge resection of the liver.

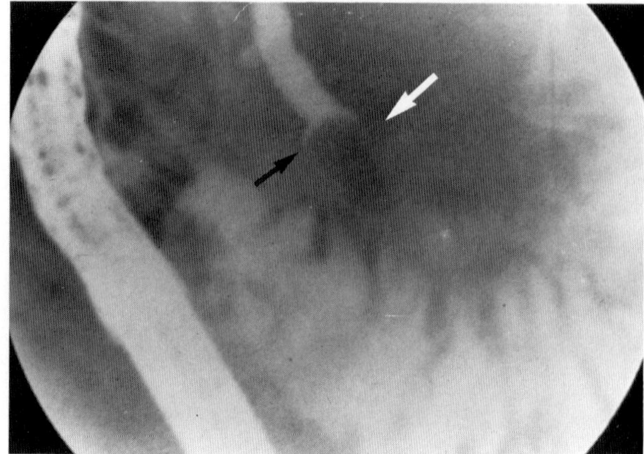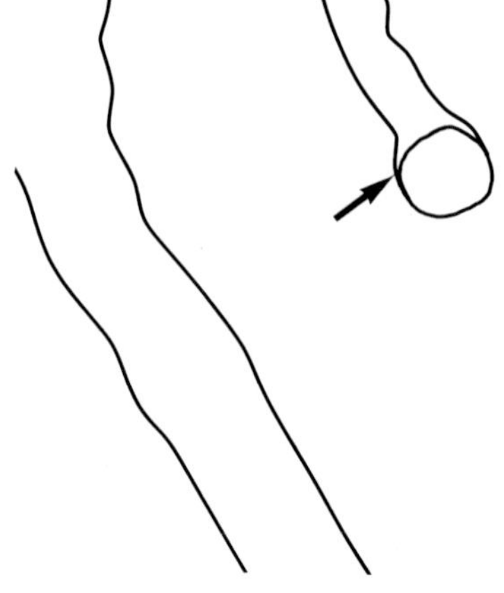

Figure 189.   Retrograde endoscopic X-ray of common bile duct showing obstruction due to an impacted gallstone.

Treatment: sphincterotomy (endoscopically).

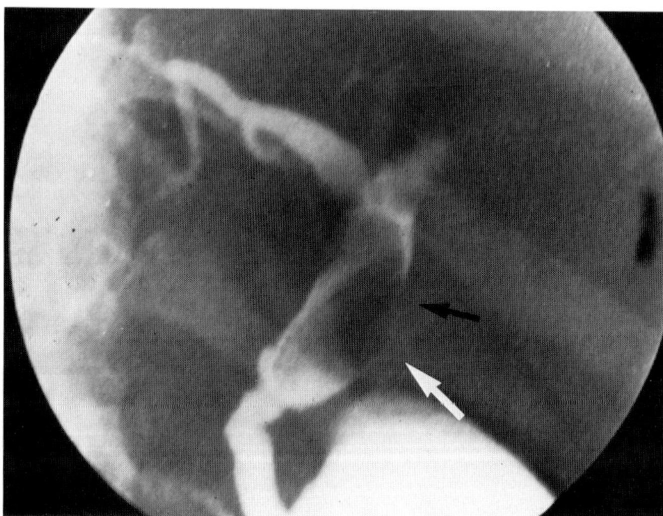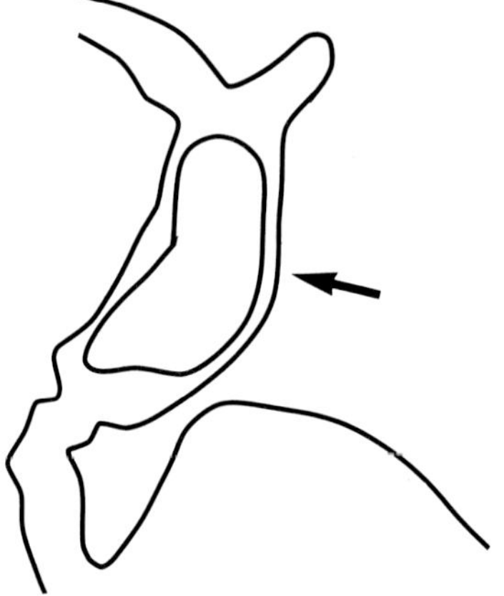

Figure 190.   Retrograde endoscopic X-ray of the common bile duct showing large gallstone impacted in common duct.

Treatment: surgical removal.

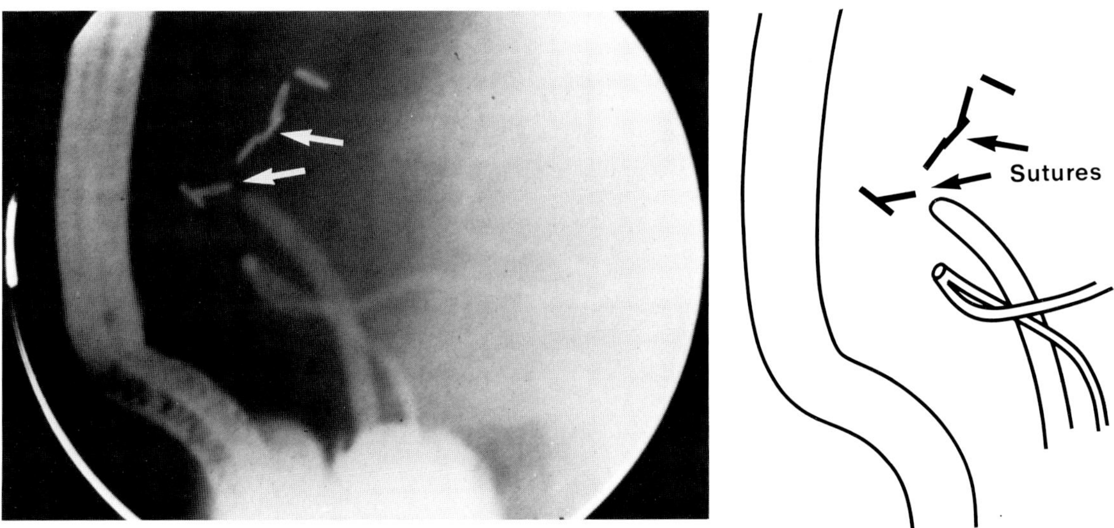

Figure 191.   Retrograde endoscopic X-ray showing postoperative stricture caused by injudious application of metallic clips. Treatment: surgical excision of stricture with end-to-end anastomosis.

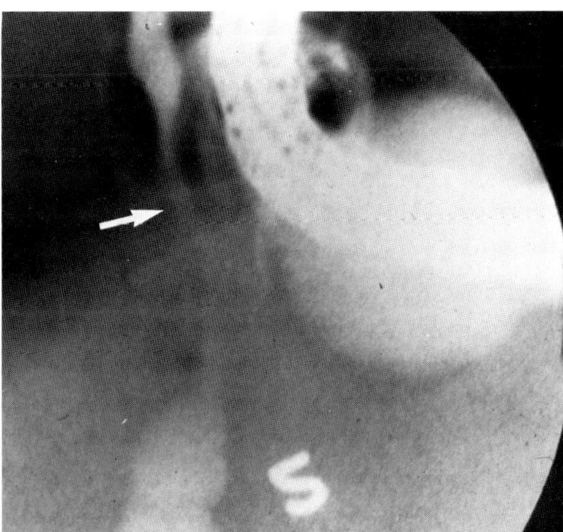

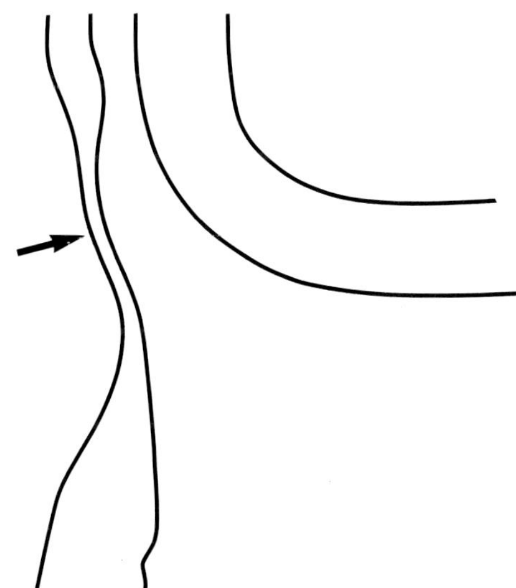

Figure 192.   Retrograde endoscopic X-ray of the common bile duct showing metastic carcinoma. Treatment: surgical exploration; inoperable.

may fail to visualize a stone or stones in the biliary system. ERCP may find a papilla of Vater with a patulous opening; this suggests that the stones have passed into the duodenum. As in T-tube cholangiography, the visualizing dye must not be too concentrated. In attempting to visualize small gallstones, the endoscopist should employ a diluted dye (see "Cholangiography" in Chapter 5); a concentrated dye may obliterate the outline of the stones. A large gallstone may ultimately break up into smaller stones. If air bubbles enter the duct, they can be detected by fluoroscopy. The air bubbles may coalesce, disappear, or float upward, especially when the body's position is changed. *It should be kept in mind that a carcinoma or a benign lesion of the duct may coexist with a stone; this combination must not be overlooked.*

EXTRINSIC COMPRESSION OF THE COMMON BILE DUCT

This form of common bile duct compression may be caused by:

1. Acute (edematous) pancreatitis
2. Chronic (fibrotic) pancreatitis
3. Pancreatic pseudocyst
4. Lymphomas, i.e., Hodgkin's disease and other forms of lymphomatous diseases

Vennes states that a benign obstruction produced by extrinsic pressure is characterized by a smooth contour, a symmetrical pattern, and a bile duct that may or may not be dilated. A pancreatogram may, on occasion, show obstruction of the bile duct and the pancreatic duct at the same level. This "double duct" sign usually suggests invasive carcinoma rather than chronic pancreatitis. Carcinoma of the bile duct, as a rule, does not involve the pancreatic duct. An obstructive jaundice may be produced by Hodgkin's disease, in which case infiltration of the biliary ductal system produces extrahepatic duct obstruction. Ochoa and Keene[6] have reviewed 52 patients with lymphoma over a 10-year period and have found that 20% of their diagnosed patient's with Hodgkin's disease developed jaundice. Obstructive jaundice caused by Hodgkin's disease must be considered in the differential diagnosis of extrahepatic jaundice.

INTRINSIC STRICTURES RECOGNIZED BY ERCP

Carcinoma of the common duct is revealed by a narrow, irregular, fuzzy filling defect.

Ampullar carcinoma (papillary stenosis) usually produces stricture at the terminal end of the bile duct, with obstruction and proximal duct dilatation. This type of neoplastic lesion is most often discovered by ERCP.

Papillary stenosis often results in poor or delayed emptying. According to Vennes, the emptying time is usually longer than 45 minutes, the latter being the limitation of normal. The Nardi test, which attempts to determine the response of the sphicter to drugs, has correlated unsatisfactorily with the use of such drugs as morphine and neostigmine.

Lesions found in the hepatic ducts or in the hilus are more likely to prove malignant. There are exceptions, such as infestations with *Clonorchis senensis* associated with secondary infections. Most malignant growths of the bilary tree appear fuzzy or irregular in outline and tend to be more completely obstructive. Benign strictures of the bile duct are almost invariably iatrogenic, i.e., related to previous biliary surgery. These lesions, contrary to the irregularity of carcinoma, are smooth in outline, more symmetrical, and, as a rule, not completely obstructive. The benign strictures are found predominantly proximal to the cystic duct or at the site of an improperly ligated cystic duct.

Sclerosing cholangitis is frequently found in patients with inflammatory disease of the bowel. Extrahepatic ducts may also be involved, and all the ducts take on varied shapes and sizes. Abnormal liver function studies may correlate well with the X-ray findings; this is not so with inflammatory bowel disease. The intrahepatic ductal patterns become varied and sharply outlined, such as alternating strictures with sacculations; cholangiocarcinoma may coexist with sclerosing cholangitis.

Postoperative biliary tract pain and dyspepsia may challenge the internist and surgeon. If cholangiographic studies (ultrasonic and IV cholangiogram) show the calculus, ERCP is indicated and will substantiate the existence of the leftover stone. During ERCP the endoscopist must rule out coexisting pancreatic disease. Sphincterotomy may be indicated in order to free the impacted stone and avoid secondary surgery.

A reminder to the surgeon and internist: In the final analysis, one must realize that lithotripsy (to fracture the gallstone) is like ERCP and chenodeoxycholic deoxycholic acid, in which the stone is removed or dissolved; only the gallstone was dealt with—not the diseased gallbladder. The leftover gallbladder is now capable of reforming stones becoming inflamed, perforating with fictula and silent carcinoma. Cholecystectomy is the ideal prophylaxis against cancer of the gall bladder. Now–with more gallbladders left in—there is greater chance for increasing the 1% incidence of cancer of the gallbladder.

Recommended Reading

Anderson RE, Priestly JT: Observations on the bacteriology of choledochal bile. *Ann Surg* 33:4786, 1951.

Bordley J, White TT: Causes for 340 reoperations on the extrahepatic bile ducts. *Ann Surg* 189:442, 1979.

Cotton PB: Endoscopic management of bile duct stones (apples and oranges). *Gut* 25:587, 1984.

Cotton PB, Vallon AG: British experience with duodenoscopic sphincterotomy for removal of bile duct stones. *Br J Surg* 68:373, 1981.

Cremer M, Gulbis A, Toussaint J, et al: Endoscopic papillotomy in Belgium, in Demling L, Classen M (eds): *Endoscopic Sphincterotomy of the Papilla of Vater.* Stuttgart, Thieme, 1978, p 90.

Escourrou J, Cordova JA, Lazorthes F, et al: Early and later complications after endoscopic sphincterotomy for biliary lithiasis with and without gallbladder "in situ." *Gut* 25:598, 1984.

Flemma RJ, Flint LM, Osterhout S, et al: Bacteriologic studies of biliary tract infection. *Ann Surg* 166:563, 1967.

Gregg JA, Girolama PD, Carr-Locke DL: Effects of sphincteroplasty and endoscopic sphincterotomy on the bacteriologic characteristics of the common bile duct. *Am J Surg* 149:668, 1985.

Jones SA: The prevention and treatment of recurrent bile duct stones by transduodenal sphincteroplasty. *World J Surg* 2:473, 1978.

Jordan L Jr: Choledocholithiasis. *Curr Prob Surg* 19:722, 1982.

Lygidakis NJ: Surgical approaches to recurrent choledocholithiasis. *Am J Surg* 145:633, 1983.

Neoptolemos JP, Carr-Locke DL, Fraser I, et al: The management of common bile duct calculi by endoscopic sphincterotomy in patients with gallbladders in situ. *Br J Surg* 71:69, 1984.

Reiter JJ, Yet HB, Mennicken C, et al: Results of endoscopic papillotomy: A collective experience from 9 endoscopic centres in West Germany. *World J Surg* 2:505, 1978.

Rosch W, Riemman JF, Lux G, et al: Long-term follow-up after endoscopic sphincterotomy. *Endoscopy* 31:152, 1981.

Rosenberg, N: Role of sphincter of Oddi in etiology of peptic ulcer. I. Evidence from review of literature. *Arch Surg* 71:239, 1955.

Rosenberg N: Role of sphincter of Oddi in etiology of peptic ulcer. II. Effects of sectioning sphincter of Oddi on resistance of cats to histamine-induced peptic ulcer. *Arch Surg* 71:246, 1955.

Rosseland AR, Osnes M, Kruse A: Endoscopic sphincterotomy in patients with Billroth II gastrectomy. *Endoscopy* 13:19, 1981.

Rubin JR, Beal JM: Diagnosis of choledocholithiasis. *Surg Gynecol Obstet* 156:16, 1983.

Safrany L: Endoscopy and retrograde cholangiopancreatography after Billroth II operation. *Endoscopy* 4:198, 1972.

Safrany L: Endoscopic treatment of biliary disease. *Lancet* 2:983, 1978.

Safrany L, Cotton PB: Endoscopic management of choledocholithiasis. *Surg Clin North Am* 62:825, 1982.

Safrany L, Neuhaus B, Portocarrero G, et al: Endoscopic sphincterotomy in patients with Billroth II gastrectomy. *Endoscopy* 12:16, 1980.

Siegel JH: Endoscopic papillotomy in the treatment of biliary tract disease: 258 procedures and results. *J Dig Dis.*

Tweedle DEF, Martin DF: Choledocholithiasis: Surgical or endoscopic lithotomy. *Gut* 22:A888, 1981.

Urakami Y: Endoscopic pancreatocholangiography after Billroth II operation. *Stomach Intestine* 10:969, 1975.

Vallon AG, Cotton PB, Holton J: Clinical endoscopic follow-up after duodenoscopic sphincterotomy. *Gut* 22:A889, 1982.

Walters W: Postcholecystectomy dyskinesia with pancreatitis, sphincteritis, and choledocholithiasis as causes. *JAMA* 160:425, 1956.

Way LW, Admirand WH, Dunphy JE: Management of choledocholithiasis. *Ann Surg* 176:347, 1972.

Winstanley PA, Ellis WR, Hamilton I, et al: Medium-term complications of endoscopic biliary sphincterotomy. *Gut* 26:730, 1985.

References

1. Vennes JA, Jacobson JR: Endoscopic cholangiography for biliary system diagnosis. *Am Instit Med* 80:61, 1974.

2. Endoscopic retrograde balloon dilatation. *GI Endoscopy* 28:149, 1982.

3. Satake K, Cho K, Tatsumi S, et al: Evaluation of cholangiographic procedures in diagnosis of obstructive jaundice. *Ann Surg* 47:387, 1981.

4. Block MA, Brush ME, Ponka JL, et al: Diagnosis of postcholecystectomy biliary stones; a comparison of biliary drainage and IV cholangiography. *Arch Surg* 73:694, 1956.

5. Kune GA, Sali A: *The Practice of Biliary Surgery;* ed 2. Oxford, Blackwell, 1980, chap 6.

6. Ochoa JA, Keene WR: Destructive jaundice in Hodgkins' disease due to infiltration of the biliary ducts. *J Fla Med Assoc* 57(12):21, 1970.

Endoscopic Sphincterotomy

ERCP is a diagnostic and therapeutic modality that is constructed to sever the sphincter of Oddi by an electrocautery wire. Severance of the sphincter should include the sphincter fibers, papilla, and intramural duct, but not the duodenal wall. The main indications for ERCP and sphincterotomy are:

1. Postoperative residual stone in the common bile duct
2. Recurrent common duct stones
3. Stenosis of the sphincter of Oddi

Vennes[1] recommends a preliminary study with cholangiograms to outline the problem (stones or pathology) in advance. He then studies the size of the stone, the length of the intramural duct, and the extent of a safe anticipated sphincterotomy. The pancreatic duct must not be encroached upon; Vennes recommends a routine pancreatogram. The sphincterotome is made up of a wire that takes the shape of a string on a bow, and its length is controlled. The greater the bend, the shorter the wire. The sphincterotome is within the canal of the papilla, and when the radiofrequency current is passed along the wire, the sphincter is severed. This cut must be carefully directed away from the pancreatic stoma. The best positioning of the wire is toward the patient's right or at 10 o'clock. At this point, the gallstone may fall out or may be removed by employing either the long-arm Dormia basket or the ballon catheter. If the stone is not retrieved at once, approximately 1 week may be allowed for it to pass out spontaneously. A transnasal bile duct catheter may be left in for drainage and for subsequent cholangiography. After several days, X-ray studies will reveal whether or not the common duct is cleared of all stones. Sphincterotomy failures may be related to improper positioning of the papillotome within the ampulla, incomplete severance of the sphincter, failure to extract a large stone, or an existing anatomical anomaly.

The complication rate varies from 7 to 10% or higher, depending upon the experience and dexterity of the endoscopist. The complications include possible gram-negative septicemia, which is usually amenable to proper antibiotic therapy. It is not uncommon for the serum amylase level to rise after the procedure, but this problem usually corrects itself. The pancreatic duct may suddenly become overdistended, resulting in shock. Carcinoma of the common duct may be vulnerable to perforation during the endoscopic procedure. Hemorrhage and cholangitis not infrequently complicate this procedure. A serious sepsis may follow when the basket and the trapped stone become caught or incarcerated during withdrawal and cannot easily be removed. Seifert[2] reported a series of 955 patients; 731 had choledocholithiasis. Of the 955 patients, 86% passed the stone spontaneously; of the remaining 16%, extraction was required in 28%. Where endoscopic sphincterotomy was employed, there was a 92.1% success rate. The complication rate was 7.3%. Seifert reported a 1.2% mortality rate. An emergency laparotomy had to be done in 2.5% of the patients. This implies that it would be wise for the hospital to keep a surgeon and the operating room on a 24-hour alert for such a contingency.

Cutaneous transhepatic cholangiography is an equally acceptable preoperative method for differentiating extrahepatic from intrahepatic obstructive causes, but it is not without certain serious complications. Some prefer to do the ERCP first and, as a second choice, percutaneous transhepatic cholangiography. One should know that in selecting to do a percutaneous transhepatic cholangiography, it is wise to have a surgeon and the operating room scheduled for standby emergency surgery. This writer feels that this precaution also pertains to the ERCP procedure, especially in view of Seifert's statistics: 1.2% mortality, and 2.5% emergency laparotomy.

References

1. Vennes JA, Jacobson JR: Endoscopic cholangiography for biliary system diagnosis. *Am Inst Med* 80:61, 1974.
2. Seifert E, Gail K, Weismuller J, et al: Langzeitresultate nach Endoskopisher Sphinkterotomie. *Dtsch Med Wochenschr* 107:610, 1982.

Surgical Sphincterotomy

The essential anatomical feature of sphincterotomy is that the pancreatic duct joins the terminal portion of the common bile duct in the lower third of the second portion of the duodenum and then forms a common opening, an exit for the two systems, biliary and pancreatic. The bile flows through the common duct and is usually joined by the pancreatic juice at a lower level; together they flow through the terminal portion of the common bile duct, through the ampulla of Vater, and into the duodenum. There are variations of this anatomy in which the duct of Wirsung, the main duct for pancreatic external secretion, may attach at various levels to the common duct from approximately a half-inch above the ampullary opening to anywhere down to the opening of the ampulla and independently enter into the duodenum (see "A Practical Review of Surgical Anatomy" in Chapter 2).

From a clinical standpoint, all diseases that develop from this anatomy, i.e., the pancreatic duct junction with the common bile duct, is based on what follows an obstruction of this ductal outlet. Obstruction that occurs beyond the junction of the pancreatic and bile ducts causes a regurgitation of these two secretions back into their respective systems. For example, pancreatic juice will be refluxed into the pancreas, and bile will be refluxed into the common bile duct. An even more serious situation occurs when the pancreatic juice mixes with the bile within the pancreatic gland; the bile activates the preenzymes of the pancreatic juice, particularly trypsinogen and amylopsin, and activates them to proteolytic trypsin and fat-digesting lipase. Trypsin digests the very pancreatic parenchyma that creates it. This process leads to pancreatitis, either acute edematous pancreatitis or the more serious acute hemorrhagic pancreatitis.

The latter pathological process depends upon the infringement of the pancreatic blood supply and the chronicity of the disease. A reflux of bile resulting from an obstruction to the ampulla of Vater from whatever cause results in a back pressure of bile into the common duct and gallbladder, and then further back into the liver. In each instance, a separate problem will result. In the gallbladder, the bile and activated pancreatic juice may produce a marked inflammatory process, i.e., acute cholecystitis, and then further back into the liver, the canaliculi become distended and inflamed (cholangiolitis). Ultimately, the back pressure causes the canaliculi to rupture, with destruction of the liver parenchyma itself.

Besides stones, mud, and gravel, a fibrous ring stenosis and spasm can produce obstruction. A neoplastic growth also causes obstruction and leads to any one of the pathological problems mentioned. Therefore, the surgeon must know the precise cause of the obstruction and deal with it appropriately at the time of surgery.

This writer believes that the most common cause of ampullary obstruction is the stone or stones in the common duct; the stone remains impacted and probably induces a local irritation sufficient to produce edema and further fixation of the stone. The site of impaction may produce fibrosis even after the stone is removed and later serves as an obstruction (stenosis) at the ampullary end of the common duct. Pancreatitis, which so commonly accompanies this disease process, is most often relieved when the obstructing stone is removed or the stenosis corrected.

There are other causes of pancreatitis, such as chronic alcoholism, but we will not deal with them here. Instead, we will focus on the mechanical and pathological factors that develop locally in the area of the sphincter itself. It is possible that in many cases of acute pancreatitis and acute cholecystitis both pathological problems may be related to one common etiological factor. Pancreatic juice has been found in the gallbladder and bile has been found in the pancreas, and we know that they are interrelated and dependent upon each other in their respective digestive functions.

It is most likely that biliary disease precedes pancreatic disease, except for the type of pancreatitis caused by primary chronic alcoholism (chronic pancreatitis). It is conceivable that even during a spastic episode concentrated bile from the gallbladder passing through the common duct is unable to properly empty into the duodenum. The bile when it admixes with the pancreatic juice stimulates cholecystokinin at the time of reflux into the pancreatic duct, (duct of Wirsung). The mixture (bile, pancreatic juice, and cholecystokinin) causes digestive and pressure changes within the pancreas itself and causes the finest radicles of the pancreas to rupture and/or be digested by the very activated enzymes of the pancreatic juice.

Hypertrophy of the sphincter of Oddi is also a possibility and has been shown to be associated with chronic spasm similar to that found in hypertrophic pyloric stenosis. The commoner causes are usually stones in the common duct, with debris impacted at the same site. The latter often coexist with spastic sphincter and pancreatitis, but more often than not, scarring with fibrosis reduces the main opening of the sphincter with a progressive contracture.

Patients who come to surgery with cholecystitis and cholelithiasis and have concomitant stenotic sphincters caused by fibrosis or stone impaction should, in the writer's opinion, be treated not only by stone removal but by the dilatation of the stenotic sphincter. When necessary, a sphincterotomy is the best supplemental procedure to prevent recurrence of obstruction.

Sphincterotomy is performed transduodenally to remove an impacted, obstructive calculus from the ampulla. The sphincter of Oddi is sectioned in a vertical and slightly oblique plane. The obstructive stone is released, and the biliary flow from the liver improves immediately; the flow of pancreatic juice is similarly relieved, and the flow returns to normal. If there is no evidence of scar formation in the ampulla of Vater, dilatation with Bakes dilators is the usual practice and ordinarily suffices. However, if it is suspected that the sphincter's obstructive fibrosis has produced a dilatation of the common duct, the surgeon would be wise to do a supplemental sphincterotomy to prevent recurrent obstruction with harmful back pressure of bile into the common bile duct, pancreas, and liver.

In 1956 Doubilet and Mulholland[1] reported on an 8-year study of 400 patients with recurrent pancreatitis in whom they had performed sphincterotomies. They claimed that 90% of their patients were improved. It is a physiological fact that whenever the sphincter closes down, for whatever reason, the obstruction forces the bile to reflux back into the pancreatic duct. The latter is a reality that must be considered in every case of gallbladder disease where offending signs and symptoms suggest concomitant pancreatitis. It is difficult to prove what benefits a sphincterotomy would offer for pancreatitis coexistent with chronic cholecystitis and cholelithiasis. After the gallbladder is removed, the common duct explored, and stones removed, it is not easy to conclude that it was the sphincterotomy that contributed toward relief of the pancreatitis. It must, however, be assumed that a better bile flow will follow, and that reflux of bile with pancreatic juice will not reflux into the pancreas. Any improvement in pancreatic function with the disappearance of signs and symptoms formerly attributed to pancreatitis must be assumed to be the result of the combined cholecystectomy, removal of the common duct stone, and sphincterotomy.

Whenever a calculus is impacted in the lower common bile duct and cannot be freed or dislodged by probing or spooning from above, or even by being milked upward, the only alternative is to resort to a transduodenal approach to enlarge the sphincteric stoma with a sphincterotomy, which allows the stone to fall out or be extracted. While sphincterotomy is a procedure for removing an impacted stone and relieving lower ductal obstruction, it also prevents residual stones from falling back into the hepatic ductal system and later impacting the common bile duct, thus causing recurrent biliary obstruction. These dropped stones pass more easily through the sphincterotomy, especially with a good flow of bile.

Sphincterotomy to date has failed to prove its effectiveness for primary pancreatitis, i.e., when the latter is not associated with cholecystitis. There is no question that we are dealing with changes that involve more than an obstruction to the outlet of pancreatic juice. The writer feels that the greatest single factor in pancreatitis is alcoholism; therefore, restriction of alcohol intake would be a most effective prophylactic measure.

TECHNIQUE

It is best to mobilize the duodenum first; this can best be accomplished with a Kocher maneuver, namely, to incise the portion of the peritoneum along the lateral curvature of the duodenum and, with the fingers, bluntly dissect up the duodenum. The retroduodenal area is usually an avascular area with a line of cleavage that offers no difficulty in freeing up the second and third portions of the duodenum and allowing this organ to be reflected medially or to the left. This maneuver also exposes the posterior aspect of the common duct, as well

as the head of the pancreas, and thus allows better visualization and easier handling. With the forefinger and thumb around the common bile duct, the surgeon palpates for stones or for any abnormal growth. Finding a stone and milking it back up to the choledochotomy stoma is an effective maneuver. However, if the stone is impacted and cannot be managed from above, a flexible metal probe can be inserted to find and indicate the lowest point that can be reached in the common bile duct. A flexible cervical probe with more rigidity can also be utilized to find the lowest portion of the common duct site of obstruction. Knowing where the stone is impacted and knowing precisely where the obstructive level is may assist the surgeon to find the ampulla of Vater after a duodenotomy.

Once the site for the ideal transduodenal opening has been found, the ampulla of Vater is more easily recognized. An appropriate vertical incision is made into the duodenum, the edges are retracted, and hemostasis is secured. The area is kept dry and under good visualization. Almost invariably a bulge will be found, indicating that the stone is protruding through the wall of the common duct. If sphincterotomy is to be avoided, a retrograde technique for displacing the stone from below may be employed. With Glassman's fine, flexible metal blunt-tipped probe, the stone can be disimpacted and displaced upward toward the choledochostomy stoma (see the discussion of the retrograde stone extraction technique in Chapter 11). Alternatively, on finding the ampulla, the surgeon employs a groove director into its lumen and incises it with a small knife vertically, with a slight obliquity toward the right. This procedure releases the impacted stone by widening the opening and allowing the trapped bile under pressure to force the stone to drop out.

The duodenal wall on both sides of the ampulla can be elevated, using a delicate Glassman-Allis 8-inch noncrushing forceps. This is better than a traction suture and less traumatic. This maneuver permits elevation of all the cut edges of the ampulla and simplifies suturing of the edges. The groove director is inserted carefully and more than 6 to 8 mm should be cut, using a small knife or angulated sharp scissors. Carefully cut the ampulla with small snips at a time to avoid damaging the posterior wall of the duodenum and creating a fistulous tract that can result in a serious complication. If necessary, the ampullary opening can be further enlarged by Bakes dilators. This step is usually not necessary because the common duct can be probed again through the choledochotomy and further irrigated with saline to make sure that all debris, sludge, and residual smaller stones are washed out into the duodenum.

When this is finally accomplished, the surgeon should approximate the cut mucosal surfaces. That is, the cut duodenal mucosa should be carefully approximated with the common bile duct mucosa, using (00000) silk. The approximation of the edges helps to prevent the formation of a stenotic ring. Another acceptable method is to insert the long-arm T-tube of Cattell[2] modified by Glassman, i.e., the distal one-third has been multiply perforated to prevent the complication that everyone fears—pancreatic duct obstruction with resulting pancreatitis. These multiple openings allow free pancreatic passage despite the fact that the tube extends into the duodenum. Still another advantage of Cattell's long-arm T-tube is that it can be shut off early, since the flow of bile into the duodenum is assured, and the patient is allowed to make a faster recovery with better conservation of body fluids, bile salts, and electrolytes. Fear that the extended area of the T-tube passing through the ampullary stoma will necrose the mucosa has proved unfounded in the writer's experience. *One should be careful not to employ a long arm T-tube whose diameter is too large for the common duct lumen.*

At this stage, having accomplished a complete sphincterotomy, it is necessary to close the duodenum. This is best accomplished with a two-layer closure in a transverse axis. A transverse closure supposedly prevents a narrowing of the duodenal lumen, though some surgeons close the duodenotomy vertically without any serious obstructive consequences. This author prefers the transverse closure and closes with a first row of chromic catgut (00) with a continuous lock; the second row is sewn interruptedly, using (000) black silk, with an intestinal-type atraumatic needle. The sutures are carefully placed to be sure that no fistula will subsequently complicate the closure.

The choledochotomy stoma is closed around the external long arm of the T-tube in the same manner as it would be around a short-arm T-tube. It should be hermetically sealed, tested to make sure that it is watertight, and brought out with a Penrose (wick) drain through a subcostal stab incision, as in regular common duct procedures. It should be removed several weeks to months later to assure that no stenosis smaller than the size of the tube will develop. Throughout this period the external arm of the T-tube may remain closed; the bile continues to flow through the T-tube directly into the duodenum.

Nothing has yet been said about neoplasia. It is possible that after a duodenostomy is performed, instead of finding a stenotic lesion, one finds a polyp or an outright adenocarcinoma of the ampulla of Vater. This problem is discussed in greater detail in terms of procedures such as pancreaticoduodenectomy, or excision of the polyp and sphincter together. In most instances, the lesion of the papilla will not be carcinoma; rather, it will be of the benign features discussed, namely, stones, stenosis, impaction with mud, gravel, and sludge, hypertrophy, and, often, sphincter spasm. After the sphincterotomy, this writer recommends a biopsy so that the exact nature of the histology is known in the postoperative period. Sphincterotomy is not to be employed as a routine procedure; it should be used only where specific indications exist.

There is no proof that routine sphincterotomy produces excellent results; in fact, there have been complications that have raised the morbidity and mortality. There will be times when a sphincterotomy is not possible but, because of the continued persistence of retained stones regardless of thorough irrigations, marked dilatation of the duct, the age of the patient, the extended length of the operation, and the possibility of recurrent obstruction which the patient will not tolerate, a choledochoduodenostomy is indicated and preferred. It is possible that stones dropping down from a higher level of the hepatic ductal system will find their way out through the common duct into the duodenum more easily. This procedure is a good precaution against threatening recurrence and serious reoperation.

At times, the most thorough search of the common bile duct and hepatic duct radicles may be insufficient to reveal the existence of high-lying residual smaller stones that may drop down at a later date. Choledochoduodenostomy is a procedure that has repeatedly proved to be effective and safe, especially when another bout of obstructive jaundice cannot be tolerated in the postoperative period. With choledochoduodenostomy, there is no fear of ascending cholangitis. This writer has not seen any cholangitis following choledochoduodenostomy other than that which occurs after indiscretions in the patient's way of living.

After a 6- to 8-mm sphincterotomy is made, exploration again from above is good practice because new probing and further irrigations may reveal stones not recognized previously. So, it is wise to reexplore the common duct routinely after sphincterotomy, and again probe from below as well as from above, to finally cleanse the entire duct with copious saline irrigations. When the sphincterotomy is open, it is not a bad idea, to search out the opening of the duct Wirsung, using the Glassman fine blunt-tipped, flexible silver probe, and explore the duct of the pancreas to assure its patency.

It should be mentioned that this writer does not prefer the Connell suture when closing the duodenum, because intraluminal bleeding is possible and can take place unrestrictedly and unknowingly within the lumen of the duodenum. To avoid this problem, the writer sews over and over with the edges everted; for the second layer of sutures, interrupted black silk (000) is used. Suturing with a second row of silk sutures prevents internal or external bleeding because it is a hemostatic stitch closure. Sphincteroplasty, unlike sphincterotomy, is not a recommended procedure because too much of the common duct is left open and an unduly patulous opening results. Too large an opening is totally unnecessary and carries a much higher risk of reflux into the common bile duct, as well as leakage from the duodenum, creating a serious fistula. Sphincterotomy is a safe procedure, especially when indicated and done carefully; fistulous formation, pancreatitis, and postoperative stenosis should be carefully avoided.

Recommended Reading

Allen AW, Wallace RH: Surgical management of stone in common bile duct: Follow-up studies with special reference to graded dilation of sphincter of Oddi. *Ann Surg* 111:838, 1940.

Brush BE, Ponka JL, Damazo F, et al: Evaluation of dilatation of sphincter of Oddi. *Arch Surg* 70:766, 1955.

Rosenberg N: Role of sphincter of Oddi in etiology of peptic ulcer. I. Evidence from review of literature. *Arch Surg* 71:239, 1955.

Rosenberg N: Role of sphincter of Oddi in etiology of peptic ulcer. II. Effects of sectioning sphincter of Oddi on resistance of cats to histamine-induced peptic ulcer. *Arch Surg* 71:246, 1955.

Walters W: Postcholecystectomy dyskinesia with pancreatitis, sphincteritis, and choledocholithiasis as causes. *JAMA* 160:425, 1956.

References

1. Doubilet H, Mulholland JH: Eight-year study of pancreatitis and sphincterotomy. *JAMA* 160:521, 1956.
2. Cattell RB, Colcock BP: Fibrosis of sphincter of Oddi. *Ann Surg* 137:797, 1953.

Disadvantages of Sphincterotomy

The following are considered disadvantages of sphincterotomy:

1. Immediate obstructive relief is transient, and sustained benefits are not predictable.
2. It is not uncommon for a sphincterotomy to restricture, with a recurrence of obstructive signs and symptoms.
3. Sphincterotomy by ERCP may cause complications, i.e., hemorrhage, pancreatitis, cholangitis, sepsis, and perforation. ERCP in good hands generally has a reported mortality of 2–3%. Interventional emergency surgery may have to be carried out in these patients. The OR should be alerted to stand by.

This writer prefers choledochoduodenostomy over sphincterotomy or sphincteroplasty because it is a more logical anatomical approach and permits a direct visual procedure. Each suture is placed under direct vision, and the stoma is established without much risk. Decompression and drainage are complete, and if the stoma has been made 2 to 2.5 cm in length, it rarely strictures. If a stricture does develop, ERCP permits effective and safe dilatation of the stoma in most instances. For the surgeon, there should be little hesitation in selecting choledochoduodenostomy over sphincterotomy in most cases.

18

WHAT'S NEW IN BILIARY SURGERY

Use of the Laser in Biliary Surgery

Carpenter et al., quoted by Dixon,[1] describe a patient with carcinoma at the junction of the hepatic ducts that had been drained through a percutaneous transhepatic catheter. Bleeding developed along the tube, and angiography demonstrated hepatic artery erosion by the carcinoma. A small endoscope was inserted along the fistulous tract and the bleeding site coagulated with an Nd YAG laser. The obstructing lesion was vaporized and gave the patient relief and drainage.

Brunetand et al.[2] used an Nd YAG laser via an endoscope to make an incision into the bulging duodenal common duct wall and to relieve a distal obstruction of the ampulla of Vater.

Ori[3] employed endoscopic laser fragmentation of very large stones in the common duct. Through a T-tube fistulous tract, the endoscope was inserted and the fiber was brought in close proximity to the stone. Multiple applications resulted in fragmentation of a large stone in six patients. Mixed and pigmented gallstones were easy to fragment; cholesterol stones were more difficult. Cholesterol stones (white/yellow) permit only minimal absorption of laser energy, while pigment easily absorbs laser energy.

Benign strictures, stenotic anastomoses, and webs have benefited by laser techniques. This writer recommends that for the present-laser best be employed by those expert in its use.

Recommended Reading

Carpenter CM, Bowers JH, Dixon JA: Neodymium YAG laser treatment of hemobilia: Instrumentation via percutaneous biliary catheter tract. *Radiology*. In press.

Nichioka NS, Kelsey PB, Abdul-Ghani-Kibbi, et al: Recanalization of occluded biliary endoprosthesis with pulsed laser radiation. *Laser Surg Med* 7:391, 1987.

Kohler B, Riemann JF, Brown BP: Incidence of bacteremia after endoscopic laser treatment of stenosing processes in upper gastrointestinal tract. *Am J Gastroenterol* 8:1026, 1982.

Anand VK, Herbert J, Robert F, et al: Is an anesthesiologist justified during therapeutic laser endoscopy? *Laser Surg Med* 7:273, 1987.

References

1. Dixon JA: Surgical applications of lasers. *Bull Am Coll Surg* 67:4, 1982. ·
2. Brunetand JM, Biserte J, Charlier J: Therapeutic applications of argon ion and neodymium YAG lasers, in Asumi K (ed): *Laser Tokyo '81*. Tokyo, Intergroup, 1981, pp 25–27.
3. Ori K: Lithotomy of bile stones by YAG laser with choledochofiberscope, in Asumi K (ed): *Laser Tokyo '81*. Tokyo, Intergroup, 1981, pp 23–29.

Electrohydraulic Lithotripsy in Choledocholithiasis

Tanaka et al.[1] of Kyushu University in Fukuoka, Japan, have researched the use of electrohydraulic lithotripsy on gallstones in the common bile duct. They have reported the results of their animal experiments and their clinical experiences with the duodenoscope and percutaneous transhepatic electrohydraulic lithotripsy on these stones. They believe that this method is a safe and effective way to break up stones in the common duct. They have used it in three patients with choledocholithiasis in whom they found stones that were not removable. Electrohydraulic lithotripsy was used via a T-tube and duodenoscope, and was found to be safe and effective. These researchers state that it can be used effectively on large stones in the common duct that cannot be removed otherwise unless broken up into several smaller pieces and removed piecemeal by ERCP in multiple sessions.

Tanaka et al. have used a surge current generator manufactured by Lithatron, Waltz Elektronic Gmbh. Rohrdorf of West Germany. The instrument produces a high-voltage shock impulse (1000 to 2000 V) of 2–4 μsec duration between two electrodes placed at the tip of the catheter in the presence of a liquid medium. The intensity of the discharge is set at one, two, three, or four, with a frequency of 10, 20, 40 or 80/second. The duration of a pulse current at one ignition is 3 seconds by foot switch. The electrodes must be in touch with the stone during the application of discharge sparks. Saline solution is instilled via the vinyl catheter attached to the probe to ensure an aqueous medium around the electrodes. Tanaka et al. recommend two approaches:

1. Sphincterotomy by duodenoscope (ERCP) followed by lithotripsy.
2. In the fragile patient, percutaneous transhepatic lithotripsy.

This writer feels that this new method has merit but should presently be employed only by researchers in the field. There is a possibility of a serious complication: burning and perforation of the biliary wall.

This author wishes to remind the reader again that removal of gallstones does not cure the patient of the primary disease process—namely, chronic cholecystitis—and that even after successful stone dissolution, reformation of stones is highly probable. Recurrences of acute cholecystitis and its attendant complications still present a serious challenge. At best, dissolution of gallstones by chenodeoxycholic acid or its derivatives has serious drawbacks (see Scott M. Grundy, Chapter 3), and for extracorporeal shock-wave therapy to depend so heavily upon dissolution is a questionable form of supplemental therapy.

Today, cholecystectomy and common duct exploration must be considered the therapy of choice in acute and chronic cholelithiasis and choledocholithiasis. The exceptions are the over-aged, the very weak and the high risk patients.

Surgical intervention in most instances of cholelithiasis and choledocholithiasis still offers the best chance for lasting relief, while offering the only prophylaxis against cancer of the biliary tract.

Reference

1. Tanaka, Yoshimoto, Ikeda, et al: Electrohydraulic lithotripsy on gallstones in common duct: Kyushu University, Fukuoka, Japan.

Magnetic Resonance Imaging

Magnetic resonance imaging (MRI) is a recent addition to the medical and surgical armamentarium. It is presently used most often in visualizing tissues such as the brain and spinal cord. The images created are available for immediate reading and can be stored.

A very brief explanation of MRI is as follows: During scanning, the hydrogen atoms within the patient align in the powerful magnetic field. A series of radio frequency waves are introduced. The radio frequency pulses cause the patient's hydrogen atoms to emit resonance energies or radio waves. The radio signals are measured and fed into a high-speed computer, creating a two-dimensional image on the video screen and then on film. The examination by MRI may require 30–60 minutes; no physical sensations are felt. Rhythmic thumping sounds may be heard during the examination, but they are harmless and produce no aftereffects.

MRI is considered the technique of choice for brain and spinal cord problems. It replaces myelograms and arteriograms because it is less risky. MRI may complement the computed tomography (CT) scan or any other diagnostic procedure. In aseptic necrosis of the hip and in multiple sclerosis, MRI is now the procedure of choice.

The advantages of MRI are:

1. No ionizing radiation
2. No biological hazards
3. No pain
4. Produces multiple images without moving the patient
5. Superior contrast resolution compared to that of other techniques
6. Vascular structures and blood flow visualized
7. No contrast injection (iodinated solutions) required

Accepted indications for MRI studies are:

A. Head and neck—tumors
   1. Multiple sclerosis
   2. Other demyelinating diseases
   3. Pituitary lesions
   4. Abnormalities of the posterior fossa and brain stem
   5. Cranial nerve tumors, e.g., acoustic neuroma
   6. Staging head and neck tumors
   7. A double check on a CT scan
B. Chest and pulmonary system
   1. Heart and pericardial diseases
   2. Aortic aneurysms
   3. Liver abnormalities
C. Abdomen
   1. No advantages observed
   2. Detects early liver abnormalities
D. Pelvis
   1. Staging of pelvic tumors
   2. Prostatic tumors
   3. Lymphadenopathy
   4. Gynecological pathology
E. Musculoskeletal system
   1. Bone and joint abnormalities
   2. Meniscal and ligamentous damage
   3. Bone marrow abnormalities

Martinez states that MRI provides a specific advantage in biliary disease. It can safely evaluate gallbladder physiology. In addition, it can safely be incorporated into clinical studies (see Chapter 5-MRI).

MRI does not replace CT scanning sonography, scintigraphy, or IV cholangiography in gallbladder and biliary tract diseases.

References

1. Hricak H, Filly RA, Margulis AR, et al: Nuclear magnetic resonance imaging of the gallbladder. *Radiology.* 147:481, 1983.

Lithotripsy

Since the development of the lithotriper for kidney stones in 1980, about 500,000 patients have been treated with extracorporeal shock-wave lithotripsy (ECSWL). Newer versions of the machine are now being used to crush gallstones. One of the leading exponents of this new treatment is Tilman Sauerbruch of Munich, West Germany. He and his colleagues[1] treated nine carefully selected patients with functioning gallbladders. The gallbladders contained one to three symptomatic radiolucent stones about 25 mm in size. They also treated five patients with diagnosed stones in the common bile duct that retrograde endoscopy failed to remove. The patients with gallbladder stones received a combination of chenodeoxycholic acid and ursodeoxycholic acid. All gallbladder stones disintegrated into sludge or fragments smaller than 8 mm in diameter. In six of the nine patients, the fragments disappeared in 1 to 25 weeks.

In four of the five patients with common duct stones, shock-wave treatment brought about stone fragmentation, which enabled retrograde endoscopy to remove them. Some disintegrated stones passed out spontaneously. The authors believe that shock-wave therapy for gallstone disease can ultimately be carried out without producing serious adverse effects.

Rigid Criteria of Selection for Extracorporeal Shock-wave Therapy

Of 152 patients with gallbladder disease, only 9 were selected for shock-wave therapy. The reasons were (1) excessively large, i.e., a diameter greater than 25 mm; (2) calcified stones; (3) nonfunctioning gallbladder; (4) inability to visualize the bile ducts with retrograde cholangiography; (5) concurrent common bile duct stones; (6) inadequate localization of stones with an ultrasonic search; (7) physical status of the patient; and (8) refusal of the procedure by the patient. Thirty-two eligible but not ideal patients were placed on a waiting list, to be treated at a later date.

Results of Shock-wave Therapy in 5 Selected Patients

Shock-wave therapy was used in five patients with impacted common duct stones that did not allow bypass by the Dormia basket at surgery. Two patients were jaundiced, and one had septic cholangitis. In one instance, the stone was too large for endoscopic removal. In several instances where post-shock-wave therapy merely fragmented the stone, postoperative endoscopy and sphincterotomy were required to eliminate post-shock-wave persistent biliary pain and, in one instance, the pain of pancreatitis.

Complications of Shock-wave Therapy in 5 Selected Patients

The authors reported good tolerance without evidence of organ damage. They believe that extracorporeally generated shock waves can be effective in disintegrating gallbladder and common duct stones. No hepatocellular injury or malfunction was reported. In some patients kidney damage resulted in hematuria, but no organic damage followed. The writers recommended that in those instances where the stones were only fragments, supplemental dissolution therapy should be instituted.

Disadvantages of Shock-wave Therapy; Required Ancillary Therapy

These workers depended on ERCP and sphincterotomy to finally extract the resistant stone fragments. They admitted that it is impossible to fragment radiopaque stones and unrecognized cholesterol-mixed stones. Pigmented stones also resist fragmentation and lithotherapy. Sauerbruch et al. also admit that after stone fragmentation, biliary pain and complications such as cholecystitis, biliary obstruction, cholangitis, and/or pancreatitis may occur. Where some stones were fragmented and pulverized, other stones required full courses of dissolution treatments with ursodexycholic acid. This combined treatment of lithotripy and chemotherapy will become increasingly popular with more failures of shock wave treatments alone. Pretreatment demonstration is strongly recommended to indicate that endoscopy and sphincterotomy are possible. The writers felt that besides stone composition, the size and number of stones can be important causes of failure with this form of therapy.

Brown[2] and Loening et al.[3] have recently reported 2 patients with biliary disease who met the criteria for being accepted for extracorporeal shock-wave (ECSWL). Both patients were considered too high-risk for surgery.

CASE 1

The patient was a 69-year-old male alcoholic with ascites and jaundice. He had had previous cholecystectomy for cholelithiasis. Physical examination revealed a cachectic-looking male with obvious abdominal distention (ascites) and jaundice. Abdominal aspirate revealed a bacterial infection. The patient received antibiotics. The endoscopic cholangiogram showed a fixed intrahepatic stone that was resistant to removal.

ECSWL was decided upon. Although the patient improved after the therapy, an X-ray still revealed small fragmentations in the same area. The authors noted that drainage had improved, and the patient left the hospital after 45 days. There was no follow-up.

CASE 2

A 76-year-old male 2 years after cholecystectomy suddenly became jaundiced, with some pancreatitis. Lithotripsy was recommended. Two sessions of shock-wave therapy were given under local anesthesia. Fragmentation of his stones was accomplished, and the fragmented pieces were removed endoscopically with the Dormia basket. Later a sphincterotomy was necessary to correct a stenosing papillitis. The patient left the hospital in good condition. There was no follow-up.

Brown et al. concluded that ECSWL does fragment gallstones and that the fragments can be removed endoscopically.

This writer believes that the criteria for lithotripsy therapy were justified in the two cases presented. Unfortunately, there was no follow-up. At this stage of lithotripsy development, the loss of patient follow-up is most unfortunate. This is another example of why the Food and Drug Administration (FDA) has ordered a controlled study of 600 patients by qualified personnel experienced in this type of therapy. Until the results of this controlled study are completed and published, lithotripsy of gallstones should be practiced with restraint.

This writer reviewed the work of other researchers in the field of lithotripsy and was able to make the following observations:

OBSERVED COMPLICATIONS

1. Tissue damage, believed due to excessive shock waves, possibly over 1500 shocks.
2. Pancreatitis, mild to moderate.
3. Continued episodes of biliary pain; recurrent cholecystitis.
4. Bile duct obstruction caused by fragments of stone.
5. Infection; ascending cholangitis.
6. Hemorrhage—hematuria.

CRITERIA FOR USE

Only about 10% of the gallstone population are accepted candidates for lithotripsy. The required criteria are:

1. Cholelithiasis must be symptomatic, and the stones must be composed of cholesterol.
2. There must not be more than three stones in the gallbladder, with a size no greater than 2.5 cm.
3. Patients with mixed or calcified stones are not considered good subjects. These stones are not fragmented by lithotripsy.
4. The patient should be evaluated for the possibility of postoperative sphincterotomy and stone extraction by the Dormia basket.

INDICATIONS FOR USE

1. Patients with chronic cholecystitis and cholelithiasis who are symptomatic; also, the patient should preferably be over 60 years of age and be considered a poor risk for cholecystectomy. Such patients usually reveal varying forms of pulmonary and cardiovascular-renal problems.
2. Patients who refuse or cannot tolerate surgery.
3. Patients who have had multiple abdominal surgeries, such as cholecystectomy and choledochotomy, and who have most likely developed extensive adhesions and distortions of their abdominal organs. Patients in this category would most likely benefit from ECSWL. How-

ever, if lithotripsy and supplemental chemotherapy (i.e., chenodeoxycholic acid and ursodeoxycholic acid) fail to fragment or shrink the stone, surgical intervention may become mandatory—even with the presenting risks.

This writer believes that lithotripsy today is in its early formative stages and that in the next 5 years physicians will find more indications for its use. The present 10% of the gallbladder population presented accepted for ECSWL will probably be increased to 20%.

It is imperative that carefully controlled studies be carried out by experienced workers and that the recorded data be explicit and honest. To this end, the FDA has appointed 10 medical centers to study lithotripsy in 600 gallbladder patients and to determine its usefulness and safety, as well as to decide who among the 20 million gallstone sufferers would benefit from lithotripsy.

Finally, this writer wishes to add a point that has not been adequately stressed by the writers on lithotripsy and chenodeoxycholic acid and its derivatives. In the final analysis the roentgenologists, the surgeon, and the gastroenterologist must realize that the above-mentioned gallstone therapies deal only with the gallstone per se; little or no attention has been paid to the residual pathological gallbladder. The gallstone represents only a complication of chronic cholecystitis; after all, it is not the primary disease. The gallstone is still capable of moving, perforating, and obstructing, but the leftover pathological gallbladder can continuously reproduce more stones, become inflamed again (cholecystitis), and produce new complications such as fistula formation and obstruction of the cystic duct, with resulting hydrops and empyema. But most important, the gallbladder can, at long last (despite the low incidence of about 1%), develop carcinoma. To reiterate: *removal or dissolution of stones is temporary, and the transient result is not curative. The primary disease process, chronic cholecystitis, remains, with its potential of re-creating new calculi with their attending complications, as well as allowing the underlying pathological process to progress. It is conceivable that with the preservation of more diseased gallbladders we may, in time, see a rise in the statistical incidence of 'silent' carcinoma of the gallbladder.*

Recommended Reading

Allen MJ, Borody TJ, Bugliosi TF, et al: Rapid dissolution of gallstones by methyl tert-butyl ether: Preliminary observations. *N Engl J Med* 312:217, 1985.

Bachrach WH, Hofmann AF: Ursodeoxycholic acid in the treatment of cholesterol cholelithiasis. *Dig Dis Sci* 27:737, 1982.

Chaussy C, Schmiedt E, Jocham D, et al: First clinical experience with extracorporeally indiced destruction of kidney stones by shock waves. *J Urol* 127:417, 1982.

Chaussy C, Schmiedt E, Jocham D, et al: Extracorporeal shock-wave lithotripsy (ESWL) for treatment of urolithiasis. *Urology* 23(suppl):59, 1984.

Erlinger S, Le Go A, Husson JM, et al: Franco–Belgian cooperative study of ursodeoxycholic acid in the medical dissolution of gallstones: A double-blind, randomized, dose–response study, and comparison with chenodeoxycholic acid. *Hepatology* 4:308, 1984.

Neubrand M, Sauerbruch T, Stellaard F, et al: In vitro cholesterol gallstone dissolution after fragmentation with shock waves. *Digestion* (in press).

Norrby S, Schoenebeck J: Long-term results with cholecystolithotomy. *Act Chir Scand* 136:711, 1970.

Ruppin DC, Dowling RH: Is recurrence inevitable after gallstone dissolution by bile-acid treatment? *Lancet* 1:181, 1982.

Sauerbruch T, Holl J, Kruis W, et al: Dissolution of gallstones by methyl tert-butyl ether. *N Engl J Med* 313:385, 1985.

Schoenfield LJ, Lachin JM, et al: Chenodiol (chenodeoxycholic acid) for dissolution of gallstones; the National Cooperative Gallstone Study: A controlled trial of efficacy and safety. *Ann Intern Med* 95:257, 1981.

Thistle JL, Carlson GL, Hofmann AF, et al: Monooctanoin, a dissolution agent for retained cholesterol bile duct stones: Physical properties and clinical application. *Gastroenterology* 78:1016, 1980.

References

1. Sauerbruch T, Delius M, Paumgartner G, et al: Fragmentation of gallstones by extracorporeal shock waves. *N Engl J Med* 314:818, 1986.
2. Brown BP: Fractionation of biliary tract stones by lithotripsy using local anesthesia. *Arch Surg* 123:91–93 1988.

Addendum

In the *New England Journal of Medicine* in February 1988, Sauerbruch et al. published their latest experience with ECSWL. They substantiated their last results, published in 1986 in the same journal.[1] Thus far, they have treated 175 select patients in whom they found radiotranslucent gallstones. Chenodeoxycholic acid and ursodeoxycholic acid were given as adjuvant medical therapy. These writers claim that all gallstones disintegrated except one. In 30% they completely disappeared, (35 patients) of all patients treated with lithotripsy, 48%; (82 patients) after 2–4 months; and 91% (157 patients) after 12–18 months.

The writers list their adverse findings as follows:

1. Cutaneous petichiae occurred in about 14% of the patients.
2. Transient gross hematuria occurred in about 3% of the patients.
3. One-third of the patients had one or more episodes of biliary colic. Colic attacks occurred so long as the stone fragments existed.
4. Two patients developed pancreatitis, which necessitated endoscopic spincterotomy (ERCP). In one patient in whom the stone did not fractionate, cholecystectomy was required.

When all the complications are counted, they amount to more than 50%. This finding compares unfavorably with the findings in the same uncomplicated patients selected for cholecystectomy. However, this writer still recognizes the advantages that lithotripsy offers the high-risk patients.

This writer does not wish to appear too critical at this stage of lithotripsy's development; he would rather remain expectantly cautious and reserve his opinion until after all the medical centers selected complete and combine their results and make them known. Until then, this writer will continue to advocate the use of conventional and accepted surgical techniques for surgically indicated gallbladder diseases.

Recommended Readings

Brendel W, Enders G, et al: Shock waves for gallstones: Animal studies. *Lancet* 1:1054, 1983.
Delius M, Enders G, et al: Biological effects of shock waves: Lung hemorrhage by shock waves in dogs—pressure dependence. *Ultrasound Med Biol* 13:61, 1987.
Owens WD, Felts JA, et al: ASA physical status classifications; A study of consistency of ratings. *Anesthesiology* 49:239, 1978.

Reference

1. Sauerbruch T, Delius M, Paumgartner G, et al: Fragmentation of gallstones by extracorporeal shock waves. *N Engl J Med* 314:818, 1986.

Index